Urolithiasis
and Related
Clinical Research

Urolithiasis and Related Clinical Research

Edited by

Paul O. Schwille

University Hospital
Erlangen, Federal Republic of Germany

Lynwood H. Smith

Mayo Clinic
Rochester, Minnesota

William G. Robertson

The General Infirmary
Leeds, England

and

Winfried Vahlensieck

University Hospital
Bonn, Federal Republic of Germany

Springer Science+Business Media, LLC

Library of Congress Cataloging in Publication Data

International Symposium on Urolithiasis and Related Clinical Research (5th: 1984: Garmisch-Partenkirchen, Germany)
  Urolithiasis and related clinical research.

  "Proceedings of the Fifth International Symposium on Urolithiasis and Related Clinical Research, held April 1–5, 1984, in Garmisch-Partenkirchen, Federal Republic of Germany" —T.p. verso.
  Includes bibliographies and index.
  1. Calculi, Urinary—Congresses. I. Schwille, P. O. (Paul O.) II. Title. [DNLM: 1. Urinary Calculi—congresses. W3 IN924XD 5th 1984 / WJ 100 I615 1984u]
  RC916.I578 1984   616.6'22   85-3582
  ISBN 978-1-4684-7274-5   ISBN 978-1-4684-7272-1 (eBook)
  DOI 10.1007/978-1-4684-7272-1

Proceedings of the Fifth International Symposium on Urolithiasis and Related
Clinical Research, held April 1–5, 1984, in Garmisch-Partenkirchen,
Federal Republic of Germany

Advisory Committee:
O. Bijvoet, B. Danielson, J. Dirks, B. Finlayson, H. Fleisch, J. Lemann, G. Nancollas, C. Pak,
W. Robertson, A. Rose, J. Sallis, L. Smith, W. Vahlensieck, and N. Zöllner

Secretary:
P. Schwille

Jacket: *Cover photo of bladder stone consisting of calcium oxalate monohydrate (COM),
         courtesy of W. Bausch, Institute of Mineralogy, University of Erlangen*

© Springer Science+Business Media New York 1985
Originally published by Plenum Press, New York in 1985
Softcover reprint of the hardcover 1st edition 1985

PREFACE

Urolithiasis is a common disorder which is recognised in most
parts of the world and occurs in both man and animals. The
multifactorial nature of the problem requires an interdisciplinary
approach which has always been a feature of this series of
International Symposia which started in Leeds in 1968 and has
progressed at four-yearly intervals through Madrid, Davos and
Williamsburg. The latest Meeting, at Garmisch-Partenkirchen in
April 1984, involved 302 participants from all five continents.

The major emphasis of the Meeting was to blend the basic and
clinical research on urolithiasis. Comprehensive reviews of the
major areas of current research were presented by invited speakers,
all internationally recognized experts in their fields. From more
than 250 submitted abstracts, 18 were selected for oral presentation
and the remainder presented at three afternoon poster sessions which
provided an opportunity for informal and more lengthy discussions
of the work on display. The Meeting also included three ad hoc
Evening Discussions on how to approach various unsolved questions in
the clinical and laboratory evaluation of stone patients and four
Round Table Discussions involving specialists in the field who
debated the theoretical aspects of stone formation in the urinary
tract, the measurement of inhibitory activity of urine, the
treatment of idiopathic stones with drugs, and the nature and
treatment of stones arising from urinary tract infection.

Thus the Symposium covered the environmental, nutritional and
genetic factors related to stone disease, the gastrointestinal,
metabolic, renal aspects of the disorder, the physico-chemical
aspects of stone-formation, the mode of action of drugs to prevent
stones and recent developments in the surgical removal of stones.
This volume contains the Proceedings of the Symposium and includes
the majority of oral and poster presentations along with the reports
from three of the Round Table Discussions.

The Meeting would not have been possible without the generous
financial support from the National Institutes of Health and the
Deutsche Forschungsgemeinschaft, and also from firms such as

Deutsche Wellcome, Dr Madaus, Hoyer and various other drug
companies.   To all of them we owe our deepest gratitude.   We are
also very grateful to our co-workers and colleagues in the field
whose ongoing efforts combined to ensure the success of this
Symposium and to Mrs Shirley Rutter for typing the entire
Proceedings.

Paul O. Schwille
Lynwood H. Smith
William G. Robertson
Winfried Vahlensieck

Garmisch-Partenkirchen
1-5 April, 1984

ACKNOWLEDGEMENTS

This Symposium was supported by:

The National Institutes of Arthritis, Diabetes and
Digestive and Kidney Diseases, National Institutes of Health,
Department of Health and Human Services
Bethesda, Maryland, USA.
Deutsche Forschungsgemeinschaft, Bonn, FRG.
University Hospital Research Funds, Erlangen, FRG.
Deutsche Wellcome, Burgwedel, FRG.
Hoyer, Neuss, FRG.
Madaus, Cologne, FRG.
Plenum Publishing Corporation, London, England.
Dornier System, Friedrichshafen, FRG.
Temmler, Marburg, FRG.
Pfrimmer, Erlangen, FRG.
TAD, Cuxhaven, FRG.
Sigma, Munich, FRG.
Beckman, Munich, FRG.
Smith, Kline & Grench, Munich, FRG.
Hoechst, Frankfurt, FRG.
Cyanamid, Wolfratshausen, FRG.
Bayer, Leverkusen, FRG.
Boehringer, Mannheim, FRG.
Grünenthal, Stolberg, FRG.
Byk Gulden, Konstanz, FRG.
Zeiss, Munich, FRG.

CONTENTS

I. GENERAL ASPECTS

GENETICS

III. RENAL PHYSIOLOGY AND PATHOPHYSIOLOGY

IV. METABOLISM

V. CLINICAL UROLITHIASIS

VI. TREATMENT

DIETARY THERAPY

DRUG TREATMENT

SURGICAL TREATMENT

VII. ANALYTICAL METHODS

URINE AND PLASMA ANALYSIS

STONE ANALYSIS

INHIBITORS AND PROMOTERS

IX. ANIMAL MODELS

I. GENERAL ASPECTS
GENETICS

INBORN ERRORS OF METABOLISM COMPLICATED BY UROLITHIASIS -

EXAMPLES FROM PURINE METABOLISM

N. Zöllner

Medizinische Poliklinik, 8000 München 2, F.R.G.

INTRODUCTION

Everyone is familiar with inborn errors of metabolism and most physicians realize that inborn errors do occur in their particular speciality. However, they regard these as "rarities", not likely to be encountered in their own clinical experience. This in turn leads to a general lack of knowledge as well as curiosity, diagnostic vigilance and clinical screening for these abnormalities. To quote from another clinical field, only a minority of cardiologists is aware that the incidence of familial hypercholesterolemia is nearly 1% and that this inborn error accounts for more than 5% of all coronary heart attacks that occur before the age of sixty. In urology the situation is probably similar; there may be more inborn errors causing urolithiasis than we think today. The problems are present but experience and initiative to attack them may be lacking.

GENERAL CONSIDERATIONS

In a recent report, the number of individual inborn errors of metabolism was estimated at approximately 700. This may be an underestimate. Indeed, individuality or at least the physical, inborn part of it, the so-called biochemical individuality, is due to the unique properties of an individual's genes. One speaks of gene defects as if an anomoly of a DNA leads to disease. However, it must be realized that the particular case of the inborn error is only the end of a continuous spectrum, the other end of which is occupied by extremely healthy people. In between there is the majority of us including a great number of stone-formers.

3

At present it is not possible apparently to elucidate minor deviations from normal metabolic pathways favouring stone formation. This is why we must turn to established inborn errors. These as such are interesting enough. Although they - or most of them - are rarities, recent discoveries suggest that there are more of them to be found and that clinical acumen plus reliable screening techniques may lead to further discoveries. However, the great importance of inborn errors for urology lies in the fact that they are monocausal diseases, of which the basic mechanisms are known.

It was Garrod who clearly saw that in his inborn errors of metabolism a single Mendelian trait was operative and that therefore all symptoms of his patients must be due to a single cause. Garrod was a man of great vision; he predicted that his discovery would further investigations in many fields of medicine, even in fields that were very new in the year of 1906. However, upon rereading the Croonian lectures as well as the Lessons from Alcaptonuria, it is amazing how little Garrod thought of applications. It was a chemist-physician of the then famous Munich school, Otto Neubauer, who used a patient with alcaptonuria to study the metabolism of aromatic amino acids. At that time Munich was full of famous, Nobel prize-winning chemists; but it took a man with understanding of pathology and chemistry to grasp the significance of inborn errors for general research into physiology and pathophysiology.

Meanwhile, inborn errors have come of age. On the clinical side we have learned of the incredible range of consequences a single defect may have. Let me quote a few. In Marfan's syndrome we find skeletal, ocular and cardiovascular manifestations; familial hypercholesterolemia leads to xanthomata of skin and tendons, coronary disease, involvement of heart valves and corneal arcus; and Lesch-Nyhan syndrome is characterized by choreoathetosis, self-mutilation and renal disease.

On the biochemical side we can spot the gene defect within the DNA, and we can infer what this may mean to the product protein, be it globin, collagen, an enzyme, a transport or a receptor protein. And of course we are certain that one gene defect is responsible for only one defective protein, i.e. that in any given inborn error all pathology has one common cause. This applies also to inborn errors associated with stones.

Inborn errors as models for the genesis of stones are experimenta naturae, but we are on safer grounds than Harvey because we are certain that we observe an experiment with only one variable, the ideal of every scientist. It still may be difficult enough to understand nature's experiments, and this applies particularly to disorders of tubular function.

4

Stone formation in the urinary tract may be due to a number of reasons. Overexcretion, changes in solubility by changes of the properties of the solvent, and changes in concentration at any given site along the nephron are the most important factors. If considered in detail, the situation may become even more complex. I have selected a few diseases to illustrate some points and I shall draw my examples from purine metabolism; it is with regret that I omit such interesting items as tubular acidosis, cystinuria and primary hyperoxaluria from my agenda. Now let us look at some interesting genocopies of the common disease urolithiasis.

DISORDERS OF PURINE METABOLISM

Stanbury et al list 8 inborn errors of purine metabolism. At least 4 of them are associated with stones. In my opinion a further syndrome must be included making a total of 5 stone-producing purine disorders. They can be separated into two categories, 3 with a net overproduction of a metabolite and 2 with a derangement of tubular transport.

Table 1. Inborn Disorders of Purine Metabolism Associated with Urolithiasis

"Transport Defect"	"Overproduction"
Gout	HGPRT-Deficiency
Inborn Renal Hypouricemia	APRT-Deficiency
	Hereditary Xanthinuria

To understand pathogenesis and therapy, only a few points of normal purine metabolism are important.

(i) Uric acid in the body comes from two sources: endogenous, so-called de novo purine synthesis and dietary purines. Endogenous uric acid is a rather constant amount; however it increases under conditions of augmented cell turnover, e.g. in most leukemias. Exogenous uric acid varies widely depending on the purine content of food, particularly its content of RNA. (Thus, growing plants deliver (per unit energy) as much purines as meat.) Currently in central Europe, exogenous uric acid amounts to as much as the endogenous component.

(ii) There is no oxidation of uric acid in the metabolism of man.

(iii) Excretion occurs by way of the kidney and the gut. The kidney plays the predominant role, excreting 70 to 80% of the uric acid produced.

(iv)   The most common cause of overproduction of uric acid is an increase of dietary purines.   However there are possibilities for overproduction in metabolism at the level of PRPP-synthesis, purine salvage and oxipurine oxidation.

(v)   The renal excretion of urate is the resultant of glomerular filtration, tubular reabsorption and tubular secretion.   Even if the sequence of reabsorption and secretion along the tubule is not yet known in complete detail, it is quite obvious that a derangement of any one mechanism may lead to abnormal concentrations of urate at certain levels of the tubule.

With these 5 facts in mind let us now look at the stone-producing inborn errors. I shall discuss gout only briefly.   In primary familial gout the amount of uric acid produced de novo is normal; however urate clearance at any given plasma level is low. Therefore urate concentrations in the glomerular filtrate are high. Due to high plasma levels, renal interstitial urate concentrations must also be high.   The basic defect is probably one of urate secretion.   Obviously, high purine intakes aggravate this unfavourable situation.   The reasons for stone formation are probably high urate concentrations in the upper nephron, possibly interstitial tophi.   Therapy must consist of lowering the urate concentration in the glomerular filtrate through dietary restriction or allopurinol administration.   A high fluid intake may help by increasing flow along the nephron; alkali will dissolve micro-deposits of urate.

Table 2.   Gout

Pathogenesis	Defective tubular urate secretion leading to hyperuricemia and high urate concentrations in the upper nephron
Stones	5 to 50%
Therapy of urolithiasis	Allopurinol, low purine diet (High fluid intake, alkali?)

Inborn renal hypouricemia is a rare disorder (Table 3), termed the "Dalmatian Dog Mutation" in man by Seegmiller, but most often described by Sperling, seems to occur particularly in Jews or people of oriental extraction.   Here, the tubular defect is one of reabsorption which may increase uric acid clearance manyfold up to the glomerular filtration rate.   As in gout, this leads to high urate concentrations in the upper nephron.   Therefore diet and allopurinol are again the treatment of choice.

Table 3.   Inborn Renal Hypouricemia

Pathogenesis	Defective tubular urate reabsorption leading to high urate concentrations in the upper nephron
Stones	Apparently common
Therapy of Urolithiasis	Allopurinol, low purine diet (high fluid intake)

There are two diseases associated with deficiencies of HGPRT; both affect only men. In these deficiencies, the reutilization of hypoxanthine and guanine is decreased or absent and they must be oxidized to uric acid. Also, the amount of unused PRPP builds up and may induce de novo synthesis of purines. Thus we have an example of endogenous urate over-production, a genocopy of the situation in leukemia. Analogous to leukemia, it is not surprising that stones may precede gout for years. Our own cases have all had stones and kidney disease (Table 4).

Diet is not effective in the therapy of this disorder and allopurinol is the treatment of choice. However, the doses required may be large. It is worthwhile to emphasize that in this disorder, therapy and treatment are often unnecessarily delayed.

Table 4.   Deficiency of HGPRT

Pathogenesis	Overproduction of uric acid due to insufficient reutilization of hypoxanthine, guanine and phosphoribosylpyrophosphate
Therapy of Urolithiasis	Allopurinol in high doses

While most stones derived from purine metabolism consist of urates, other constituents occur. Unfortunately material from these stones gives a positive murexide test and this may prevent diagnosis.

In the deficiency of APRT, renal disease is the only consequence. Stones or gravel lead to colic, hematuria, urinary tract infection and dysuria. The stones consists of 2,8-dihydroxyadenine. This is the end product of adenine metabolism via xanthine oxidase when adenine from polyamine metabolism cannot be reutilized via APRT.

The disease is considered to be rare but a relatively high frequency of heterozygosity (0.4 to 1.0%) has been reported. Administration of allopurinol inhibits xanthine oxidase. Some 8-hydroxyadenine is still formed, but adenine becomes the major urinary component.

Table 5.   Deficiency of APRT

Pathogenesis	Inability to reutilize adenine which is oxidized to 2,8-dihydroxyadenine
Stones	Stones may lead to the discovery of the metabolic defect
Therapy of Urolithiasis	Allopurinol, low purine diet, no alkali

Xanthine stones were recognized as early as 1817 by Marcet. However not all patients with these stones suffer from hereditary xanthinuria which is characterized by a gross deficiency of xanthine oxidase.   The diagnosis is made from a jejunal biopsy or by measuring oxypurine excretion which is highly elevated.   It can be suspected if serum urate and urinary urate excretion are very low. The disease is probably not as rare as generally considered.   On the basis of preliminary screenings, there may be about 200 cases in Bavaria.   Since allopurinol is useless in the therapy of this disorder, the diagnosis must be carefully established or excluded in all murexide-positive calculi.   It is worthwhile knowing that a phenocopy of the disease may be produced by administering allopurinol to leukemia patients under chemotherapy.   Although in this particular clinical situation urate stones predominate and are properly treated by allopurinol, occasionally xanthine stones occur not in spite but because of this therapy.

Table 6.   Hereditary Xanthinuria

Pathogenesis	Deficiency of xanthine oxidase leading to xanthine accumulation
Stones	30 to 50%
Therapy of Urolithiasis	High fluid intake

UROLITHIASIS IN A LARGE KINDRED DEFICIENT IN ADENINE

PHOSPHORIBOSYLTRANSFERASE (APRT)

M. H. Gault, T. O'Toole, J. M. Wilson, R. H. Payne,
T. H. Ittel, A. Simmons, D. N. Churchill, and J. Morgan

Memorial University and the General Hospital, St. John's
Newfoundland, Canada, The Purine Laboratory, Guy's
Hospital, London, U.K. and the Purine Research Center
University of Michigan, Ann Arbor, Michigan, U.S.A.

INTRODUCTION

Dihydroxyadenine urolithiasis was first described in 1974 by
Cartier et al[1] and confirmed by Simmonds et al.[2]. The subject has
been recently reviewed[3,4]. The poorly soluble purine,
2,8-dihydroxyadenine, appears in urine when there is a homozygous
deficiency of adenine phosphoribosyltransferase (APRT). Calculus
formation, crystal type nephrotoxicity and renal failure have been
described, mainly in children. Of 20 patients reported with
dihydroxyadenine calculi[3-8], including the family to be discussed,
the onset of symptoms was under 4 years in 11 and under 10 years in
all but 4, 3 of whom were from Japan. Patients commonly present
with symptoms of urinary obstruction such as abdominal or flank
pain, but also with frequent passage of small stones,
macrohematuria, urinary tract infection and renal failure[3,4].

Dihydroxyadenine stones give falsely positive reactions for
uric acid with standard wet chemical colorimetric procedures such as
with phosphotungstate and murexide, and are typically radiolucent,
making radiological diagnosis more difficult. Diagnosis may be
suggested by spherical, rosette-like birefringent crystals on
microscopic examination of urine[3,7], and confirmed by infrared
analysis, mass spectroscopy or X-ray spectroscopy[9]. Infrared
spectroscopy has provided identification in the majority.
Additional diagnostic features include the virtual absence of APRT,
the excretion of adenine, 8-hydroxyadenine and particularly
2,8-dihydroxyadenine in urine[3].

The defect is inherited as an autosomal recessive trait. In
European and North American families, those heterozygotes studied

have neither had calculi nor have they excreted adenine,
8-hydroxyadenine or 2,8-dihydroxyadenine[3]. However, 5 patients
have been reported from Japan with 2,8-dihydroxyadenine calculi in
association with a partial deficiency of APRT[3,5-7] (30, 28, 19, 10
and 9% of normal activity). No blood transfusions were noted to
suggest that these APRT values might be factitious and suggests that
2,8-dihydroxyadenine urolithiasis may be genetically heterogenous.
The incidence of heterozygosity has been estimated at 0.4 to 1.1%,
suggesting a homozygosity of about one in 100,000[3].

APRT catalyzes the conversion of adenine to adenosine
monophosphate. The only other metabolic route available for
urinary excretion in the absence of APRT is oxidation of adenine to
8-hydroxyadenine and 2,8-dihydroxyadenine by xanthine oxidase.
Apart from problems related to the urinary tract, homozygotes are
well, without evidence of immunodeficiency or an increased incidence
of gout[3]. Thus, it appears that unlike its companion salvage
enzyme, hypoxanthineguanine phosphoribosyltransferase, a homozygous
deficiency of which is associated with gross overproduction of uric
acid and the Lesch-Nyhan syndrome, APRT is not involved in the
overall control of purine and uric acid production in humans.

METHODS

We have studied APRT in 18 subjects from 3 generations of a
Newfoundland family including 12 of 13 members of the second
generation (Fig. 1). Both maternal and paternal sides of the
family came to Newfoundland from England and the marriage was non-
consanguineous. The parents were heterozygotes with values for
erythrocyte APRT of 20 and 22% of controls. Inheritance was
autosomal recessive. Two of the 12 were homozygotes with virtual
absence of erythrocyte APRT activity. One presented at age 42 with
2,8-dihydroxyadenine urolithiasis established by infrared and mass
spectrographic analysis[9]. Adenine compounds comprised 16% of total

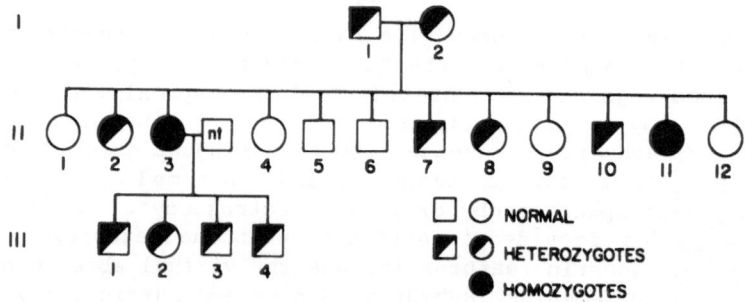

Fig. 1. Pedigree of Newfoundland Family, nt = not tested

urine purines with a urinary 2,8-dihydroxyadenine of 0.13 mmol/24h
in spite of a daily dose of 300 mg (5 mg/kg) of allopurinol.   The
second homozygote was a 24-year-old woman with no past or present
evidence of urolithiasis or renal disorder.   She had normal renal
function and excreted 0.18 mmol of adenine, 0.02 of 8-hydroxyadenine
and 0.54 mmol 2,8-dihydroxyadenine per 24h.   Adenine compounds
represented 45% of total purines excreted.   These values are
similar to those found in other untreated homozygotes.   None of the
10 heterozygotes has any past or present evidence of urolithiasis or
impairment of renal function.

RESULTS AND DISCUSSION

For the 10 heterozygotes, the mean value for APRT enzyme
activity in erthyrocyte hemolysates was 28% of controls,
substantially less than the expected 50%[10].   The reduced APRT
activity in erythrocytes compared with lymphoblasts in heterozygotes may be related to active synthesis of 'hybrid' diamers
composed of one normal and one mutant subunit, the latter existing
even though they are abnormally labile, whereas in erythrocytes the
putative 'hybrid' is not seen because this labile protein is
degraded too rapidly.   Alternatively, there may be a compensatory
increase in the normal allele in lymphoblasts, something not
possible in erythrocytes.   Molecular variants of peptidase A and C
and of isocitrate dehydrogenase are other examples where expression
is not observed in erythrocytes but is in other tissues[10].

The APRT locus has been assigned by somatic hybridization
studies to the long arm of chromosome 16[11].   The commonly
polymorphic serum protein haptoglobin, in part determined by the
gene HPA, is also located on chromosome 16[12].   This family is
informative for the common HPA polymorphism.   One APRT heterozygote
parent (I-1) is homozygous for HPA^2 and the other (I-2) is a
HPA^1/HPA^2 heterozygote.   APRT may be syntenic with HPA^1 in I-2 as
this gives a minimum number of crossovers (3 in 12, RF = 0.25 $\pm$
0.13).   Hence, linkage between haptoglobin (α-submit) and APRT
suggest a minimum map distance of 27.5 (SE = +22, -15) centimorgans
between these two chromosome 16 loci.

Treatment with increased fluid intake and a low purine diet is
recommended in homozygotes with urolithiasis and probably should be
used in asymptomatic homozygotes[3].   Allopurinol (10 mg/kg/day) has
eliminated 2,8-dihydroxyadenine in most cases[3].   However, total
adenine compounds excreted in urine remain little changed as there
is rearrangement of the proportion so that the more soluble adenine
becomes the major urinary component.   A lower dose of allopurinol
may be indicated in renal failure because of retention of its
metabolite oxypurinol which may also cause stones and depress the
bone marrow.

In conclusion, urolithiasis related to homozygous APRT deficiency may present in middle age and some adults may have no detectable evidence of urolithiasis. This phenomenon is not due to a lower excretion of dihydroxyadenine. Inheritance of APRT deficiency in this family was clearly autosomal recessive and, as in European case reports, no urolithiasis has occurred in any hetero-zygote. Erythrocytes may give inappropriately low values for APRT compared with lymphoblasts.

REFERENCES

1. P. Cartier and M. Hamet, C.R. Acad. Sci. (Paris), 297:883 (1974).
2. H. A. Simmonds, K. J. Van Acker, J. Cameron, and W. Snedden, Biochem. J. 157:485 (1976).
3. H. A. Simmonds and K. J. Van Acker, in":"Metabolic Basis of Inherited Disease", 5th ed. J. B. Stanbury, J. B. Wyngaard, D. S. Fredrickson, J. L. Goldstein, and M. S. Brown, eds., McGraw-Hill, New York (1983).
4. F. R. Witten, J. W. Morsan, J. G. Foster, and J. F. Glenn, J. Urol. 130:938 (1983).
5. H. Takeughi, T. Tomoyoshi, Y. Takahashi, O. Yoshida, M. Uchda, and T. Nakamura, Acta Urol. Jap. 27:189 (1981).
6. K. Sakamoto, Y. Fujisawa, A. Ohmori, K. Minoda, H. Yamanaka, and K. Nishioka, Urol. Int. 36:274 (1981).
7. H. Yamamoto, Personal Communication, 1981.
8. T. Nakamoto, H. Nakatsu, T. Kishi, N. Sakura, T. Usui, and H.Nihira, J. Urol., 130:580 (1982).
9. M. H. Gault, H. A. Simmonds, W. Snedden, D. Dow, D. N. Churchill, and H. Penney, New Engl. J. Med. 305:1570 (1981).
10. T. M. O'Toole, J. M. Wilson, M. H. Gault, and W. N. Kelley, Biochem. Gen. 21:1121 (1983).
11. J. A. Tischfield and F. H. Ruddle, Proc. Nat. Acad. Sci. 71:45 (1974).
12. E. B. Robson, P. E. Polani, S. J. Dart, A. A. Jacobs, and J. H. Renwick, Nature 223:1163 (1967).

UROLITHIASIS IN HEREDITARY RENAL HYPOURICEMIA

O. Sperling

Dept. of Clinical Biochemistry, Beilinson Medical
Center, Petah-Tikva, and Dept. of Chemical Pathology
Tel-Aviv University, Tel-Hashomer, Israel

INTRODUCTION

Urolithiasis due to excessive excretion of insoluble urinary
components, is an important clinical manifestation of several inborn
errors of metabolism in man.   In some of these disorders the
excessive excretion is due to a metabolic defect, such as in primary
hyperoxaluria, xanthinuria, hypoxanthine-guanine phosphoribosyltransferase (HGPRT) deficiency and phosphoribosylpyrophosphate
(PRPP) synthetase over-activity, whereas in other disorders, it is
due to a renal tubular transport abnormality, such as in cystinuria.
Hereditary hypouricemia, due to an isolated defect in renal tubular
urate reabsorption, is a relatively new disorder, which should be
classified with the inborn transport disorders associated with stone
formation.   Renal hypouricemia of the isolated type was first
described by Praetorius and Kirk[1], but no evidence was adduced for
genetic transmission.   The first case of inborn renal hypouricemia[2]
was reported in 1972.   Since 1974 we have encountered 7 Israeli
familes with renal hypouricemia in whom the tubular abnormality
pertained to urate handling only[3-8].   Three of the 7 propositi, as
well as the propositus reported by Greene et al[2], were found to have
stones and urolithiasis is a common manifestation of the syndrome.
The study of the affected Israeli families contributed to the
characterization of the physiological, clinical and genetic aspects
of this rare inborn transport error[9].

CHARACTERIZATION OF THE RENAL TUBULAR TRANSPORT DEFECT

The nature of the renal tubular defect causing the increase in
renal urate clearance, manifest in the hypouricemia, has not yet

13

been clarified. The possibility that the renal tubular abnormalities may be either the expression of a generalized impairment of transport of uric acid across cell membranes[10], or secondary to an abnormal metabolite produced elsewhere in the body has been investigated. We could not demonstrate a defect in urate transport through the erythrocyte membrane and the intestinal wall in the propositus of a renal hypouricemic family[11]. Furthermore, our preliminary studies failed to detect an abnormal uricosuric agent in the plasma of several renal hypouricemic subjects. This suggests that renal hypouricemia is indeed the result of a primary urate transport defect in the renal tubules.

The present concept of urate handling by the kidney proposes a 4-component model involving glomerular filtration, pre-secretory reabsorption, tubular secretion and post-secretory reabsorption[12]. It is acccepted that filtered urate is reabsorbed almost totally in the proximal tubule, that urate is secreted also at a proximal site, and that some of the secreted urate is reabsorbed at a post-secretory site. Renal hypouricemia may thus be caused by defective pre- or post-secretory reabsorption or a combined reabsorption defect. The pyrazinamide (PZA) suppression test[12] was performed in

Table 1. Data on Propositi with Inborn Isolated Renal Hypouricemia.

Propositus Sex	Age	Lowest Plasma Urate (mg/dl)	Highest Urinary Urate (mg/24h)	$\frac{C_{Ur}}{C_{Cr}}$ (%)	Response to PZA	Associated condition
M	53	0.6	691	60	Attenuated[3]	Hypercalciuria, decreased bone density
F	37	1.1	662	36	Attenuated[4]	Kidney stone (unidentified)
M	48	1.2	750	38	Attenuated[5]	
M	53	1.0	1000	48	Attenuated[6]	Hypercalciuria, uric acid stone
M	37	1.0	1000	45	Attenuated[6]	Hypercalciuria, uric acid stone
M	8	0.7	355	36	See text[7]	Moderate hypercalciuria
M	10	1.5	286	36	Attenuated[8]	Moderate hypercalciuria

an attempt to characterize the abnormality in renal handling of urate causing the hypouricemia. The PZA response is believed to reflect mainly the inhibitory effect of the drug on tubular urate secretion, although its magnitude may not be an exact measure of urate secretion[9]. In normal subjects PZA administration results in almost total suppression of urate excretion[12]. Three types of renal hypouricemia were classified, according to the response of urate excretion to PZA administration to such subjects. In defective proximal pre-secretory renal tubular reabsorption of uric acid the PZA response is attenuated, while in defective post-secretory reabsorption, PZA markedly decreases uric acid excretion, resembling the response in normal subjects. When the reabsorption defect is combined, the clearance ratio of urate to creatinine is greater than 1.0 and PZA administration reduces the clearance ratio to about 1.0. In all subjects studied in our laboratory (Table 1), the C_{Ur}/C_{Cr} ratio was < 1 and in all but one propositus and PZA administration resulted in an attenuated decrease in urate excretion. These results are in accordance with a pre-secretory defect in urate reabsorption.

CLINICAL SIGNIFICANCE

The hypouricemia has no clinical significance. On the other hand, 3 out of the 7 propositi with inborn isolated renal hypouricemia studied in our laboratory, had urinary tract stones (Table 1), 2 composed of uric acid and one of unidentified composition. The patient studied by Greene et al[2] had a calcium oxalate stone. In the 2 with uric acid stones[6] the hypouricemia was associated with a marked hyperuricosuria, exceeding 1000 mg/day. Hyperuricosuria, although moderate, was also present in many other hypouricemic propositi[9]. No evidence could be obtained in our hypouricemic-hyperuricosuric subjects of purine overproduction. Indeed, there is no known reason for purine overproduction in renal hypouricemia. On the other hand, it is very likely that in the patients with renal hypouricemia, the hyperuricosuria reflects diversion of intestinal urate elimination to urinary urate excretion, consequent to the hypouricemia. The low plasma urate concentration undoubtedly results in reduced secretion of urate into the intestine, decreasing the availability of urate for bacterial degradation. Apparently this fraction of urate, which in normal subjects would have been eliminated by the intestinal bacteria, is excreted by the kidneys in patients with renal hypouricemia[13].

Hypercalciuria was found in 5 of the propositi (Table 1). In all except one[8] in whom the hypercalciuria could be attributed to immobilization, there was no detectable etiology for the hypercalciuria, which should therefore be classified as "idiopathic". In 3 of our propositi[3,6], the hypercalciuria was due to increased intestinal absorption of unexplained origin. None of these patients had evidence for a primary abnormality in renal calcium handling. Furthermore, in all propositi, careful studies refuted the presence of other tubular transport abnormalities, such as aminoaciduria or glycosuria. Thus the renal tubular defect leading to hypouricemia may be considered to be an isolated tubular abnormality.

GENETIC CONSIDERATIONS

Altogether, in the 7 families studied, 21 subjects (13 males and 8 females) were found to be affected with renal hypouricemia. In 4 families, both males and females were affected, whereas in 3 families only males could be found affected. The youngest hypouricemic subjects was a 2-year-old boy[7], the oldest a 65-year-old female[3]. In the family described by Sperling et al[3], an autosomal recessive mode of inheritance was proven and in all other families the mode of inheritance was compatible with such a pattern. A point of interest is that all 7 familial cases of renal hypouricemia reported from Israel are non-Ashkenazi Jews, 5 Iraqis, one Lybian and one Turk.

REFERENCES

1. E. Praetorius and J. E. Kirk, J. Lab. Clin. Med. 35:865 (1950).
2. M. L. Green, R. Marcus, G. D. Aurbach, E. S. Kazam, and J. E. Seegmiller, Am. J. Med. 53:361 (1972).
3. O. Sperling, A. Weinberger, I. Oliver, U. A. Liberman, and A. deVries, Ann. Intern. Med. 80:482 (1974).
4. D. Benjamin, O. Sperling, A. Weinberger, J. Pinkhas, and A. de Vries, Nephron 18:220 (1977).
5. D. Benjamin, O. Sperling, A. Weinberger, and J. Pinkhas, Biomed. 29:54 (1978).
6. M. Frank, M. Many, and O. Sperling, Br. J. Urol 51:88 (1979).
7. R. Weitz and O. Sperling, J. Pediat. 96:850 (1980).
8. M. Garty, A. Nitzan, and O. Sperling. Is. J. Med. Sci. 17:295 (1981).
9. A. de Vries and O. Sperling, Biomed. 30:75 (1979).
10. T. F. Yü, A. B. Gutman, L. Berger, and C. Kaung, Am. J. Physiol. 220:973 (1971).
11. O. Sperling, P. Boer, A. Weinberger, and A. Vries, Biomed. 23:157 (1975).
12. R. E. Rieselbach, Adv. Exp. Med. Biol. 76B:1 (1977).
13. O. Sperling, M. Frank, and M. Many, Adv. Urol. Nephrol. 14:67 (1979).

FAMILIAL XANTHINURIA IN A LARGE KINDRED: PURINE METABOLITES IN

PLASMA AND URINE OF XANTHINURICS, SIBLINGS AND NORMAL SUBJECTS

J. Costello, E. Al-Dabagh, M. Bentley, N. Fituri,
A. Watson, and B. Keogh

The Irish Stone Foundation Meath Hospital, Dublin
Eire, and The Renal Research Laboratory, Allegheny
General Hospital, Pittsburgh, Pennsylvania, U.S.A.

INTRODUCTION

Xanthinuria is a rare hereditary defect where there is a gross
deficiency of the enzyme xanthine oxidase. This results in hypouricemia, hypouricosuria and increased serum and urinary xanthine
and hypoxanthine. More than forty cases have now been reported in
the literature[1,2] and these have recently been reviewed[2]. We
report a further 3 cases of xanthinuria, 2 brothers and a sister.
The discovery of a case of familial xanthinuria provided a unique
opportunity to study purine metabolism in the patients, their
parents and siblings.

PATIENTS AND METHODS

The index case is an 8-year-old male who presented with
recurrent attacks of renal colic associated with macroscopic
hematuria. Biochemical investigations showed a urinary urate of 25
µmol/24 h and a plasma urate of 0.29 µmol/100 ml. Further analysis
revealed a urinary oxypurine excretion of 1345 µmol/24. The
patient had a kidney stone removed some 2 years earlier which on
analysis was unidentified. We suspect that it may have been a
xanthine calculus. Screening the parents and 6 siblings, we
identified a further 2 siblings, one male and one female, with this
metabolic defect. Neither of these 2 siblings had any history of
renal disease.

Urinary and plasma urate of normal subjects and urinary urate
of xanthinurics were determined as described by Praetorius and
Poulsen[3]. A modification of the method of Klinenberg et al[4] was

17

used for determination of urinary oxypurines in normal subjects. The uric acid in a 200 µl aliquot of urine was removed enzymically by action of uricase which was then inactivated by NaOH[5]. Plasma oxypurines of all subjects and plasma urate of xanthinurics were determined in the ultrafiltrate. Plasma was ultrafiltered through a PM-30 membrane using an Amicon Model 52 cell. Plasma oxypurines and uric acid of xanthinurics were determined on 500 µl of ultrafiltrate[4]. In normal subjects oxypurines were determined in 2.0 ml of ultrafiltrate after enzymic removal of uric acid[5]. Correction for losses on ultrafiltration were made by use of tracer ^{14}C-xanthine and hypoxanthine, and for uric acid by recovery of carrier urate. Urinary oxalate was determined by the method of Costello et al[6].

The 3 xanthinurics were studied while on a low purine diet as in-patients in the hospital. After 2 days on a normal hospital diet (control) they received a low purine diet (< 20 mg purine/day) for 3 days. Twenty-four-hour urine collections, containing 10 ml toluene, were made throughout the 5 days. Samples were analyzed for urate, oxypurines and oxalic acid. These metabolites were also studied in parents, siblings and normal subjects.

RESULTS AND DISCUSSION

Plasma and urinary excretion values for xanthinurics, parents, siblings and normal subjects are shown in Table 1. Parents and two siblings had plasma oxypurine values above normal (normal range 0.309 to 0.488 µmol/100 ml). Oxypurine excretion decreased dramatically (53.0 - 82.0%) in all 3 patients on a low purine diet while uric acid excretion increased 3.7- to 6.0-fold. Renal clearance of oxypurines was 74.0, 55.5 and 58.3 ml/min and for uric acid 5.4, 11.7 and 4.7 ml/min respectively for M.M., F.M. and Maj.M. while the oxypurine:creatinine clearance ratios were 2.2, 1.8 and 2.1.

Findings of hypouricemia, hypouricosuria, along with raised plasma urinary oxypurines (Table 1) confirmed 3 siblings to be xanthinuric. Xanthine accounted for 73 to 83% of the urinary oxypurines in agreement with others[1,7,8]. The plasma oxypurine values for normal subjects are lower than many earlier findings[1,7,8] but in agreement with the concentration of Yamanaka et al[9], who determined oxypurines by high performance liquid chromatography. The modified procedure of the present study, assaying 2.0 ml of plasma ultrafiltrate, makes these results more reliable. Both parents and siblings J.M. and S.M. had plasma oxypurines above our normal range while D.M. and C.M. had values close to the upper limit of normal. Raised plasma oxypurine levels in siblings or parents of xanthinurics have not been previously reported and may be indicative of carriers of a gene for xanthinuria. The xanthinuric patients had a somewhat higher renal clearance for oxypurines than

Table 1. Summary of Biochemical Features of Normal and Xanthinuric Subjects.

| | Age | Plasma (μmol/100 ml) | | Urine (μmol/24 h) | | | |
		Urate	Oxypurines	Uric Acid	Oxypurines	Creatinine	Xanthine (%)
Normal Adults [a]	–	21.6 ± 7.6	0.41 ± 0.06[b]	3047 ± 871	98.8 ± 34.1		
Normal Children [a]	(4–10)			1044 ± 425	57.4 ± 37.4		
Xanthinuric M.M.	8	0.290	1.23	22.5	1311	4199	82.3
Xanthinuric F.M.	7	0.089	1.94	15.0	1549	4384	73.0
Xanthinuric Maj.M.	5	0.372	1.20	25.0	1010	3182	83.0
Parents Js.M.	43	27.7	0.892	6017	99.8	–	–
Parents E.M.	41	23.6	0.601	2512	86.9	–	–
Siblings S.M.	14	16.6	0.517	1494	59.8	–	–
Siblings C.M.	13	21.7	0.476	1935	84.2	–	–
Siblings D.M.	11	20.2	0.446	3208	53.6	–	–
Siblings J.M.	4	16.3	0.708	1017	55.9	–	–

[a] Mean ± SD of ten subjects with exception of [b]; [b] Mean ± SD of seven subjects
(range 0.309 – 0.488 μmol/100 ml)

19

found by Engelman et al[7] and their oxypurine/creatinine clearance ratio exceeded unity, signifying tubular secretion of oxypurines. Higher clearance values for uric acid were also obtained.   Our higher clearance values are probably in part due to lower and more reliable plasma concentrations obtained for these metabolites using a large assay sample volume (500 μl of ultrafiltrate).

While on a low purine diet ($<$20 mg purine/day), urinary oxypurine excretion decreased dramatically in all 3 patients while uric acid excretion increased 3.7- to 6.0-fold.   These findings are in contrast to those of Ayvazian and Skupp[10] who found no decrease in oxypurines in their xanthinuric patient on a similar diet.   The increase in urinary uric acid when oxypurines decreased supports the hypothesis that oxypurines and uric acid compete for renal tubular secretory sites[7].   The decreased oxypurine excretion indicates that a low purine intake would be helpful to these patients in reducing the risk of xanthine crystal deposition in the tissues and renal stone formation.

Urinary oxalate excretion for the xanthinurics was in the normal range, decreasing somewhat on a low purine diet.   These observations are in accord with those of Gibbs and Watts[11] and suggest that xanthine oxidase is not essential for the glyoxylate to oxalate conversion in the intact human subject.

REFERENCES

1. R. A. Frayha, I. S. Salti, A. Arnaout, A. Khatchadurian, and S. M. Uthman, Nephrol. 19:328 (1977).
2. J. E. Seegmiller, in:"Metabolic Control and Disease", P. K. Bondy and L. E. Rosenberg, eds., W. B. Saunders, Philadelphia (1980).
3. E. Praetorius and H. Poulsen, Scand. J. Clin. Lab. Invest. 5:273 (1953).
4. J. R. Klinenberg, S. Goldfinger, K. H. Bradley, and J. E. Seegmiller, Clin. Chem. 13:834 (1967).
5. S. Jorgensen and H. E. Poulsen, Acta. Pharmacol. Toxicol. 11:223 (1955).
6. J. Costello, M. Hatch, and E. Bourke, J. Lab. Clin. Med. 87:903 (1976).
7. K. Engelman, R. W. E. Watts, J. R. Klinenberg, A. Sjoerdsma, and J. E. Seegmiller, Am. J. Med. 37:839 (1964).
8. H. J. Castro-Mendoza, L. Cifuentes Delatte, and A. Rapado Errazti, Rev. Clin. Esp. 124:341 (1972).
9. H. Yamanaka, K. Nishioka, T. Suzuki, and K. Kohno, Ann. Rheum. Dis. 42:684 (193).
10. J. H. Ayvazian and S. Skupp, J. Clin. Invest. 44:1248 (1965).
11. D. A. Gibbs and R. W. E. Watts, Clin. Sci. 31:285 (1966).

HEREDITY, SERUM PHOSPHATE AND URINARY CALCIUM IN CALCIUM UROLITHIASIS

B. Wikström, U. Backman, B. G. Danielson, B. Fellström,
K. Holmgren, G. Johansson, and S. Ljunghall

Dept. of Internal Medicine, University Hospital
S-751 85 Uppsala, Sweden

INTRODUCTION

Familial patterns of renal calcium stone disease have been reported[1,2]. Familial hypercalciuria has also been described[3]. The question as to whether or not other risk factors besides urinary calcium are inherited has not been extensively studied. Since stone formers often have low serum phosphate values[4] we designed a study to examine if low serum phosphate or hypercalciuria was a familial feature of stone formers.

PATIENTS AND METHODS

Our first series of stone patients in this study consisted of 380 stone formers, 253 males with a median age of about 50 years and 127 females with a median age of about 40 years. During a visit to our out-patient stone clinic these patients answered questions about their family history of stones. Low serum phosphate was defined as serum phosphate concentrations less than 0.80 mmol/l, and hypercalciuria as a urinary calcium excretion >7.5 mmol/day in males and >6 mmol/day in females.

RESULTS

A family history of stones was found in 56% of the stone formers. There was no difference between stone formers with low or normal serum phosphate. When we looked at the stone formers with low serum phosphate we found the same distribution of family history of stones in male and female patients. Analysis of the occurrence

21

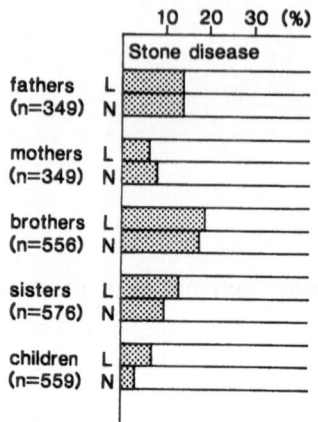

Fig. 1. Stone prevalence in relatives of stone patients.

Table 1. Distribution of the Different Relatives of the 18 Stone
         Formers in the Family Study.

4	Fathers
9	Mothers
15	Brothers
19	Sisters
14	Children
79	Subjects

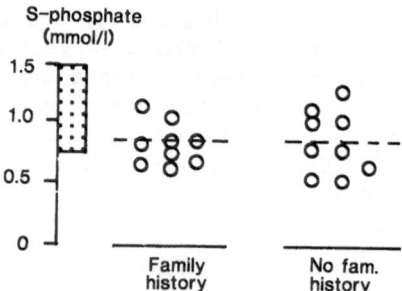

Fig. 2. Serum phosphate and family history of renal stones in a
         metabolic family study.

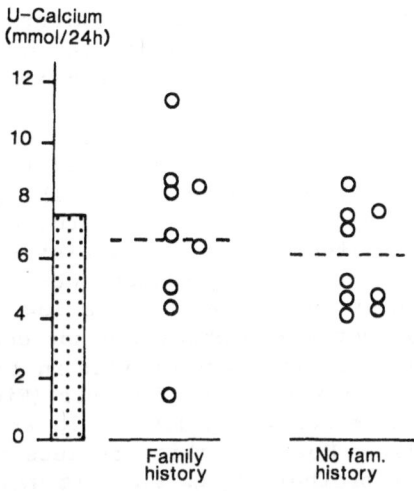

Fig. 3. Urinary calcium and family history of stones in a metabolic
family study.

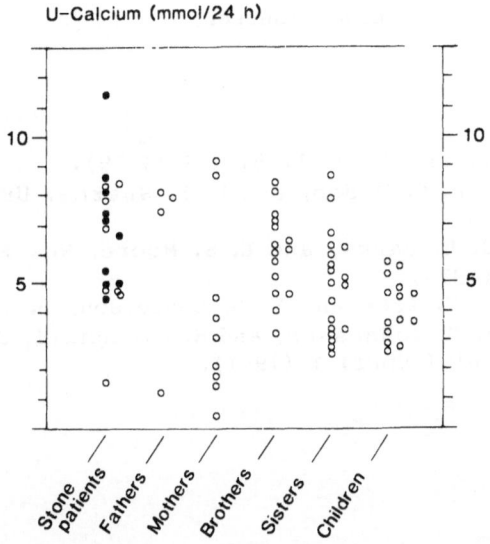

Fig. 4. Distribution of urinary calcium and serum phosphate in
the families of 18 stone patients.

of stone disease in relatives of stone patients showed that the prevalence of stone disease in the relatives was independent of the serum phosphate concentrations of the probands (Fig. 1).

Eighteen randomly selected patients and 61 of their first-degree relatives were studied in more detail in terms of their serum phosphate and urinary calcium excretion. The distribution of different relatives is shown in Table 1. Serum phosphate levels were not related to the existence of a family history of stones in the patients (Fig. 2). Such a family history was evident in 9 of the 18 stone formers. Ten of the patients had a low serum phosphate. In their relatives, low serum phosphate was noticed only occasionally. Also urinary calcium excretion was similar in the two patient groups with and without a family history of stones (Fig. 3). As might be expected, calcium excretion was generally lower in relatives compared to patients. However, this was less pronounced in siblings, especially brothers (Fig. 4). It was also noted that a low serum phosphate was not related to hypercalciuria.

DISCUSSION

This study has revealed that there is a familial tendency to calcium stone formation. Low serum phosphate and high urinary calcium were common findings in stone patients. However, first-degree relatives generally had normal serum phosphate and urinary calcium levels. Although low levels of serum phosphate or high levels of urinary calcium are common in stone formers, they are not familial features of stone disease.

REFERENCES

1. S. Ljunghall, Br. J. Urol. 51:249 (1979).
2. R. K. Marya, R. C. Dadoo, and N. K. Sharma, Urol. Int. 36:245 (1981).
3. F. L. Coe, J. H. Parks, and E. S. Moore, New Engl. J. Med. 300:337 (1979).
4. B. Wikström, U. Backman, B. G. Danielson, B. Fellström, K. Hellsing, G. Johansson, and S. Ljunghall, Scand. J. Urol. Nephrol. 61 (Suppl):1 (1981).

THE SIGNIFICANCE OF THE SEXUAL DEPENDENCY OF LITHOGENIC
AND INHIBITORY SUBSTANCES IN URINE

A. Hesse, A. Classen, K. Klocke, and W. Vahlensieck

Urologische Universitåtsklinik Bonn, D-5300 Bonn, F.R.G.

INTRODUCTION

Early studies indicated that the ratio of males:females among urolithiasis patients was 3:1. More recent studies, however, have shown that an increasing number of women suffer from stones. In our own study in 1980 of more than 10,000 persons the ratio of males:females was 1:1.2. For calcium oxalate urolithiasis, the age maxima are approximately the same for men and women, although weddellite stones are found more frequently in young people.

METHODS

In order to compare the urinary composition of men and women, 26 healthy persons (13 men, 13 women) and 71 calcium oxalate stone patients (52 men, 19 women) were examined on a normal free diet and during a 10-day period of standard food intake.

RESULTS AND DISCUSSION

Healthy men and women showed no differences in their urine volume, pH or specific gravity on either diet (Table 1). Similarly the stone patients did not show any significant differences in these parameters, although the men always had a larger urine volume than the women (Table 2). The excretion of oxalic acid, calcium and uric acid did not differ between healthy men and women. The trend towards an increased excretion of inorganic phosphorus observed in healthy men on a free diet was significant on the standard diet (Table 1).

Table 1. Sex Dependency of Urinary Excretion in 13 Health Controls (mean ± SD).

Urinary Factor (mmol/24 h)	Free Diet		Standard Diet	
	Females	Males	Females	Males
Volume 1/24h	1.23 ± 0.51	1.5 ± 0.62	2.67 ± 0.20	2.57 ± 0.14
pH	6.24 ± 0.49	6.24 ± 0.32	6.55 ± 0.29	6.52 ± 0.17
SG	1.015 ± 0.005	1.014 ± 0.006	1.006 ± 0.002	1.005 ± 0.002
Oxalic acid	0.40 ± 0.13	0.40 ± 0.15	0.38 ± 0.07	0.38 ± 0.07
Ca	3.71 ± 1.99	4.83 ± 2.18	3.99 ± 2.67	3.11 ± 1.16
Ca^{++}	1.23 ± 0.69	1.77 ± 1.02	0.63 ± 0.46	0.53 ± 0.37
P	24.8 ± 9.6	28.3 ± 9.0	19.4 ± 3.4	28.8* ± 6.8
Uric acid	3.22 ± 1.03	3.32 ± 1.10	2.52 ± 0.73	2.71 ± 0.44
Citric acid	3.18* ± 1.30	2.01 ± 1.05	4.27* ± 1.51	2.93 ± 0.94
Mg	3.54 ± 1.58	4.28 ± 2.51	4.44 ± 1.81	4.54 ± 1.68
SO_4	19.9 ± 6.6	22.8 ± 8.7	18.5 ± 7.3	23.9 ± 16.3
Na	140.1 ± 71.9	150.1 ± 65.0	113.8 ± 40.3	100.3 ± 40.3
K	40.4 ± 13.1	41.0 ± 19.9	35.5 ± 9.9	32.3 ± 9.3
Relative Superaturation	7.70 ± 4.74	7.91 ± 4.40	2.75 ± 1.37	2.59 ± 0.88

*$P < 0.05$

Table 2. Sex Dependency of Urinary Excretion of Calcium Oxalate Stone Formers (Mean ± SD).

Urinary Factor (mmol/24h)	Free Diet		Standard Diet	
	Females	Males	Females	Males
Volume 1/24h	1.52 ± 0.57	1.84 ± 0.7	2.45 ± 0.32	2.35 ± 0.33
pH	6.09 ± 0.60	6.07 ± 0.42	6.43 ± 0.43	6.54 ± 0.34
SG	1.012 ± 0.005	1.012 ± 0.005	1.006 ± 0.002	1.007 ± 0.002
Oxalic acid	0.38 ± 0.12	0.63* ± 0.42	0.38 ± 0.98	0.53 ± 0.36
Ca	4.14 ± 2.24	7.17* ± 3.30	4.14 ± 2.38	5.98 ± 4.49
Ca^{++}	1.59 ± 0.99	2.26* ± 1.16	0.74 ± 0.44	1.21 ± 1.08
P	27.1 ± 10.3	36.4 ± 10.3	21.6 ± 4.5	27.9* ± 6.5
Uric acid	3.57 ± 1.48	4.37 ± 1.57	2.61 ± 0.66	3.06 ± 1.37
Citric acid	2.18 ± 0.71	2.52 ± 1.23	3.74 ± 0.84	3.35 ± 1.48
Mg	4.49 ± 1.92	5.15 ± 2.19	4.00 ± 1.50	4.86 ± 2.70
SO_4	16.9 ± 7.5	24.1* ± 7.9	12.5 ± 4.3	17.1* ± 5.3
Na	163.4 ± 67.0	225.4* ± 71.1	110.2 ± 22.9	124.0 ± 35.3
K	26.3 ± 9.8	41.9* ± 19.0	32.5 ± 32.5	43.2* ± 19.4
Relative Supersaturation	6.52 ± 3.67	11.10 ± 8.11	3.71 ± 2.38	6.30 ± 5.23

*$P < 0.05$

In calcium oxalate stone patients, however, we found a significant sex dependence in the excretion of lithogenic substances. On a free diet there was a significant difference in oxalic acid, calcium (ionized calcium) and inorganic phosphorus. For oxalic acid and inorganic phosphorus the significance still remained after 7 days on the standard diet. However, there was a clear decrease in values on the standard diet in men and to some extent also in women so that the nutritional influence is obvious (Table 2).

In healthy women the excretion of citric acid was significantly higher than in men. This difference was not found in stone patients. However, for the urinary inhibitors (other than citric acid), the men had higher excretions than the women.

The calculation of the complex chemical interactions between the measured parameters and the relative supersaturation of calcium oxalate was carried out using the EQUIL computer program of Finlayson. Table 1 summarizes the results for healthy men and women. This shows that there is no difference between these groups on either dietary regime. The high relative supersaturation on the free diet is clear. For the stone patients, however, the results obtained were different (Table 2). Men have a significantly higher relative supersaturation than women and therefore a higher risk of calcium oxalate stone-formation.

We also compared calcium oxalate stone patients and healthy test persons on each of the dietary regimes. Female stone-formers had significantly lower potassium and citric acid excretions than normals. The male stone-formers had significantly higher excretions of sodium, calcium, phosphorus, uric acid and oxalic acid in their 24-h urine than normals on a free diet. Different results, however, were obtained on the standard diet. Under these conditions it is clear that the urine volume of stone patients is lower than that of healthy persons. This means that on a standard fluid intake, the stone patients must have a higher loss of fluid outside the kidneys. As a result the specific gravity of urine is higher in male stone patients than in healthy persons. Moreover, the excretions of potassium and calcium and relative supersaturation are significantly higher in men. In the female stone patients chloride and sulphate are significantly lower.

EPIDEMIOLOGY

INCIDENCE OF RENAL STONES IN WESTERN COUNTRIES

S. Ljunghall

Dept. of Internal Medicine, University Hospital
S-751 85 Uppsala, Sweden

INTRODUCTION

Since 1970 we have carried out a number of studies of the occurrence of renal stones in the unselected population in different types of health surveys[1-7]. This brief review summarizes some of the experiences from these investigations. It also includes results from a recent study in which almost 2000 60-year-old men were re-assessed 10 years after their initial evaluation[8], to enable us to estimate prospectively the natural history of stones.

It became apparent early in the course of these studies that hospital admission rates grossly underestimate the prevalence of stones in the population. For example, the data showed that about 14% of all middle-aged men experienced at least one renal stone and the annual incidence of stones in these age groups was around 1%. Yet, only between 2 and 3 patients per 1000 had been admitted to the hospital annually. Worldwide comparison of hospital statistics shows that Sweden, in fact, appears to have a rather low frequency of stones.

This discrepancy obviously arose because many patients with renal colic who subsequently passed their stone(s) spontaneously, did not seek medical care even when readily available[4]. Unless the hospital admission rates reflect the pattern of stone formation in the unselected population in a constant way they can therefore not be used for close estimations of the true occurrence and changes of frequency of stones in the population. At our own hospital, the admission rates for upper urinary tract stones have decreased considerably during the last decade (Fig. 1). This might give the impression that there has been a decrease in the incidence of stones

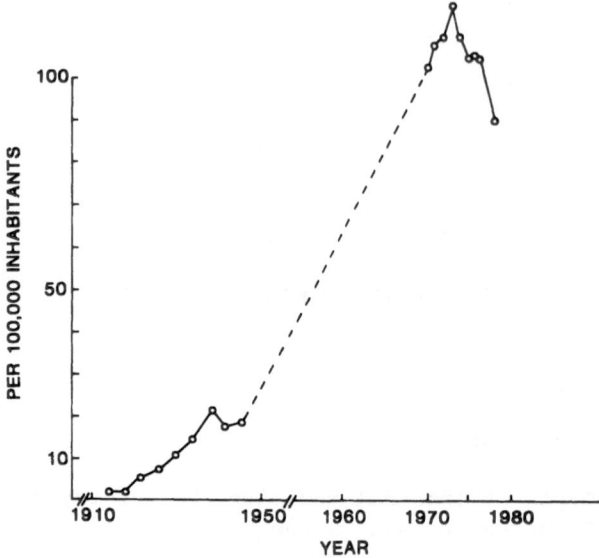

Fig. 1. Hospital admission rates for upper urinary tract stones
in Uppsala.

during this period. However, as will now be shown, evidence from
studies of unselected populations indicates that this is not the
case. A more likely explanation is that small change in the
criteria for admission have influenced the admission rates.

PREVALENCE OF RENAL STONE DISEASE

In a cross-sectional study of the population it is clear that
renal stones aflict mainly men and that the highest figures are
obtained in the middle-aged (Table 1). If frequency figures are to
be compared they must therefore refer to populations of similar age-
and sex-distributions.

In Rochester, Minnesota, a study was carried out on the
epidemiology of renal stones over a period of 25 years[9]. The
prevalence of stones was estimated to increase to a peak level of
about 12% in men over the age of 70. The equivalent rate in
females was less than 5%. It should be noted, however, that
clinical symptoms of stones diagnosed by a physician were required
in order for an individual to be included. Similar criteria were
used in a large study from the northern California region[10] where
3.2% of all males and 2.1% of all females had ever been informed by
a doctor that they had urinary tract stones. The annual incidence
rate of stones in males around the age of 50 was 0.36% and in

Table 1. Prevalence of Renal Stones (%) in a Swedish Health Survey.

Age (years)	35	40	45	50	55	60	65
Males	5.0	6.4	8.0	8.4	8.2	8.6	8.6
Females	2.9	2.0	2.3	3.3	3.1	2.0	2.2

females 0.15%. A large survey in West Germany[11] recorded a prevalence of urolithiasis of 6% of the men and 4% of the women of all ages. Stone prevalence increased with age and reached 7 to 8% in the group over 50 years of age. The annual occurrence was found to be 0.54% in all ages with a male to female ratio of 2:1. In a smaller sample Tschöpe et al[12] found an average prevalence of 6.9% with the highest value in 50 to 65 year-old men among whom 20% had a history of stones.

All studies referred to so far, including our own, have required symptomatic stone disease. The magnitude of asymptomatic, "silent", stones in the population has been studied in both autopsy and radiograph surveys of the population. Schumann[13], in a large autopsy series over several decades, found an increasing prevalence of urolithiasis with advancing age reaching 2% around the age of 50 and no difference between the sexes. In a radiographic survey of a random sample of the population in a new town in Scotland[14] a figure of 3.8% of calcified stones were found in 2000 subjects with an almost equal male to female ratio. A radiographic study with a similar design in the Netherlands[15] disclosed "silent" stones in 1% of the participants (1.6% of the males and 0.7% of the females). In addition 5.5% of all males and 3.4% of the females gave a history of previous stones.

These findings lend support to the conclusions from the epidemiological studies[1-7] that stones affect a considerable proportion of the population. The intriguing question of whether or not there are geographical variations and, if so, what are the reasons for the variable distribution of stones, is not completely answered. The studies cited above, give quite different prevalence figures that might cause speculation on whether or not there are significant geographic variations. However, the criteria for inclusion of individuals in the different studies and the techniques used have varied to such an extent that the differences in prevalence figures, although of an order of 2 to 3, cannot be definitely considered as significant. The intriguing question concerning the cause of any geographic variation might therefore have to await a definite answer until more directly comparable studies have been carried out. Based on the material presently available, it cannot be ruled out that inhabitants in Western countries share the most important environmental factors relevant to stone formation.

RISK OF RECURRENCE

Few prospective studies have been performed where patients have been followed regularly after their first stone incident. Johnson et al[9] in their detailed study from the Mayo Clinic found that 14 years after the first stone almost 50% of the males and 30% of the females had experienced at least one more stone (in both instances a physician's diagnosis was required for inclusion). These figures agree well with those obtained from retrospective evaluations of health surveys[2] and also in a 10-year follow-up study of middle-aged men[8]. Similarly, in a follow-up of patients presenting with their first stone, we recently found that, within 8 years, half of them had a recurrence of stones, the risk being almost twice as high in males as in females[16].

In several studies of various forms of medical treatment, control groups of recurrent stone patients have been followed either on placebo[17] or, in open studies, without attempts at specific treatment[18,19]. Among these patients the recurrence rate was even higher and amounted to 50% within 3 to 4 years. The risk of recurrence appears to be greatest during the years immediately after the first stone[9] but first recurrences can appear also more than 20 years later[5].

Naturally, it would be desirable to be able to predict the risk of recurrence after the patient first forms a stone. There have, however, been no reports where risk may be predicted with any greater degree of certainty from laboratory findings, although statistically a high urinary excretion of calcium and oxalate is related to an increased stone episode rate[16,20].

Individuals with an early onset of stone disease are slightly more prone to recurrence than those who do not experience stones until later in life, but the difference is not particularly impressive[8]. In the population studies the only notable factor that appeared to be related to the risk of stones and to frequent recurrence was a positive family history of stones[1]. The risk of stones was almost doubled in males with a family history of stones, i.e. stones in a first-degree relative. More detailed analysis showed that among these relatives there was a preponderance of stones in fathers and brothers of the prepositi. Similar findings have been reported from large studies in the USA[21] and Canada[22], where it was concluded that there was evidence of polygenic inheritance of renal stones. Later it was reported that, in some families, the inherited trait is idiopathic hypercalciuria[23]. We

34

were unable, however, to detect any differences in urinary calcium excretion between stone-formers with and without a family history of stones and also between non-stone-forming individuals classified as to whether or not they had a family history of stones[1].

Possibly the preponderance of stones in certain families could be due to factors other than genetic predisposition. It has been reported that the spouses of stone formers have a higher urinary calcium excretion than that of spouses from non-stone-forming house-holds and that, consequently, dietary factors are likely to be of importance[24]. In accordance with this observation, we found that the wives of those stone formers who had a family history of stones, had more than twice the incidence of stones observed in the wives of stone patients without stones among their relatives[1].

In a recent study we have attempted to analyze the family history of stones in a stone population investigated in some detail[25]. Almost 400 recurrent stone formers who had been submitted for evaluation were included, about 50% of whom had a positive family history of stones. This was more common among those who had frequent recurrences of stones particularly so in the females. In this study urinary calcium did not discriminate between the groups. A remarkable feature, however, was that subtle renal tubular defects, particularly appearing as incomplete renal acidification disturbances[26], were related to a family history of stones. Such defects, which can only be detected by ammonium chloride loading, occur in 15 to 20% of all stone formers. More than 80% of these patients, where there was a female dominance, had a positive family history of stones, and almost 40% of parents were affected. Only a few families have been investigated with acid-loading tests and it is not definite that the relatives of the patients with tubular defects also formed stones because of such defects. However, such a hypothesis seems attractive, particularly as it is well known that the complete acidification defects can be inherited.

Studies on the possible genetic factors of importance in calcium stone formation are hampered, however, by the large number of stones that seem to be caused by non-specific factors related to the affluence of our society. These dominate the field to such an extent that the subgroups with more specific causes, e.g. genetic, are overshadowed.

TIME DEVELOPMENT

It seems apparent from the frequency figures presented so far that there has been a marked increase in the incidence of renal stones during the recent few decades. This rise appears to be closely related to changes in life-style[26,27]. Without a prospective study it is difficult to ascertain if the increase is still continuing. There are indications from the population studies that we have not yet reached the peak of the "stone wave". Thus, at comparable ages the individuals of younger age classes generally have a higher prevalence of renal stones than the older ones. For example, in one study[5] the prevalence of stones in 40-year-old men was around 6%, whereas in the 20-year older age group at the same age the cumulated prevalence was only 2%. For female age groups the corresponding figures were 3.5% and 1%, respectively. Naturally we do not know for certain whether or not this tendency will continue in the future.

In conclusion, most studies attempting to measure the incidence of renal stones in unselected Western populations, have arrived at similar estimates. The life-time risk for males is at least of the order of 10% and that of females 1/3 to 1/2 of this. Insufficient data prevent analysis of possible geographical variations and environmental influences. The recurrence rate is high and in individuals with a long follow-up more common than single stones. In the multifactorial background of stone formation an inherited propensity could be of importance in some patients, particularly young females with an early onset of stone disease.

REFERENCES

1. S. Ljunghall, Br. J. Urol. 51:249 (1979).
2. S. Ljunghall, Eur. Urol. 4:424 (1978).
3. S. Ljunghall, Br. Med. J. 1:439 (1978).
4. S. Ljunghall, Scand. J. Urol. Nephrol. 41(Suppl):6 (1977).
5. S. Ljunghall, T. Christensson, and B. Wengle, Scand. J. Urol. Nephrol. 41(Suppl):39 (1977).
6. S. Ljunghall and H. Hedstrand, Acta Med. Scand. 199:481 (1976).
7. S. Ljunghall and A. U. Waern, Scand. J. Urol. Nephrol. 41(Suppl):55 (1977).
8. S. Ljunghall, E. Skarfors, and H. Lithell, (Submitted for publication).
9. C. M. Johnson, D. M. Wilson, W. M. O'Fallon, R. S. Malek, and L. T. Kurland, Kidney Int. 16:624 (1979).
10. R. A. Hiatt, L. G. Dales, G. D. Friedman, and E. M. Hunkeler, Am. J. Epidemiol. 115:255 (1982).
11. E. W. Vahlensieck, D. Bach, and A. Hesse, Urol. Res. 10:161 (1982).
12. W. Tschöpe, E. Ritz, M. Haslbeck, H. Mehnert, and H. Wesch, Klin. Wochenschr. 59:411 (1981).
13. H.-J. Schuman, Z. Urol. Nephrol. (1964).
14. R. Scott, R. Freeland, W. Mowat, M. Gardiner, V. Hawthorne, R. M. Marshall, and J. G. Yves, Br. J. Urol. 49:589 (1977).
15. H. van Geuns "Urinary tract calculi", Van Gorcum, Assen (1978).

16. S. Ljunghall and B. G. Danielson, Brit. J. Urol. (1984) (in press).

17. B. Ettinger, Am. J. Med. 61:200 (1976).

18. F. L. Coe, Ann. Intern. Med. 87:404 (1977).

19. S. Ljunghall, U. Backman, B. G. Danielson, B. Fellström, G. Johansson, and B. Wikström, Scand. J. Urol. Nephrol. 53 (Suppl):239 (1980).

20. W. G. Robertson, M. Peacock, R. W. Marshall, D. H. Marshall, and B. E. C. Nordin, New. Engl. J. Med. 194:249 (1976).

21. M. I. Resnick, D. P. Pridgen, and H. O. Goodman, New Engl. J. Med. 278:313 (1968).

22. D. N. Churchill, C. M. Maloney, J. Bear, D. G. Bryant, G. Fodor, and M. H. Gault, J. Chron. Dis. 33:727 (1980).

23. F. L. Coe, J. H. Parks, and E. S. Moore, New Engl. J. Med. 100:337 (1979).

24. R. W. White, R. D. Cohen, F. P. Vince, G. Williams, J. Blandy, and C. G. Tresidder, in:Proceedings of the Renal Stone Research Symposium", A. Hodgkinson and B. E. C. Nordin, eds., Churchill Livingstone, London (1969).

25. S. Ljunghall, B. G. Danielson, B. Fellström, K. Holmgren, G. Johannson, and B. Wikström (Submitted for publication 1984).

26. W. G. Robertson, M. Peacock, P. J. Heyburn, and F. A. Hanes, Scand. J. Urol. Nephrol. 53(Suppl):15 (1980).

27. W. G. Robertson, M. Peacock, P. J. Heyburn, F. A. Hanes, and R. Swaminathan, in:"Urinary Calculus", J. G. Brockis and B. Finlayson, eds., PSG Publishing Co., Littleton, Mass. (1981).

UROLITHIASIS - EPIDEMIOLOGICAL DATA FROM THE SOUTH OF PORTUGAL

J. M. Reis-Santos

Dept. of Urology, Curry Cabral Hospital and Faculty of
Medical Science, New University of Lisbon, Portugal

INTRODUCTION

Before treating patients with stones we must have
epidemiological and pathophysiological data to justify the type of
therapy given.   Priority areas or groups should be identified.   We
must also take into account the intrinsic and extrinsic factors
which, when combined with the abnormal excretion of one or more
urinary constituents, determine the "stone risk"[1].

PATIENTS AND METHODS

In an attempt to standardize the clinical history of patients
seen in the out-patient stone clinic, we have followed a fixed
protocol since 1975[2].   There are now 1452 patients in this survey,
756 males and 696 females.   To avoid variation due to climate, we
have only included patients living in Lisbon for more than 5 years
(67%) or in the south of Portugal (33%).   Age, sex and positive
family history were analyzed as intrinsic factors.

RESULTS

In 287 patients (19.8%) there was a family history of lithiasis
predominantly in brothers and sisters (91) or fathers (89);a history
of stones in mothers (32), aunts and uncles (27) was less common.
The majority of these patients were men with calcium oxalate stones.
Climate, passage through equatorial regions, profession, diet,
ingestion of liquids, urinary volume, disorders and drugs conducive
to lithiasis were considered to be extrinsic factors. The south

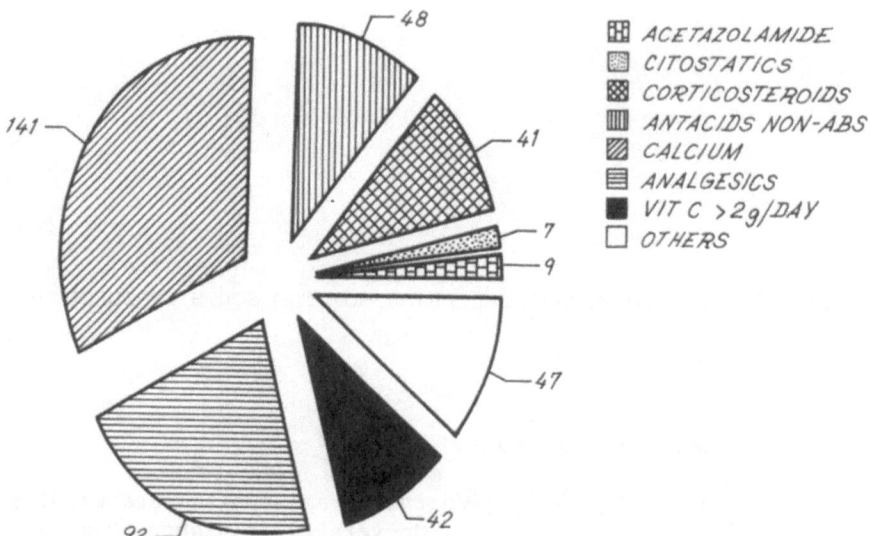

Fig. 1. Distribution of drugs possibly leading to stone-formation in 427 patients.

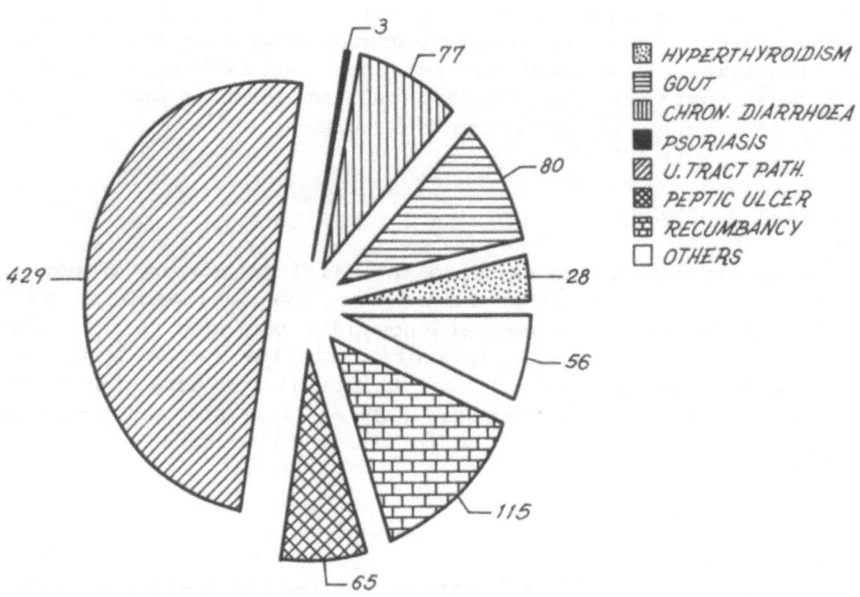

Fig. 2. Distribution of disorders predisposing to stone formation in 853 patients.

of Portugal is hot and sunny most of the year and it is uncommon to find people who drink a lot of water. As a result many patients on their first visit to our clinic have a total daily urine volume of less than 1000 ml. This chronic dehydration is aggravated if the patient has spent some time in the tropics. This was the case in 15.2% of our patients and 75% of their stone episodes, usually the first stone, occurred during this period. The majority of the group were young men doing military service in Angola, Mozambique and Guinea.

Only 2.6% of the total had an occupation which might lead to chronic dehydration. On classifying the patients according to profession we found that 9.9% were considered active, 83% sedentary and 7.1% could not be classified. In 29.3% of the cases there was a history of drug ingestion leading to stone formation (acetazolamide 0.6%, cytostatics 0.5%, uricosuric drugs 0.3%, corticosteroids 2.8%, ACTH 0.2%, non-absorbable antacids + milk 3.3%, vitamin D 0.4%, calcium 9.7%, analgesics 6.3%, vitamin C (+ 2 g/day) 2.9%, others 2.3%) (Fig. 1). A history of disorders known to cause stone formation (Fig. 2) was found in 58.7% of the patients (hyperthyroidism 1.9%, gout 5.5%, psoriasis 0.2%, chronic diarrhoea 5.3%, upper urinary tract obstruction 7.6%, lower urinary tract obstruction 1.7%, history of urinary tract infection 15.5%, genito-urinary tuberculosis 4.7%, peptic ulcer 4.5%, prolonged recumbency 7.9%, and others 3.9%).

A diet history was taken from all the patients to evaluate eating and drinking habits and to determine their total daily caloric intake. We also tried to estimate the daily intake of protein, carbohydrate and lipid. The daily intake of fibre was particularly noted. We found 4.8% had a hypocaloric diet, 36.2% a hypercaloric diet and 59% a normal caloric diet. Only 2.4% had a high fibre intake compared with 73.5% with a low fibre intake and 24.1% with a normal fibre intake.

A total of 1320 calculi were collected from these patients and analysed by crystallography; 64.5% consisted of calcium oxalate, 14% of magnesium ammonium phosphate, 19% of uric acid, 0.9% of cystine, and 1.5% formed the remainder. It was possible to identify the constituents of the nucleus in 67% of the stones. Whewellite accounted for 29%, uric acid 3.5%, brushite 2.9%, cystine 0.4% and ammonium acid urate 0.4%.

DISCUSSION

In our survey the ratio of male to female patients is almost equal. This is probably because our unit deals only with complicated cases and therefore we tend to get a disproportionate number of women with infected stones, rather than young men who pass their first stone spontaneously. Lisbon and the south of Portugal have a warm, sunny climate most of the year and, generally speaking, people drink very little water. This leads to "chronic dehydration". It is quite common to see patients with total daily urine volumes of between 500 and 1000 ml. It is interesting to note the high percentage of patients who had lived in the tropics and the relationship between this and the formation of stones[3]. Hereditary factors were more common among male patients[4]. The majority of our patients had sedentary occupations and only a few had active jobs. A tiny majority worked under conditions leading to chronic dehydration[3]. In many cases we found a history of drug ingestion that might have been responsible for stone formation[5].

The high calcium intakes were associated with the prescription of calcium to patients with tuberculosis and during pregnancy. Amongst the disorders related to urolithiasis, urinary pathology, upper urinary tract obstruction, a history of urinary infection and genito-urinary tuberculosis were the most common. (Genito-urinary tuberculosis is found frequently in our clinic). Obesity and a hypercaloric diet, either separately or together, were often found in our patients, usually in association with a high consumption of sugar-containing drinks and refined carbohydrates[6,7]. Few people ate green vegetables, either cooked, in soup, or raw in salads and fruit was nearly always peeled. Wholemeal bread was seldom eaten. Hence, it is not surprising to find that the daily fibre intake was low in 75% of our patients[3]. Crystallographic analysis of the calculi show calcium oxalate stones to be the most common[8]. Uric acid stones were commonly found in the south of Portugal.

REFERENCES

1. W. G. Robertson and M. Peacock, in:"Scientific Foundations of Urology", G. D. Chisholm and D. I. Williams, eds., Heinemann, London (1982).
2. J. M. Reis-Santos and A. Matos-Ferreira, Acta Med. Portuguesa (1984) (in press).
3. N. J. Blacklock, in:"Scientific Foundations of Urology", G. D. Chisholm and D. I. Williams, eds., Heinemann, London (1982).
4. S. Ljunghall and H. Hedstrand, Acta Med. Scand. 197:439 (1975).
5. G. A. Rose, "Urinary Stones:Clinical and Laboratory Aspects", MTP Press, Lancaster (1982).
6. O. Zechner and V. Scheiber, in:"Urolithiasis:Clinical and Basic Research", L. H. Smith, W. G. Robertson, and B. Finlayson, eds., Plenum, New York (1981).
7. W. G. Robertson, M. Peacock, P. J. Heyburn, R. Speed, and F. Hanes, Fortshr. Urol. Nephrol. 11:5 (1978).
8. B. I. Otnes and D. Montgomery, Invest. Urol. 17:314 (1980).

EPIDEMIOLOGICAL ASPECTS OF UROLITHIASIS IN A GERMAN COUNTY

B. Ulshöfer

Urologische Universitätklinik und Poliklinik Marburg
D-3550 Marburg a.d. Lahn, F.R.G.

INTRODUCTION AND METHODS

Factors other than those measured in the laboratory may be important for stone formation[1-7]. Using a routine laboratory program[8], more than 1200 stone patients were investigated over 3 years. Additional information concerning the age, sex, occupation, education and stone history of the patients was collected. The majority of stone formers in the Marburg area within a set time have been recorded. Statistics were provided by the local records department[9] and stone incidence was calculated from their records and from the urology clinic records.

RESULTS

Fig. 1 shows that stone incidence ranged from 0.012% in young adults to over 0.3% in the elderly ($P < 0.001$). Differences between males and females were established in the 35 to 49 year-old ($P < 0.025$), the 50 to 64 year-old ($P < 0.001$) and the over 64 year-old age groups ($P < 0.001$). Fig. 2 shows the incidence of calcium and uric acid stones in males in relation to age. The pattern of stone composition in various socio-economic groups, consisting of 44 farmers, 493 workers, 233 employees and 48 graduates, is shown in Fig. 3. The prevalence of uric acid-containing stones was lower in graduates than in the other groups (farmers $P < 0.005$, workers $P < 0.025$, employees n.s.). Indeed, no pure uric acid stones were found in this group. Workers and graduates also differed with respect to the age of onset of calcium stone formation (Fig. 4). Most of the graduates were between 25 and 34 and the workers between 50 and 64 years old ($P < 0.001$).

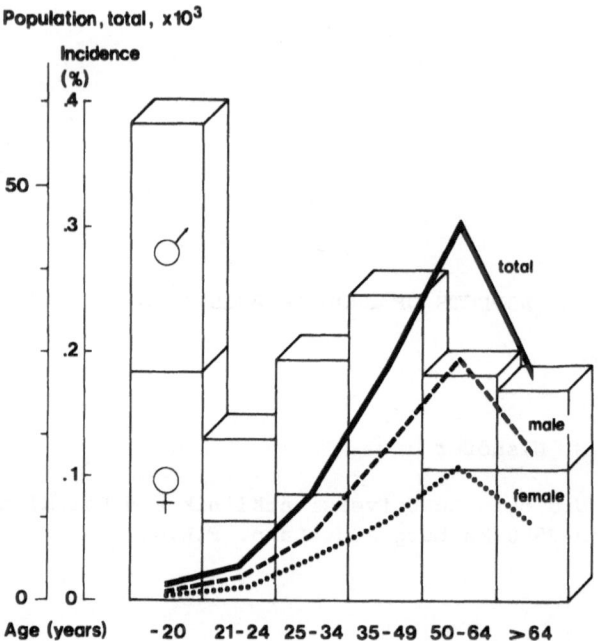

Fig. 1. Stone incidence in a German county.

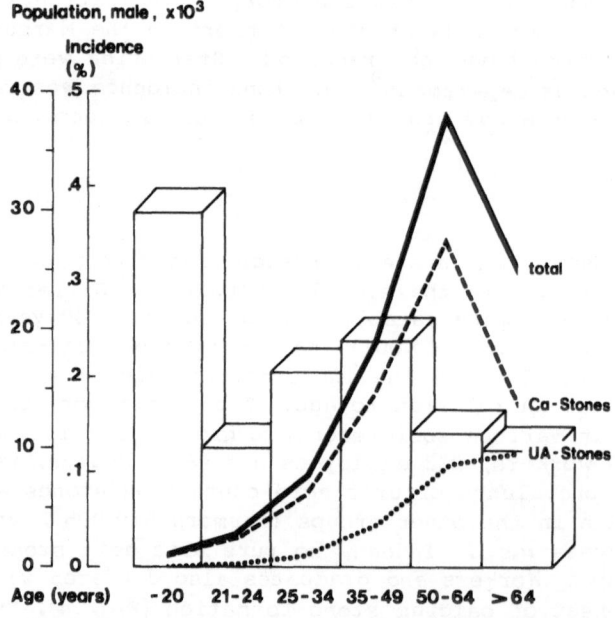

Fig. 2. Incidence of calcium and uric acid stones in males in a Germany county.

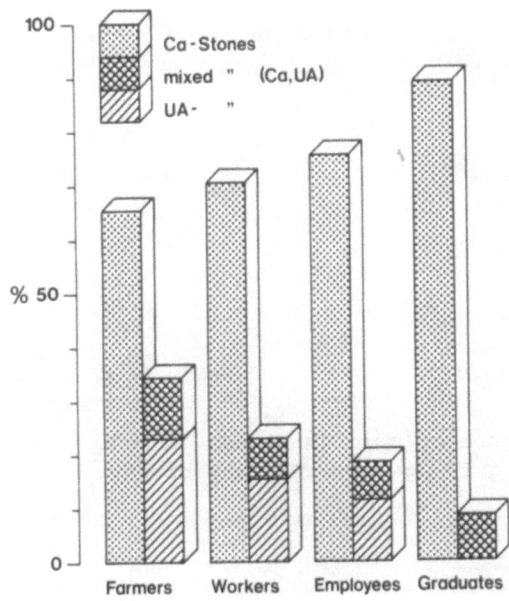

Fig. 3. Frequency of stone types in different socio-economic
groups in a German county.

DISCUSSION

     In the area described the actual incidence of stone formation
depends more on age and sex than on calcium and uric acid excretion,
at least up to the age of about 64 years. The decrease in the over
64-year-old group is explained to some extent by a lowered excretion
of lithogenic substances. The sharp increase over 35 years and the
difference between males and females cannot be explained entirely
from our laboratory results. It is concluded that where there is
similar urinary composition the risk of forming stones depends
mainly on sex and age.

     Standard of living seems to be another factor influencing the
risk of urinary stones[3,10]. Socio-economic (s-e) grouping takes
education, occupation and income into consideration. Stone composition is related to s-e group[3]. The higher incidence of uric acid
stones in the "lower" groups is not explained by uric acid excretion
or urinary pH. Calcium excretion was elevated in the calcium
stone-formers in all groups, but there was no difference in uric
acid excretion. So the pattern of stone composition agreed with
previous findings over the centuries and in various countries[11].

     The different ages at which stone formation occurs in the
different s-e groups, particularly workers and graduates, has not
been reported before. Stone formation in the latter occurs about

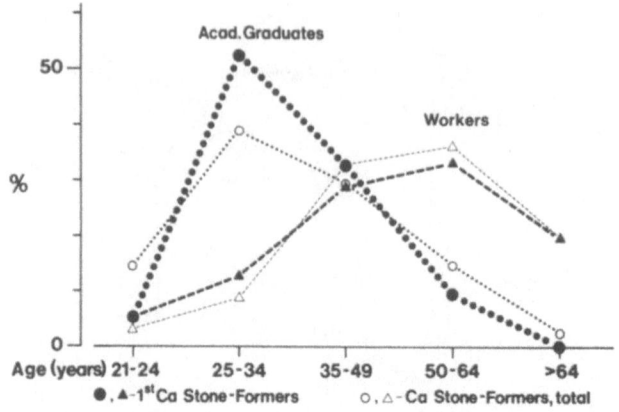

Fig. 4. Occurrence of calcium stones in male workers and graduates acording to age in a Germany county.

20 years earlier than in the former (P<0.001). Previous studies have shown that stress, within the 2 years before the first attack of renal colic, may be a promoter of the first calcium stone in males[7]. It is suggestive that living conditions and the problem of obtaining or keeping a job along with somatic or psychosomatic illness[12] may influence the age at which stones form.

REFERENCES

1. H.-J. Schneider and E. Hienzsch, in:XVIII Congress of the International Society of Urology", Paris (1979).
2. W. Vahlensieck, A. Hesse, and W. Bach, Urologe B 20:273 (1980).
3. W. G. Robertson, M. Peacock, and P. J. Heyburn, Fortschr. Urol. Nephrol. 14:105 (1979).
4. B. Ulshöfer, Klin. Wschr. 62:191 (1984).
5. P. Brundig, W. Berg, and H.-J. Schneider, Urol. Int. 36:265 (1981).
6. H. Toggenburg, C. Horica, and K. Bandhauer, Fortschr. Urol. Nephrol. 17:15 (1981).
7. B. Ulshöfer, G. Paar, and B. Cramer, Verhandlungsber. 34 Tagung Dtsch. Ges. fur Urologie, Springer-Verlag, Berlin (1983).
8. B. Ulshöfer, Helv. Chir. Acta, 47:345 (1980).
9. Statistisches Handbuch Marburg-Biedenkopf, Marburg (1978).
10. O. Zechner and V. Scheiber, in:"Urolithiasis - Clinical and Basic Research", L. H. Smith, W. G. Robertson, and B. Finlayson, eds., Plenum, New York (1981).
11. R. Asper, Urol. Res. 12:1 (1984).
12. J. Siegrist, Nervenarzt 51:313 (1980).

EPIDEMIOLOGY OF UROLITHIASIS AND CALCIUM METABOLISM

IN HUMAN DIABETES MELLITUS

W. Tschöpe, E. Ritz, M. Haslbeck, H. Mehnert, and
D. Deppermann

Depts. of Internal Medicine, University of Heidelberg
Diabetes Research, Municipal Hospital, Munchen-
Schwabing, and Internal Medicine, Ludwigshafen, F.R.G.

INTRODUCTION

It has been shown in man[1] and dogs[2] that, in the presence of a
constant blood glucose level, administration of insulin results in
an exaggerated urinary excretion of calcium and increased tubular
reabsorption of phosphorus. In the diabetic state (established
insulin deficiency) the hypocalciuric effect of insulopenia
counteracts the hypercalciuric effect of glucose-induced osmotic
diuresis[3]. In the present epidemiological study the prevalence of
urolithiasis and hypercalciuria have been determined in diabetics
and controls.

PATIENTS AND METHODS

A total of 339 diabetics (169 male, 179 female) and 317
controls (171 male, 156 female) were examined. All were
interviewed by one examiner with a standardized questionnaire. In
addition, 24-h urines were collected. The exclusion criteria were
renal insufficiency (plasma creatinine 1.4 mg/dl), immobilisation,
chronic intestinal diseases, parenteral nutrition, malignant
diseases, nephrological problems, and steroid treatment. The
controls were non-diabetic patients, admitted to the Departments of
Dermatology or Surgery of the Municipal Hospital of Munich.

RESULTS

Since the menopause may influence urinary calcium, the age
groups (20 to 40 years and 45 and 65 years) were analysed separately

47

Table 1. Data on 20 to 4-Year-Old Diabetics and Controls (Mean+SD).

	Diabetics		Controls	
	Male	Female	Male	Female
Number	57	54	72	63
Age (years)	30.5 ± 6.0	30.0 ± 6.3	31.0 ± 6.0	30.0 ± 5.7
Weight (kg)	69 ± 9	62 ± 10	71 ± 10	62 ± 15
UV Cr (mmol)	13.0 ± 5.6	10.9 ± 5.6	13.4 ± 5.2	10.3 ± 4.3
UV Ca (mmol)	4.6 ± 2.8	3.5 ± 1.9	3.5 ± 2.6	3.5 ± 2.1
UV Na (mmol)	175 ± 92	140 ± 68	116 ± 69	104 ± 50
UV Gluc (mmol)	205 ± 227	125 ± 159	–	–

Table 2. Data on 45 to 65-Year-Old Diabetics and Controls (Mean+SD).

	Diabetics		Controls	
	Male	Female	Male	Female
Number	36	43	37	32
Age (years)	52.6 ± 6.8	50.0 ± 6.0	52.0 ± 5.6	53.0 ± 6.0
Weight (kg)	70 ± 10	66 ± 12	75 ± 9	68 ± 10
UV Cr (mmol)	12.3 ± 4.3	10.0 ± 3.2	13.2 ± 6.7	9.4 ± 2.4
UV Ca (mmol)	4.5 ± 3.7	3.9 ± 2.5	3.5 ± 2.6	2.7 ± 1.6
UV Na (mmol)	169 ± 79	139 ± 81	142 ± 78	118 ± 50
UV Gluc (mmol)	67 ± 69	137 ± 203	–	–

Table 3. Calcium Excretion and Mode of Therapy in Diabetic Patients (Median (range)).

	Oral	Insulin		
		1 year	10 years	10 years
Age (years)	49 (22-63)	39 (20-64)	36 (20-64)	37 (23-63)
Weight (kg)	75 (49-106)	65 (45-101)	64 (49-53)	65 (50-88)
UVCr (mmol)	11.7 (7.0-218)	10.7 (6.4-17.5)	11.8 (3.4-26)	12.3 (0.5-28.4)
UVCa (mmol)	4.2 (0.2-11.5)	52.5 (0.2-11.5)	3.7 (0.7-15.6)	3.7 (1.0-13.5)
UVNa (mmol)	112 (35-109)	151 (20-278)	144 (34-448)	153 (19-343)
UVGluc (mmol)	29 (0.7-412)	74 (0.3-907)	116 (0.5-833)	76 (0.2-724)

(Tables 1 and 2). Diabetics had significantly higher urinary volumes than controls, but showed no increase in urinary calcium. There were slightly higher calcium excretions in the younger male diabetics than in the controls (Table 1;$P<0.05$) but this was associated with a high urinary sodium excretion. Since the mode of therapy (oral or insulin) could be important in determining urinary calcium, all diabetics in the age group 20 to 65 years were analysed according to therapy (Table 3): 26 patients had been treated with oral anti-diabetic medication, 35 with insulin for less than one year, 59 for between 1 and 10 years, and 57 for more than 10 years. As shown in Table 3, only the insulin-treated subgroups were comparable in terms of age and weight. There were no differences in urinary calcium or sodium between these 3 groups. After correction for lean body mass there was no difference in urinary calcium between the orally- and insulin-teated groups, though diabetics on oral treatment excreted markedly less sodium and glucose and calcium excretion. In addition, urinary calcium was not correlated with the form of therapy, duration of treatment or length of disease.

A group of 34/339 (10%) diabetics had a history of renal stone disease. In controls, the prevalence of nephrolithiasis was not different (32/337 (9.8%)). A total of 13.9% of the male diabetics and 9.9% of the male controls gave a history of stone disease: in women this percentage was slightly lower (diabetics 12.3%, controls 7.1%). A total of 3.8% of the diabetic population and 2.7% of the controls had been operated on because of stone disease. In the 15 to 65 year-old group, the prevalence rates of renal stone formation in non-diabetic patients (6.7%) and diabetic patients (6.8%) were identical. The calculated stone incidence in the combined populations was approximately 0.6% per year[6].

DISCUSSION

Though the presence of osteopenia in diabetics has been proven histomorphologically[4], no increased risk of skeletal fractures in diabetics has been found[7]. In a study on vitamin D metabolism in diabetics[8] there was no difference in iPTH, 25-H-HCC or 1,25-DHCC levels between treated diabetics and their age- and sex-matched controls. These findings contrast with the experimental diabetes mellitus of the insulin-deficient rat, in which in the presence of normal renal function 1,25-DHCC levels are markedly suppressed[9]. The observation[4] that, in severely ketotic diabetics, hypercalciuria is common, is not inconsistent with the present findings, since chronic insulin treatment leads to normalisation of urinary calcium and 1,25-DHCC[10]. The present data show, that even in the presence of very high urinary glucose levels (>180 g/24 h) there is no hyper-calciuria. The slightly higher urinary calcium of the younger male diabetics might be of dietary origin, since they also had higher urinary sodium excretions. Form of therapy, length of disease, duration of insulin treatment and degree of hyperglycosuria were not correlated with urinary calcium.

It is difficult from the present epidemiological study to explain diabetic osteopenia on the basis of the renal loss of calcium. In addition, the comparable calcium excretions in diabetics and controls is consistent with the observation that diabetics do not have a higher prevalence of urolithiasis. It can be concluded that the risk of renal stone disease in diabetics is comparable with that in non-diabetics despite their glucosuria and increased prevalence of urinary tract infection, since the degree of hypercalciuria is correlated with the prevalence of nephrolithiasis[11].

REFERENCES

1. R. A. DeFronzo, M. Goldberg, and Z. A. Agus, J. Clin. Invest. 58:83 (1976).
2. R. A. DeFronzo, C. R. Cooke, R. Andres, G. R. Faloona, and P. J. Davis, J. Clin. Invest. 55:845 (1975).
3. P. Raskin, M. R. M. Stevenson, D. E. Barilla, and C. Y. C. Pak, Clin. Endocrinol. 9:329 (1978).
4. J. D. Ringe, F. Kuhlencordt, and J. Kuhnau, Dtsch. Med. Wschr. 101:280 (1976).
5. L. Sachs, "Angewandte Statistik", Springer, Berlin (1978).
6. W. Tschöpe, E. Ritz, M. Haslbeck, H. Mehnert, and H. Wesch, Klin. Wschr. s59:411 (1981).
7. H. Heath, L. J. Melton, and C. Chu, New Engl. J. Med. 303:567 (1980).
8. H. Heath, P. W. Lambert, F. J. Service and S. B. Arnaud, J. Clin. Endocrinol. Metab. 49:462 (1979).
9. B. E. Walker, and H. P. Schedl,. Proc. Soc. Exp. Biol. Med. 161:149 (1979).
10. J. M. Gerner, V. W. Tamborlande, R. L. Horst, R. S. Sherwin, P. Feelig, and M. Genel, J. Clin. Endocrinol. Metab. 50:862 (1980).
11. S. Ljunghall, Scand. J. Urol. Nephrol. (Suppl) 41:5 (1977).

NUTRITION

URINARY CALCIUM EXCRETION AND NET ACID EXCRETION: EFFECTS OF DIETARY PROTEIN, CARBOHYDRATE AND CALORIES

J. Lemann

Nephrology Section, Dept. of Medicine and Clinical
Research Center, Medical College of Wisconsin
Froedtert Memorial Lutheran Hospital, Milwaukee
Wisconsin 53226, U.S.A.

INTRODUCTION

The incidence of kidney stones composed of calcium oxalate and apatite is increased among the populations of developed nations[1,2]. This increased frequency may be related to the dietary intake of animal protein[3]. Dietary protein intake is a determinant of endogenous fixed acid production, renal net excretion and external acid balance[4,5]. In turn, acid production, renal net acid excretion and acid balance are determinants of urinary Ca excretion and Ca balance[6]. Increased rate of urinary Ca excretion is one of the risk factors for Ca stone formation.

NET FIXED ACID PRODUCTION, RENAL NET ACID EXCRETION AND ACID BALANCE

The chemical reactions resulting in the addition of acid or base to body fluids can be indirectly quantitated[7]. Normal diets contain actual or potential base, reflecting net addition of base to body fluids that can be quantitated as the unmeasured anion of the diet ($\sum$ [Na + K + Ca + Mg, mEq/day] − [Cl, mEq/day + 1.8 PO_4, mmol/day]). The feces also contain potential base reflecting net addition of acid to (or loss of potential base from) body fluid, that can be similarly quantitated by estimation of the fecal unmeasured anion. The quantities of inorganic sulfate in the urine and of organic anion in the urine also reflect reactions leading to the net addition of acid to the body. The sum of these reactions (urinary $SO_4^=$ + O.A.⁻ + fecal UA − diet UA, mEq/day) provides an estimate of acid production.

53

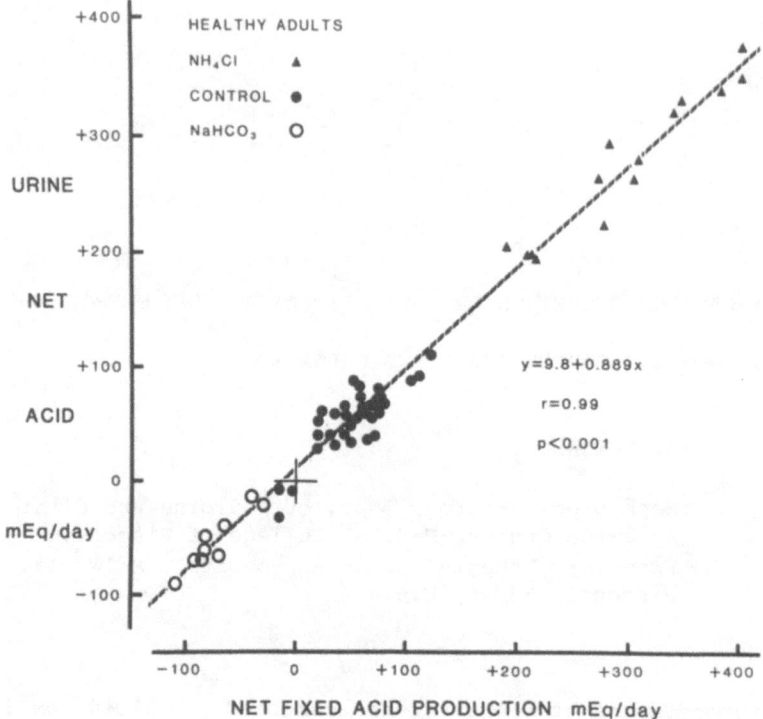

Fig. 1. Renal net acid production as a function of net fixed acid production[4,6-10].

Net renal hydrogen ion or acid excretion can be quantitated as the sum of the secreted hydrogen ion appearing in the urine buffered by filtered buffer, chiefly phosphate (tritratable acidity) and buffered by secreted (ammonium) less any filtered bicarbonate that escapes renal tubular reabsorption (i.e. $TA + NA_4^+ - HCO_3^-$, mEq/day).

The difference between net acid production and renal net acid excretion is an estimate of external acid balance. When acid production in 16 healthy adults averaged 63 mEq/day and ranged from 20 to 120 mEq/day, net acid excretion was virtually identical so that acid balance was indistinguishable from zero[7] averaging -1 ± 12 mEq/day (n = 16). In the chronic steady state, the kidney possesses an enormous capacity to augment either net acid excretion or bicarbonate excretion in response to changes in acid production achieved either by altering dietary protein intake, administering NH_4Cl or $NaHCO_3$. Thus, as shown in Fig. 1, net acid excretion varies directly with acid production. However, the slope of the relationship is significantly less than one (P<0.001). Consequently, acid balance varies directly with the rate of fixed

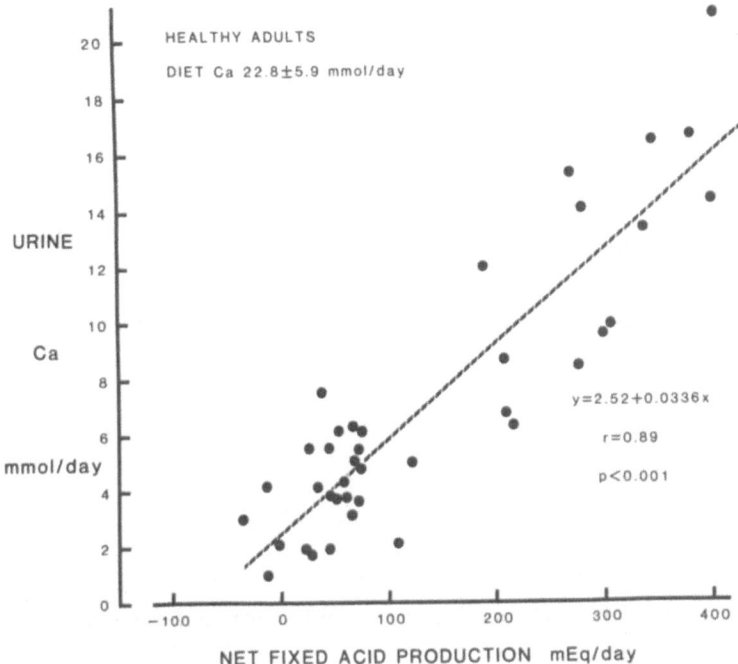

Fig. 2. Urinary calcium excretion as a function of net fixed acid production[4,6,7,9,10].

acid production (Acid Balance, mEq/day = - 9.7 + 0.104 Net Fixed Acid Production, mEq/day; r = 0.65; P<0.001). Acid balance will, on the average, be positive when acid production exceeds about 90 mEq/day.

RELATIONSHIPS OF URINARY CALCIUM EXCRETION AND CALCIUM BALANCE TO ACID PRODUCTION AND ACID BALANCE IN HEALTH

As shown in Fig. 2, when dietary Ca intake (mean ± SD) is normal averaging 22.8 ± 5.9 mmol/day, urinary Ca excretion is directly related to acid production. However, on the average, urinary Ca excretion does not exceed 7.5 mmol/day, the generally accepted upper limit of normal, until acid production exceeds about 140 mEq/day. Urinary Ca excretion obviously is also directly related to net acid excretion: UCaV, mmol/day = 2.67 + 0.037 net acid excretion, mEq/day; r = 0.91; P<0.001, n = 48 [4,6,9,10] but on the average urinary Ca excretion will not exceed 7.5 mmol/day unless net acid excretion exceeds about 130 mEq/day. Increased rates of acid production, net acid excretion and urinary Ca excretion are not, however, accompanied by a compensatory increase in intestinal Ca absorption either when acid production is augmented by the

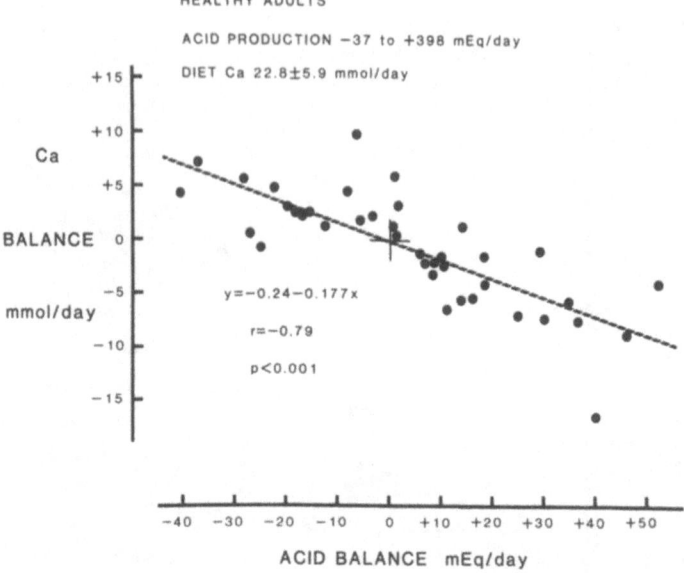

HEALTHY ADULTS

ACID PRODUCTION −37 to +398 mEq/day

DIET Ca 22.8±5.9 mmol/day

$y = -0.24 - 0.177x$

$r = -0.79$

$p < 0.001$

Fig. 3.   Calcium balance as a function of acid balance[4,6,9,10].

administration of NH_4Cl[11] or by increasing dietary protein[12-15].
Thus, as shown in Fig. 3, Ca balance is inversely related to acid
balance as acid balance ranges from −37 to +52 mEq/day in healthy
subjects eating diets providing normal quantities of Ca.   The
augmented Ca losses into the urine that result in negative Ca
balances when acid production is increased are thus ultimately
derived from bone[6].

THE COMPONENTS OF ACID PRODUCTION IN HEALTH

    The diet is a major determinant of acid production[4,6,7,9,10].
Urinary SO_4 excretion is directly correlated with dietary protein
intake and the sulfur content of the protein.   Egg white contains
20 mg S/g protein[16] or 1.25 mEq potential SO_4/g protein while mixed
dietary proteins provide about 9 mg S/g protein or 0.57 mEq
potential SO_4/g protein.   Urinary organic anion also increases by
about 9 mEq/100 g protein as dietary protein is increased using meat
as the additional protein[17].   Since the administration of base as
$NaHCO_3$ reduces net fixed acid production[8,18], diets containing
significant quantities of potential base, chiefly as potassium salts
of metabolizable organic acids in vegetables and fruits will reduce
net fixed acid production and thus limit urinary Ca losses.
Potassium itself appears to have an additional effect on reducing
urinary Ca excretion[19].

ACID PRODUCTION, NET ACID EXCRETION AND URINARY CALCIUM EXCRETION IN
PATIENTS WITH NEPHROLITHIASIS

Acid balances have not, apparently been measured in Ca stone
formers.   However, despite hypercalciuria in about one-half of this
group, they are not known to exhibit reduced serum bicarbonate
concentrations or obvious defects in renal net acid excretion.
Moreoever, they do not exhibit significant bone disease which would
be expected if chronically positive acid balances were a determinant
of hypercalciuria.   Daily urinary net acid excretion in relation to
urinary urea-nitrogen excretion, as an estimate of protein intake,
is similar among stone formers and among healthy adults when both
groups were studied while eating their usual self-selected home
diets (for both groups: Net acid excretion, mEq/day = 6 + 5 Urine
urea nitrogen, g/day).   This observation suggests both groups eat
comparable mixed diets.   However, since most stone formers are men
with greater body weights, some stone formers will thus eat more
protein and exhibit higher rates of net acid excretion.   To the
extent that high protein diets are also accompanied by increased
oxalate excretion[20] and increased net acid excretion may be

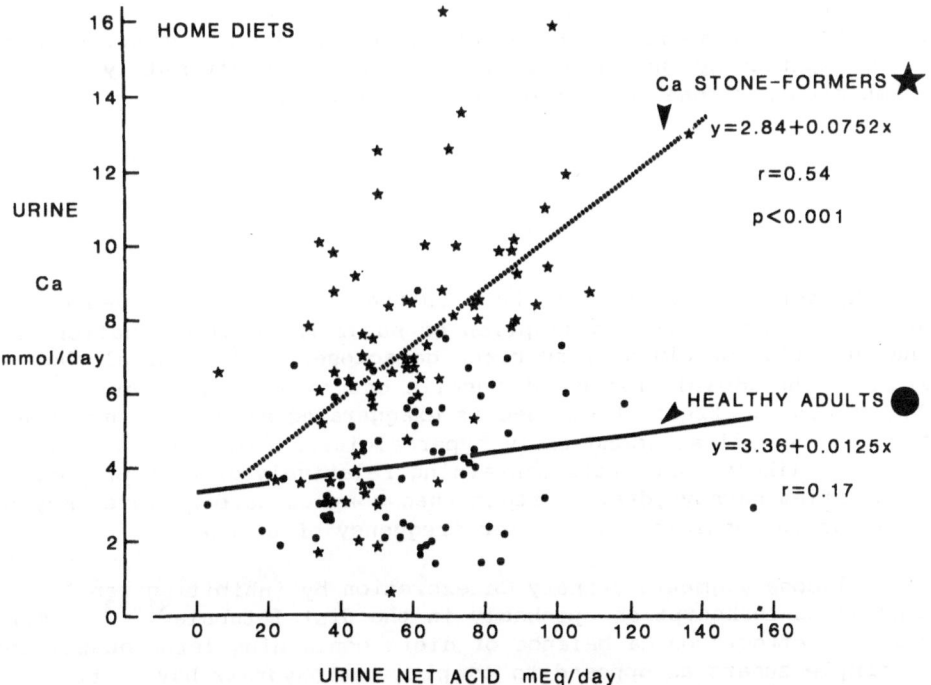

Fig. 4.   Daily urinary Ca excretion as a function of urinary net
          acid excretion in healthy adults and in Ca stone formers
          eating their home diets.

accompanied by a reduced citrate[21] as well as increased Ca excretion, crystallization of Ca oxalate would be favored. Fig. 4 illustrates daily urinary Ca excretion in relation to net acid excretion for healthy subjects and for Ca stone formers when both groups were eating their usual self-selected home diets. Urinary Ca excretion is not correlated with net acid excretion among normal subjects indicating that other factors such as dietary Ca intake and the efficiency of intestinal Ca absorption as determined by the prevailing serum $1,25-(OH)_2$-D concentrations, are more important. Among the stone formers eating their customary diets, urinary Ca excretion was significantly, although not closely, correlated with net acid excretion. Many stone formers exhibit hypercalciuria despite normal rates of net acid excretion and exhibit increased rates of intestinal Ca absorption, either primarily or secondary to a renal Ca leak[22,23]. Thus, such factors are the principal determinants of hypercalciuria which is then aggravated when increased rates of net acid excretion are superimposed.

The augmentation of urinary Ca excretion in response to NH_4Cl or increased protein intake is the consequence of reduced renal tubular reabsorption of filtered Ca[15,24,25], an effect that is independent of PTH[24,26]. Reabsorption of Ca relative to reabsorption of Na is impaired in the distal tubule, a defect that is acutely corrected by the administration of bicarbonate, suggesting that distal delivery of bicarbonate may be a major factor[26]. The mechanism by which chronic metabolic acidosis that is accompanied by increased urinary Ca excretion ultimately stimulates net bone resorption remains unknown.

SUGAR

Epidemiological studies have indicated that the incidence of stones rises with the consumption of sugar in developed nations[3]. The ingestion of glucose, sucrose, galactose, protein or alcohol as well as the administration of insulin causes acute calciuria[27-29]. The calciuric effect of glucose is exaggerated among calcium stone formers as well as among their hypercalciuric relatives[30]. Thus, it seems likely that diets containing relatively greater proportions of purified carboyhydrate, rather than complex carbohydrate, may be a factor responsible for greater frequency of stones.

Glucose augments urinary Ca excretion by inhibiting renal tubular Ca reabsorption, probably in the distal tubule[31-33]. The relative effects on Ca balance of diets containing large quantities of simple sugars as opposed to complex carbohydrate have not, apparently, been evaluated.

58

CALORIC INTAKE AND SERUM 1,25-$(OH)_2$-D

In a retrospective review of studies of healthy adults fed constant diets[34], we have observed that serum 1,25-$(OH)_2$-D levels are directly related to estimated caloric intake/kg/day; serum 1,25-$(OH)_2$-D, pmol/l = -51 + 3.1 caloric intake, kcal/kg/day; r = 0.39; P = 0.01.   Serum 1,25-$(OH)_2$-D levels fell promptly within a day or two as these subjects lost weight.   Speculatively, therefore, total caloric affluence among the populations of developed nations may establish higher serum 1,25-$(OH)_2$-D levels leading to an enhanced intestinal Ca absorption, hypercalciuria and an increased incidence of kidney stones, a process that would be aggravated if such high calorie diets contain more protein and refined carbohydrates.

ACKNOWLEDGMENTS

This work was supported in part by grants USPHS RR-00058 and AM 15089.

REFERENCES

1. D. A. Andersen, in:"Proceedings of the Renal Stone Research Symposium", A. Hodgkinson and B. E. C. Nordin, eds., Churchill, London (1968).
2. C. M. Johnson, D. M. Wilson, W. M. O'Fallon, R. S. Mulch, and L.T. Kurland, Kidney Int. 16:624 (1979).
3. W. G. Robertson, M. Peacock, P. J. Heyburn, R. Speed, and F.Hanes, Fortschr. Urol. Nephrol. 11:5 (1978).
4. N. D. Adams, R. W. Gray, and J. Lemann, Jr. Calc. Tiss. Int. 27:233 (1979).
5. M. Hegsted and H. M. Linkswiler, J. Nutr. 111:244 (1981).
6. J. Lemann, Jr., J. R. Litzow, and E. J. Lennon, J. Clin. Invest. 45:1608 (1966).
7. E. J. Lennon, J. Lemann, Jr., and J. R. Litzow, J. Clin. Invest. 45:1601 (1966).
8. J. Lemann, Jr., E. J. Lennon, A. D. Goodman, J. R. Litzow, and A. S. Relman, J. Clin. Invest. 44:507 (1965).
9. H. P. Weber, R. W. Gray, J. H. Dominguez, and J. Lemann, Jr., J. Clin. Endocrinol. Metab. 43:1047 (1976).
10. J. Lemann, Jr. Unpublished observations.
11. J. Lemann, Jr., N. D. Adams, and R. W. Gray, New Engl. J. Med. 301:535 (1979).
12. C. R. Anand and H. M. Linkswiler, J. Nutr. 104:695 (1974).
13. Y. Kim and H. M. Linkswiler, J. Nutr. 109:1399 (1979).
14. L. H. Allen, E. A. Oddoye, and S. Margen, Am. J. Clin. Nutr. 32:741 (1979).

15. S. M. Schuette, M. B. Zemel, and H. M. Linkswiler,
    J. Nutr. 110:305 (1980).
16. A. A. Paul and D. A. T. Southgate, "The Composition of Foods,
    4th Edition", Elsevier, Amsterdam (1978).
17. E. J. Lennon, J. Lemann, Jr., and A. S. Relman, J. Clin. Invest.
    41:637 (1962).
18. A. S. Relman, E. J. Lennon, and J. Lemann, Jr., J. Clin. Invest.
    40:1621 (1961).
19. K. Sakhaee, M. Nicar, K. Hill, and C. Y. C. Pak, Kidney Int.
    24:348 (1983).
20. W. G. Robertson, P. J. Heyburn, M. Peacock, F. A. Hanes, and
    R.Swaminathan, Clin. Sci. 57:285 (1979).
21. D. P. Simpson, Am. J. Physiol. 244:F223 (1983).
22. F. L. Coe and M. J. Favus, in:"The Kidney", 2nd edn.
    B. M. Brenner and F. C. Rector, Jr., eds., W. B. Saunders,
    Philadelphia (1981).
23. J. Lemann, Jr., in:"Contemporary Issues in Nephrology", Vol. 5,
    F. L. Coe, guest ed., B. M. Brenner and J. H. Stein, eds.,
    Churchill Livingstone, New York (1980).
24. J. Lemann, Jr., J. R. Litzow, and E. J. Lennon, J. Clin. Invest.
    46:1318 (1967).
25. A. Hodgkinson and F. W. Heaton, Clin. Chim. Acta 11:354 (1965).
26. R. A. L. Sutton, N. L. M. Wong, and J. H. Dirks, Kidney Int.
    15:520 (1979).
27. R. D. Lindeman, S. Adler, M. J. Yiengst, and E. S. Beard,
    J.Lab. Clin. Med. 70:236 (1967).
28. J. M. Kalbfleisch, R. D. Lindeman, H. E. Ginn, and W. O. Smith,
    J. Clin. Invest. 42:1471 (1963).
29. R. A. DeFronzo, C. R. Cooke, R. Andres, G. R. Faloona, and
    P. J. Davis, J. Clin. Invest. 55:845 (1975).
30. J. Lemann, Jr., W. F. Piering, and E. J. Lennon,
    New Engl. J. Med. 280:232 (1969).
31. J. Lemann, Jr., E. J. Lennon, W. F. Piering, E. L. Prien, Jr.,
    and E. S. Ricanati, J. Lab. Clin. Med. 75:578 (1970).
32. E. J. Lennon, J. Lemann, Jr., W. F. Piering, and L. S. Larson,
    J. Clin. Invest. 53:1424 (1974).
33. E. J. Lennon and W. F. Pering, J. Clin. Invest. 49:1458 (1970).
34. J. Lemann, Jr., R. W. Gray, W. J. Maierhofer, and N. D. Adams,
    Calc. Tiss. Int. 36:139 (1984).

DIETARY FACTORS IMPORTANT IN CALCIUM STONE-FORMATION

W. G. Robertson

MRC Mineral Metabolism Unit, The General Infirmary
Leeds LS1 3EX, U.K.

INTRODUCTION

One of the major debates in the field of primary calcium stone-formation is centered round the role of diet in the causation of the disorder. Indeed, since the time of Hippocrates various dietary factors have been suggested to be important in causing stones, including lime-rich water, soft water, high amounts of dairy foods, high oxalate, high sugar, high salt, low salt, low fibre and high protein. The suggestions are as numerous and as heterogeneous as the patients with the disorder. This review sets out to assess the evidence as it stands at the present time.

DIETARY COMPOSITION

Fig. 1 reviews the intakes of a number of nutrients assessed from diet histories taken by a single dietitian from 103 male primary recurrent calcium stone-formers and 54 healthy male control subjects. The date for refined carbohydrate (sugars)[1] and the normal data for fibre consumption[2] are taken from the literature. Although there was a tendency towards an increased intake of calcium, phosphorus and fat in the stone-formers, these small differences were not significant. Sugar consumption also was not significantly different between the groups. Significant differences were noted, however, in the consumption of oxalate ($P < 0.001$), fibre ($P < 0.001$), and protein ($P < 0.001$). The last-mentioned difference was almost entirely due to an increased consumption of animal protein which, in turn, was attributable almost entirely to an increase in flesh protein. There were no differences in the intake of either dairy or vegetable protein.

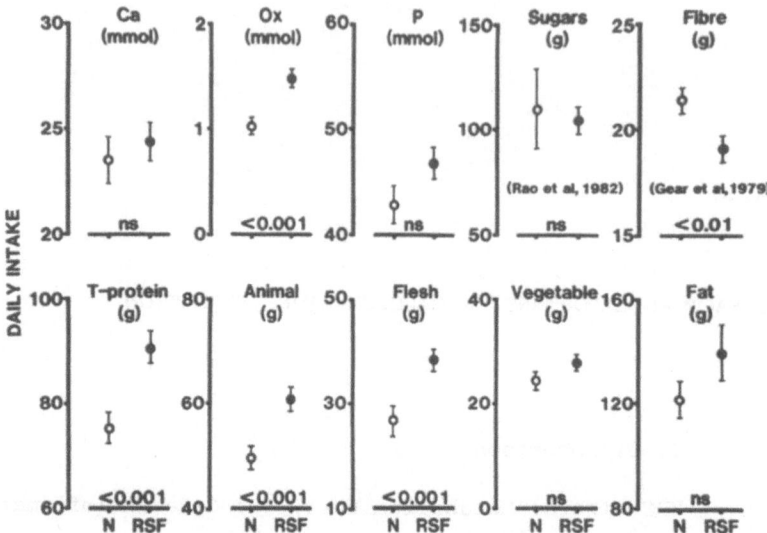

Fig. 1.   The mean daily intake of a number of nutrients in normal
men and in male, recurrent primary calcium stone-formers.

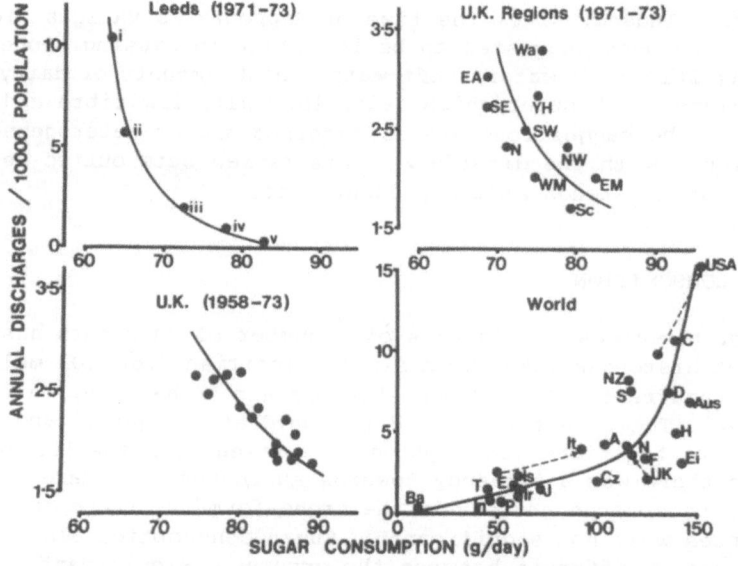

Fig. 2.   The annual hospital discharge rate for urinary stone
disease in relation to daily total sugar consumption (i) in
men in Leeds according to social class, (ii) in the various
administrative regions of the UK, (iii) in the UK as a
whole for each year between 1958 and 1973 and (iv) in
various countries of the world.

REFINED SUGARS

It has been suggested that an increased consumption of refined carbohydrate increases the risk of stone disease[3,4]. Fig. 2 shows, however, that epidemiologically even if such a difference exists it cannot be a major factor in determining the risk of stones in the population. At 3 out of the 4 population levels studied, there is actually an inverse relationship between hospitalisation for stones and sugar consumption. Only on the much broader world scale of sugar consumption (from which data Andersen[3] drew up his original hypothesis on the role of sugar intake in stone disease) is there a positive correlation with the risk of stones. Together with the negative evidence in Fig. 1, this suggests that a high sugar consumption is not a major risk factor for stone disease. Studies on the biochemical effects of a high sugar diet are equally unconvincing since it does not increase either urinary calcium or oxalate significantly[5], although there is a suggestion that a small proportion of stone-formers respond more sensitively than others[6]

FIBRE

Fig. 1 suggests that stone-formers consume less fibre in their diet than normal subjects. Epidemiologically this is supported by the data in Fig. 3 which shows that at 4 separate demographic levels

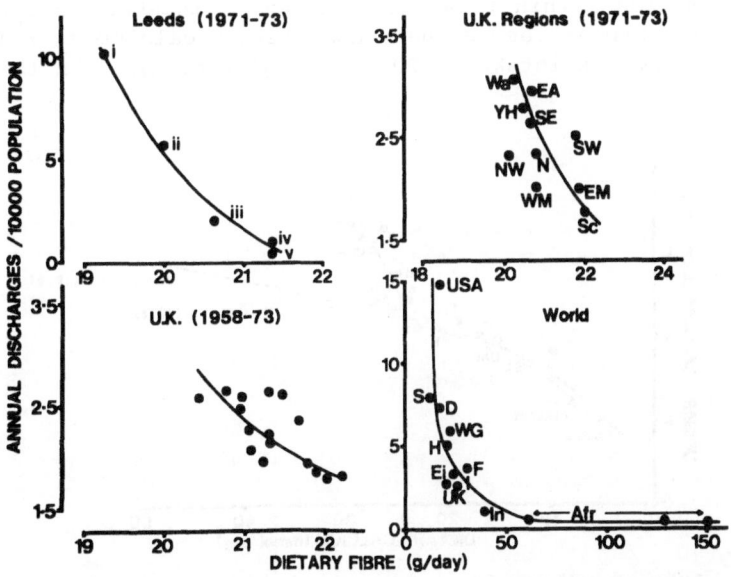

Fig. 3. The annual hospital discharge rate for urinary stone disease in relation to daily fibre consumption (Key as in Fig. 2).

there is a consistent but weak inverse relationship between
hospitalization for stones and dietary fibre consumption.   Thus a
high risk of stones appears to be associated with a low dietary
fibre intake.   Biochemically there is a weak inverse relationship
between urinary calcium and fibre intake suggesting that fibre,
possibly through its phytate content, binds calcium either
chemically or mechanically in the intestine and renders it less
available for absorption[7,8].   However, chemical binding of calcium
will result in a release of oxalate within the intestine and this
may be passively absorbed and excreted in the urine.   Mechanical
binding of calcium (as calcium oxalate), on the other hand, would
not have this effect.   The situation is further complicated by the
fact that different high fibre foodstuffs contain different amounts
of oxalate (unpublished data).   Thus wheat-based bran appears to
have a high oxalate content whereas soya bran contains little
oxalate.   Studies on fibre must take this into account.

CALCIUM

     Hypercalciuria has been long considered to be a feature of many
calcium stone-formers.   Fig. 1 shows, however, that stone-formers
do not have a higher intake of calcium than normal and thus excess
calcium in the diet cannot be a major cause of their hypercalciuria.
Epidemiologically there is a relationship between hospitalization
for stones and dietary calcium up to an intake of 23 to 25 mmol/day;
thereafter, however, the curve rises vertically[9].   Thus an
excessive calcium intake is not the cause of the sharp rise in
stone-formation within this narrow range of intake.   Furthermore,
the relationship between urinary and dietary calcium is relatively
flat[10,11] above an intake of 20 mmol/day (Fig. 4).   In the majority

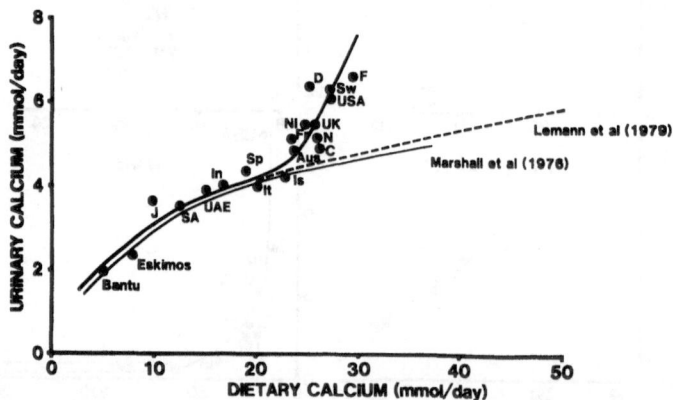

Fig. 4.   Average values for urinary calcium in normal men in various
          countries of the world in relation to dietary calcium.

of hypercalciuric patients the high calcium excretion is due to increased intestinal absorption[11,12] secondary to an increased plasma level[13] of 1,25-(OH)$_2$ vitamin D$_3$. Thus the hypercalciuria is partly due to a hypersensitivity of response to a given (normal) dietary stimulus. At intakes below 15 mmol/day, urinary calcium falls rapidly, suggesting that a low calcium intake might be useful in the prevention of urinary stones. However, when dietary calcium is reduced without a concomitant reduction in dietary oxalate, urinary oxalate increases significantly and this may more than offset the beneficial effect of a fall in urinary calcium[14].

OXALATE

Fig. 1 indicates that stone-formers ingest slightly but significantly, more oxalate than normals. However, this cannot be a major contributory factor in the causation of the mild hyperoxaluria observed in these patients[15] since the relationship between urinary and dietary oxalate is relatively flat up to an intake of about 2 mmol/day (our own unpublished results). Only above this intake does urinary oxalate increase rapidly in relation to intake. However, at all levels of dietary oxalate (except in the fasting state) stone-formers have a significantly higher urinary oxalate than normals suggesting that, during the day, either they absorb more oxalate from the diet or they ingest more oxalate-producing nutrients or they metabolise a greater proportion of oxalate-producing nutrients than normals. This question remains to be answered.

ANIMAL PROTEIN

Fig. 4 also shows the average urinary calcium excretion in normal men in a number of countries in relation to the mean calcium intake in that country. Clearly the urinary data lie along the "Lemann/Marshall" line, obtained from calcium-loading studies, until a dietary calcium of approximately 25 mmol/day is reached. Above that figure, urinary calcium rises sharply for a very small increase in dietary calcium. Why? One possible explanation derives from the data in Fig. 5. This shows the relationship between dietary animal protein and dietary calcium in various countries of the world. The plot appears to consist of two sections - a linear relationship between dietary animal protein and calcium within the range 5 to 25 mmol/day calcium, where dairy produce is the main source of both calcium and animal protein, and then a rapid increase in animal protein over the calcium range 25 to 28 mmol/day, where meat takes over as the main source of animal protein. Fig. 5 strongly suggests that the upward "kick" in the curve of urinary versus dietary calcium in Fig. 5 is attributable to the higher intake of flesh protein in the more affluent countries of the world.

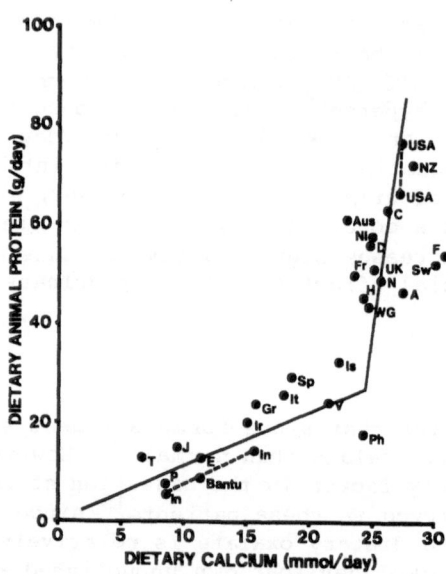

Fig. 5. Dietary intake of animal protein in various countries of the world in relation to dietary calcium.

Table 1. Biochemical Effects of a High Animal Protein Diet.

Urinary factor	Possible mechanism
↓pH	↑Acid ash diet
↑Calcium	↑Acid→↓Tubular reabsorption of calcium→ ↑Bone resorption or ↑Calcium absorption ↑Methionine (?); ↑Lysine (?)
↑Oxalate	↑Calcium absorption→ ↑Oxalate absorption ↑Metabolic production from ↑glycine, phenylalanine, tyrosine, tryptophan, hydroxyproline;↑Purine (?); ↑Fat (?)
↑Uric acid	↑Purine

    Does then a high animal protein intake, partly through its apparent ability to increase urinary calcium, increase the risk of stones in the population?   Epidemiologically there is a consistent relationship at 4 demographic levels between stone disease and animal protein consumption[9].   Moreover, temporal changes in the hospitalisation rate for stones and days lost from work owing to renal colic correlate well with changes in animal protein consumption within the UK.   There are no such strong relationships with dietary calcium, oxalate, fibre or sugars.   Furthermore, stone-formers ingest more animal protein than non-stone-formers (Fig. 1).   Biochemically a high animal protein diet not only increases urinary calcium, but also urinary oxalate and uric acid[16]. Thus 3 out of 6 urinary risk factors for stones are affected adversely by such a diet. Conversely, reducing animal protein intake to levels taken by vegetarians decreases both the biochemical risk[17] and the prevalence rate[18] of stones.

Some of the suggested mechanisms responsible for the adverse biochemical changes produced by a high animal protein diet are shown in Table 1. It may be that a proportion of stone-formers are biochemically sensitive to a dietary stimulus, such as a high animal protein intake, and that this pushes them into a high risk region of one or more of the urinary risk factors for stones[19,20].

Table 2. Dietary Factors of Importance in Calcium Stone Disease.

Dietary factor	Effect on urine	
	Adverse	Beneficial
↑Calcium	↑Calcium	↓Oxalate
↑Oxalate	↑Oxalate	–
↑Phosphorus	↑Phosphorus	↓Calcium; ↑Pyrophosphate
↓Magnesium	↓Magnesium	–
↓Vitamin B$_6$	? ↑Oxalate	–
↑Vitamin C	? ↑Oxalate	–
↑Refined carbohydrate	↑Calcium;?↑oxalate	–
↓Fibre	↑Calcium; ↑oxalate	–
↑Animal protein	↑Calcium; ↑oxalate	↓pH
↑Purine	↑Uric acid	–
↑Fat	↑Oxalate	–
↑Sodium	↑Calcium	–

OTHER DIETARY CONSTITUENTS

Table 2 summarises the current knowledge on the adverse and beneficial effects of changing the amount of various nutrients in the diet. Most have already been discussed. Of the remainder there is no good evidence that a consistently low magnesium diet or a high vitamin C diet cause stones in man, although they may aggravate the problem. Indeed, the increase in urinary oxalate allegedly produced by the latter must be in some doubt in the light of the observations that a high urinary vitamin C may be converted to oxalate during the storage period prior to analysis and/or during the analytical procedure itself. Chronic pyridoxine deficiency may lead to stones in a few individuals but cannot be a major cause of the disorder. The higher fat and salt intakes associated with a high animal protein diet may aggravate some of the biochemical changes produced by the animal protein itself.

REFERENCES

1. P. N. Rao, V. Prendiville, A. Buxton, D. G. Moss, and
    N. J. Blacklock, Br. J. Urol. 54:578 (1982).
2. J. S. S. Gear, A. Ware, P. Fursdon, J. I. Mann, D. J. Nolan,
    A. J. M. Brodribb, and M. P. Vessey, Lancet 1:511 (1979).
3. D. A. Andersen, in:"Urinary Calculi", L. Cifuentes Delatte,
    A. Rapado, and A. Hodgkinson, eds., Karger, Basel (1973).
4. N. J. Blacklock, in:"Scientific Foundations of Urology",
    2nd edn, G. D. Chisholm and D. I. Williams, eds., Heinemann,
    London (1982).
5. J. A. Thom, J. E. Morris, J. E. Bishop, and N. J. Blacklock,
    Br. J. Urol. 50:459 (1978).
6. P. N. Rao, C. Gordon, D. Davies, and N. J. Blacklock,
    Br. J. Urol. 54:575 (1982).
7. P. J. R. Shah, N. A. Green, and G. Williams, Br. Med. J. 2:426
    (1980).
8. P. N. Rao, I. L. Jenkins, W. G. Robertson, M. Peacock, and
    N. J. Blacklock, in:"Urolithiasis and Related Clinical
    Research", P. O. Schwille, L. H. Smith, W. G. Robertson,
    and W. Vahlensieck, eds., Plenum, London (1985).
9. W. G. Robertson, M. Peacock, P. J. Heyburn, R. Speed, and
    F. Hanes, Fortschr. Urol. Nephrol. 11:5 (1978).
10. D. H. Marshall, B. E. C. Nordin, and R. Speed, Proc. Nutr. Soc.
    35:163 (1976).
11. J. Lemann, N. D. Adams, and R. W. Gray, New Engl. J. Med.
    301:535 (1979).
12. B. E. C. Nordin, M. Peacock, and R. Wilkinson, Clin. Endocrinol.
    Metab. 1:169 (1972).
13. R. W. Gray, D. R. Wilz, A. E. Caldas, and J. Lemann, J. Clin.
    Endocrinol. Metab. 45:299 (1977).
14. R. W. Marshall, M. Cochran, and A. Hodgkinson, Clin. Sci. 43:91
    (1972).
15. W. G. Robertson and M. Peacock, Nephron 26:105 (1980).
16. W. G. Robertson, P. J. Heyburn, M. Peacock, F. Hanes, and
    R. Swaminathan, Clin. Sci. 57:285 (1979).
17. W. G. Robertson, M. Peacock, P. J. Heyburn, F. Hanes,
    A. Rutherford, E. Clementson, R. Swaminathan, and P. B. Clark,
    Br. J. Urol. 51:427 (1979).
18. W. G. Robertson, M. Peacock, and D. H. Marshall, Europ. Urol.
    8:334 (1982).
19. B. Arora, P. L. Selby, R. W. Norman, M. Peacock and
    W. G. Robertson, in:"Urolithiasis and Related Clinical
    Research", P. O. Schwille, L. H. Smith, W. G. Robertson, and
    W. Vahlensieck, eds., Plenum, London (1985).
20. W. G. Robertson and M. Peacock, in:"Urolithiasis and Related
    Clinical Research", P. O. Schwille, L.H. Smith,
    W. G. Robertson, and W. Vahlensieck, eds., Plenum, London
    (1985).

DIETARY FACTORS AS CAUSES OF THE SO-CALLED RENAL LEAK OF

CALCIUM IN IDIOPATHIC STONE FORMERS

P. Jaeger, L. Portmann, and P. Burckhardt

Dept. of Internal Medicine, University Hospital
1011 Lausanne, Switzerland

INTRODUCTION

In 1972, Coe et al postulated the existence of a renal tubular leak of calcium to account for the hypercalciuria of some idiopathic stone formers[1]. More recently, it has been suggested that such patients have an overall defect in the proximal tubular reabsorption of fluid and electrolytes[2]. To shed more light on this controversial topic, we have examined the question as to whether or not the apparent renal leak of calcium is due to dietary factors, or to some general renal tubular dysfunction.

PATIENTS AND METHODS

A group of 108 male patients with idiopathic renal stone disease were enrolled in the study. They were classified according to their urinary excretion of calcium[3]; 40 were normocalciuric (<280 mg/24 h) on a free diet and 78 hypercalciuric. In 41 of the latter sub-group, hypercalciuria persisted after 5 days on a diet containing no dairy produce.

Two studies were carried out. First, in the 41 patients with hypercalciuria on the low Ca diet, 24 h urine was analyzed for Na, urate and creatinine, and a fasting blood sample analyzed for insulin and glucose. This study was aimed at detecting the potential causes of the apparent renal leak of Ca. Second, 66 of the 118 idiopathic stone formers were selected at random and their renal tubular function evaluated. A 2-h fasting morning urine was analyzed for lysozyme, ɤ-glutamyl transpeptidase (ɤ-GT), glucose and insulin, and the fractional excretion (FE) of the latter 2 variables calculated. The FE of HCO_3 was also measured in a 2-h fasting morning urine obtained after 3 days on a standard load of alkali (Ca lactate and gluconate 15.7 g/day + Ca carbonate 2.4 g/day).   Values were compared with those obtained in 36 male healthy volunteers, the normal limits being defined as the mean $\pm$ 2SD.   In this second study, the hypercalciuric patients were subdivided into 3 groups, 13 with absorptive hypercalciuria (HC)[3], 6 with renal HC, defined in the restricted sense (see below), and 28 with HC secondary to dietary factors i.e. HC apparent only on a free diet or HC on a low Ca diet associated with identifiable nutritional factors.

RESULTS

In 20 of the 41 patients who were hypercalciuric after 5 days on the diet containing no dairy produce, the degree of hypercalciuria was considered appropriate to the level of urinary sodium. Indeed, their calcium excretions fell within the 99.7% confidence limits of urinary calcium ($U_{Ca}V$) plotted against urinary sodium ($U_{Na}V$), in 27 healthy male volunteers on the low calcium diet where $U_{Ca}V = 0.414\ U_{Na}V + 83.233$ (r= 0.530, P<0.01).   In the remaining 21

Table 1. Search for Potential Causes of the Apparent Renal Leak of Ca in 21 ISF with UCaV out of Proportion to UNaV.

Patient	U Urate >800 mg/24 h	% of Ideal Weight >120	Fast. plasma Insulin >15 µU/ml	Final Diagnosis
1	+			
2	+			
3	+			
4	+	+		
5	+		+	
6	+	+	+	
7	+	+	+	Dietary
8	+	+	+	idiopathic
9	+	+	+	hypercalciuria
10		+	+	
11		+	+	
12		+	+	
13		+	+	Medullary
14				sponge kidney
15				
16				
17				
18				Renal
19				idiopathic
20				hypercalciuria
21				

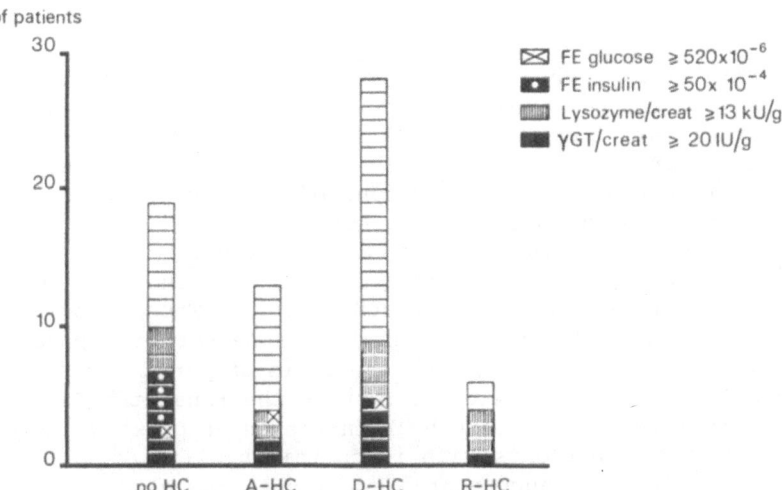

Fig. 1. Number of idiopathic stone formers of each subgroup
presenting with one or more signs of renal tubular
dysfunction. Each box represents one patient. no-HC:
without hypercalciuria; A-HC : absorptive hypercalciuria;
D-HC : dietary hypercalciuria; R-HC : renal hypercalciuria.

patients with persistent hypercalciuria, the increased urinary
calcium was out of proportion to sodium excretion. In the majority,
the hypercalciuria on the low calcium diet could be explained by
other factors (Table 1), in 9 cases, by a high intake of animal
protein (as reflected by hyperuricosuria with concomitant normal
plasma level of urate), in 8 cases by obesity with concomitant
fasting hyperinsulinemia, in 2 cases by medullary sponge kidney
which until that time had remained undiagnosed. Thus, in only 7
cases did the hypercalciuria on the low calcium diet remain
unexplained. This was defined as "renal" hypercalciuria.

The urinary excretions of lyosozyme and γ-GT and the fractional
excretions of glucose and insulin measured in the fasting state in
66 idiopathic stone formers showed that 27 (40%) had one or two
indices of renal tubular dysfunction. However, as shown in Fig. 1,
these signs of tubular defects were encountered with equal frequency
in each of the 4 subgroups of idiopathic stone formers, i.e. the
normocalciuric stone formers and those with absorptive, dietary and
renal hypercalciuria. Measurement of the fractional excretion of
bicarbonate after a load of alkali gave similar results. It was
greater than normal (5000×10^{-6}) in 9/17 (53%) of the normocalciuric
stone formers, in 5/11 (45%) , 13/24 (54%) and 1/5 (20%) of the
patients with absorptive, dietary and renal hypercalciuria
respectively.

DISCUSSION

This study shows that in 41 of the 78 patients with idiopathic hypercalciuria, the hypercalciuria persisted on a low calcium diet, suggesting that they had a renal leak of calcium. In 33 of these, however, nutritional factors such as a high intake of sodium, or animal protein or obesity with concomitant hyperinsulinemia, all of which have been shown to lead to hypercalciuria[4-9], might account for the disorder. In addition, a renal tubular leak of calcium can also indicate unrecognized medullary sponge kidney[10]; this was the case in two patients of the present study. Thus, a true primary tubular leak of calcium in idiopathic stone formers appears to be much rarer than was thought on the basis of persistent hyper-calciuria on low Ca intake. A test of the renal tubular function showed that there is a very high incidence of proximal tubular defects amongst patients with idiopathic urolithiasis. Moreover, these disorders are encountered equally in the various groups of patients, suggesting that, rather than being a primary cause of stone-formation, they might result from the urolithiasis itself.

ACKNOWLEDGMENTS

We are grateful to Ms A. F. Jacquet and Ms E. Maeder for technical assistance. This work was supported by the Swiss National Science Foundation (grant no. 3.816.0.81).

REFERENCES

1. F. L. Coe, J. M. Canterbury, J. J. Firpo, and E. Reiss, J.Clin. Invest. 52:134 (1972).
2. R. A. L. Sutton and V. R. Walker, New Engl. J. Med. 302:709 (1980).
3. P. Jaeger, L. Portmann, J. M. Bugnon, A. F. Jacquet and P. Burckhardt, Schweiz. Med. Wschr. 112:1975 (1982).
4. F. P. Muldowney, R. Freaney and M. F. Moloney, Kidney Int. 22:292 (1982).
5. N. A. Breslau, J. L. McGuire, J. E. Zerwekh, and C. Y. Pak, J. Clin. Endocrinol. Metab. 55:369 (1982).
6. J. Silver, D. Rubinger, M. M. Friedlaender, and M. M. Popovtzer,Lancet ii:484 (1983).
7. J. Lemann, N. D. Adams, and R. W. Gray, New Engl. J. Med. 301:535 (1979).
8. R. D. Lindenman, S. Adler, M. J. Yengst, and E. S. Beard, J.Lab. Clin. Med. 70:236 (1967).
9. A. Ulmann, J. Aubert, A. Bourdeau, C. Cheynel, and C. Bader, J. Clin. Endocrinol. Metab. 54:1063 (1982).
10. E. R. Yendt, New Engl. J. Med. 306:1106 (1982).

DIETARY HISTORY AND DIETARY RECORDS IN RENAL STONE PATIENTS

AND CONTROLS

B. Fellström, B. G. Danielson, B. Karlström, H. Lithell,
S. Ljunghall, and B. Vessby

Dept. of Internal Medicine and Geriatrics, University
Hospital, 751 85 Uppsala, Sweden

INTRODUCTION

Dietary factors have been suggested to be important in the
increase in renal calcium stone disease in Western countries.   It
has been shown that dietary animal protein is the nutrient best
related to the frequency of stone disease between various
countries[1].   Animal protein has also been shown to cause an
increased excretion of urinary constituents important for calcium
stone formation[2-6].   In another controlled study on dietary habits,
however, based on interviews with stone formers and controls, no
difference could be found regarding the major nutrients, except for
a higher intake of fibre among healthy controls[7].   These
conflicting reports prompted us to make the present study.

MATERIALS AND METHODS

Twenty stone patients attending our out-patient stone clinic
were included.   They were 16 males and 4 females with an average
age of 44+13 years.   The control group was obtained by asking the
stone patients to select a person of the same age and sex and with a
similar socio-economic status and working habits as themselves, but
without renal stone disease.

The stone patients and the controls were all asked to make a
4-day record of their dietary intake and were also interviewed by a
dietitian who took a dietary history from each individual.   Using
computerized food composition data[8], the nutrient contents of the
dietary records and histories were calculated.   During the study
period the patients and the controls also collected urines during

73

two 24-h periods. The urines were analyzed for constituents believed to be important for stone disease.

Conventional statistical methods were used for calculating means, standard deviations and linear correlations and Student's t-test was employed for comparison of mean values. Discriminant analysis was performed, on urinary excretions or dietary nutrients, using a model based on the measure of the generalized squared distance between the groups.

RESULTS

The dietary intake of protein, sodium, phosphate and potassium in the 4-day records and in the dietary histories were compared with the urinary excretions of total nitrogen, sodium, phosphate and potassium in order to compare the two methods for estimating the dietary intake of nutrients. It was found that the dietary data from the 4-day records correlated very well with the urinary excretions, whereas the data obtained from the diet histories did not correlate with the corresponding urinary excretions. Furthermore, data obtained by dietary histories were on an average 15% higher than the 4-day records. For this reason 4-day dietary records were used in all subsequent calculations.

There was no difference in the dietary intake of the major nutrients in stone formers compared with controls, except for a higher intake of vitamin C in the controls (Table 1). The consumption of alcohol was not different in the two groups although

Table 1. Daily Dietary Intake of Nutritions (4-Day Records) in Stone Formers and Controls (Mean $\pm$ SD).

Nutrient	Stone Formers	Controls	P
Protein (g)	85 $\pm$ 74	84 $\pm$ 15	0.87
Fat (g)	106 $\pm$ 27	106 $\pm$ 27	0.98
Carbohydrate (g)	263 $\pm$ 72	287 $\pm$ 70	0.33
Fibre (g)	14.0 $\pm$ 4.5	15.3 $\pm$ 4.2	0.38
Purine (mg)	169 $\pm$ 68	147 $\pm$ 59	0.39
Alcohol (g)	9.4 $\pm$ 10.0	6.6 $\pm$ 9.2	0.39
Sodium (g)	2.3 $\pm$ 0.6	2.4 $\pm$ 0.6	0.54
Potassium (g)	3.2 $\pm$ 0.8	3.2 $\pm$ 0.6	0.86
Calcium (g)	0.88 $\pm$ 0.39	1.05 $\pm$ 0.30	0.13
Phosphate (g)	1.38 $\pm$ 0.41	1.48 $\pm$ 0.26	0.34
Iron (mg)	20 $\pm$ 6	20 $\pm$ 5	0.97
Vitamin C (mg)	80 $\pm$ 41	121 $\pm$ 55	0.01

Table 2. Daily Urinary Excretion (mmol/24 h) of Various Ions
in Stone Formers and Controls (Mean ± SD).

	Stone Formers	Controls	P
Calcium	6.5 ± 1.5	4.7 ± 2.0	0.005
Phosphate	37 ± 13	27 ± 7	0.008
Sodium	192 ± 49	149 ± 40	0.007
Potassium	75 ± 16	67 ± 15	0.12
Urate	4.2 ± 1.0	3.6 ± 0.8	0.07
Citrate	3.5 ± 1.3	3.3 ± 0.7	0.49
Oxalate	0.40 ± 0.10	0.35 ± 0.10	0.16
Urea	362 ± 79	322 ± 98	0.21
Nitrogen	817 ± 173	731 ± 209	0.20

there were 8 consumers of hard liquor among the stone formers
compared with only 4 among the controls.   Three stone formers never
consumed alcohol compared with 6 controls.

Expected differences regarding the urinary excretion of
potential risk factors were found (Table 2).   Stone formers
excreted more calcium than the controls but tended to have a lower
intake of calcium (Table 1).   The quotient of urinary excretion/
dietary intake of calcium was 19 ± 10 in controls and 36 ± 22% in
stone formers (P<0.005).

The discriminant analysis based on the intakes of vitamin C,
calcium, purine, phosphate and fibre gave a correct classification
of 26/37 subjects (P<0.05).   Based on the urinary excretion of
calcium, sodium, phosphate, urate and oxalate the discriminant
function gave a correct classification of 25/35 subjects (P<0.02).

DISCUSSION

It has been shown previously that an excess of dietary animal
protein causes unfavourable changes in the urinary composition with
respect to the risk of stone formation[2-6].   According to the
present results, where the dietary habits in stone patients were
compared with those of carefully selected controls, no differences
in the major nutrients could be found.   A higher intake of vitamin
C in the controls, probably reflects a higher consumption of fruit
and vegetables.   The low level, 80 to 120 mg daily, probably does
not influence the production rate of oxalate.

The urinary excretion of potential risk factors was, however,
in accordance with previous findings, despite the absence of major
dietary differences.   Whether or not there are other differences in
nutrient intake, requires further study.

According to the discriminant analysis, based on the 5 nutrients with the lowest P-values comparing stone formers and controls, a discriminant function could be calculated, which classified 2/3 of the patients correctly ($P < 0.05$), but as 11/37 individuals were misclassified the usefulness of this discriminant function is doubtful. When the discrimination was based on the urinary constituents with the lowest P-values, the discrimination was slightly better but still 10/35 patients were misclassified.

ACKNOWLEDGEMENTS

This work was supported by the Swedish Medical Research Council (nos. 2329, 6354), the Swedish Society of Medical Sciences and the Tore Nilsson Foundation.

REFERENCES

1. W. G. Robertson, M. Peacock, P. J. Heyburn, F. A. Hanes, and R. Swaminathan, in:"Urinary Calculus", J. G. Brockis and B. Finlayson, eds., PSG Publishing Co., Littleton, Massachusetts (1981).
2. F. L. Coe, E. Moran, and A. G. Kavalich, J. Chron. Dis. 29:793 (1976).
3. W. G. Robertson, P. J. Heyburn, M. Peacock, F. A. Hanes, and R. Swaminathan, Clin. Sci. 57:285 (1979).
4. B. Fellström, B. G. Danielson, B. Karlström, H. Lithel, S.Ljunghall, and B. Vessby, Clin. Sci. 64:399 (1983).
5. B. Fellström, B. G. Danielson, H. Lithell, S. Ljunghall, and H.Vessby, Fortschr. Urol. Nephrol. 17:112 (1981).
6. B. G. Danielson, B. Fellström, H. Lithell, S. Ljunghall, and B. Vessby, Fortschr. Urol. Nephrol. 17:96 (1981).
7. H. M. Griffith, B. O'Shea, J. P. Kevany, and J. S. McCormick, Br. J. Urol. 53:416 (1981).
8. Swedish National Food Administration, "Food Composition Tables", Liber Tryck, Stockholm (1978).

UROLITHIASIS IN SOUTHERN RAJASTHAN: CONTRIBUTION OF DIETARY

OXALATE TO URINARY OXALATE

P. P. Singh, A. K. Pendse, and A. K. Jain

Depts. of Biochemistry and Surgery, R.N.T. Medical
College, Udaipur, Rajasthan, India

INTRODUCTION

The incidence of urinary stones is high in this Western part of
India and has been increasing progressively during the last few
years[1,2].   Our studies have shown that hyperoxaluria is one of the
most significant etiologic factors in the local population[3].   Singh
et al[4] have reported previously that oxalate intake is quite high in
some sections of the local population.   However, the contribution
of dietary oxalate to urinary oxalate has not been studied.
Various reports indicate that 2 to 12% of dietary oxalate can be
absorbed and is excreted in the urine[5].   Since the consumption of
oxalate-rich vegetables, especially spinach, is very high in this
area, we have undertaken the present study to define the effect of a
dietary oxalate load on urinary oxalic acid in normal individuals
and stone formers.

MATERIALS AND METHODS

In the present study, 14 healthy individuals and 14 radiologically confirmed stone formers admitted to our surgical ward were
included.   The normal subjects were kept on their routine diet,
except that oxalate-rich foods were excluded for the two days prior
to and during the study.   The stone formers were kept on a low
oxalate hospital diet for the same period.   Both groups were given
the same number of cups of tea during this period.   None of the
subjects was given parenteral fluid and they were asked to take the
same amount of fluid per day during the period of study.   The first
basal 24-h urine sample (from 08.00 to 08.00) was collected in a
bottle containing 10 ml concentrated HCl.   Next day at 08.30, 200 g

of boiled, minced spinach was given to each individual. The urine during the next 24 h was collected in the same way. The 24-h urine volume before and after spinach ingestion was measured. Oxalate, by the method of Hodgkinson and Williams[6], and calcium, by the method of Gindler and King as described by Varley[7], were estimated.

RESULTS AND DISCUSSION

In our series, one normal and one stone former had an oxalic acid excretion 50 mg/24 h. The 200 g of spinach contributed an additional intake of oxalic acid varying from 1508 to 2155 mg. In the normals, the mean 24-h urinary oxalate excretion before spinach ingestion was 22.0 $\pm$ 4.6 mg (Table 1). This increased to 45.1 $\pm$ 5.9 mg after the spinach ingestion (P<0.001). This increase in oxalic acid represented 1.19% $\pm$ 0.24 (0.2 to 3.3%) of administered oxalic acid from spinach.

In the stone formers the mean oxalic acid excretion was higher than in the normal subjects (31.7 $\pm$ 6.8 mg), before spinach ingestion and increased to 77.0 $\pm$ 26.1 mg after the spinach ingestion (P<0.05). The increase in oxalic acid excretion in this group was 2.24 $\pm$ 0.95 (0.2 to 11.4%) of the administered oxalic acid. In two stone formers the absorption (10.3 and 11.4%) was much higher than in the rest. In the first, the 24-h urinary oxalic acid excretion before and after spinach ingestion was 32.0 mg and 252.1 mg respectively, while in the latter it was 113.6 and 350.7 mg respectively. Thus, these two stone formers were distinctly hyperabsorbers of oxalic acid. Except in these 2 patients, however, the contribution of the oxalic acid from the ingested spinach to urinary oxalic acid in both normal subjects and stone formers was lower than in other reports[8-14]. This we cannot explain.

Hodgkinson[13] has reported that, under normal dietary conditions, the increased excretion of oxalic acid is associated with an increased excretion of calcium. Our observations corroborate his findings. In all 28 subjects the increase in urinary oxalic acid was accompanied by an increase in calcium excretion, although the individual variations were wide. The mean increase in 24-h urine calcium was 61.6 $\pm$ 11.6 mg in normal subjects and 44.1 $\pm$ 8.3 mg in stone formers.

In 13 out of the 14 normals, the 24-h urine volume was increased after spinach ingestion, as found by others[19,20], while in stone formers it increased in only 7 out of 14 cases. This failure to increase diuresis may be important for stone-formation.

Table 1. Biochemical Data before and during Spinach Load (mean ± SEM).

	Urinary Oxalic Acid		Urinary Calcium	
	Excretion	Mean Difference	Excretion	Mean Difference
Normals				
Preload (mg/dl)	2.4 ± 0.4	1.5 ± 0.4 **	13.8 ± 3.7	4.8 ± 1.9 *
Postload (mg/dl)	3.9 ± 0.6		18.7 ± 4.9	
Preload (mg/24h)	22.0 ± 4.6	23.1 ± 5.3 **	100.6 ± 21.0	61.6 ± 11.6 ***
Postload (mg/24h)	45.1 ± 5.9		162.2 ± 20.6	
Stoneformers				
Preload (mg/dl)	2.4 ± 0.3	3.3 ± 1.2 *	9.4 ± 1.1	5.07 ± 1.4 ***
Postload (mg/dl)	5.8 ± 1.2		14.5 ± 6.8	
Preload (mg/24h)	31.7 ± 6.8	45.3 ± 20.9 *	108.2 ± 12.1	44.1 ± 8.4 ***
Postload (mg/24h)	77.0 ± 26.1		152.3 ± 16.7	

* $p < 0.05$; ** $p < 0.01$; *** $p < 0.001$.

REFERENCES

1. A. K. Pendse, A. K. Shrivastava, J. L. Kumawat, H. S. Sharma, R. Ghosh, A. Goyal, and P. P. Singh. Bull. Int. Cong. Surg. 188 (1982).

2. S. G. Kabra, S. S. Gaur, S. S. Sharma, M. K. Patni, and P. Banerji, Indian J. Surg. 34:309 (1972).

3. P. P. Singh, A. K. Pendse, R. Ghosh, and A. Goyal, Asian Med. J. (in press).

4. P. P. Singh, L. K. Kothari, D. C. Sharma, and S. N. Saxena, Am. J. Clin. Nutr. 25:1147 (1972).

5. M. Menon and C. J. Mahle, J. Urol. 127:148 (1982).

6. A. Hodgkinson and A. Williams, Clin. Chim. Acta 36:127 (1972).

7. H. Varley, A. H. Gowenlock, and M. Bell. "Practical Clinical Biochemistry", Vol. I, Heinemann, London (1976).

8. J. C. Dunlop, J. Pathol. Bacteriol. 3:389 (1896).

9. H. E. Archer, A. E. Dormer, E. F. Scowen, and R. W. E. Watts, Clin. Sci. 16:405 (1957).

10. P. M. Zarembski and A. Hodgkinson, Clin. Chim. Acta 25:1 (1969).

11. R. W. Marshall, M. Cochran, and A. Hodgkinson. Clin. Sci. 43:91 (1972).

12. V. S. Chadwick, K. Modha, and R. H. Dowling, New Engl. J. Med. 289:172 (1973).

13. A. Hodgkinson, Clin Sci Mol. Med. 46:357 (1974).

NUTRITION AND CALCIUM OXALATE UROLITHIASIS

R. A. J. Conyers, A. M. Rofe, and W. Bais

Metabolic Research Group, Division of Clinical
Chemistry, Institute of Medical and Veterinary Science
Adelaide, SA 5000, Australia

INTRODUCTION

In affluent societies urolithiasis is a major cause of morbidity
and calcium oxalate is a major constituent in over 70% of the stones
examined[1]. Our data confirm this figure[2]. Much attention has
been paid to the role of calcium but a number of investigators now
consider oxalate excretion to be the most critical factor in urine
for determining the risk of formation of calcium oxalate stones[3].
Diet has traditionally been viewed as the major source of oxalate
for the formation of urinary tract stones but, in more recent times,
it has become accepted that approximately 90% of the oxalate appearing in urine comes from endogenous sources[1]. Two possible dietary
sources of endogenous oxalate are refined carbohydrates and animal
proteins[4-6].

Metabolic studies provide strong support for a role for dietary
refined carbohydrate in the genesis of urinary tract stones.
Clinically, more than 50 cases of tissue oxalosis have been reported
in the literature in association with the intravenous use of the
sugar alcohol, xylitol[7]. Increased oxalate production is
associated with xylitol infusions in rats[8-10] and with xylitol
metabolism in isolated rat hepatocytes[11,12] and liver homogenates
from humans, rats, mice and guinea pigs[13]. Radioisotopic studies
confirm that xylitol gives rise to oxalate directly[10-13].
Xylulose, formed from xylitol, can be phosphorylated to xylulose
1-phosphate by fructokinase and then cleaved by aldolase to produce
glycolaldehyde, a known oxalate precursor[7,13,14]. The observed
conversion (<1%) of xylitol to oxalate is biologically significant
when considered in models of renal clearance based on a one-
compartment kinetic model for oxalate metabolism[15].

METABOLIC STUDIES

It is tempting to consider xylitol as a special case but other carbohydrates, such as fructose, are good oxalate precursors in isolated rat hepatocytes[12] and in liver homogenates[14]. Fructo-kinase and aldolase are also important enzymes in the proposed path-way[12] (Fig. 1). A study in which rats were given 1% (v/v) ethylene glycol in their drinking water and fed diets containing 20% (w/w) starch, glucose, sucrose, fructose, galactose, xylitol or sorbitol for 21 days, showed that the fructose, xylitol and sorbitol diets caused twice the renal deposition of CaOx that occurred with the starch, sucrose and galactose diets. The renal deposition in the glucose-fed rats was less than half that of the starch-fed rats.

Can we extrapolate from these metabolic studies to postulate a role for dietary nutrients in urolithiasis? In human dietary studies[6], 8 healthy volunteers consumed 3 different test diets each for a period of 3 days. The protein, fat, carbohydrate and alcohol contents (MJ%) of the diets were as follows: normal diet, 15:38:42:5; high protein-high fat diet, 25:70:5:0; high sucrose diet, 13:10:77:0; and high starch diet, 20:36:44:0. The sucrose content of the diets was 12, 0, 70 and 0, respectively. For each subject, each test diet was isocaloric with respect to his normal diet. Within the 3 test diets, the animal protein (beef and chicken) content (g/day) was 128.6 (73.1), 76.4 (73.1) and 79.6 (73.1), the Ca content (mmol/day) was 46.6, 3.2 and 14.3, and the oxalate content (mmol/day) was 0.76, 0.41, 0.16, respectively. For all the diets the mean urinary Ca excretion (mmol/day) was 5.3, 8.0, 2.6 and 4.0; and the oxalate excretion (mmol/day) was 0.38, 0.33, 0.29 and 0.45, respectively. Ca excretion correlated with Ca, protein and fat intakes. No simple relation was observed between oxalate excretion and oxalate, calcium, protein, animal protein, fat or carbohydrate intake. The urinary CaOx relative supersaturation indices (RSSI) for the four diets were calculated[16] to be 7.08, 6.09, 1.72 and 7.82, respectively.

In a similar study in the rat, animals were fed isocaloric diets (20 g/day) containing mouse cubes (calcium content, 188 μmol/g; oxalate content 4.8 μmol/g) and added carbohydrate (50:50 w/w) for 21 days. These diets provided the same protein, fat, total carbohydrate, Ca and oxalate intakes for all animals. The added carbohydrates were starch, glucose, sucrose and fructose. The mean urinary Ca excretion (μmol/day) was 55.3, 23.4, 31.6 and 97.1, the oxalate excretion (μmol/day) was 9,7, 6.0, 6.5 and 12.8, and RSSI was calculated to be 20, 26, 20 and 58; and the % oral dose of U - ^{14}C-oxalate excreted/day was found to be 4.35, 2.80, 3.10 and 2.60, respectively. The addition of 5% (w/w) glycine to these diets increased the Ca excretion of the glucose and sucrose-fed rats and appeared to ameliorate the effect of dietary fructose on Ca and oxalate excretion. The progressive replacement of sucrose by casein (Ca content, 16 μmol/g; oxalate content, 0 μmol/g) increased Ca excretion but had no effect on oxalate excretion. The addition of glycine and, in particular, casein to the diet reduced the RSSI in urine. In rats fed mouse cubes alone, decreases in the total energy intake decreased the excretion of CaOx.

In the mouse study, animals (28 per dietary group; approximately 32 g each) were meal-fed mouse cubes for 3 h/day but given free access to water or a 20% (w/w) solution of glucose, sucrose, fructose, xylitol or sorbitol for 5 months. In this study the total food enerlgy intakes/day were in the proportions 1.0, 1.3, 1.3, 1.1, 0.7 and 0.6 and the urinary excretion of oxalate 1.0, 1.5, 2.0, 1.5, 1.0 and 0.5, respectively. (In all these studies, calcium was measured by either atomic absorption spectrometry[6] or EGTA titration[6] and oxalate by either a modified colorimetric assay[17] or immobilized oxalate oxidase in a continuous-flow system[17]).

DISCUSSION

Obviously, the metabolic approach to the problem of urolithiasis can demonstrate oxalate production from individual carbohydrates by specific metabolic pathways. The simple nutritional approach, however, leads to confusion in that, for example, sucrose diets do not appear to increase the risk of urolithiasis in humans but a diet of fructose, a component of sucrose, does so in rats. The mouse study, on the other hand, suggests that the total food energy intake is the most important risk factor. This confusion probably arises from the fact that most diet studies of urolithiasis are based largely on the measurement of physico-chemical characteristics in urine. We suggest that a more appropriate model for the role of nutrition in calcium oxalate urolithiasis would be one that takes account of the gastrointestinal absorption of calcium and oxalate, the hepatic production of oxalate, the renal handling of calcium and oxalate and the dietary-induced hormonal milieu. Dietary refined carbohydrates are known to have effects at all these levels[4-7]. Such a model would mean that the role of nutrition in calcium oxalate urolithiasis would have to be assessed not in the simple terms of a specific nutrient but in terms of the various proportions of nutrients and the total energy intake of the diet.

REFERENCES

1. A. Hodgkinson, "Oxalic Acid in Biology and Medicine", Academic Press, New York (1977).
2. A. M. Rofe, R. A. J. Conyers, and D. W. Thomas, Med. J. Aust. 2:158 (1981).
3. W. G. Robertson and M. Peacock, Nephron 26:105 (1980).
4. W. G. Robertson, M. Peacock, and A. Hodgkinson, J. Chron. Dis. 32:469 (1979).

5. P. N. Rao, V. Prendiville, A. Buxton, D. G. Moss, and
   N. J. Blacklock, Br. J. Urol. 54:578 (1982).
6. R. A. J. Conyers, A. G. Need, A. Bracken, M. Meyler, R. Bais,
   A. M. Rofe, N. Potezny, and M. Guerin, Int. J. Vit. Nutr. Res.
   (1984) (in press).
7. R. A. J. Conyers, A. M. Rofe, R. Bais, H. M. James,
   J. B. Edwards, D. W. Thomas, and R. G. Edwards, Int. J. Vit.
   Nutr.Res. (1984) (in press).
8. B. Hannett, D. W. Thomas, A. H. Chalmers, A. M. Rofe,
   J. B. Edwards, and R. G. Edwards, J. Nutr. 107:458 (1977).
9. D. W. Thomas, B. Hannett, A. Chalmers, A. M. Rofe,
   J. B. Edwards, and R. G. Edwards, Int. J. Vit. Nutr. Res.
   (Suppl.) 15:181 (1976).
10. A. M. Rofe, R. A. H. Conyers, R. Bais, and J. B. Edwards,
    Aust. J. Exp. Biol. Med. Sci. 57:171 (1979).
11. A. M. Rofe, D. W. Thomas, R. G. Edwards, and J. B. Edwards,
    Biochem. Med. 18:440 (1977).
12. A. M. Rofe, H. M. James, R. Bais, J. B. Edwards, and
    R. A. J. Conyers, Aust. J. Exp. Biol. Med. Sci. 58:103
    (1980).
13. H. M. James, S. G. Williams, R. Bais, A. M. Rofe, J. B. Edwards,
    and R. A. J. Conyers, J. Vit. Nutr. Res. (1984) (in press).
14. H. M. James, R. Bais, J. B. Edwards, A. M. Rofe, and
    R. A. J. Conyers, Aust. J. Exp. Biol. Med. Sci. 60:117 (1982).
15. R. A. J. Conyers, T. W. Huber, D. W. Thomas, A. M. Rofe,
    R. Bais, and R. G. Edwards, J. Vit. Nutr. Res. (1984)
    (inpress).
16. J. R. Burns and B. Finlayson, Invest. Urol. 18:167 (1980).
17. N. Potezny, R. Bais, P. O'Loughlin, J. B. Edwards, A. M. Rofe,
    and R. A. J. Conyers, Clin. Chem. 29:16 (1983).

THE EFFECT OF AN INCREASED INTAKE OF VARIOUS CONSTITUENTS
OF A HIGH ANIMAL PROTEIN DIET ON THE RISK OF CALCIUM OXALATE
STONE FORMATION IN MEN

B. Arora, P. L. Selby, R. W. Norman, M. Peacock, and
W. G. Robertson

MRC Mineral Metabolism Unit
The General Infirmary, Leeds LS1 3EX, U.K.

INTRODUCTION

The prevalence of calcium oxalate stone disease is rising in
affluent societies[1]. The major dietary changes in these societies
shown so far are a high consumption of animal protein[2], sugar[3] and
depletion of fibre[4]. Analysis of the diets of various population
groups has shown that the factor which correlates best with
affluence and stone disease is a high consumption of animal
protein[2]. Animal protein contains a higher amount of certain amino
acids, and is associated with a higher fat[5] and purine[6] content in
the diet than vegetable protein. The objective of this
investigation is to study the biochemical changes produced by
increasing the consumption of these constituents and to assess the
effect of these changes on the risk of stone formation.

MATERIALS AND METHODS

Groups of normals were studied under their home conditions for
one week during which they were advised to maintain a constant diet.
During the following week, the same diet was supplemented with one
of the following constituents: methionine (2.5 g/day), glycine (4
g/day), hydroxyproline (0.45 g/day), RNA (2 g/day), or fat (100
g/day). The number of volunteers studied in each group were 6, 6,
5, 3, 13 respectively. The quantities of the constituents to be
tested were selected with a view to doubling the normal daily intake
of these in the diet. These were divided and taken with meals. The
effect of methionine and glycine was also tested on 12 stone formers
in a metabolic ward on a constant diet and fluid intake.

Twenty-four-hour urines were collected with preservative on the last 3 days of the basal and experimental weeks. These were analysed for calcium, oxalate, pH, volume, phosphorus, uric acid, creatinine and alcian blue precipitable polyanions (ABPP). The averages of the 3 days' excretions were calculated and the differences of both weeks tested statistically using the paired 't' test in which every volunteer acted as his own control.

Fasting blood and urine samples were also taken on the last day of each week. Calcium, pH, phosphorus and creatinine were estimated in a fasting urine sample. Blood was analysed for calcium, ionized calcium, phosphate, creatinine and uric acid. Ultrafilterable calcium, glomerular filtration rate (GFR) and tubular reabsorption maxima for calcium (TmCa) were calculated.

RESULTS

Of all the constituents tested, methionine caused a 14% increase in urinary excretion of calcium ($P<0.05$) in normals (Fig. 1). Five out of the 6 patients studied also showed a marked increase (26%) in urinary calcium, but the overall effect was non-significant because of the large variation in response.

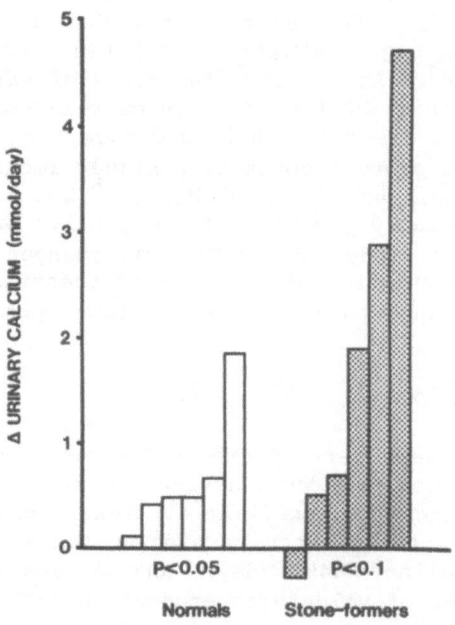

Fig. 1. The effect of 2.5 g/day methionine on urinary calcium in stone-formers and normals.

86

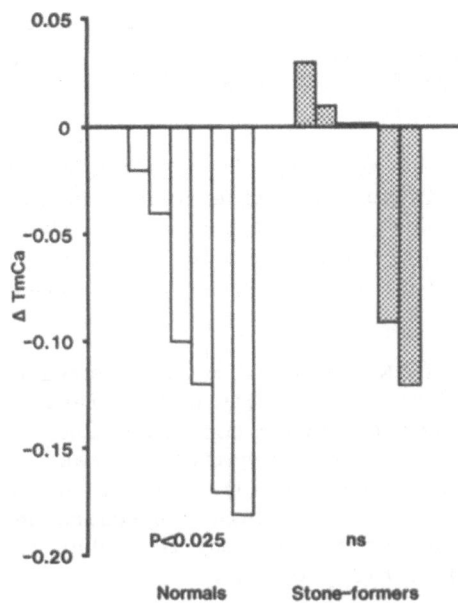

Fig. 2. The effect of 2.5 g/day methionine on TmCa in stone-formers
and normals.

Glycine, hydroxyproline, RNA and fat caused a variable increase
in oxalate in some volunteers, but the effect was non-significant.
However, as expected, RNA produced a dramatic increase in uric acid
in all the volunteers studied (P<0.001).

DISCUSSION

It has been shown that a diet containing a high proportion of
animal protein and purines aggravates the risk of calcium oxalate
stone formation by increasing the urinary excretion of calcium,
oxalate and uric acid. The present investigation confirms that
methionine, 70% of which is derived from animal foods, is an
important cause of the hypercalciuria due to a high protein diet as
shown in earlier studies. Although the mechanism of the
hypercalciuric effect of methionine is not yet clear, estimation of
various parameters of renal handling shows that there is no effect
on GFR, ultrafilterable calcium and the amount of filtered calcium,
but there was a significant (P<0.025) decrease in TmCa (Fig. 2)
which suggests that the increase in urinary excretion might be due
to reduced tubular reabsorption of calcium. It has been suggested
that sulphate (a breakdown product of methionine) forms a complex
with calcium which is poorly reabsorbed in the renal tubule[7].
Alternatively, the significant decrease in urinary pH in both
normals (P<0.001) and patients (P<0.005) suggests that mild

metabolic acidosis (resulting from the two equivalents of hydrogen ions which are produced per mol of oxidized sulphur, when methionine is metabolized) might be the cause of the reduced tubular reabsorption of calcium[8].

Fat, glycine and hydroxyproline in the amount given did not increase any risk factor for stone formation. Our inability to demonstrate the effect may have been due to the small amount of amino acids used in the test, but our investigation was designed to evaluate the effect of the amounts which realistically might be consumed per day.

Consumption of RNA caused a marked increase in uric acid excretion and confirms the results demonstrated by previous investigators[9]. Thus the study concludes that animal protein increases the risk of stone formation at least in part by the combined effect of methionine and purines. Research is in progress on the effect of tryptophan, lysine, tyrosine and phenylalanine, other amino acids which are present in higher concentrations in animal than in vegetable proteins.

ACKNOWLEDGEMENTS

We acknowledge the finacial help given to B.A. by the Kellogg Company of Great Britain and by the British Council.

REFERENCES

1. W. G. Robertson, M. Peacock, P. J. Heyburn, R. Speed, and F. Hanes, Fortschr. Urol. Nephrol. 11:5 (1978).
2. W. G. Robertson, M. Peacock, and A. Hodgkinson, J. Chron. Dis. 32:469 (1979).
3. T. L. Cleave, "The Saccharine Disease", John Wright, Bristol (1974).
4. D. P. Burkitt and H. C. Trowell, "Refined Carbohydrate Foods and Disease. Some Implications of Dietary Fibre", Academic Press, London (1975).
5. A. A. Paul and D. A. T. Southgate, "Composition of Foods", H.M.S.O., London (1978).
6. A. J. Clifford and D. L. Story, J. Nutr. 106:435 (1976).
7. M. Walser, Am. J. Physiol. 201:769 (1961).
8. J. Lemann, J. R. Litzow, and E. J. Lennon, J. Clin. Invest. 46:8 (1967).
9. J. Bowering, D. H. Colloway, S. Margen, and N. A. Kaufman, J. Nutr. 100:249 (1970).

CALCULOGENIC POTENTIAL OF THE DIET -   A NEW CONCEPT

Y. M. Fazil Marickar, D. Joseph, and
P. B. Abraham

Medical College Hospital, Trivandrum, S. India

INTRODUCTION

The role of diet is one of the most controversial topics in
any discussion on the epidemiology of urolithiasis.   Dietary
studies are complicated by the practical problem of assessing the
pattern of intake in the individual. The difference between the
dietary pattern of the individual and that of his family or
community in which he lives[1] and the variation in the nutritional
content of the same foodstuffs cultivated in different areas are
some of the complicating factors. Prescription of a diet for the
stone patient is riddled with inconsistencies. Many foodstuffs
contain a combination of calculogenic as well as anticalculogenic
agents. The present study aims at identifying the net potential of
a number of foodstuffs to promote or inhibit calculogenesis.

MATERIALS AND METHODS

A procedure was devised to identify the calculogenic status
of the diet based on the nutritional values of the diets, taking
into account the previously recognised physico-chemical principles
of promotion and inhibition of calculogenesis. The nutritional
analysis of some common foodstuffs published by the Indian
Council of Medical Research[2] was taken into consideration,
supplemented by other reports. The contents of protein, uric
acid, citrate, oxalate, calcium, magnesium, chloride, sodium,
vitamins A, D, B_1, and pyridoxine, and the ratio of oxalate to
calcium and calcium to phosphate were assessed. The calculogenic
potential of each nutrient was defined by allotting positive or
negative points to each ingredient. The value of points ranged

from 0 to +32 or 0 to -32 according to the content of the ingredients in the foodstuff (Table 1). Thus the calculogenic potential (C.P.) was calculated as equal to the total value of protein (0 to -8) + uric acid (0 to +32) + citrate (0 to -12) + oxalates (0 to +20) + oxalate:calcium ratio (0 to +10) + calcium (0 to +12) + calcium:phosphorus ratio (0 to +20) + magnesium (0 to -4) + chloride (0 to -4) + sodium (0 to -32) + vitamin A (0 to -16) + vitamin D (0 t +12) + vitamin B_1 (0 to -4) + pyridoxine (0to -8).

Calculation of the Dietetic Index of the patients was made after identifying the average weight of each nutrient ingested by the patient, and calculating the positive and negative potentials of the diet according to the formula:

$$\text{Dietetic Index (D.I.)} = \frac{\text{Total positive points}}{\text{Total negative points}} \times 100$$

Dietetic Index over 100 was considered to be calculogenic and an Index below 100 to be non-calculogenic. A dietetic study was carried out in 342 patients and 50 controls.

RESULTS

The calculogenic potentials of some common foodstuffs are detailed in Table 2. The value of potential ranged from the lowest for salt (-32) to the highest for spinach (+49).

The average value of the Dietetic Index of the urinary stone patients was 97, compared with 93 for the control group. The difference was not statistically significant. However, some of the patients showed a markedly high Index. In these patients, it was possible to reduce the Index by appropriate dietetic advice.

DISCUSSION

In this study, an assessment of the total calculogenic property of the diet has been attempted. It has been found to be useful for providing proper dietetic advice for the stone patients. Even though the mean Dietetic Index of the stone patients was not significantly different from that of the controls, it was possible to reduce the Index in these patients. Furthermore, using this technique, it was possible to study the stone-forming propensity of the diet and to advise intake of diets with a lower calculogenic potential. Such advice has been found to have a beneficial effect on the progression and recurrence of stone-formation.

Table 1. The Calculogenic Potential of Various Nutrients.

| Nutrient | Range of contents | | | |
	Low range points	Moderate range points	High range points	Very High range points
Protein (g)	0-4(-1)	5-8 (-2)	9-16(-4)	17-32(-8)
Uric acid(mg)	0-50(+4)	51-100(+8)	101-200(+16)	201-400(+32)
Citrate(mg)	0-100(-2)	101-200(-3)	201-400(-6)	401-800(-12)
Oxalates(mg)	0-100(+3)	101-200(+5)	201-400(+10)	401-800(+20)
Ox:Calcium	1:2(0)	1:1(+2)	2:1(+10)	
Calcium(mg)	1-100(+2)	101-200(+3)	201-400(+6)	401-800(+12)
Ca:P	1:2(0)	1:1(+5)	2:1(+20)	
Magnesium(mg)	0-30(0)	31-60(-1)	61-125(-2)	126-250(-4)
Chloride(g)	0-0.8(0)	0.8-1.5(-1)	1.5-3.0(-2)	3.0-6.0(-4)
Sodium(g)	0-1.25(-4)	1.25-2.5(-8)	2.5-5.0(-16)	5.0-10.0(-32)
Vitamin A (10000 IU)	0.04(-2)	0.4-0.75(-4)	0.75-1.5(-8)	1.5-3.0(-16)
Vitamin D (IU)	0-15(+2)	16-25(+3)	26-50(+6)	51-100(+12)
Vitamin B_1(mg)	0.0.3(0)	0.3-0.6(-1)	0.7-1.5(-2)	1.6-3(-4)
Pyridoxine(mg)	0-40(-1)	41-75(-2)	76-150(-4)	151-300(-8)

Table 2. Calculogenic Potential of Common Foodstuffs.

Foodstuff	Points	Foodstuff	Points	Foodstuffs	Points
Rice	- 2	Ginger	- 2	Prawns	- 6
Wheat	- 7	Gooseberries	+10	Chicken	- 7
Black gram	-12	Lemon	+ 2	Mutton	- 7
Bengal gram	-14	Onion	+ 2	Beef	+11
Green gram	-11	Cashew nuts	+ 1	Pork	+ 9
Peas	- 4	Ground nuts	- 7	Liver	+ 9
Cabbage	- 5	Pepper	+36	Lard	+11
Spinach	+49	Cardamom	- 2	Coconut oil	0
Drumstick leaf	+23	Apple	- 1	Vegetable oil	- 1
Cauliflower	- 4	Banana	- 4	Eggs	- 4
Carrots	- 3	Mango	- 1	Cow's milk	- 1
Potatoes	-12	Orange	- 4	Buffalo's milk	+ 1
Radish	+ 2	Mulberries	- 1	Goat's milk	+ 1
Tapioca	+ 2	Papaya	- 1	Ghee	- 1
Yam	+ 2	Pineapple	-12	Sugar	0
Beans	- 2	Dates	+ 2	Jaggery	+ 1
Tomatoes	- 9	Grapes	- 1	Salt	- 3
Chillies	- 3	Sardines	- 5	Tea, coffee	+ 5
Garlic	+ 1	Mackerel	+13	Beverages	0

REFERENCES

1. G. W. Drach, in:"Campbell's Urology", 4th edition, W. B. Saunders Co. Philadelphia, (1979).
2. W. R. Arkroyd, in:"Nutritional analysis of Indian Foodstuffs", I.C.M.R. Special report series No. 42, p.88 (1966).

TEA DRINKING - A RISK FACTOR FOR UROLITHIASIS?

D. N. Churchill, J. Morgan, and M. H. Gault

Faculty of Health Sciences, McMaster University
Hamilton, Ontario, and Memorial University
St John's, Newfoundland, Canada

INTRODUCTION

A small increase in urinary oxalate concentration produces a considerable increase in supersaturation with respect to calcium oxalate[1]. Although dietary oxalate is responsible for only 10-15% of total urinary oxalate[2], ingestion of oxalate-rich foods (e.g. rhubarb, spinach, chocolate) causes a marked increase in urinary oxalate excretion[3]. Tea, a major source of oxalate, is a popular beverage and, therefore, could be a clinically important risk factor for calcium oxalate urolithiasis. We have used a case control design to estimate this risk.

METHODS

The cases were 117 stone formers identified among 1112 adults in a population survey for urolithiasis in Newfoundland[4]. A person was defined as a stone former if a stone had ever been passed, had been removed at operation or had been visualized by X-ray. The control subjects were 117 persons matched for sex, district and age $\pm$ 4 years. Sibling matches were excluded. Tea consumption at the time of the survey was recorded. The mean difference in tea consumption between paired cases and controls was analyzed by the paired "t" test. The null hypothesis of no difference between paired cases and controls for the exposure factor, tea drinking, was analyzed by McNemar's test. The extent of tea drinking was graded by cups per day as mild (0 to 2.5), moderate (3.0 to 5.0) and strong ($>$ 5). To test the null hypothesis of no difference between paired cases and controls for ordered exposure to 3 categories of tea drinking, the x^2 derived by Fleiss and Everitt was used[5].

RESULTS

The mean ages for male stone formers and control subjects were 47.04 and 47.02 years; for female stone formers and controls 47.49 and 47.46 years ($P>0.10$ in each case). The mean number of cups of tea consumed daily was 4.00 for stone formers and 4.18 for controls ($P>0.10$). The null hypothesis of no difference in the proportion of tea drinkers between stone formers and paired controls was not rejected ($x^2 = 0.45$; $P>0.10$). The null hypothesis of no difference between pairs with increasing exposure to tea drinking was not rejected ($x^2 = 0.00$; $P>0.10$).

DISCUSSION

Inferences based on the results of case-control study must include consideration of the potential biases to which this design is susceptible. The cases were identified by history and will therefore contain a proportion with stones other than calcium oxalate. In Newfoundland, more than 85% of stone formers have calcium oxalate stones and while the risk conferred by tea drinking is possibly higher than suggested by this study, the difference is unlikely to change the result significantly. Cases may have decreased their tea ingestion after diagnosis. This is unlikely as no subject, in an open-ended question, identified tea drinking as a possible cause of kidney stones.

The mean oxalate content of a cup of tea (3 g tea bag immersed in recently boiled water for 5 min) was 21 mg[6]. If only 2 to 3% of ingested oxalate were absorbed, as occurs with oxalate ingested as rhubarb, spinach and chocolate, this would provide only an additional 0.5 mg per cup of tea ingested. We have found no evidence to support the suggestion that tea drinking is a risk factor for calcium oxalate urolithiasis.

REFERENCES

1. W. G. Robertson and M. Peacock, Nephron 26:105 (1980).
2. A. Hodgkinson, "Oxalic Acid in Biology and Medicine", Academic Press, London (1977).
3. A. Strenge, A. Hesse, D. Bach, and W. Vahlensieck, in:"Urolithiasis, Clinical and Basic Research", L. H. Smith, W. G. Robertson, and B. Finlayson, eds., Plenum, New York (1981).
4. D. N. Churchill, C. M. Maloney, J. Bear, D. G. Bryant, G. Fodor, and M. H. Gault, J. Chron. Dis. 33:727 (1980).
5. J. L. Fleiss and B. S. Everitt, Br. J. Math. Stat. Psychol. 24:117 (1971).
6. J. Fraser and D. J. Campbell, Clin. Biochem. 5:99 (1972).

ENVIRONMENT

INFLUENCE OF WATER QUALITY ON UROLITHIASIS

W. Vahlensieck

Urologische Universitätsklinik, 5300 Bonn 1, F.R.G.

FLUID INTAKE

In order to prevent the recurrence of urinary stone formation, there is general agreement on the value of a high fluid intake[1,2]. Pak et al[3] have demonstrated the satisfactory response of patients treated with only an increased fluid intake and dietary modification. Hosking et al[4] have shown that the "stone clinic effect" (defined as a high intake of fluid with avoidance of dietary excesses) in patients with idiopathic calcium urolithiasis and indeterminate metabolic activity brought about metabolic inactivity without further stone formation after a mean follow-up of 62.2 months in 58.3% of their patients. The patients were advised to increase their fluid intake to achieve a daily urine output of $\geqslant$ 2500 ml. Specifically, an oral fluid intake of approximately 8 ounces (240 ml) hourly while awake was recommended, with at least half of the fluid being water.

Such advice guarantees that patients will have a daily water consumption of at least 1500 ml to 2000 ml. With this level of water intake the question arises as to whether or not the quality of the water can influence urinary stone formation or growth. In considering this question, the hardness of water is often discussed, i.e. the content of the alkaline earth ions, calcium, magnesium, strontium and barium. In any study on the influence of water intake on urolithiasis, however, it is also necessary to look into the other constituents of drinking water. Furthermore, we have to distinguish between tap, natural and artificial water since the composition, especially the calcium content, may vary considerably.

CALCIUM CONTENT OF WATER

Studies on the content of calcium in tap water in the different districts of the Federal Republic of Germany[5] show that there are only two small regions where the calcium content is more than 150 mg/l. Although it should be remembered that tap water often has a higher content of calcium than ground water because of the addition of calcium hydroxide to the ground water to adjust pH.

A daily intake of tap water of 1500 ml to 2000 ml in the Federal Republic of Germany would mean that the intake of calcium from the water would be less than 300 mg/day. This would lead to hypercalciuria only if the intake of calcium in food was already >800 mg/day. This may provide a special problem for hyperabsorbers where increased fluid intake will not achieve adequate dilution of calcium in the urine to prevent supersaturation of the calcium salts in urine.

The importance of such complex environmental factors became evident from the study of Sierakowski et al[6] who found in the United States a negative correlation between the geographical distribution of hospital discharges for stone disease and water hardness within. Recently Shuster et al[7] have shown on a microgeographical scale that after adjusting for environmental factors, tap water hardness is of minor importance with respect to urinary stone formation. Churchill et al[8,9] stated in a study of the prevalence of kidney stone formers and the relationship of genetic factors and drinking water composition in 6 districts in Newfoundland that the range of water hardness values (7 to 89 ppm $CaCO_3$) was relatively narrow and that there was no detectable association between district urinary stone prevalence (male or female) and the mean district drinking water hardness.

With the consumption of natural or artificial mineral water we have often a different situation. As we already have shown, the diet history of 72 recurrent stone formers who had been told by their doctor to have a high fluid intake revealed that 61% of these patients drank mineral water every day[10]. Of these patients, 45% reported a daily consumption up to 400 ml, 39% up to 700 ml and 16% between 1000 ml and 1400 ml of mineral water. At that time we did not look at the content of calcium of the mineral waters consumed, but Fuss et al[11] reported that 9% of their patients consumed water with a calcium content between 100 mg/l and 200 mg/l and 15% between 200 mg/l and 500 mg/l.

In this connection it is of interest to examine the calcium content of the different mineral waters. In the Federal Republic of Germany we identified 57 mineral waters with a calcium content between 9 mg/l and 150 mg/l which compares with tap water. In 43 other mineral waters, however, the calcium content ranged from

152 mg/l to 281 mg/l. Furthermore, we found 23 mineral waters with a calcium content between 312 mg/l and 491 mg/l, as well as 21 with a very high calcium content, between 510 mg/l and 893 mg/l. Consumption of mineral water with such a high calcium content must be taken into account when considering the total intake of calcium.

We measured the calcium excretion in normals on the fifth day of a standard diet with a daily calcium ingestion between 700 and 800 mg and a total fluid intake of 2000 ml. The next day we replaced 1 litre of hip tea with 1 litre of mineral water with a calcium content of 497 mg/l. This was drunk as 500 ml at 09.00 and 11.00. We found an elevated calcium excretion following this load with a peak between the 13th hour and the 16th hour.

Shuster et al[7] have noted the relatively higher risk of consuming water from a private well as compared to using public water. Also Jaeger et al[12] have shown that the consumption of water with a calcium content of 597 g/l may render stone formers markedly hypercalciuric, particularly those with calcium hyper-absorption. These results emphasize the importance of knowing the calcium content of the local tap water and of the mineral water preferred by the patient. This knowledge allows instruction of the patient in terms of how much water he should drink daily and what other dietary modalities will be necessary to prevent hypercalciuria.

We found a markedly elevated oxalate excretion after an intake of 200 mg spinach. If a patient in such a situation also became hypercalciuric following consumption of water with a high content of calcium, then in spite of the dilution effect there would be a risk of increasing the calcium oxalate activity product and the tendency toward stone formation in the patient.

MAGNESIUM CONTENT OF WATER

With the consumption of high quantities of water the intake of magnesium also becomes important. Sierakowski et al[6] stated that 2 litres of very hard water will supply 106 mg of magnesium. In the Federal Republic of Germany, there are only a few districts with tap water containing more than 30 mg/l magnesium. The situation is similar with natural or artificial mineral waters, but we have here waters with a magnesium content up to 735 mg/l. Apart from these exceptions the ingestion of magnesium with water is not sufficient to reach the daily requirement of 240 mg demanded by the German Association of Nutrition[13]. On the other hand, it was shown that the magnesium intake of adult persons is up to 25 to 60% higher than required[13]. This infers that magnesium is sufficiently absorbed from bread and other baked goods ($\sim$22%), alcoholic (male 14%) and non-alcoholic beverages (13%), milk and milk products ($\sim$8.5%) and potatoes ($\sim$8%). In keeping with this, it is important to note that in many studies the magnesium excretion was similar in normal subjects and stone formers[14-17].

In this context the findings of Churchill et al are difficult to explain[5,6]. They found in areas of soft drinking water that the mean urine magnesium excretion was lower than otherwise reported. They thought that the excessive loss of magnesium from foods cooked in soft water could produce a decrease in magnesium ingestion despite an apparently adequate diet. With these observations in mind it is important to consider the possible reasons for magnesium deficiency. Bach et al[14] as well as Churchill et al[8,9] found a reduced magnesium excretion in women compared with men. If a low magnesium excretion pre-disposes to urinary stone formation, then more stones should occur in women. Since this is not the case and taking the other findings into account, the magnesium content of water must be of minor importance for urinary stone formation and growth.

PHOSPHATE CONTENT OF WATER

Of further interest is the phosphate content of water. The orthophosphate content of tap water in the different districts of the Federal Republic of Germany, is relatively low (only a few regions have more than 0.25 mg/l). This is due to the fact that, in the formation of ground water, phosphates are retained in the ground. If surface water is prepared for drinking water, the increased existing phoshates are retained by the purification procedure. We did not measure the content of phosphate in natural or artificial mineral waters and this has yet to be examined.

Such studies may be of special interest in view of the variable clinical results of prophylactic treatment with phosphate and the associated basic research[2,18,19]. Wikström et al[20] found a significant increase in the urinary excretion of phosphate and pyrophosphate and a corresponding decrease in calcium excretion during orthophosphate treatment. On the other hand, Smith et al[21] have shown that hydroxyapatite is the predominant crystal present in freshly voided urine of patients with idiopathic calcium urolithiasis and primary hyperparathyroidism and that hydroxyapatite, as small crystals with a large surface area or in association with matrix, may induce the heterogenous nucleation of calcium oxalate in these patients. Furthermore, Nancollas et al[22] noted that the formation of concretions of calcium phosphate is complicated by the precipitation of precursors during the overall crystallization process.

SULFATE CONTENT OF WATER

The content of sulfate in the drinking water of the different districts of the Federal Republic of Germany generally lies between 25 mg/l and 150 mg/l. A high sulfate content is found in regions where the water has passed over sediments of calcium and sulfate. Usually waters with a high content of sulfate also have a high content of calcium. Until now we have not looked at the content of sulfate in all mineral waters, but in the analysed mineral waters, sulfate ranged between 12.6 mg/l and 1085 mg/l. According to Michalk[23] there is little information on the intestinal absorption of free sulfate ions. Up till now the effect of the sulfate content of water on the urinary excretion of sulfate has not been examined. This question is of interest since free sulfate ions and free calcium ions present in urine combine as soluble complexes thereby decreasing the free calcium ion activity[24]. This, in turn, reduces the urine supersaturation with calcium salts.

OTHER FACTORS IN WATER

It is helpful to have information on the acidity and the content of other ions in the local drinking water. We do not have any information of the content of aluminium, iron, and copper ions because they are precipitated or complexed during the analytical determination for hardness. However, Churchill et al[9] have stated that copper, iron, manganese, silica, and zinc have no influence on the prevalence of urinary stones. On the otherhand, Anasuya and Narasinga Rao[25] have shown that silica accelerated mineralization in vitro.

No information is available on the content of fluoride in tap water or in mineral waters in the Federal Republic of Germany. This may be important since Summers and Keitzer[26] noted the prevalence of fluoride in calcium oxalate stones and Juuti and Heinonen[27,28] found the highest urinary stone incidence in a region with a high fluoride content in the ground water. Jolly et al[29] have reported an increased urinary excretion of fluoride in fluorotic patients. The urinary stones from patients residing in an endemic fluorotic area revealed a significantly higher fluoride content compared to calculi from persons from a non-endemic area. Anasuya[30] proved that ingestion of excess fluoride facilitates calcium oxalate crystalluria and promoted the formation of bladder stones in rats. Using an in vitro mineralizing system Anasuya and Narasinga Rao[25] have shown that fluoride accelerated calcium uptake. On the other hand, Luoma et al[31] could prevent nephrocalcinosis which normally resulted from a diet void of magnesium, by giving fluoride. Hering et al[32] noted that low fluoride concentrations in urine retarded crystalluria while higher concentrations in urine intensified crystalluria. Apart from the endemic fluorotic areas, this problem is also important for regions where fluoridation of drinking water is performed to prevent dental caries.

REFERENCES

1. K. Sakhaee, J. E. Zerwekh, and C. Y. C. Pak, in:"Urolithiasis: Clinical and Basic Research", L. H. Smith, W. G. Robertson, and B. Finlayson, eds., Plenum, New York (1981).
2. L. H. Smith, C. J. Van Den Berg, and D. M. Wilson, N. Engl. J. Med. 298:87 (1978).
3. C. Y. C. Pak, P. Peters, G. Hurst, M. Kadesky, M. Fine, D. Reisman, F. Splann, C. Caramela, A. Freeman, F. Britton, K. Sakhall, and N. A. Breslau, Am. J. Med. 71:615 (1981).
4. D. H. Hosking, S. B. Erickson, C. J. Van Den Berg, D. M. Wilson, and L. H. Smith, J. Urol. 130:1115 (1983).
5. K. Aurand, U. Hasselbarth, and G. Muller, "Atlas Zur Trinkwasserqualität der Bundesrepublik Deutschland", Schmidt-Verlag, Berlin (1980).
6. R. Sierakowski, B. Finlayson, and R. Landes, Urol. Res. 7:157 (1979).
7. R. Sierakowski, B. Finlayson, R. Scheafter, R. Sierakowski, J. Zoltek, and S. Dzegede, J. Urol. 128:422 (1982).
8. D. N. Churchill, D. P. Black, C. M. Maloney, and M. H. Gault, in:"Urolithiasis:Clinical and Basic Research", L. H. Smith, W. G. Robertson, and B. Finlayson, eds., Plenum, New York (1981).
9. D. N. Churchill, C. M. Maloney, J. C. Bear, D. G. Bryant, G. Fador, and M. H. Gault, in:"Urolithiasis:Clinical and Basic Research", L. H. Smith, W. G. Robertson, and B. Finlayson, eds., Plenum, New York (1981).
10. E. W. Vahlensieck, A. Strenge, and A. Hesse, in:"Urinary Stone", R. Ryall, J. G. Brockis, V. Marshall and B. Finlayson, eds., Churchill Livingstone, Melbourne (1984).
11. M. Fuss, J. Simon, N. Fontinoy, and E. Coussaert, Eur. Urol. 5:97 (1979).
12. P. Jaeger, L. Portmann, A. F. Jacquet, and P. Burckhardt, Eur. Urol. 10:53 (1984).
13. Deutsche Gesellschaft fur Ernahrung e.V., Frankfurt. "Ernahrungsbericht 1980", Henrich, Frankfurth (1980).
14. D. Bach, A. Hesse, A. Strenge, and W. Vahlensieck, in:"Urolithiasis:Clinical and Basic Research", L. H. Smith, W. G. Robertson, and B. Finlayson, eds., Plenum, New York (1981).
15. G. Johansson, U. Backman, B. G. Danielson, B. Fellström, S. Ljunghall, and B. Wikström, in:"Urolithiasis:Clinical and Basic Research", L. H. Smith, W. G. Robertson, and B. Finlayson, eds., Plenum, New York (1981).
16. M. J. Resnick, D. Munday, and W. H. Boyce, Urology 4:385 (1982).

17. H.-G. Tiselius, XIX Int. Congr. Intern. Assoc. Urol.,
    San Francisco, 1982.
18. B. Ettinger, Am. J. Med. 61:200 (1976).
19. P. J. Heyburn, W. G. Robertson, and M. Peacock, Nephron 32:314
    (1982).
20. B. Wikström, U. Backman, B. G. Danielson, B. Fellström,
    G. Johansson, and S. Ljunghall, Fortschr. Urol. Nephrol. 22:
    480 (1984).
21. L. H. Smith, A. D. Jenkins, J. W. L. Wilson, and P. G. Werness,
    Fortschr. Urol. Nephrol. 22:193 (1984).
22. G. H. Nancollas, M. H. Salimi and J. F. de Rooig,
    Fortschr. Urol. Nephrol. 22:198 (1984).
23. D. V. Michalk, "Der Stoffwechsel von Sulfat und Taurin und seine
    Veranderung in der Uramie", Med. Hab.-Schrift, Erlangen
    (1982).
24. A. Hamper, E. Hanisch, P. O. Schwille, and A. Sigel, Forschr.
    Urol. Nephrol. 22:83 (1984).
25. A. Anasuya, and B. S. Narasinga Rao, Biochem. Med. 30:145
    (1983).
26. L. J. Summers and W. A. Keitzer, Ohio State Med. J. 781:25
    (1975).
27. M. Juuti and O. P. Heinonen, Acta Med. Scand. 206:397 (1979).
28. M. Juuti and O. P. Heinonen, Scand. J. Urol. Nephrol. 14:181
    (1980).
29. S. S. Jolly, O. P. Sharma, G. Garg, and R. Sharma Patiala,
    Fluoride 13:10 (1980).
30. A. Anasuya, J. Nutrition 112:1787 (1982)
31. H. Luoma, T. Nunja, Y. Collan, and P. Nummikoski, Calc. Tiss.
    Res. 20:291 (1976).
32. F. Hering, R. Brunner, T. Briellmann, H. Seiler, and
    G. Rutishauser, Fortschr. Urol. Nephrol. 22:44 (1984).

DRINKING WATER QUALITY AND UROLITHIASIS

P. M. Ilievski and S. S. Ilievska

Medical Center of Bitola, 97000 Bitola, Yugoslavia

INTRODUCTION

A negative correlation between water hardness and lithiasis has been demonstrated in Czechoslovakia, in the south eastern part of the United States, in some regions of the United Kingdom and in Yugoslavia[1-10]. From these investigations we conclude that regions with soft drinking water have a higher incidence of urolithiasis than regions with hard drinking water.

METHODS

Water hardness is normally measured using American, English, French or German scales of hardness. We measured water hardness using the German system (grade one is equivalent to 10 mg/l calcium oxide or 7.19 mg/l magnesium oxide). On this scale the hardness of the drinking water in our area is 0.45 (2.2. mg/l calcium oxide and 1.6 mg/l magnesium oxide). Apart from these cations, other constituents of our water include chloride (5.0 mg/l) and silicate (between 1.5 mg/l to 25 mg/l) at a pH of 6.6. Thus our drinking water is very soft and we have a high rate of stone disease.

RESULTS

We carried out a statistical study involving 1240 operations for stones performed over a period of 35 years in an area whose population is 138,000. In addition to the statistical study, we analysed urine from 20 stone formers after chemical analysis of water quality had been done. Operations for stones constitute the best recorded data on this disorder over a long period of time but, in our opinion, these cases make up only a small percentage of those with urolithiasis in this area where 75% of patients admitted to the Dept. of Urology have stone disease. Of these 1240 operations, the highest number, 496 (40%), was carried out on the kidney, 228 (18.4%) on the ureter, 462 (37.25%) on the bladder and 54 (4.35%) on the urethra. Thus upper urinary tract stones made up 724 or 58.40% of all stones. Bladder and urethral stones may develop in the kidneys and pass down to the bladder and urethra or they may originate in the bladder. Our investigations show that the right side is more affected than the left and that the male to female ratio is 1:1:07. In the last 5 years, 75% of stones in our area contained calcium oxalate as the main constituent.

Biochemical investigations were performed on 20 stone formers (14 male and 6 females). The mean ($\pm$ SD) 24-h excretion of calcium was 6.16 ($\pm$ 2.64) mmol and magnesium was 3.43 ($\pm$ 1.01) mmol. The magnesium/calcium ratio was 0.59 $\pm$ 0.19. Hypercalciuria (that is calcium >7.5 mmol/24 h in men and >6.25 mmol/24 h in women) was found in only 3 cases (15%).

DISCUSSION

We consider that the mineral content of the drinking water has an influence on the aetiology of calcium oxalate urolithiasis through its effect on the magnesium/calcium ratio of urine. Our results show a reduced magnesium/calcium ratio (0.59) in the urine of stone-formers compared with normal. A relatively low percentage of the cases had hypercalciuria, which further emphasises that a reduced urinary magnesium is an important predisposing factor for stone formation. Furthermore, a low level of calcium in the drinking water enables better intestinal absorption of oxalate whose concentration in urine is very important for stone formation[7].

A correlation between the % contribution of magnesium to the total hardness of drinking water and the prevalence of urolithiasis is evident from data in the United States. The magnesium in tap-water in the Rockies is more than double that in the Carolinas yet the number of discharges for stone disease per 1000 hospital discharges in the Rockies is less than half that in the Carolinas. A similar correlation between the percentage of magnesium hardness and the rate of nephrolithiasis occurs in both the coastal and inland parts of Yugoslavia. In the coastal areas the rate of nephrolithiasis is double that in inland areas whereas the percentage of magnesium hardness in inland areas is more than double that in the coastal areas. Whether these findings on the magnesium hardness of drinking water and the prevalence of urolithiasis are related or spurious should be investigated further. The importance of a low magnesium in water and the consequent low magnesium in urine is that it competes with calcium for binding to oxalate. In our area the drinking water has a very low level of magnesium and there is a high prevalence of urolithiasis. This is consistent with the hypothesis that drinking water which has a low content of calcium and magnesium leads to a high prevalence of urolithiasis.

REFERENCES

1. D. Churchill, D. Bryant, G. Fodor, and M. H. Gault, Ann. Int. Med. 88:513 (1978).
2. R. Sierakowski, B. Finlayson, and G. Hemp, in:"Colloquium on Renal Lithiasis", B. Finlayson and W. C. Thomas, eds., University Presses of Florida, Gainesville (1976).
3. R. Sierakowski, B. Finlayson, R. Landes, C. Finlayson, and N.Sierakowski, Invest. Urol. 15:438 (1978).
4. D. Derzic, M. Zebec, Lj. Cecuk, and N. Kulcar, XVIII Congrès de la Société Internationale D'Urologie, Paris (1979).
5. R. Sierakowski, B. Finlayson, and R. Landes, Urol. Res. 7:157 (1979).
6. L. Baker and W. Mallinson, Br. J. Urol. 51:181 (1979).
7. M. Menon and C. Mahle, J. Urol. 127:148 (1982).
8. H. Rushton and M. Spector, J. Urol. 127 (597 (1982).
9. J. Shuster, B. Finlayson, R. Scheaffer, R. Sierakowski, J. Zoltek, and S. Dzegede, J. Urol. 128:422 (1982).
10. P. Ilievski, I. Vlaski, R. Nakovski, and S. Ilievska, XIX International Congress of the International Society of Urology, San Francisco (1982).

II. GASTROINTESTINAL PHYSIOLOGY
AND PATHOPHYSIOLOGY

INTESTINAL ABSORPTION OF CALCIUM: BASIC ASPECTS

F. Bronner

Dept. of Oral Biology, University of Connecticut
Health Center, Farmington, CT 06032, U.S.A.

Intestinal calcium absorption is the resultant of two types of movement: peristaltic movement by the chyme from stomach to colon and movement across the epithelium of solubilized calcium all along the intestine. Transepithelial movement in turn involved two processes: (i) a saturable process that requires metabolic energy and by which calcium is moved across the mucosal cell, and (ii) a concentration-dependent, non-saturable process that does not appear regulated. The saturable process is encountered in the proximal portion of the intestine, mostly the duodenum. The non-saturable process prevails throughout the intestine. Thus, in the duodenum and upper jejunum calcium moves transepithelially by a combination of saturable and non-saturable processes, in the lower jejunum and ileum, calcium moves across the epithelium largely by the non-saturable, concentration-dependent process[1-4].

To demonstrate this, one can exteriorize the intestine and tie off segments, fill the segments with buffer containing varying concentrations of calcium and measure the amount absorbed. In the duodenum (Fig. 1) the amount of calcium absorbed can be described as a sum of a saturable component (J_{max}) and a linear, non-saturable component. In the ileum, on the other hand, (Fig. 1) there is no evidence for the occurrence of a saturable component, the amount absorbed at all concentrations being linearly proportional to the amount instilled. In the upper jejunum, the situation is intermediate, with some calcium being absorbed by the saturable and most by the non-saturable route (Fig. 1).

The saturable component can be reasonably thought to be regulatable. An obvious candidate for regulating saturable calcium absorption is vitamin D or its active metabolite, 1,25-dihydroxy-

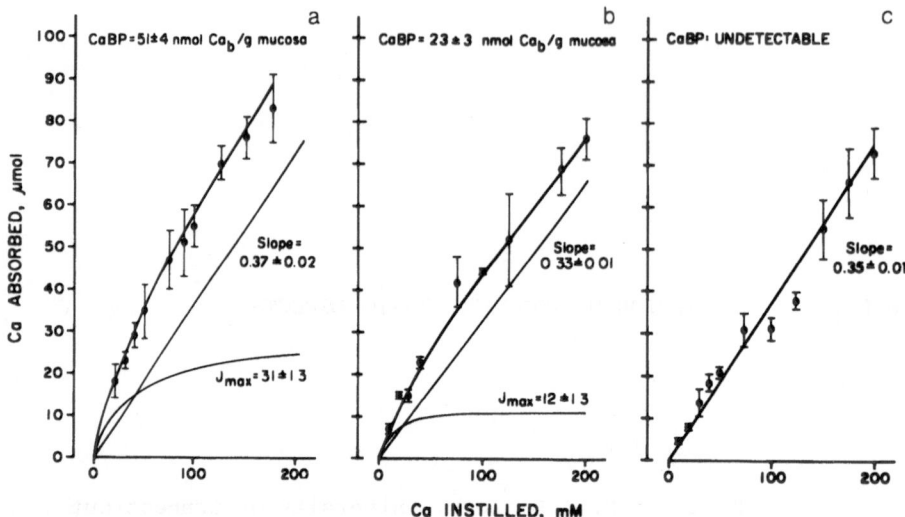

Fig. 1. Transumural calcium absorption in rat duodenum, upper
jejunum and distal ileum, evaluated by an in situ loop procedure[4].
The general absorption function is:

$$J_{m \to s} = J_{max} \left[Ca^{2+} \right] / (K_T + \left[Ca^{2+} \right]) + P \left[Ca^{2+} \right]$$

Where $J_{m \to s}$ = calcium absorbed (μmol), J_{max} = maximum saturable
calcium flow from lumen to blood, $\left[Ca^{2+} \right]$ = luminal calcium
concentration, K_T = luminal calcium concentration at which $J_{max}/2$ is
attained, and P = diffusivity constant (slope).
Note that when $J_{max} = 0$, $J_{m \to s} = P \left[Ca^{2+} \right]$.
CaBP = tissue content of the cytosolic, vitamin D-dependent
calcium-binding protein. Its content varies linearly with J_{max}[2,3].

vitamin D_3 (1,25-(OH)$_2$-D_3). Fig. 2 shows that in vitamin D-
deficient animals the saturable component of calcium absorption in
the duodenum was lost, so that calcium was absorbed only by the non-
saturable route, with no difference in ileal and duodenal calcium
absorption. When, however, the vitamin D-deficient animals were
treated with 1,25-(OH)$_2$-D_3, the saturable component of calcium
absorption was induced in the duodenum in a matter of 12 h, whereas
the non-saturable component was unchanged (Fig. 2). Thus, the
former is vitamin D-dependent and occurs largely in the duodenum.

To study the mechanism of the transcellular, active process of
calcium absorption, we utilized the everted sac procedure[5]. By
modifying the experimental conditions suitably, we have been able to
differentiate between the calcium that enters the tissue from the
mucosal side, termed "calcium in transit", the net amount

112

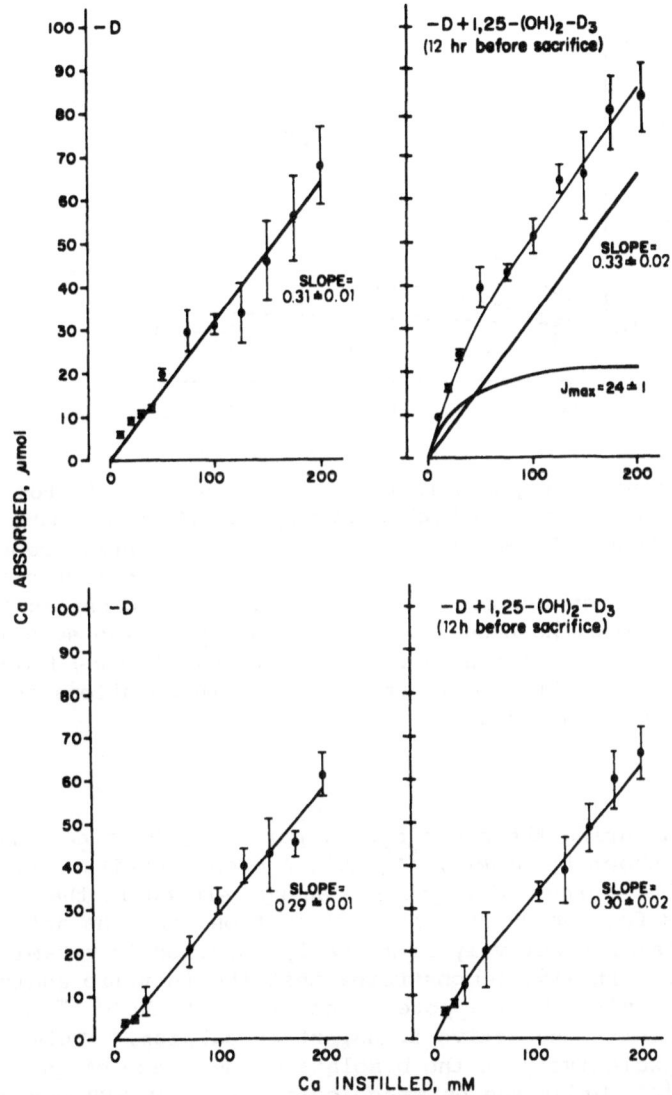

Fig. 2. Calcium absorption in duodenum and ileum of vitamin D-deficient rats[4] before and after treatment with $1,25-(OH)_2D_3$.
Left-hand panels: Ca absorption (in situ loop procedure) in duodenum and ileum of vitamin D-deficient animals; Right-hand panels: Ca absorption in duodenum and ileum of vitamin D-deficient rats that had received 3 μg $1,25(OH)_2-D_3$ by i.p. injection 12 h before sacrifice.

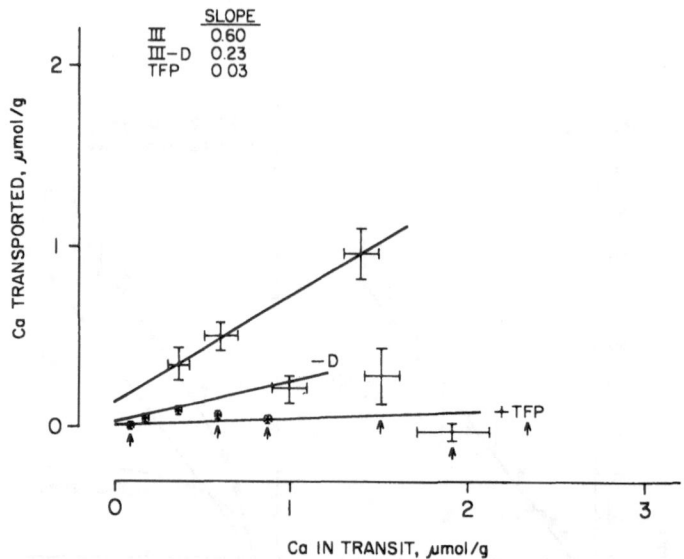

Fig. 3. Calcium absorption in everted duodenal sacs[7] from male Sprague-Dawley rats on a high-calcium diet (1.5% Ca, 1.5% P) with (III) or without (III-D) vitamin D_2. "Ca in transit" represents the calcium associated with the thoroughly rinsed sac tissue at the end of the experiment (90 min); "Ca transported" represents the amount of calcium above the base level found in the inside solution after 90 min. In the experiment labeled TFP (arrows), sacs from animals on diet III were filled with and immersed in solutions containing 400 µM trifluroperazine.

transported during the experimental period of 90 min. As previously shown by others, [5,6] this process requires oxygen and utilizes the sources of metabolic energy stored in the tissue. Fig. 3 confirms[6] for the everted sac preparation that the ability to transport calcium actively is markedly impaired in vitamin D-deficiency. It also demonstrates that the in vitro addition of trifluoroperazine (TFP) a potent inhibitor of the Ca^{2+}-Mg^{2+}-ATPase, totally inhibits the active transport of calcium. This enzyme is localized exclusively at the basolateral membrane of the enterocyte[7]. While the pharmacologic action of TFP may go beyond inhibiting the Ca^{2+}-Mg^{2+}-ATPase, the results shown in Fig. 3 point to the major importance of the $Ca^{2+}Mg^{2+}$-ATPase in the process of transcellular Ca movement.

In order for calcium to cross the intestinal cell, it must enter the brush-border, move across the cell in a manner so as not to raise the intracellular free calcium concentration to levels that threaten the life of the cell, and finally be extruded. Studies utilizing the brush-border preparation in the form of right side-out vesicles[8-10] have clarified aspects of calcium entry. These are

Table 1. Characteristics of Ca^{2+} Uptake by Brush-Border Membrane Vesicles from Rat Duodenum.

Saturable kinetics	Half-maximal activity: 1.1 mM Ca^{2+} pH optimum: 7.5 - 8.0 No metabolic energy required Sensitive to ionic composition of medium Inhibited by Na^+ or K^+
Uptake	Translocation and binding to inner side of vesicle membrane
High affinity site	$K_a = 6.3 + 3.3 \times 10^5$ M^{-1} Binds $\overline{0.8} + 0.1$ nmol Ca/Mg protein Ca^{2+} selectivity Phosphoprotein or protein-phospholipid complex May be part of Ca^{2+} channel
Low affinity site	K_a $2.8 + 0.3 \times 10^2 M^{-1}$ Binds $\overline{33} \pm 3.5$ nmol Ca/mg protein Membrane protein sites, mainly phospholipids

summarized in Table 1. Functionally, the high affinity Ca^{2+}-specific binding site of the brush border membrane may be part of a Ca^{2+}-channel and involved in channel gating[10], though its vitamin D-dependence is less clear[11,12].

Details of the movement of calcium inside the intestinal cell are not well known. Many potential sites of calcium movement and transient storage exist[1], but how these are involved in the vectorial movement of calcium across the cell is not understood.

At the basolateral membrane, two mechanisms for calcium extrusion have been postulated, a Na^+/Ca^{2+} exchanger and a Ca^{2+}-Mg^{2+}-ATPase. Direct demonstrations of the existence of a Na^+/Ca^{2+} exchanger in the enterocyte are few[13] and there is controversy about the functional significance of this route. Agreement seems to be emerging[14] that the major mechanism for active Ca^{2+} extrusion by the enterocyte is the Ca^{2+}-Mg^{2+}-ATPase, as suggested also by the data in Fig. 3. Vitamin D-dependence of the $Ca^{2+}Mg^{2+}$-ATPase has been demonstrated generally[15] and specifically[16]. However, the nature of the vitamin D dependence is not known. The Ca^{2+}-Mg^{2+}-ATPase of the intestinal cell, like that of other cells, is stimulated by calmodulin[17]. Since, however, intestinal calmodulin is not vitamin D-dependent[18], one might postulate that another regulator molecule, similar to calmodulin but dependent on vitamin D, contributes to regulation of the Ca^{2+}-Mg^{2+}-ATPase. A possible candidate is the cytosolic calcium-binding protein (CaBP, $M_r \approx 9000$) which has amino acid sequences homologous with those of calmodulin[19].

Since only part of calcium absorption is regulated, there is no simple way to decrease calcium absorption below that due to the non-saturable process. The latter probably averages 25 to 30%. This estimate is based on the average slope of non-saturable transport in older rats[3] and available estimates of calcium absorption in menopausal middle-aged women[20], in whom the saturable component of absorption is likely to be small.

One way to increase calcium absorption is to give large amounts of vitamin D or appropriately smaller amounts of $1,25(OH)_2-D_3$. True calcium absorption was found to be increased in two normal post-menopausal women by 50% after 8 weeks of daily treatment with 150,000 IU vitamin D[21]. However, because urinary calcium excretion increased by an amount approximately equal to the increased absorption, there was no change in net calcium balance.

The conversion of 25-hydroxyvitamin D_3 to $1,25-(OH)_2-D_3$ is enhanced by parathyroid hormone, though the mechanism is unknown. Consequently, hyperparathyroidism might be thought to be associated with hyperabsorption of calcium. Although this does occur, it is not an inevitable consequence of hyperparathyroidism. Patients with known or suspected hyperparathyroidism should be checked for the level of calcium absorption. This is most conveniently done by the urine test[22]. Patients with high calcium absorption could then be treated by dietary means, e.g. by diminishing total calcium intake.

There is no relationship in terms of mechanism between calcium and phosphate absorption. A high intake of inorganic phosphate decreases the availability of calcium, and a high intake of calcium accompanied by a low phosphate intake augments calcium utilization. It is unclear, however, whether or not the saturable component of calcium absorption is altered under these conditions.

Studies on the interrelationship between magnesium and calcium absorption have not so far yielded clearly interpretable results, but they do not appear to share a common active transport mechanism[23].

As for hormonal effects on calcium absorption, the only proven direct effect is that of $1,25-(OH)_2-D_3$. No in vitro studies have been published testing the effect of other vitamin D metabolites. In vivo studies with various metabolites cannot be interpreted readily, as it is difficult to exclude the conversion of some metabolites to a compound hydroxylated at the 1-carbon. Moreover, there is controversy as to whether the kidney mitochondrion is the only site where hydroxylation of the 1-carbon can occur and whether in the anephric organism other tissues can take over this function, at least in part.

116

Most other hormones have in some way or other been implicated in the modification of calcium absorption[24,25] but the absence of appropriate in vitro systems has made it difficult to differentiate direct from indirect effects. On the other hand, if a hormone or other agent were to alter calcium absorption unequivocally by an indirect route, this could have great clinical significance, provided the indirect action did not involve a compromised kidney.

In conclusion, intestinal calcium absorption involves a saturable and non-saturable route. The saturable route is clearly transcellular, involves entry and extrusion steps and is subject to regulation by vitamin D. Events that regulate vitamin D metabolism therefore also indirectly regulate calcium absorption. The nature of the non-saturable route is less well understood, as it is unclear whether it is solely or only partly paracellular. By definition the non-saturable route is unregulated, as least acutely. Long-term regulation, such as implied in the aging of tissue, may occur, but has not been studied in detail.

In clinical practice, the existence of the non-saturable route is of importance, as it provides a way for increasing calcium absorption by augmenting dietary intake. Increasing calcium intake has practical and theoretical limitations, but is relatively safe and easy to accomplish. For example, if in an anephric patient who ingests 300 mg Ca/day and absorbs about 75 mg Ca/day it is desired to double calcium absorption, it suffices to raise intake to 600 mg/day; this is the equivalent of 1 glass (250 ml) of milk or skim milk. Pills containing that amount of calcium are also available. Similarly, if it is desired to lower calcium intake and absorption, this is readily accomplished by cutting down on dairy or milk-enriched foods, as three-quarters of the dietary calcium in Western-style diets is derived from dairy products.

REFERENCES

1. F. Bronner, in:"Membrane Transport of Calcium", E. Carafoli, ed., Academic Press, London (1982).
2. D. Pansu, C. Bellaton, and F. Bronner, Am. J. Physiol. 240:G32 (1981).
3. D. Pansu, C. Bellaton, and F. Bronner, Am. J. Physiol. 244:G20 (1983).
4. D. Pansu, C. Bellaton, C. Roche, and F. Bronner, Am. J. Physiol. 244:G695 (1983).
5. D. K.Martin, and H. F. DeLuca, Am. J. Physiol. 216:1351 (1969).
6. D. Schachter, and S. M. Rosen, Am. J. Physiol. 196:357 (1959).
7. W. E. J. M. Ghijsen, M. E. DeJong, and C. H. Van Os, Biochim. Biophys. Acta 689:327 (1982).

8. A. Miller, and F. Bronner, Biochem. J. 196:391 (1981).

9. W. Haase, A. Schafer, H. Murer, and R. Kinne, Biochem. J. 172:57 (1978).

10. A. Miller, S.-T. Li, and F. Bronner, Biochem. J. 208:773 (1982).

11. S. Kowarski, and D. Schachter, J. Biol. Chem. 255:10834 (1980).

12. A. Miller, T.-H. Ueng, and F. Bronner, FEBS Lett, 103:319 (1979).

13. H. Murer, and B. Hildmann, Am. J. Physiol. 240:G409 (1981).

14. H. N. Nellans, and J. R. Popovitch, in:"Epithelial Calcium and Phosphate Transport:Molecular and Cellular Aspects", F. Bronner and M. Peterlik, eds., Liss, New York (in press).

15. H. Schiffl, and U. Binswager, Am. J. Physiol. 238:G424 (1980).

16. W. E. J. M. Ghijsen, and C. H. Van Os, Biochim. Biophys. Acta.689:170 (1982).

17. H. N. Nellans, and J. E. Popovitch, J. Biol. Chem. 256:9932 (1981).

18. M. Thomasset, A. Molla, C. O. Parkes, and J. Gemaille, FEBS Lett. 127:13 (1981).

19. C. Desplan, O. Heidman, J. W. Lillie, C. Auffray, and M.Thomasset, J. Biol. Chem. 258:13502 (1983).

20. R. P. Heaney, R. R. Recker, and P. D. Saville, Am. J. Clin. Nutr. 30:1603 (1977).

21. B. D. Hall, D. R. MacMillan, and F. Bronner, Am. J. Clin. Nutr. 22:448 (1969).

22. F. Bronner, Nutritio et Dieta 3:22 (1962).

23. C. S. Anast, and D. W. Gardner, in:"Disorders of Mineral Metabolism", Vol. 3 F. Bronner and J. W. Coburn, eds., Academic Press, New York (1981).

24. B. S. Levine, M. W. Walling, and J. W. Coburn, in:"Disorders of Mineral Metabolism", Vol. 4. F. Bronner and J. W. Coburn, eds., Academic Press, New York (1982).

25. R. Rude and F. Singer, in:"Disorders of Mineral Metabolism", Vol.2. F. Bronner and J. W. Coburn, eds., Academic Press, New York (1982).

NEPHROLITHIASIS ASSOCIATED WITH INTESTINAL DISEASE

J. W. Dobbins

Dept. of Internal Medicine, Yale University
New Haven, CT 06510, U.S.A.

INTRODUCTION

It has been noted since the 1960's that there is an increased incidence of nephrolithiasis in patients with idiopathic inflammatory bowel disease and in individuals who have undergone jejuno-ileal bypass for obesity[1-14]. In patients with inflammatory bowel disease, prior surgical treatment increases the risk of nephrolithiasis[7,9,10]. The incidence of nephrolithiasis in patients with Crohn's disease who have undergone an ileal resection is approximately 10%. The large majority of these stones, when analyzed, are composed of calcium oxalate. The incidence of nephrolithiasis in patients with ulcerative colitis who have undergone an ileostomy is also approximately 10%. Uric acid stones, however, make up a significant proportion of the calculi in these patients[1-3]. The incidence of nephrolithiasis in patients who have undergone jejuno-ileal bypass for obesity is 20% or more.

Examination of the urine in these patients (Table 1) reveals a number of abnormalities[15-17]. Urine volume, sodium and chloride are low, indicating dehydration and extracellular volume deficit. Urine pH and CO_2 content are low and the ammonia concentration is high, indicative of metabolic acidosis, though, as will be discussed later, other factors control urinary citrate levels. Magnesium and pyrophosphate levels are also low. Magnesium, pyrophosphate and citrate are considered inhibitors of calcium oxalate stone formation because they form stable complexes with calcium or oxalate. Urinary oxalate excretion is normal in patients who have undergone a total colectomy or have an ileostomy whereas it is elevated in patients who have undergone an ileal resection and have either all or part of the colon in the alimentary stream or who have undergone a jejunoileal bypass for obesity. As a general rule, we can conclude that all of these urinary abnormalities, except for oxalate, are due to the malabsorption of water, electrolytes and alkali (accounting for the acidosis and hypocitraturia). The increased absorption of oxalate is the sole exception and, as will be discussed, it is primarily due to the increased absorption of dietary oxalate. In the following sections we will discuss how intestinal disease, resection or bypass can result in the urinary abnormalities listed in Table 1.

Table 1. Urinary Changes Following By-Pass Resection or Ileostomy.

Urinary Constituents	By-pass Resection (n = 15)	Ileostomy (n = 32)
Volume	Normal	↓
pH	Normal	↓
NH_4	↑	↑
CO_2	↓	↓
NaCl	Normal	↓
K	↓	↓
Calcium	Normal	Normal
Mg	↓	↓
Pyrophosphate	↓	↓
Citrate	↓	↓
SO_4	↓	Normal
PO_4	↓	↓
Oxalate	↑	Normal
Urate	Normal	Normal

From Smith et al [15-17].

ENTERIC HYPEROXALURIA

Hofmann et al initially described the occurrence of increased urinary oxalate excretion in patients with inflammatory bowel disease in 1970[18]. In 1973, in an eloquent study performed by Chadwick et al, the increased oxalate was shown to be primarily, if not totally, due to increased absorption of dietary oxalate[19]. Recently, Hofmann et al have suggested that part of the hyperoxaluria in patients with jejuno-ileal bypass for obesity is due to dietary intake of protein[20]. This protein source of oxalate, however, accounts for only a small fraction of the hyperoxaluria. It is not clear from these studies whether the hyperoxaluria results from the endogenous production of oxalate from protein or from bacterial conversion of the dietary protein to oxalate in the colon. Two theories have arisen to explain the occurrence of increased absorption of dietary oxalate.

120

Solubility Theory

The solubility theory can be stated as follows: In the normal intestine calcium binds to oxalate preventing the absorption of oxalate; in diseased or resected intestine, unabsorbed fatty acids bind to calcium leaving oxalate in solution and available for absorption. The evidence for solubility theory is as follows: (i) when a long chain fatty acid such as sodium oleate is added to a solution containing precipitated calcium oxalate, the amount of oxalate in solution increases with the amount of fatty acid added[21,22]; (ii) several investigators have found a direct correlation between urinary oxalate excretion and fecal fat excretion[23-25]. It should be noted, however, in these studies, that there are some patients who have hyperoxaluria without steatorrhea; (iii) the oral administration of calcium has been shown to decrease urinary oxalate excretion and to decrease the urinary oxalate excretion and to decrease the urinary excretion of orally administered ^{14}C-oxalate[22,26-29].

Permeability Theory

The permeability theory states that unabsorbed fatty acids and bile acids (resulting from disease, resection or bypass) increase the permeability of the colon to oxalate. Ordinarily, fatty acids and bile acids are absorbed in the small intestine. When the colon is exposed to dihydroxy bile acids or long chain fatty acids, either in vivo or in vitro, increased absorption (mucosal to serosal movement) of oxalate occurs[30-34]. This increased absorption or movement of oxalate is probably due to an increase in the permeability of the intercellular tight junctions. The main reason for suspecting the tight junction as the site of increased movement is because bile acids and fatty acids increase the movement of substances such as mannitol, PEG and inulin which are thought to traverse only the extracellular pathway[34-36]. A direct correlation between oxalate and PEG movement and between Na and mannitol movement after exposure to bile acids has been observed, suggesting that oxalate is moving via the extracellular pathway and that there is nothing specific about the increase in permeability, since it occurs for cations such as sodium[34,35]. Considering both the ability of bile acids and fatty acids to chelate calcium and the importance of calcium in maintaining the integrity of the intra-cellular tight junctions, it is likely that the increase in colonic permeability induced by bile acids and fatty acids is a result of chelating calcium in the tight junctions[35]. It should be noted that medium chain fatty acids do not bind calcium nor increase the permeability of the colon to oxalate.

"Active" Transport of Oxalate

Recently, there have been some data suggesting that the transcellular transport of oxalate also occurs in the colon. Two groups have reported that net oxalate absorption occurred in the rat colon and rabbit colon in vitro under short circuit conditions[37-39]. Net transport under these conditions usually indicates an active transport or secondary active transport process. Further, net absorption in the rat colon was inhibited by the metabolic inhibitor dinitrophenol and abolished by SITS, an anion exchange inhibitor[39]. These results suggest that transcellular transport of oxalate occurs in the colon and an anion exchange process may be involved. Further studies will need to be done to determine the clinical significance, if any, of this transcellular transport process.

Role of the Colon

Table 1 shows that increased urinary oxalate excretion is not seen in patients with an ileostomy. This observation suggests that the increased absorption of dietary oxalate occurs in the colon. It has been demonstrated by numerous investigators that patients with an ileostomy rarely have increased urinary oxalate excretion and do not have increased absorption of orally administered ^{14}C-oxalate, even when they have marked steatorrhea[23,25,28,40]. The colon as the site of increased oxalate absorption is quite compatible with the permeability theory which states that unabsorbed fatty acids and bile acids spill into the colon inducing permeability changes in that organ. Conversely, the absence of hyperoxaluria in patients without a colon strongly suggests that increased colonic permeability is an important component in determining enteric hyperoxaluria, since removal of the colon would not be expected to affect the solubility of the oxalate. Further, the presence of hyperoxaluria in patients with jejuno-ileal and jejunal-colonic bypass for obesity virtually exclude the small bowel as a site of increased oxalate absorption since practically the entire small intestine has been bypassed with these procedures. Finally, although bile acids and fatty acids have been shown to increase the permeability of the colon to oxalate and other substances, bile acids and fatty acids do not increase the permeability of the small intestine to oxalate[33,34].

HYPOCITRATURIA

Profound hypocitraturia has been noted in patients with intestinal resection and bypass. This hypocitraturia is multi-factorial in origin. Acidosis is known to decrease urinary citrate and these patients have a metabolic acidosis secondary to bicarbonate loss in diarrheal stool. Urinary magnesium excretion has a profound effect on urinary citrate and since hypomagnesuria is common in these patients, hypocitraturia is undoubtedly related to this problem[41]. Rudman et al suggested that malabsorption of citrate may play a role in hypocitraturia in these patients[41]. This suggestion was based on their observation that these patients had a relatively flat "citrate tolerance test" when given oral citrate by mouth and serum levels were measured. However, Rudman has subsequently demonstrated that removal of citrate from the diet has no effect on urinary citrate in normal subjects and that patients on total parenteral nutrition have normal urinary citrate levels even though they receive no citrate in their intravenous feedings[41,42]. Thus, it appears that dietary citrate is unnecessary for the maintenance of a normal urinary citrate excretion.

HYPOMAGNESURIA

Normal magnesium absorption is not well understood, therefore, our understanding of the role of the intestine in hypomagnesuria associated with intestinal resection and bypass is poor. It is known that fatty acids and bile acids can precipitate magnesium and some magnesium malabsorption probably occurs on this basis. It appears likely that when there is extensive resection or bypass that some magnesium is malabsorbed because of loss of intestinal surface area and finally, some magnesium malabsorption may be obligatory simply because of the volume of the diarrheal stool.

THERAPY

The goal of treatment should be to reverse all the urinary abnormalities listed in Table 1. This, of course, can be a difficult task when there is extensive resection or when there has been jejuno-ileal bypass. Hyperoxaluria can be treated in a variety of ways. The first thing to do is to place the patient on a low oxalate diet. This maneuver alone will result in a substantial reduction in urinary oxalate excretion in the majority of patients. If steatorrhea is present, a low fat diet can be instituted. A low fat diet can impose caloric restrictions which may be a problem in a patient with extensive resection. In this situation medium change triglycerides can be added to the diet. It should be remembered that medium chain fatty acids do not increase the colonic absorption of oxalate[31]. Medium chain fatty acids do not chelate calcium and probably do not chelate magnesium[43].

If dietary maneuvers are not sufficient, then an anion binding agent should be added to the regimen. Anion binding agents serve a dual purpose: (i) they bind oxalate preventing its absorption and (ii) they bind fatty acids and bile acids preventing these agents from increasing colonic permeability to oxalate. Anion binding agents include cholestyramine, calcium, aluminum, magnesium and bismuth. These agents may worsen the steatorrhea by binding bile acids and fatty acids. Use of magnesium as an anion binding agent has the advantage of increasing urinary magnesium excretion although worsening diarrhea is clearly a problem. Aluminum toxicity, which is occasionally seen with long-term use of this agent, must be kept in mind. I prefer to use the agent Camalox[R] which is composed of calcium carbonate, aluminum hydroxide and magnesium hydroxide. Diarrhea is not usually a major problem with this antacid and magnesium is provided as well as alkali.

Hypocitraturia should be corrected by increasing urinary magnesium excretion as much as possible and as administering alkali such as calcium carbonate or sodium bicarbonate. Citrate can be given orally but probably has no advantage over giving alkali.

Urine volume, sodium, chloride and potassium excretion can be increased by decreasing the diarrhea. Treatment of diarrhea in general is beyond the scope of this review but includes treating the underlying disease using opiates, etc. Obviously, adequate fluid intake is essential.

The final therapeutic modality is surgical. If the patient has had a jejuno-ileal bypass for obesity, then this procedure can be reversed and will result in correction of all the urinary abnormalities seen in Table 1. We have, on one occasion, removed a small portion of remaining colon in a patient with Crohn's disease, thereby correcting the hyperoxaluria.

REFERENCES

1. A. W. Badenoch, Br. J. Urol. 32:374 (1960).
2. R. I. Breuer, E. A. Gelzayd, and J. K. Kirsner, Gut 11:314 (1970).
3. J. J. Deren, J. G. Porush, M. F. Levit, and M. T. Khilnani, Ann. Intern. Med. 56:843 (1962).
4. S. S. Dickstein and B. Frame, Surg. Gyn. Obst. 136:259 (1973).
5. R. H. Dowling, G. A. Rose, and D. J. Sutor, Lancet 1:1103 (1971).
6. E. Fikri and R. R. Cassella, Ann. Surg. 179:460 (1974)
7. E. A. Gelzayd, R. I. Breuer, and J. B. Kirsner, Am. J. Dig. Dis. 13:1027 (1968).
8. J. G. Gregory, E. B. Starkloff, K. Miyai, and H. Schoenberg, J. Urol. 113:521 (1975).
9. M. S. Grossman and F. W. Nugent, Am. J. Dig. Dis. 12:491 (1967).
10. Z. Maratka and J. Nedbal, Gut 5:214 (1964).

11. J. P. O'Leary, W. C. Thomas and E. R. Woodward, Am. J. Surg. 127:142 (1974).
12. K. Dharmsathaphorn, D. H. Freeman, H. J. Binder, and J. D. Dobbins, Dig. Dis. Sci. 17:401 (1982).
13. E. Hylander, S. Jarnum, and I. Frandsen, Scand. J. Gastroenterol. 14:475 (1979).
14. C. P. Bambach, W. G. Robertson, M. Peacock, and G. L. Hill, Gut 22:257 (1981).
15. L. H. Smith, P. G. Werness, and D. M. Wilson, in"Oxalate in Human Biochemistry and Clinical Pathology", G. A. Rose, W. G. Robertson, and R. W. E. Watts, eds., Wellcome Foundation, London (1979).
16. L. H. Smith, in:"Contemporary Issues in Nephrology", Vol. 5, F. L. Coe, B. M. Brenner, and J. H. Stein, eds., Churchill Livingstone, New York (1980).
17. L. H. Smith, Personal communication.
18. A. F. Hofmann, P. J. Thomas, L. H. Smith and J. T. McCall, Gastroenterol. 58:960 (1970).
19. V. S. Chadwick, K. Modha, and R. H. Dowling, New Engl. J. Med. 289:172 (1973).
20. A. F. Hofmann, M. F. Laker, K. Dharmsathaphorn, H. P. Sherr, and D. Lorenzo, Gastroenterol. 84:293 (1983).
21. H. J. Binder, Gastroenterol. 67:441 (1974).
22. D. L. Earnest, H. E. Williams, and W. H. Admirand. Trans. Assoc. Am. Physns. 88:224 (1975).
23. E. Hylander, S. Jarnum, H. J. Jensen, and M. Thale, Scand. J. Gastroenterol. 13:577 (1978).
24. H. Andersson, R. Jagenburg, Gut 15:360 (1974).
25. D. L. Earnest, G. Johnson, H. E. Williams, and W. H. Admirand, Gastroenterol. 66:1114 (1974).
26. E. Hylander, S. Jarnum, and K. Nielsen, Scand. J. Gastroenterol. 15:349 (1980).
27. W. F. Caspary, J. Tonissen, and P. G. Lankisch, Acta Hep. Gastroenterol. 24:193 (1977).
28. R. Modigliani, D. Labayle, C. Aymes, and R. Denvil, Scand. J. Gastroenterol. 13:187 (1978).
29. H. Pedersen, J. Steen, Scand. J. Gastroenterol.14:97 (1979).
30. V. A. Chadwick, E. Elias, G. D. Bell, R. J. Dowling, in:"Advances in Bile Acid Research", S. Matern, J. Hackenschmidt, P. Back and W. Gerok, eds., Schattauer Verlag, Stuttgart (1975).
31. J. W. Dobbins and H. J. Binder, Gastroenterol. 70:1096 (1976).
32. P. D. Fairclough, T. G. Feest, U. S. Chadwick, and M. L. Clark, Gut 18:240 (1977).
33. D. R. Saunders, J. Sillery, and G. B. McDonald, Gut 16:543 (1975).
34. R. Davies, J. Laurenson, H. J. Binder, and J. W. Dobbins (Submitted for publication)
35. R. W. Freel, M. Hatch, D. L. Earnest, and A. M. Goldner, Am. J. Physiol 245:G816 (1983).

36. P. Bright-Asare and H. J. Binder, Gastroenterol. 64:81 (1973).

37. S. C. Kathpelia, M. J. Favus, and F. L. Coe, Clin. Res. 29:777A
    (1981).

38. R. W. Freel, M. Hatch, D. L. Earnest, A. M. Goldner, Biochim.
    Biophys. Acta 600:838 (1980).

39. M. Hatch, R. W. Freel, A. M. Goldner, and D. L. Earnest,
    Gut (1984) (in press).

40. J. W. Dobbins and H. J. Binder, New Engl. J. Med. 296:298
    (1977).

41. D. Rudman, J. L. Dedonis, M. T. Fountain, J. B. Chandler,
    G. G. Gerron, G. A. Fleming, and M. H. Kutner, New Engl. J.
    Med. 303:657 (1980).

42. D. Rudman, M. H. Kutner, S. C. Redd, W. C. Waters, G. G. Gerron,
    and J. Bleier, J. Clin. Endocrinol. Metab. 55:1052 (1982).

43. G. Gacs and D. Barltop, Gut 18:64 (1977).

INTESTINAL ABSORPTION OF CALCIUM, MAGNESIUM, PHOSPHATE AND

OXALATE: DEVIATION FROM NORMAL IN IDIOPATHIC UROLITHIASIS

C. Y. C. Pak, M. J. Nicar, and G. J. Krejs

Division of Mineral Metabolism, Dept. of Internal
Medicine, SW Medical School, University of Texas
Health Science Center, Dallas, TX 75235, U.S.A.

INTRODUCTION

There is increasing evidence that intestinal absorption of
stone-forming substances may be disturbed in many patients with
calcium nephrolithiasis. This disturbance in intestinal absorption
in such patients is usually metabolic in origin, although it may be
modified by dietary aberrations. The resulting aberration in
urinary composition may lead or contribute to stone formation.

In this communication, we shall first discuss normal intestinal
handling of calcium, magnesium, phosphate and oxalate, in order to
provide the background for comparison of results in "idiopathic"
calcium nephrolithiasis. Because of the important effect of
vitamin D on intestinal ionic transport and proposed pathogenetic
role of vitamin D in calcium nephrolithiasis, the direct action of
$1,25-(OH)_2$ vitamin D_3 on absorption of above substances in different
segments of the bowel will be reviewed. The specific derangements
in ionic absorption encountered in the two major forms of idiopathic
calcium nephrolithiasis will then be considered.

NORMAL INTESTINAL ABSORPTION OF STONE-FORMING SUBSTANCES

The introduction of segmental perfusion technique has allowed
us to describe transport kinetics and to measure ion movement in
different segments of the bowel in man in vivo[1]. The method
entails measurement of ionic absorption or unidirectional ion fluxes
from defined segments of the bowel during perfusion with solutions
of varying ionic concentrations.

127

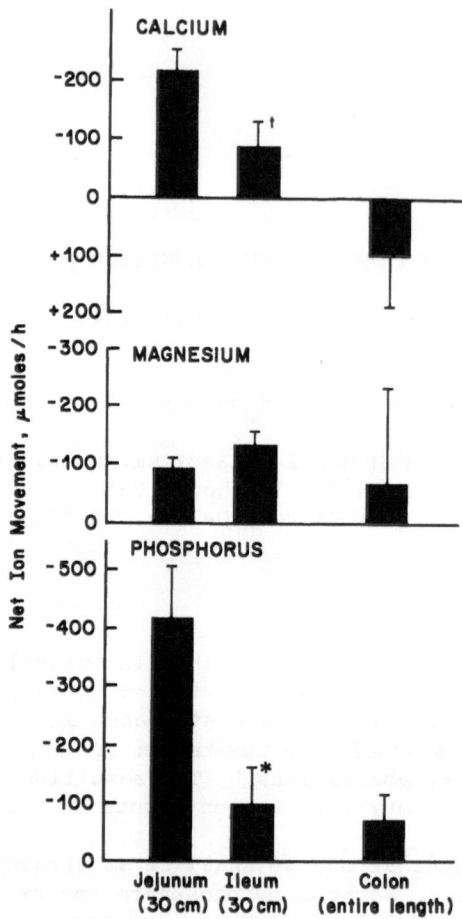

Fig. 1. Comparison of net Ca, Mg and P movement in 30-cm segments of
jejunum and ileum and in the entire colon. Perfusates
contained either 5 mM Ca or Mg, or 2.5 mM P. Results are
mean $\pm$ SEM in 10 healthy subjects except for P absorption
in the jejunum and ileum which was studied in 5 subjects
and Mg movement in the jejunum and ileum which was studied
in 27 and 20 subjects, respectively. *P<0.05, +P<0.001
refer to the difference between jejunal and ileal mineral
ion movement.   Negative signs indicate absorption,
positive signs denote secretion.   Ca and P absorption are
significantly higher in the jejunum than in the ileum.
There is no significant difference between Mg absorption
rates in the jejunum and ileum.   Net movement in the colon
is not significantly different from zero for all three
mineral ions.

Such studies have shown that calcium absorption occurs by both active and passive processes[2]. In the basal state (with an estimated calcium intake of 1000 mg/day), there is net calcium absorption in the jejunum and ileum, since the lumen-to-plasma flux exceeds the plasma-to-lumen flux[3]. Net calcium absorption is significantly higher in the jejunum than in the ileum (Fig. 1). In the colon of healthy subjects, calcium movement is not significantly different from zero (small net luminal gain)[4] (Fig. 1).

Magnesium absorption also occurs by both active and passive processes[5]. Net magnesium absorption occurs in both segments of the small bowel but not in the colon[3,5].

Phosphate absorption can occur independently of calcium absorption since both active and passive phosphate transport may be demonstrated from solutions devoid of calcium[6]. The net phosphate absorption in the jejunum is more prominent than that occurring in the ileum (Fig. 1). There is no net absorption of phosphate in the colon[4].

Oxalate absorption probably occurs passively, since the luminal oxalate concentration usually exceeds the low plasma concentration. It has been suggested that the colon is the principal site of oxalate absorption, since the hyperoxaluria may be corrected when the colon is rendered non-functional in patients with enteric hyperoxaluria. However, available perfusion data suggest that oxalate absorption also occurs in the jejunum of normal subjects, although to a small degree. The rapid appearance in urine (within 2 h) of orally administered oxalate supports the participation of proximal bowel in oxalate absorption[7].

Various intraluminal factors influence the absorption of calcium, magnesium, phosphate and oxalate. Although the pH of the jejunum is typically less than 6, that in the ileum and colon may be alkaline. Thus, the absorption of calcium and magnesium in distal segments may not be prominent because of increased dissociation of phosphate (owing to the alkaline pH), and consequent complexation by phosphate. Intraluminal fatty acids or bile salts may also bind divalent cations and interfere with their absorption. Conversely, oxalate absorption is critically dependent on the intraluminal content of divalent cations which bind oxalate and dictate the amount of available oxalate[8]. Finally, intestinal ionic absorption is dependent on the physical state of feces in which the ionic constituents are contained. It is expected that less ionic constituents would be available for absorption when they are present in a more solid fecal state in distal segments. These intraluminal factors may override the intrinsic capability of a given segment for ionic absorption.

There are scanty data concerning the absorption of citrate and uric acid, two other substances of considerable importance in calcium stone formation. Citrate is probably absorbed efficiently. However, the absorbed citrate does not directly contribute substantially to renal citrate excretion; rather, its metabolism to alkali leads to increased urinary loss via alkali-induced changes in the renal handling of citrate. The principal dietary determinant of uric acid excretion is the amount of purine which provides substrate for in vivo urate synthesis, and not the uric acid content. Orally-administered uric acid is almost completely destroyed by bacterial enzymatic action in the intestinal tract.

ACTION OF $1,25-(OH)_2$VITAMIN D_3 ON INTESTINAL IONIC TRANSPORT

It is not our intent to review the cellular basis of vitamin D action; rather, we shall review the physiological effects on ionic transport examined in human beings. Exogenous $1,25-(OH)_2$vitamin D_3 has been shown to increase net calcium absorption in healthy subjects, principally by stimulating the active component of lumen-to-plasma flux. All three sites examined (jejunum, ileum and colon) respond to this treatment. The responsiveness is greatest in the ileum, since ileal net calcium absorption is low in the basal state. After $1,25-(OH)_2$vitamin D_3 treatment[3], jejunal and ileal calcium absorption rates become equivalent. In the colon, therapy with $1,25-(OH)_2$vitamin D_3 induces net calcium absorption[4]. However, the rate of net calcium absorption (corrected for length) is only about 1/10 that encountered in the ileum after vitamin D treatment (or 1/4 of ileal calcium absorption in the basal state)[3,4].

The treatment with $1,25-(OH)_2$vitamin D_3 also stimulates net magnesium absorption[3], again by affecting principally the active transport process. The jejunum and ileum are equally responsive, but the colon shows no net absorption despite treatment[4].

During treatment with $1,25-(OH)_2$vitamin D_3, in patients with renal failure, net phosphate absorption is increased in the jejunum owing to stimulated active transport[6]. Their phosphate absorption in ileum and colon has not been measured. In healthy subjects, exogenous $1,25-(OH)_2$vitamin D_3 has no effect in all three segments[4].

No data are available on the direct action of $1,25-(OH)_2$vitamin D_3 on oxalate absorption. However, this treatment may indirectly increase oxalate absorption by stimulating calcium absorption and reducing intraluminal calcium complexation of oxalate.

130

DEVIATION FROM NORMAL ABSORPTION IN ABSORPTIVE HYPERCALCIURIA

In absorptive hypercalciuria, the main form of idiopathic hypercalciuria and idiopathic calcium nephrolithiasis, calcium absorption from the whole intestinal tract has been shown to be increased by various techniques[9,10]. Intestinal perfusion studies have disclosed enhanced jejunal net calcium absorption but normal ileal net calcium absorption, due to increased lumen-to-plasma flux[11]. Colonic calcium absorption has not been measured.

Magnesium absorption has been shown to be normal by various techniques[11-13]. Net magnesium absorption in both segments of the small bowel are normal[11]; that in the colon is unknown. Phosphate absorption has been shown to be normal by balance techniques; segmental perfusion studies have not been performed.

Oxalate absorption, determined by the increment in urinary oxalate following an oral load of soluble oxalate (without calcium), is normal in absorptive hypercalciuria[7]. Oxalate absorption has not been measured by the intestinal perfusion technique.

Thus, absorptive hyperalciuria has a unique pattern, characterized by jejunal hyperabsorption of calcium, but normal absorption of calcium in the ileum, of magnesium in both proximal segments, of phosphate, and of oxalate (except in the presence of calcium). This picture, atypical for $1,25-(OH)_2$vitamin D_3 action previously enumerated, suggests a "primary" disturbance in calcium transport involving the jejunum (Fig. 2).

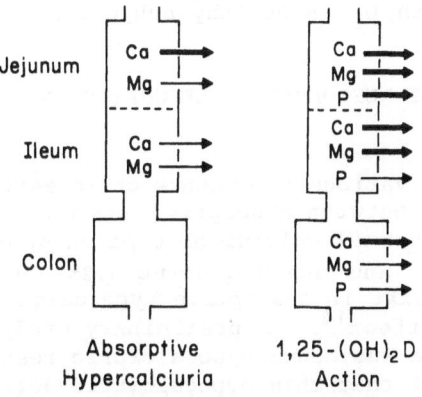

Fig. 2.   Intestinal transport profile in absorptive hypercalciuria compared to $1,25-(OH)_2$vitamin D_3 action.   Increased absorption is indicated by thick arrows.

DEVIATION FROM NORMAL ABSORPTION IN HYPERPARATHYROIDISM

Renal hypercalciuria, another form of idiopathic hypercalciuria, is also characterized by enhanced calcium absorption from the whole intestinal tract, as shown by the increment in urinary calcium following an oral calcium load and fecal recovery of orally administered radiocalcium[9,10]. A preliminary study indicates that magnesium absorption is increased, when assessed by oral magnesium load. Oxalate absorption has been shown to be normal by oral oxalate load (devoid of calcium)[7]. However, no study of phosphate absorption has been done, and intestinal perfusion for segmental absorption has not been performed.

More data are available in another hyperparathyroid state, resorptive hypercalciuria of primary hyperparathyroidism. The net calcium absorption in both jejunum and ileum is higher than in healthy subjects in the basal state, and similar to that of healthy subjects following $1,25(OH)_2$vitamin D_3 treatment (unpublished observations). Net magnesium absorption in the jejunum is considerably greater than the basal rate of control subjects and similar to that of the control group receiving $1,25(OH)_2$vitamin D_3. Moreover, magnesium absorption assessed from an oral magnesium load is significantly increased in patients with primary hyperparathyroidism[13].

The above results suggest that the disturbance in intestinal ionic transport of the hyperparathyroid state (e.g. renal hypercalciuria) may be vitamin-D dependent, accountable by stimulation of PTH-dependent $1,25-(OH)_2$vitamin D_3 synthesis. Thus, calcium absorption was increased in both jejunum and ileum and magnesium absorption was high, as might be expected from the action of $1,25-(OH)_2$vitamin D_3 in healthy subjects.

DIFFERENT TREATMENT RESPONSES OF ABSORPTIVE AND RENAL HYPERCALCIURIAS

The effect of various treatments on intestinal calcium absorption differs between absorptive and renal hypercalciurias. Thiazide restores normal calcium absorption by correcting secondary hyperparathyroidism and reducing serum $1,25-(OH)_2$vitamin D_3 in renal hypercalciuria, unlike in absorptive hypercalciuria where this treatment has no effect[14]. A preliminary study indicates that thiazide produces a sustained hypocalciuric response in renal hypercalciuria, but that this hypocalciuric action is attenuated in absorptive hypercalciuria.

In absorptive hypercalciuria, orthophosphate treatment reduces serum $1,25-(OH)_2$vitamin D_3[15]. Despite this fall, intestinal calcium absorption does not decrease in many patients. In some,

calcium absorption decreases but remains above normal[16].
Conversely, adrenocorticosteroid treatment increases serum
concentration of $1,25-(OH)_2$vitamin D_3. However, intestinal calcium
absorption remains elevated[17].

These findings suggested a vitamin D-independent process for
the increased calcium absorption in absorptive hypercalciuria,
unlike the situation in renal hypercalciuria where the high calcium
absorption is dependent on $1,25-(OH)_2$vitamin D_3.

REFERENCES

1. J. S. Fordtran, Gastroenterol. 56:987 (1969).
2. C. Y. C. Pak and J. S. Fordtran, in:"Gastrointestinal Disease",
   M. H. Sleisenger, J. S. Fordtran, and F. J. Ingelfinger,
   eds., W. B. Saunders, Philadelphia (1978).
3. G. J. Krejs, M. J. Nicar, J. E. Zerwekh, D. A. Norman,
   M. G. Kane, and C. Y. C. Pak, Am. J. Med. 75:973 (1983).
4. W. C. Grinstead, C. Y. C. Pak,and G. J. Krejs, Am. J. Physiol.
   (in press).
5. P. G. Brannan, P. Vergne-Marini, C. Y. C. Pak, A. R. Hull, and
   J. S. Fordtran, J. Clin. Invest. 57:1412 (1976).
6. G. R. Davis, J. E. Zerwekh, T. F. Parker, G. J. Krejs, C. Y. C.
   Pak, and J. S. Fordtran, Gastroenterol. 85:908 (1983).
7. D. E. Barilla, C. Notz, D. Kennedy, and C. Y. C. Pak,
   Am. J.Med. 64:597 (1978).
8. P. M. Zarembski and A. Hodgkinson, Clin. Chim. Acta 25:1 (1969).
9. C. Y. C. Pak, M. Ohata, E. C. Lawrence, and W. Snyder,
   J.Clin. Invest. 54:387 (1974).
10. C. Y. C. Pak, R. A. Kaplan, H. Bone, J. Townsend, and O. Waters,
    New Engl. J. Med. 292:497 (1975).
11. P. G. Grannan, S. Morawski, C. Y. C. Pak, and J. S. Fordtran,
    Am. J. Med. 66:425 (1979).
12. G. Johansson, U. Backman, B. Danielson, S. Ljunghall, and
    B. Wikstrom, Invest. Urol. 18:93 (1980).
13. M. J. Nicar and C. Y. C. Pak, Min. Electr. Metab. 8:44 (1982).
14. J. E. Zerwekh and C. Y. C. Pak, Metabolism 29:13 (1980).
15. D. E. Barilla, J. E. Zerwekh, and C. Y. C. Pak, Min. Electr.
    Metab. 2:302 (1979).
16. C. Y. C. Pak and J. E. Zerwekh, Proc. Symp. Clin. Disorders Bone
    Min. Metab. (in press).
17. J. E. Zerwekh, C. Y. C. Pak, R. A. Kaplan, J. L. McGuire,
    K. Upchurch, N. Breslau, and R. Johnson, J. Clin. Endocrinol.
    Metab. 51:381 (1980).

KINETIC STUDY OF THE INTESTINAL CALCIUM-BINDING PROTEIN

IN ABSORPTIVE HYPERCALCIURIA

B. Pinto, M. A. Vilanova, F. J. Ruiz-Marcellan, and J. Bernshtam

Servicio de Analisis Clinicos, Hospital Joan XXIII Tarragona and Servicio de Urologia Hospital Valle Hebron, Barcelona, Catalunya, Spain

INTRODUCTION

Hypercalciuria is found in 48.8% of recurrent stone formers[1]. Hyperabsorption, bone resorption[2] or a renal leak of calcium[3] are the possible causes of hypercalciuria. Intestinal hyperabsorption of calcium may be due to a renal leak of phosphorus followed by an increased synthesis of 1,25-dihydroxycholecalciferol (1,25-$(OH)_2D_3)$[4]. Alternatively, it has been suggested that the hyperabsorption is due to a higher calcium transport without increased synthesis of the vitamin D_3 metabolites[5], perhaps mediated by a specific protein existing in the brush border cells[6]. The purpose of this paper was to investigate the roles of the calcium-binding protein (CaBP) and 1,25-$(OH)_2D_3$ in absorptive hypercalciuric stone formers and normal control subjects.

METHODS AND MATERIALS

The control group included 12 individuals (6 males and 6 females) aged 32 $\pm$ 8.8 years. The hypercalciuric group included 18 recurrent Ca oxalate/phosphate stone formers (7 males and 11 females) aged 40 $\pm$ 13.8 years. The presence of hypercalciuria was investigated by a two-phase study. In the first stage, calcium, magnesium, phosphate, urate and creatinine were determined in plasma and 24-h urine samples. Oxalate excretion was determined in the urine[7]. In fasting 2-h urine samples, pH, ammonia and titratable acidity were also measured[7]. Calcium absorption was measured by giving orally a 250 mg calcium chloride load containing 25 uCi of ^{45}Ca while the individuals were kept on a daily 400 mg calcium diet[8]. Intestinal calcium hyperabsorption, radio-calcium

135

clearance and the calcium:creatinine ratio were determined[8]. $1,25-(OH)_2D_3$[9,10], PTH[11] and c-AMP[12] were all determined by radioimmunoassay.

The dissociation constant of the calcium-binding protein was calculated from Scatchard plots. The calcium-binding protein was obtained from the cytosol portion of human intestinal biopsies. The assay contained in a 0.1 ml final volume: 100 µg of protein from the cytosol fraction, 26 µmol of tris-HCl (pH 7.5) buffer and increasing concentrations of calcium chloride from 0 to 250 pmol, containing a tracer dose of 20×10^3 cpm of ^{45}Ca. Mixtures were incubated for 2 h at $4^\circ C$. Afterwards, the samples were diluted with 1 ml of tris-HCl buffer and pressure-filtered through a 25 mm Vs Millipore disc of 0.025 µm. The filters were dissolved in 10 ml PPO-POPOP-toluene (20 mg:2 mg:100 ml toluene).

RESULTS

The plasma phosphate levels were higher in the control than the hypercalciuric group while the phosphaturia was slightly lower (Table 1). No significant differences in $1,25-(OH)_2D_3$ plasma levels were detected between the groups; if anything they were lower in the hypercalciuric group than the controls (Table 2). The kinetic profile of the calcium-binding protein, (Fig. 1), showed a steeper line in the controls than in the absorptive hypercalciuric group. The Kd was higher in the controls whereas the number of binding sites was more numerous in the hypercalciuric group (Table 3).

DISCUSSION

The results of this study show no significant differences between the control group and the absorptive hypercalciuric stone formers in terms of the plasma levels of PTH and $1,25-(OH)_2D_3$. The urinary excretion of c-AMP was similar in both groups.

Table 1. Calcium and Phosphate Data (mean $\pm$ SD).

Group	n	Age (years)	Plasma P (mg/dl)	Urine Ca (mg/24 h)	P
Control	12	32.5 ± 8.8	3.4 ± 0.5	132 ± 47	676 ± 181
Hyper-calciuric	18	40.2 ± 13.8	3.0 ± 0.4	292 ± 70	786 ± 234
		$P < 0.05$	$P<0.05$	$P<0.05$	$P<0.05$

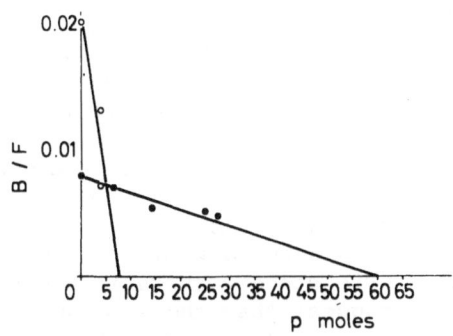

Fig. 1. Scatchard plot of the intestinal calcium-binding protein (Control (o); Stone-formers (●)).

Table 2. Parathyroid Hormone, 1,25-Dihydroxycholecalciferol and Cyclic-AMP values (mean ± SD).

Group	n	Plasma		Urine
		PTH (ng/ml)	$1,25-(OH)_2D_3$ (pg/ml)	c-AMP (pmol/mg Cr)
Control	12	0.29 ± 0.26	40.5 ± 27.7	4.24 ± 3.87
Hyper-calciuric	18	0.37 ± 0.44	19.5 ± 23.5	3.41 ± 2.03
		P<0.05	P<0.05	P<0.05

Table 3. Kinetics of Calcium-Binding by Duodenal Biopsies (mean ± SD).

Group	n	Calcium	
		Kd (10-13 mol/l)	Binding Sites (n/ng protein)
Control	12	4.0 ± 4.0	8.7
Hyper-calciuric	18	26.0 ± 2.6	29.2
		P<0.05	P<0.1

Furthermore, the $1,25-(OH)_2D_3$ levels were slightly lower in the stone-formers. Serum phosphate was slightly lower in the hypercalciuric group while the urinary excretion of phosphate was higher. These results contradict the finding of Lemann et al[3] who showed that there was an increase in $1,25-(OH)_2D_3$ levels in some recurrent stone formers. This discrepancy may be explained by the use of two different populations of stone formers or by the fact that Lemann's patients had a renal leak type of hypercalciuria. On the other hand, the Kd of the calcium-binding protein of the control group was higher than that of the absorptive hypercalciuric group. However, the number of binding sites was more numerous in the stone formers. Such findings may indicate that the calcium-binding protein of normals has a higher affinity than that of the stone formers but the total capacity to transport calcium by the absorptive hypercalciuric stone formers is higher than that of the controls. This may suggest that the absorptive hypercalciuric individuals are able to transport more calcium than the controls whose ability to transport calcium is saturated more rapidly. The absence of a difference in $1,25-(OH)_2D_3$ levels and the presence of kinetic differences in the calcium-binding protein indicate that calcium hyperabsorption can be explained through a phosphate renal leak mechanism.

REFERENCES

1. B. Pinto, F. J. Ruiz-Marcellan, and J. Bernshtam, in:"Advances in Nephrourology", M. Pavone-Macaluso and P. H. Smith, eds., Plenum, New York (1981).
2. B. E. C. Nordin and M. Peacock, in:"Urinary Calculi", L. Cifuentes-Delatte, A. Rapado, and A. Hodgkinson, eds., Karger, Basel (1973).
3. C. Y. C. Pak, in:"Litiasis Renal", B. Pinto, ed., Salvat Editions, Barcelona (1976).
4. R. W. Gray, D. R. Wilz, A. E. Caldas, and J. Lemann, J. Clin. Endocr. Metab. 45:299 (1977).
5. B. Pinto and E. Garcia-Cuerpo, in:"Urolithiasis Research", H. Fleisch, W. G. Robertson, L. H. Smith, and W. Vahlensieck, eds., Plenum, New York (1976).
6. R. H. Wasserman, in:"The Fat Soluble Vitamins", H. F. DeLuca and J. W. Suttle, eds., University Wisconsin Press, Madison (1970).
7. B. Pinto, F. J. Ruiz-Marcellan, and E. Garcia-Cuerpo, Med. Clin. 69:141 (1977).
8. B. Pinto, F. J. Ruiz-Marcellan, Rev. Esp. Fisiol. 35:311 (1979).
9. M. R. Hughes, D. J. Bayling, P. C. Jones, and M. Haussler, J. Clin. Invest. 58:61 (1976).
10. J. A. Etssman, A. J. Hamstra, B. E. Kream, and H. F. DeLuca, Science 170:1021 (1976).
11. C. D. Arnaud, H. S. Tsao, and E. T. Littledicke, J. Clin. Invest. 50:21 (1971)
12. K. C. Tovey, K. G. Oldham, and J. A. M. Whelan, Clin. Chim. Acta 56:221 (1974).

INTESTINAL FLORA AND OXALATE EXCRETION IN PATIENTS WITH ENTERIC HYPEROXALURIA

B. Nordenvall, D. Hallberg, L. Larsson, and C.-E. Nord

Dept. of Surgery, Danderyd Hospital, Dept. of Surgery
and Clinical Microbiology, Huddinge University Hospital
Karolinska Institute, Stockholm and Dept. of Clinical
Chemistry, University Hospital, Linköping, Sweden

INTRODUCTION

The commonest type of hyperoxaluria today is found in
conditions of gastrointestinal malabsorption and is designated
"enteric hyperoxaluria". It is most pronounced after intestinal
resection[1] and jejunoileal bypass[2]. Increased absorption of
oxalate is the main reason for the hyperoxaluria[3]. Most of the
absorption takes place in the colon[4], but the reason for it is not
fully known. Little is known about the role of the intestinal flora
in patients with enteric hyperoxaluria. Changes in the intestinal
flora might theoretically influence the hyperoxaluria. After
jejuno-ileal bypass the bacterial flora in the small intestine
changes towards that in the large intestine[5]. This might result in
deconjugation of bile acids and steatorrhea[6], since conjugated bile
acids are important stimulators of fat absorption. Another
possibility is that in these patients bacteria produce fatty acids
and oxalate in the colon, since the amount of nutrients available
for bacterial metabolism in the colon is increased in patients with
malabsorption.

The aim of the present study was to examine whether changes in
intestinal flora influence the degree of hyperoxaluria by studying
the effect of administration of clindamycin on urinary oxalate
excretion in patients with enteric hyperoxaluria.

MATERIALS AND METHODS

Eleven patients who had undergone jejunoileostomy because of
obesity were studied. Two surgical techniques were used: end-to-

end jejunoileostomy[7] and end-to-side jejunoileostomy with a bilio-intestinal shunt[8]. At these operations the length of the small intestine in continuity reduced to about 10% of the original. All had a stable body weight and recurrent kidney stones after the operation. The patients were studied under surgical ward conditions for 5 days. The daily average content of nutrients in the diet was unchanged during the study (100 g fat, 300 g carbohydrates, 90 g protein, 1.0 mmol oxalate, and 28 mmol calcium; energy, 10.2 MJ (2440 kcal)). During days 3, 4 and 5 clindamycin (Dalacina[R], Upjohn, USA), 1.8 g/24 h, was given parenterally in three divided doses (at 08.00, 16.00 and 24.00). Stool specimens were obtained the day before antibiotic administration (day 2), then on the last day of antibiotic administration (day 5), and 2 weeks after the administration had stopped (day 19). The specimens were collected in sterile plastic containers on the mornings of the collection

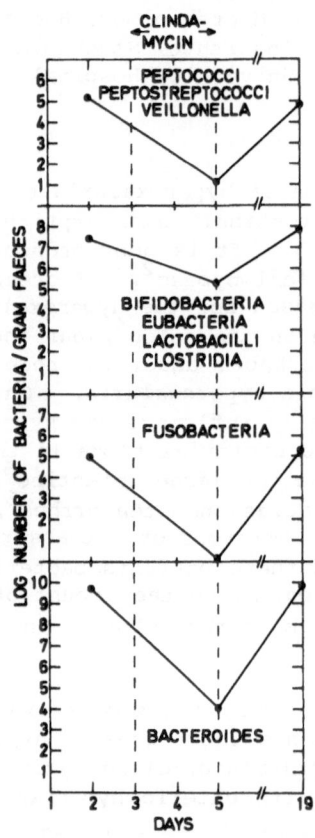

Fig. 1. Effect of clindamycin on the anaerobic flora in 11 patients. The numbers of bacteria are given in log of mean values of colony-forming units per gram faeces.

days. The time lapse between collection and plating was 1 h. A 1 g sample of faeces was homogenized in 9 ml peptone-yeast extract medium. Ten-fold serial dilutions were made to 10^{-8}. The samples were inoculated and manipulated as described by Heimdahl and Nord[9]. After incubation, total colony counts were made from the anaerobic blood agar plates. Strains belonging to Enterobacteriaceae were identified biochemically by using a test-kit system, API 20E (Analytic Products, New York). Oxidative-fermentative Gram-negative rods were identified by using another test-kit system, Oxi-Ferm (Hoffman-La Roche, N.J., USA). Urine was collected for 24 h periods (08.00 - 08.00) during the study (days 1-5). The urine was sampled in plastic bottles containing 90 mmol of hydrochloric acid to maintain oxalate in solution. Of each sample 250 ml was frozen at -20°C and analyzed at the end of the study. Oxalate was determined by the method of Hodgkinson and Williams[10]. The upper reference limit was 0.45 mmol/24 h[11]. The excretion was expressed in relation to the creatinine excretion to compensate for errors in urine collection[11]. The upper reference limit was 30 mmol oxalate/mol creatinine[11].

RESULTS

Clindamycin had no effect on the aerobic flora. The anaerobic bacteria were affected by clindamycin (Fig. 1). The number of anaerobic cocci and Gram-positive and Gram-negative rods decreased markedly during the administration period. After 2 weeks the anaerobic flora was normalized in all patients. All patients had hyperoxaluria (Table 1). The degree of hyperoxaluria did not change during administration of clindamycin.

DISCUSSION

No studies have to our knowledge been done to investigate the colonic microflora in patients with jejunoileal bypass. These patients have increased amounts of nutrients available for metabolism in the colon owing to malabsorption, and thus an abnormality in the colonic microflora might occur. However, in the present study we found that the total bacterial (aerobic and anaerobic) counts in stool specimens were in close agreement with those reported in healthy individuals[12]. The anaerobic bacteria decreased markedly during clindamycin administration. In spite of that the degree of hyperoxaluria did not change. The anaerobic flora was normalized in all patients 2 weeks after administration had stopped. The changes in colonic microflora during anti-microbial treatment are similar to those found in other patients[12]. Our patients with enteric hyperoxaluria had a normal colonic microflora. The degree of hyperoxaluria does not seem to be related to changes in the intestinal anaerobic flora.

141

Table 1. Urinary Oxalate Excretion (mmol/24 h) before and during Administration of Clindamycin.

Day	1	2	3	4	5
Nutrition		Normal diet		+1.8 g Clindamycin	
Patient					
C.J.	0.76	0.68	0.80	0.91	0.88
K.L.	1.02	1.08	1.06	0.98	1.07
A.B.	1.85	1.90	1.20	1.14	1.11
K.M.	0.78	0.79	0.75	0.61	0.82
M.R.	0.82	0.96	1.07	0.95	1.05
A.J.	0.78	0.53	1.06	0.68	0.47
G.A.	1.02	1.05	1.05	1.27	0.87
E.E.	1.38	1.08	1.11	0.94	1.19
M.S.	0.60	0.67	0.71	0.55	0.69
K.W.	0.71	0.69	0.67	0.93	1.18
L.J.	0.69	0.88	0.78	0.97	0.82
Mean±	0.95	0.94	0.93	0.90	0.92
SEM	0.11	0.11	0.06	0.07	0.07

REFERENCES

1. J. W. Dobbins and H. J. Binder, in:"Progress in Gastroenterology", Vol. 3, G. B. J. Glass, eds., Grune and Stratton, New York (1977).
2. J. Gregory, K. Park, and H. W. Schoenberg, J. Urol. 117:631 (1977).
3. B. Nordenvall, L. Backman, and L. Larsson, Scand. J. Gastroenterol. 16:395 (1981).
4. J. W. Dobbins and H. J. Binder, New Engl. J. Med. 296:298 (1977).
5. P. Dano, K. Lenz, and T. Justeson, Scand. J. Gastroenterol. 9:767 (1974).
6. M. E. Ament, S. S. Shimoda, D. R. Saunders, and C. E. Burin, Gastroenterology 63:728 (1972).
7. M. Buchwald and R. L. Varco, Surgery 70:62 (1971).
8. D. Hallberg and U. Holmgren, Acta Chir. Scand. 145:405 (1979).
9. A. Heimdahl and C. E. Nord, Scand. J. Infect. Dis. 11:233 (1979).
10. A. Hodgkinson and A. Williams, Clin. Chim. Acta 36:127 (1972).
11. H.-G. Tiselius, L. E. Almgård, L. Larsson, and B. Sörbo, Eur. Urol. 4:241 (1978).
12. L. Kager, L. Liljeqvist, A. S. Malmborg, and C. E. Nord, Antimicrob. Agents Chemother. 20:736 (1981).

RENAL TUBULAR FUNCTION IN PATIENTS FOLLOWING INTESTINAL

BY-PASS OPERATIONS

L. Backman, U. Backman, B. G. Danielson, and
B. Nordenvall

Dept. of Surgery, Karolinska Institutet, Danderyd
Hospital, Stockholm and Dept. of Medicine, University
Hospital, Uppsala, Sweden

INTRODUCTION

Patients with inflammatory bowel disease or jejunoileal by-pass have a high incidence of hyperoxaluria and an increased risk of forming renal calculi. In patients forming idiopathic calcium-containing kidney stones about 2 to 30% of the patients have been found to have renal tubular defects such as defective acidification of urine, tubular proteinuria, phosphate leak etc. The aim of the present study was to investigate a group of patients who had undergone jejunoileostomy because of obesity with respect to risk factors of calcium stone formation and renal tubular function.

MATERIALS AND METHODS

The observations were made on 16 patients who had undergone jejunoileostomy because of obesity. Two surgical techniques had been used, end-to-side jejunoileostomy[1] and end-to-end jejuno-ileostomy[2]. The operation reduced the functional length of the small intestine to about 10% of the original. The patients were studied 5 to 11 years post-operatively. They had, on average, lost 39 kg of body weight.

The clinical data are presented in Table 1. Body weight was stable in all patients. Nine patients had recurrent urolithiasis after the operation. One patient (No 1) had had stones before the intestinal by-pass operation. In addition to routine blood and urine tests, the urinary excretion of calcium, magnesium and citrate were measured. Citrate was assayed using an enzymatic method. As an indicator of tubular proteinuria, the urinary excretion of α_2-

Table 1. Data on 16 patients with Jejunoileal By-pass.

Case	Acidification Capacity	Sex	Age (yr)	Surgical Method	Renal Stone	Years after op	Present Weight (kg)	Postop Weight Loss (kg)
1	Normal	M	58	End-to-end	+	11	99	41
2	Normal	M	58	"	+	7	101	46
3	dRTA	M	34	End-to-side	+	8	100	26
4	Normal	M	28	End-to-end	+	7	104	60
5	dRTA	F	59	"	+	10	79	60
6	Normal	F	58	End-to-side	+	6	85	25
7	dRTA	F	48	End-to-end	+	7	82	40
8	dRTA	F	42	End-to-end	+	6	73	32
9	Normal	F	36	"	+	6	78	25
10	dRTA	M	47	"	0	5	95	29
11	Normal	M	39	"	0	6	105	31
12	Normal	M	34	"	0	5	98	28
13	Normal	F	60	End-to-end	0	11	93	73
14	Normal	F	51	End-to-side	0	6	77	33
15	dRTA	F	46	"	0	5	98	29
16	dRTA	F	39	End-to-side	0	7	70	46

Table 2. Renal Tubular Function on 16 Patients with Jejunoileal
          By-pass.

Case	Acidification Capacity	U-Citrate (mmol/24h)	U-α_2-microglobulin (mg/24 h)
1	Normal	0.20	0.4
2	Normal	0.76	0.5
3	dRTA	0.19	1.1
4	Normal	0.26	0.9
5	dRTA	0.40	3.2
6	Normal	0.60	0.1
7	dRTA	0.80	0.8
8	dRTA	1.20	0.1
9	Normal	0.81	0.1
10	dRTA	2.10	0.1
11	Normal	2.80	0.2
12	Normal	–	–
13	Normal	0.29	0.3
14	Normal	1.6	0.2
15	dRTA	0.64	0.2
16	dRTA	0.29	0.1
Mean $\pm$ SEM		1.86 $\pm$ 0.20	
Normal range		3.3 $\pm$ 0.2	0.4

microglobulin was measured using a radioimmunoassay (Phadebas,
Pharmacia, Uppsala, Sweden). The acidification of urine was
estimated using an ammonium chloride load, where 25 g ammonium
chloride was given in the form of crushed tablets.   Urinary pH, and
the excretion of titratable acid and ammonium ions in relation to
the acid-base status were investigated[3].

RESULTS

     The biochemical data are presented in Table 2.   Nine patients
acidified their urine normally.   Seven exhibited abnormal
acidification and had a distal renal tubular acidosis (dRTA).   One
of these patients had complete dRTA and the others the incomplete
form of the disorder.   All patients, including the normals, had a
low urinary pH before their acid load.   Citrate excretion was low
in nearly all patients and was significantly low for the group
compared with healthy controls.   For comparison with other stone
formers with idiopathic calcium stones, see Table 2.   It is obvious
that the by-pass patients as a group had a very low citrate
excretion.   An increased excretion of α_2-microglobulin was found in
5 patients, whereas 10 had a normal excretion.   Three patients with
tubular proteinuria also had a defective acidification; the other 2
acidified normally.

145

DISCUSSION

A significant portion (44%) of the investigated patients who had undergone intestinal by-pass operations because of obesity, exhibited defective acidification of the urine, indicating renal tubular defects. Low and sometimes very low citrate excretion was also found among the investigated patients. Another indication of tubular dysfunction, namely tubular proteinuria, was found in 33% of the patients compared with 8 to 10% in idiopathic stone formers[4]. Even if the number of the patients investigated is rather small, the results indicate that renal tubular defects are common in patients operated by intestinal by-pass. Clearly elevated values of other risk factors, such as a high urinary oxalate[5] and reduced urinary citrate, indicate a highly increased risk of calcium stone formation in these patients.

The changes in metabolism following intestinal by-pass operations seem to induce an increased risk of stone formation. Since several reports have been published on renal failure following bowel disease and enteric hyperoxaluria[6-9], it is essential to be aware of the potential risk of calcium oxalate deposition in the renal parenchyma and the risk of kidney failure following bowel disease as well as intestinal by-pass operations. Even if the mechanisms are not yet clear, the results of this investigation, as well as other reports, indicate an increased risk of kidney stone formation and kidney dysfunction and failure in patients with enteric hyperoxaluria caused by bowel disease or following by-pass operations.

REFERENCES

1. J. H. Payne and L. T. De Wind, Am. J. Surg. 118:141 (1969).
2. H. Buchwald and R. L. Varco, Surgery 70:62 (1971).
3. U. Backman, B. G. Danielson, and M. Sohtell, Scand. J. Urol. Nephrol. 35 (Suppl)33: (1976).
4. B. Wikström, U. Backman, B. G. Danielson, B. Fellström, G. Johansson, and S. Ljunghall, Klin. Wschr. 61:85 (1983).
5. B. Nordenvall, L. Backman, L. Larsson, and H.-G. Tiselius, Eur. Urol. 9:35 (1983).
6. K. Junker, J. B. Jensen, and H.-E. Jensen, Scand. J. Gastroentrol. 16:433 (1981).
7. J. B. Jensen, I. Nilsen, H.-E. Jenson, and B. Nielsen, Ugeskr. Laeg. 139:2742 (1977).
8. M. Vainder and J. Kelly, J. Am. Med. Soc. 235:1257 (1976).
9. H. Hey, P. Skaarup, K. Sølling, M. S. Christensen, B. Lund, O. H. Sørensen, and B. Lund, Int. J. Obesity 5:155 (1981).

MECHANISM OF SODIUM GLYCOLATE ABSORPTION IN RAT INTESTINE

H. S. Talwar, M. S. R. Murthy, S. K. Thind,
and R. Nath

Dept. of Biochemistry, Postgraduate Institute of
Medical Education and Research, Chandigarh-160012
India

INTRODUCTION

Glycolic acid is a precursor of oxalate in animals and man and the importance of it in the diet as a cause of increased urinary oxalate has recently been emphasised[1]. Under normal physiological conditions only 5% of dietary glycolate is converted to urinary oxalate, amounting to about 20 mg oxalate per day. This conversion rate, however, increases 18-fold in conditions such as pyridoxine deficiency[2,3]. Because of the wide-spread evidence of subclinical pyridoxine deficiency in the population[4,5], dietary glycolate may be enormously important as an oxalate precursor. However, no data are available on the mechanism of intestinal absorption of glycolate and its alterations in vitamin B_6 deficiency. The present study was undertaken to elucidate the mechanism of the intestinal transport of glycolate in rats and to study how it is effected by pyridoxine deficiency.

MATERIALS AND METHODS

The intestinal absorption of $1-^{14}C$-glycolate was studied using intestinal rings produced by the tissue accumulation technique[6]. The $1-^{14}C$-glycolate absorption was measured at glycolate concentrations ranging from 0 to 10 mM and at various incubation time intervals from 15 to 90 min. In all other experiments, incubation was carried out at $37^{\circ}C$ for 30 min. Effect of thiol-binding agents (p-chloromercuribenzoate 0.02 mM, and iodoacetate 1.0 mM), inhibitors of respiration (e.g. KCN 1.0 mM and 2,4-dinitrophenol (DNP) 0.5 mM), and structural analogues of glycolate (sodium glyoxylate, sodium pyruvate, sodium lactate and sodium

147

oxalate) on glycolate absorption were studied. Segmental
differences in the transport of glycolate were measured in the
duodenum, jejunum, ileum and colon of the rat.

Male Wistar weanling rats were made pyridoxine-deficient by
feeding vitamin B_6-deficient diet.   After 6 weeks the vitamin B_6-
deficient and the pair-fed controls were sacrificed and their
intestines removed to study the intestinal transport of ^{14}C-
glycolate.   The pyridoxine status of these animals was ascertained
by erythrocyte glutamate pyruvate transaminase assay[7].

RESULTS AND DISCUSSION

The effect of substrate concentration (0 to 15 μmol) on intestinal
transport of glycolate indicates that glycolate is absorbed by a
carrier-mediated process and after a linear increase in
transport up to 20 μmol, saturation was attained (Fig. 1).   The Km
for sodium glycolate was 6.25 mM at pH 7.4, while V_{max} was 5.56
μmol/30 min/g tissue.   The intestinal transport of glycolate
increased linearly for 25 min with no significant increase in the
uptake rate thereafter.   Glycolate is a negatively charged ion with
low lipid solubility; hence it may require a carrier to facilitate
its transport[8].   Thiol-binding agents showed no effect on glycolate
uptake suggesting that free thiol groups on the carrier molecule are
not involved in glycolate transport.   The respiration inhibitors,
e.g. KCN, 2,4-DNP, had no effect on glycolate transport indicating
that this process is not energy dependent (Table 1).   A marked
effect of various structural analogues on glycolate uptake was
observed.   Sodium glyoxylate showed significant inhibition (P<0.05)

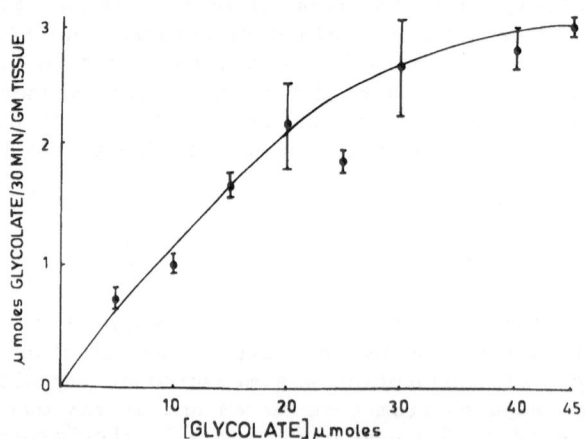

Fig. 1.   Intestinal transport of glycolate: effect of substrate
concentration.

Table 1. Effect of Various Compounds on Intestinal Glycolate Transport in Rats (Mean ± SEM).

Compound	Concentration (mM)	Glycolate (μmol/30 min/g/ wet wt)
Control	-	2.39 ± 0.06
p-Chloromercuribenzoate	0.02	2.19 ± 0.18
Iodoacetic acid	1.00	2.26 ± 0.24
KCN	1.00	2.51 ± 0.13
2,4-Dinitrophenol	0.50	2.12 ± 0.03
Sodium glyoxylate	2.00	2.03 ± 0.03
Sodium lactate	2.00	2.03 ± 0.12*
	6.00	1.72 ± 0.03**
Sodium oxalate	2.00	2.06 ± 0.14
	6.00	2.15 ± 0.10
Sodium pyruvate	2.00	2.36 ± 0.17
	6.00	2.07 ± 0.10
	10.00	2.09 ± 0.14

*$P < 0.05$; ***$P < 0.001$ compared with control.

at both 2.0 and 6.0 mM concentrations while sodium lactate showed profound inhibition at 6.0 mM ($P < 0.001$). Sodium pyruvate and oxalate did not affect glycolate absorption. Glyoxylate, in alkaline aqueous solution, exists in a hydrated form structurally similar to glycolate[9] and lactate is also an α-hydroxy acid like glycolate, which can thus compete with the glycolate-binding site on the carrier. Beneficial effects of pyruvate feeding on hyperoxaluria induced by glycolate feeding were thought to be due to the possible interference of pyruvate with intestinal glycolate absorption[10]. However, no such effect was observed in the present study at any of the pyruvate concentrations studied (2 to 10 mM). The absorption of sodium glycolate was studied in different intestinal regions. The jejunum and ileum exhibit significantly higher rates of absorption than the colon, but there were no great differences between the duodenum, jejunum and ileum.

The role of dietary glycolate as an oxalate precursor in vivo is significantly enhanced in vitamin B_6 deficiency[2]. No differences in glycolate absorption were observed between pair-fed controls and vitamin B_6-deficient rats in the present study; both showed low glycolate absorption (1.97 ± 0.06 μmol glycolate/30 min/g wet wt for pair-fed rats and 1.94 ± 09.04 μmol glycolate/30 min/g wet wt for vitamin B_6-deficient rats) owing to their low food consumption. The increased oxalate transport in the intestine of vitamin B_6-deficient rats over their pair-fed controls as reported earlier[11], suggests that the mode and regulation of oxalate absorption is different from that of glycolate.

REFERENCES

1. K. S. Harris and K. E. Richardson, Invest. Urol. 18:106 (1980).
2. T. J. Runyan and S. N. Gershoff, J. Biol. Chem. 240:1889 (1965).
3. A. M. Rofe and J. B. Edwards, Biochem. Med. 20:323 (1978).
4. J. G. Gregory, J. Nutr. 110:995 (1980).
5. M. S. R. Murthy, S. Farooqui, H. S. Talwar, S. K. Thind, R. Nath, L. Rajendran, and B. E. Bapna, Int. J. Clin. Pharmacol. Ther. Toxicol. 20:434 (1982).
6. F. Alvarado and A. Mahmood, Biochemistry 13:2882 (1974).
7. H. Kishi and K. Folkares, J. Nutr. Sci. Vitaminol. 22:225 (1976).
8. K. J. Ullrich and G. Rumrich, in:"Biochemistry of Kidney Functions", F. Morel, ed., Elsevier, Amsterdam (1982)
9. C. Iluis and J. Bozal, Biochim. Biophys. Acta 461:209 (1977).
10. F. H. C. Chow, D. W. Hamar, J. P. Boulay, and L. D. Lewis, Invest. Urol. 15, 493 (1978).
11. S. Farooqui, A. Mahmood, R. Nath, and S. K. Thind, Ind. J. Exptl. Biol. 19:551 (1981).

INTESTINAL ABSORPTION OF OXALATE IN GONADECTOMIZED RATS

S. K. Thind, V. Sharma, S. Farooqui, and
R. Nath

Dept. of Biochemistry, Postgraduate Institute of
Medical Education and Research, Chandigarh-160012
India

INTRODUCTION

Hyperabsorption of oxalate from the gut has been shown to be an important contributory factor in the production of calcium oxalate urolithiasis[1], a disease which is more prevalent in men than women[2]. Sex hormones regulate the enzymes of oxalate biosynthesis in the glycolate-glyoxylate-oxalate pathways[3,4]. To elucidate the role of sex hormones in the intestinal uptake of oxalate, male and female rats were gonadectomized and treated with estradiol and testosterone respectively.

MATERIALS AND METHODS

Oxalate uptake rate (μmol/h/g tissue wt) was determined in everted intestinal rings using the tissue accumulation method[5], in the following group of animals:male (M), castrated male (CM), castrated male administered estradiol (CM + E), female (F), castrated female (CF), castrated female administered testosterone (CF + T). Testosterone and estradiol were inserted into silastic capsules of 2 cm length and implanted subcutaneously on the dorsal side of the neck.

RESULTS

The intestinal oxalate uptake rate for the different groups of animals (using 0.5 mM oxalate in the incubation medium) (Table 1) shows that castrated male rats absorbed twice as much oxalate as normal males, and females and castrated males receiving estradiol

Table 1. Effect of Castration, Estradiol and Testosterone on
Intestinal Uptake of Oxalate in Male and Female Rats
(mean $\pm$ SEM).

Group	Oxalate uptake (μmol/h/g tissue wt)
Male (M)	0.242 ± 0.007
Castrated male (CM)	0.439 ± 0.045[a]
Castrated male + estradiol (CM + E)	0.347 ± 0.019[a,b]
Female (F)	0.341 ± 0.057[a]
Castrated female (CF) + testosterone (CF + T)	0.307 ± 0.063[a]

[a] $P < 0.001$ as compared to male.

[b] $P < 0.001$ as compared to castrated male.

absorbed 1.5 times more oxalate than males.   Oxalate uptake rates
in females, castrated females and castrated females receiving
testosterone were the same (Table 1), indicating that while
castration increases oxalate absorption from the intestine,
ovariectomy had no effect on oxalate uptake rate.   Female rats
absorbed more oxalate than males and castrated males receiving
estradiol absorbed oxalate at the same rate as females.

The intestinal oxalate uptake rate over the range 0.1 mM to 6
mM oxalate in the incubation medium is plotted in Fig. 1.   The
oxalate uptake rate increases linearly with the increase in oxalate
concentration, suggesting that oxalate is absorbed by a passive,
non-saturable process.   The slopes calculated from Fig. 1 are 0.51
for males, 1.07 for castrated males and 0.77 for castrated males
receiving estradiol.

DISCUSSION

The role of sex hormones in regulating oxalate metabolism has
been questioned by Tiselius et al[6] who found no change in the
oxalate excretion of pre- and post-orchiectomized elderly patients
with prostatic carcinoma.   From our study it appears that although
following orchiectomy endogenous oxalate synthesis might have
decreased, a parallel increase in the uptake of oxalate from the
intestine might have resulted in normal urinary levels of oxalate.

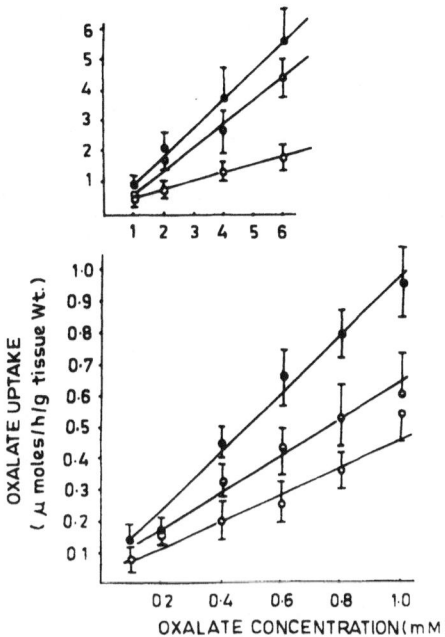

Fig. 1. Intestinal uptake of oxalate in control (o), castrated male (●) and castrated male + estradiol (⊝) rats. Each point is mean ± SEM of 8 to 10 observations. Inset: Oxalate uptake at higher concentrations.

Similarly, Menon (personal communication) has found a decline in oxalate excretion following orchiectomy, which later returns to normal. Lack of an appreciable sex difference in the urinary excretion of oxalate, despite low levels of enzymes in females, also may be due to increased absorption of oxalate from the gut. The chemical composition of the intestinal brush border membrane (BBM) preparation in rats[7] following castration, showed decreased phospholipid, cholesterol and sialic acid content of the BBM. Therefore, it appears likely that these changes in the chemical composition of the BBM may be a cause of the hyperabsorption of oxalate observed following castration.

REFERENCES

1. A. Hodgkinson, Clin. Sci. Mol. Med. 54:291 (1978).
2. T. Inada, S. Mujazaki, T. Omori, H. Nihira, and T. Hino, Urol. Int. 7:150 (1958).
3. V. Sharma, M. S. R. Murthy, S. K. Thind, and R. Nath, Biochem.Int. 3:507 (1981).

4. V. Sharma, S. K. Thind, and R. Nath, Biochem. Med. (1984)
   Inpress.
5. S. Farooqui, A. Mahmood, R. Nath, and S. K. Thind,
   Ind. J. Exptl. Biol. 19:551 (1981).
6. H. G. Tiselius, E. Varenhorst, K. Carlstrom, and L. Larsson,
   Invest. Urol. 18:110 (1980).
7. V. Sharma, S. Farooqui, S. K. Thind, and R. Nath,
   (in preparation).

EFFECT OF MALEIC ACID ON THE INTESTINAL UPTAKE OF CALCIUM AND

OXALATE IN PYRIDOXINE-DEFICIENT RATS

S. K. Thind, S. Farooqui, A. Mahmood, R. Gupta,
and R. Nath

Dept. of Biochemistry, Postgraduate Institute of
Medical Education and Research, Chandigarh, India

INTRODUCTION

Calcium oxalate is the most common lithogenic substance found
in human urinary calculi[1]. Hyperoxaluria has been observed in
pyridoxine-deficiency and is presumably due to the increased
endogenous synthesis of oxalate[2,3] or to the increased
bioavailability of dietary oxalate[4,5]. Oxalate uptake follows a
biphasic transport mechanism. In vitamin B_6-deficient rats, at low
oxalate concentrations (0.1 to 0.8 mM), a saturable oxalate
transport system (OTS) operates, while at higher concentrations of
oxalate (0.8 to 6 mM), its uptake follows a passive diffusion
mechanism[5]. Carrier-mediated OTS is inhibited by protein synthesis
inhibitors and glycolate or glyoxylate competitively inhibits
oxalate transport[4]. To understand the mechanism of this uptake
process the effect of other mono- and dicarboxylic acids on the
saturable oxalate transport system and calcium uptake in pyridoxine-
deficient rats has been investigated.

MATERIALS AND METHODS

Male albino Wistar strain rats weighing (40 to 50 g) were
divided into 3 groups of 10 rats each: Group I was fed a vitamin B_6-
deficient diet[6]; Group II was pair-fed with Group I and orally
supplemented with 100 μg pyridoxine HCl/day; Group III was given
Hindustan Lever pellet diet ad libitum. After 45 days, overnight-
fasted animals were sacrificed and the intestines removed.
Pyridoxine deficiency was confirmed by erythrocyte glutamate
pyruvate transaminase index (EGPT index)[4,5]. The intestine
(duodenum and jejunum) was everted and 0.5 cm rings incubated in

Kreb's Ringer buffer. The oxalate uptake in jejunal rings and calcium uptake in duodenal rings were measured[5]. Correction for extracellular space was made separately using ^{3}H-inulin[7]. For kinetic studies, the uptake of ^{14}C-oxalic acid/^{45}Ca was measured at various concentrations (0 to 10 mM) in the presence or absence of neutralized 1 mM maleic acid in the incubation medium. When the effect of mono- or dicarboxylic acids were tested, neutralized lactic, pyruvic or succinic acids in 0.1 ml was added to the incubation medium to attain a final concentration of 1 mM.

RESULTS AND DISCUSSION

A significant decrease in body weight, but no change in the intestine weight or length, was observed in pyridoxine-deficient rats. The pyridoxine status ascertained by the EGPT index, showed maximum stimulation (65.8 ± 5.6%) in the deficient group as compared to the pair-fed (6.8 ± 1.4%) or control (5.05 ± 0.8%) groups, indicating a depletion of pyridoxal-5'-phosphate from the tissue reserves of the deficient animals. The effect of various mono- and dicarboxylic acids (viz. pyruvate, lactate, succinate, maleate) on oxalate transport was studied in control and vitamin B_6-deficient rats. Succinate, lactate or pyruvate did not have any significant influence on the oxalate uptake rate. However, maleate significantly ($P < 0.001$) stimulated oxalate uptake in pyridoxine-deficient rats. Earlier studies from this laboratory have indicated the presence of a biphasic oxalate transport system in pyridoxine-deficiency[4,5]. Maleate stimulates the carrier-mediated oxalate transport system. Kinetic studies reveal a significant increase in the V_{max} (1.25 μmol/h/g tissue without maleic acid and 2.00 μmol/h/g tissue in presence of 1 mM maleic acid), without affecting the K_m (1.15 mM). These results suggest that maleic acid activates OTS by exposing more oxalate transport carriers thereby increasing the transport capacity. A similar concentration of maleic acid failed to enhance the passive diffusion component in control rats (unpublished observations). The oxalate uptake in the absence of maleic acid reaches a steady state value in 20 to 30 min; while in the presence of maleic acid it was achieved after only 40 to 50 min, with a 4-fold increase in the steady state ratio (0.24 ± 0.03 in the absence to 0.89 ± 0.08 in the presence of 1 mM maleic acid). The enhancement in OTS was observed in the initial period of incubation (1 to 2 min), which suggests that maleic acid activates OTS by directly interacting at the brush border membrane surface. Similar enhancement in α-methyl D-glucoside uptake by maleic acid was observed in isolated rat renal tubules[8].

Table 1. Kinetic Parameters of Calcium Uptake in Control and Vitamin B_6-Deficient Rats (Mean $\pm$ SD).

Group	Steady state value (μmol/h/g tissue)	K_m (mM)	V_{max} (μmol/30 min/g tissue)	K_i (mM)
Control	0.98 $\pm$ 0.11	4.21	3.33	
Control + 1 mM Maleic acid	0.59 $\pm$ 0.08[*]	8.00	3.33	1.11
Vitamin B_6 deficient	1.42 $\pm$ 0.28	5.92	5.71	-
Vitamin B_6 deficient + 1 mM Maleic acid	0.82 $\pm$ 0.14[•]	13.33	5.71	0.79

*$P < 0.001$ compared to control.
•$P < 0.001$ compared to vitamin B_6-deficient.

The effect of maleic acid on calcium uptake was studied at different concentrations of calcium (1 to 10 mM) in the incubation medium. The presence of 1 mM maleic acid in the incubation medium competitively inhibited calcium uptake in both control and vitamin B_6-deficient rat intestine. The results of these kinetic studies are tabulated in Table 1. The addition of maleic acid to the incubation medium increases the K_m from 4.21 mM to 8.00 mM without any profound effect on the V_{max} of the transport system. The inhibitory constant K_i was calculated from the equation: $V_{max} = v(1 + (K_m/S)(1+I/K_i))$. This gave a value of 1.11 mM. The steady state value was also decreased significantly ($P < 0.001$) in presence of maleic acid (Table 1). Vitamin B_6-deficient rats exhibited a higher calcium uptake rate. The increase in uptake was mainly due to the increase in V_{max} of the transport system (Table 1) suggesting an increase in the capacity of the calcium transport system. The aberrations produced in the chemical architecture of the brush border membrane in pyridoxine deficiency[5] could be responsible for the enhanced ^{45}Ca uptake in pyridoxine-deficient rats. Alterations in vitamin D function could also be present because increased steroid binding of the nuclear fraction in vitamin B_6 deficiency has been previously reported[9,10]. This may be compared to the mode of action of vitamin D_3 for the induction of the calcium transport carrier in enterocytes[11].

Maleic acid inhibits calcium uptake in vitamin B_6-deficient rat intestine by interacting at the calcium-binding sites on the microvillus membrane thus increasing the K_m from 5.92 to 13.33 mM without affecting the V_{max}, with the K_i of the order of 0.79. A 48% decrease in the steady state ratio was also observed in presence of 1 mM maleic acid (Table 1). These results demonstrate that maleic acid decreases the ^{45}Ca uptake by the intestinal segments from vitamin B_6-deficient rats by decreasing the affinity of the transport system without affecting the transport capacity.

REFERENCES

1. S. K. Thind and R. Nath, Ind. J. Med. Res. 57:1790 (1969).
2. J. D. Rabaya and S. N. Gershoff, J. Nutr. 109:171 (1979).
3. M. S. R. Murthy, H. S. Talwar, S. K. Thind, and R. Nath, Ann. Nutr. Metabol. 26:201 (1982).
4. S. Farooqui, A. Mahmood, S. K. Thind, and R. Nath, Ind. J. Exp. Biol. 19:551 (1980).
5. S. Farooqui, R. Nath, S. K. Thind, and A. Mahmood, Biochem. Med. (in press) (1984).
6. T. J. Runyan and S. N. Gershoff, J. Biol. Chem. 240:1889 (1965).
7. F. Alvarado and A. Mahmood, Biochemistry 13:2882 (1974).
8. K. S. Roth, S. M. Wang, and S. Segal, Biochim. Biophys. Acta 426:675 (1976).
9. D. M. Disorbo, D. S. Phelps, V. S. Ohl, and G. J. Litwack, J. Biol. Chem. 255:3886 (1980).
10. J. Holley, D. A. Bender, W. F. Coulson, and E. K. Symes, J. Ster. Biochem. 18:161 (1983).
11. D. D. Bikle, R. L. Morrissey, D. T. Zolock, and H. Rasmussen, Rev. Physiol. Biochem. Pharmacol. 89:62 (1981).

III. RENAL PHYSIOLOGY AND PATHOPHYSIOLOGY

THE RENAL HANDLING OF MAGNESIUM

E. Slatopolsky, Y. L. Chan, and K. J. Martin

Renal Division, Dept. of Medicine, Washington University
School of Medicine, St. Louis, Missouri 63110, U.S.A.

INTRODUCTION

In the last decade, the use of micropuncture and microperfusion
techniques have further advanced our knowledge of the renal handling
of magnesium in health and disease.   The purpose of this paper is
to review (i) the renal handling of magnesium, (ii) the role of
magnesium in the pathogenesis and treatment of renal calculi, and
(iii) the role of magnesium depletion in the pathogenesis of
hypocalcemia.

Magnesium is the fourth most abundant cation of the body, and
after potassium is the second most abundant intracellular cation.
Total body magnesium is approximately 2000 mEq (25 g).   As for
calcium, only a small fraction (about 1%) of the total body
magnesium is present in the extracellular fluid (ECF) compartment.
Approximately 60 to 65% of the total magnesium is found in bone.
Most of the magnesium in bone is associated with apatite crystals, a
significant amount being present as a surface-limiting ion and
freely exchangeable.   Magnesium plays an essential role as a
cofactor for a variety of enzymes, most of which utilize ATP.
Approximately 300 mg (25 mEq) of magnesium are ingested daily in the
diet.   Of the total amount ingested in the diet, about 1/3 is
eliminated in the urine and the remainder in the feces.   This
relationship is maintained constant with diets providing as much as
600 mg/day of magnesium.   Most of the magnesium is absorbed in the
small intestine.   However, there is evidence that it can also be
absorbed in the colon.   Approximately 75 to 80% of the magnesium in
serum is ultrafilterable;   the remainder is protein bound.   Most of
the ultrafiltrable magnesium is present in ionized form.

RENAL HANDLING OF MAGNESIUM

Approximately 2 g of magnesium are filtered daily by the human kidney and about 100 mg appear in the urine. Thus, 95% of the filtered load of magnesium is reabsorbed and 5% is excreted in the urine. As mentioned above, the amount of magnesium excreted in the urine is greatly influenced by the amount ingested in the diet. Clearance studies have demonstrated that the mammalian kidney is characterized by a filtration-reabsorptive system for magnesium with little evidence for magnesium secretion. However, more recent micropuncture and microperfusion studies have provided new information regarding sites and characteristics of magnesium transport in the nephron. It is clear now that in some segments of the nephron magnesium is not handled in a similar way to calcium and sodium. Thus, clearance studies are no longer sufficient to clarify all of these intricate processes occurring along the various nephron segments.

Glomerulus

Micropuncture studies of surface glomeruli in rats have shown that plasma magnesium is filtered at the glomerular membrane at a rate of approximately 80% of the total serum magnesium[1].

Proximal Tubule

The tubular fluid to ultrafilterable (TF/UF) magnesium ratio increases along the proximal tubule but to a lesser extent than that of inulin. In other words, magnesium concentration of the late tubular fluid exceeds that obtained from early puncture sites. Studies in the dog[2] and the rat[3] both reveal a TF/UF ratio of 1.5 to 1.6, indicating that only 20 to 25% of the filtered load of magnesium is reabsorbed in the proximal convoluted tubule. This is in contrast to other major cations. Recent studies[4] have further characterized the transport mechanism for magnesium in the proximal tubule. These microperfusion studies showed that this segment of the nephron is relatively impermeable to magnesium. There does not seem to be a Tm for magnesium in the proximal tubule. Magnesium concentration as high as 15 mEq/l is associated with a proportional increase in reabsorption without any evidence of saturation[4]. Also, there was very little backflux of magnesium so that transport is basically a unidirectional process. These studies confirmed early observations in the rat[5] demonstrating that the excretory pattern of ^{28}Mg when injected into the proximal tubule was the same as that of inulin, suggesting poor permeability of the tubular epithelium to magnesium.

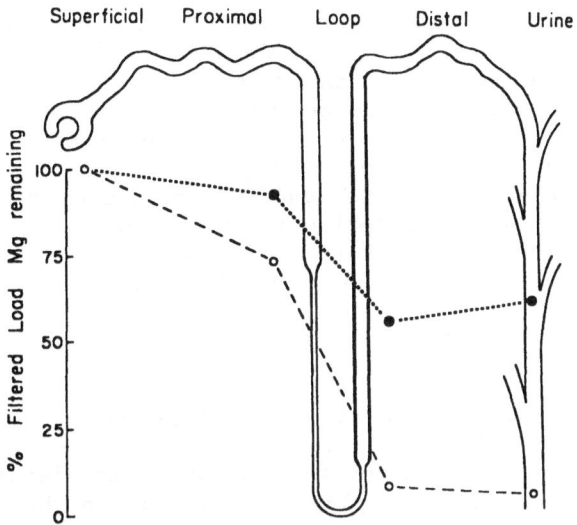

Fig. 1. Fractions of magnesium remaining along the nephron in normal conditions (o---o) and following acute $MgCl_2$ loading (•---•)[7].

Loop of Henle

Studies in Psammomys[6] revealed little transport in the descending limb of Henle's loop, and suggested that the ascending limb plays a major role in magnesium reabsorption. Tubular fluid obtained from the early distal tubule has a lower magnesium concentration than that in the glomerular filtrate. The ascending limb reabsorbs 60 to 70% of the filtered load of magnesium. The permeability of the ascending limb to magnesium is quite different from that of the proximal tubule. Urinary fractional excretion of magnesium may be as low as 1 to 2% in magnesium depletion or as high as 60 to 80% during magnesium-loading studies (Fig. 1). This remarkable difference in the behavior of the nephron represents changes in the transport capacity of the thick ascending limb of the loop of Henle. Increasing the perfusate or luminal concentration of magnesium resulted in a significant increase in net magnesium reabsorption in the thick ascending limb of the loop of Henle. On the other hand, if there is a simultaneous increase in plasma magnesium, there is a significant inhibition of magnesium reabsorption[4]. This, net and fractional reabsorption of magnesium at any perfused load is reduced by the presence of hypermagnesemia. Two mechanisms have been proposed to explain magnesium transport in the thick ascending limb of Henle[7]: (i) passive, secondary to the potential difference generated by the active transport of chloride which facilitates the entry of magnesium into the cell; and (ii) active, since the chemical concentration of magnesium in the cells is higher than in the lumen, and the potential gradient may not be great enough to explain the entry of magnesium into the cells. Diets deficient in magnesium or the administration of parathyroid hormone or cyclic AMP enhance the reabsorption of magnesium in the thick ascending limb of Henle's loop. On the other hand, diets containing large amounts of magnesium or factors that decrease the reabsorption of sodium chloride in this portion of the nephron (ECF volume expansion, or administration of furosemide or ethacrynic acid) decrease the reabsorption of magnesium.

Distal and Collecting Segments of the Nephron

The terminal segment of the nephron (late distal tubule and collecting duct) appear to play a minor role in the reabsorption of magnesium under normal conditions. Micropuncture studies[8] suggest net transport of approximately 5% of the filtered load in this segment of the nephron. Studies in the isolated perfused cortical collecting duct demonstrate significant amounts of net magnesium reabsorption and no net transport has been detected along the inner medullary collecting duct[9] or in the papillary collecting duct[10].

Factors which Alter the Renal Handling of Magnesium

As mentioned before, the amount of magnesium ingested in the diet is probably the most important factor determining the final excretion of magnesium in the urine. Most of the adaptative process is localized in the thick ascending part of the limb of Henle. This site of the nephron has the capability of reabsorbing or secreting large amounts of magnesium according to the serum magnesium and intracellular magnesium concentrations. Magnesium excretion has been demonstrated to follow closely that of sodium and calcium. Maneuvers to decrease cellular reabsorption, such as ECF volume expansion or use of diuretics, greatly enhance the amount of magnesium in the urine. Similarly, calcium competes with magnesium reabsorption and during calcium administration magnesium excretion increases in the urine. Parathyroid hormone and cyclic AMP both have a stimulatory effect on magnesium transport. It has been suggested[11] that the loop of Henle is an important site of action of PTH on magnesium transport. It would seem that physiological concentrations of calcitonin stimulate magnesium reabsorption in the presence or absence of PTH[12]. Quamme[13], utilizing an in vivo microperfusion system in rats, demonstrated that calcitonin produces hypocalcemia and a marked decrease in the fractional excretion of magnesium.

164

MAGNESIUM IN THE PATHOGENESIS AND TREATMENT OF RENAL CALCULI

Compounds which inhibit the crystallization of calcium salts have interested investigators in the field of renal urolithiasis. It has been known for over 50 years that magnesium can increase the solubility of calcium oxalate[14] presumably by forming complexes with oxalate ions that are not available for precipitation by calcium. In the early 1960s renal histological abnormalities were demonstrated in experimental magnesium-deficient rats. Light and electron microscopic studies showed that young rats that were made magnesium-deficient developed renal calcification after 4 to 6 days on a low magnesium diet and this was limited to the inner stripe of the outer zone of the medulla. It appeared to involve the thick ascending limb of Henle and less frequently the thin limb. Calcium deposition was found in lyosome-like bodies and free in the cytoplasm. Cellular calcification was never seen in the absence of luminal calcium. Collections of dilated proximal and distal convoluted tubules probably represent focal internal hydronephrosis secondary to calcification in the medulla. To characterize further the role of magnesium in the formation of calcium oxalate crystals in the urine and the % of ^{14}-C oxalate radioactivity in urine from patients on a low magnesium diet. A low urinary magnesium was induced in normal volunteers by giving cellulose phosphate, magnesium was added in vitro to yield urine samples of normal and high magnesium concentration. After rapid evaporation of the urine samples at pH 5.3, the calcium oxalate crystals were measured by microscopy and isotopic methods. Their studies showed a clear inverse correlation between magnesium concentration and calcium oxalate crystal formation. A controversial issue, perhaps unresolved at the present time, is related to the actual concentration of magnesium in the urine in patients with calcium oxalate stones. Although it is accepted that magnesium decreases the formation of calcium oxalate stones, it is not fully understood if the majority of patients with this type of stone have low concentrations of magnesium in the urine or if the magnesium/calcium ratio is decreased when compared with values obtained in normal volunteers. It would seem that in several patients with calcium oxalate stones, the actual concentration of magnesium in the urine is normal. However, the ratio magnesium/calcium is decreased. Recent studies[17] have demonstrated the beneficial effect of magnesium in patients with calcium oxalate stones. In these studies 56 patients with renal stones received magnesium hydroxide 200 mg twice a day for a period of one year and then the dose was increased to 500 mg. Most of their patients underwent treatment for at least 2 years and 45 patients have been free of recurrence or formation of new stones. The mean stone episode rate during treatment was 0.03 stones/year compared with 0.8 stones/year before treatment. The authors believe that magnesium therapy is comparable with thiazides and probably more effective than cellulose phosphate in preventing the recurrence of stones. The study

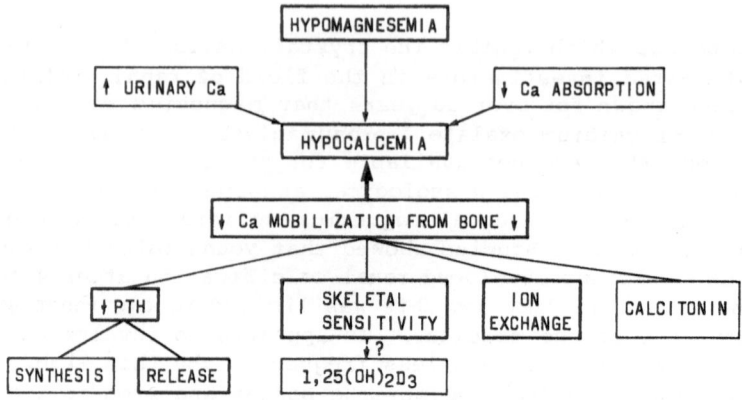

Fig. 2. Pathogenetic mechanisms responsible for the development of
hypocalcemia in magnesium depletion[26].

confirmed the beneficial effect of magnesium described earlier[18]
using magnesium oxide at a dose level of 1200 mg/day.   That there
were no changes in serum and urinary calcum or in serum magnesium.
However, as expected, there was an increase in urinary magnesium.
Therefore, the magnesium/calcium ratio increased in the majority of
patients.   In some patients, it required several months before
there was a remarkable increase in urinary magnesium.   This delay
was interpreted as magnesium depletion in some patients with calcium
oxalate stones[18].   It is obvious that the precise pathogenetic
mechanism by which magnesium interferes with the formation of
oxalate crystals is not known at the present time.

MAGNESIUM DEPLETION IN THE PATHOGENESIS OF HYPOCALCEMIA

     From a pathogenetic point of view the development of
hypocalcemia in magnesium depletion may be due to: (i) an increase
in urinary calcium excretion; (ii) a decrease in calcium absorption
from the gastrointestinal tract; and (iii) a decrease in calcium
mobilization from bone (Fig.2).   The possibility that increased
calcium excretion in the urine or decrease in calcium absorption
from the gastrointestinal tract be responsible for the development
of profound hypocalcemia in patients with hypomagnesemia is
extremely remote.   Patients with idiopathic hypercalciuria who may
be losing 300 to 400 mg calcium daily do not develop profound
hypocalcemia.   Moreover, mild malabsorption of calcium will be
compensated by secondary hyperparathyroidism, increased 1,25-
dihydroxycholecalciferol (1,25(OH)$_2$D$_3$) and PTH.   There is also
evidence that, in magnesium depletion, calcium absorption in the
gastrointestinal tract is increased.   The third and most likely
explanation for the development of hypocalcemia and magnesium

166

depletion in man is a decrease in calcium mobilization from bone. It is known that mild hypomagnesemia increases the levels of PTH in vivo or in vitro; on the other hand, profound magnesium depletion decreases the levels of PTH in blood. Several studies have shown that magnesium does not affect either the synthesis or the conversion of pro-PTH to PTH[19,20]. Studies in vivo[21] indicate that administration of magnesium intravenously to hypomagnesemic patients increases the levels of circulating PTH within 2 to 5 min suggesting that the main defect in hypomagnesemia is due to a decrease in release of PTH from the parathyroid glands. Controversy, however, exists regarding whether the response of the skeleton to exogenous PTH during magnesium deficiency is normal or reduced. As noted by Connor[22], the many variables involved, including species difference, degree of magnesium depletion, dose and preparation of PTH used, age of the subject and degree of hypocalcemia, need to be considered in attempting to reconcile the different results reported. In order to elucidate further the development of skeletal resistance in hypomagnesemia, we performed experiments in the isolated perfused bone preparation obtained from normal dogs and animals fed a low magnesium diet for a period of 4 to 6 months [23]. Our results demonstrate that the uptake of PTH by the isolated perfused bone system is remarkably decreased and a biological action of PTH in bone, i.e. an increase in cyclic AMP, is greatly diminished. The results of quantitative micromorphometric analysis of the ribs obtained from normal and magnesium-depleted dogs indicate a significant decrease in both the % of non-mineralized bone matrix (% relative osteoid volume) and the % of trabecular bone surface covered by osteoid. Because osteoid in normal animals represent sites of current bone formation, magnesium deficiency appears to suppress skeletal synthesis markedly and results in a histological picture comparable with that of skeletal inactivity. This "adynamic" appearance of bone may also play a role in the reduced immunoreactive PTH extraction by bone and blunted cyclic AMP response observed in magnesium-depleted dogs. Finally, an increase in the level of calcitonin plays no role in this syndrome. As a matter of fact, there is evidence to suggest that hypermagnesemia and not hypomagnesemia increases the release of calcitonin[24].

ACKNOWLEDGMENTS

This work was supported by U.S.P.H.S.NIADDK Grants AM-09976, AM-07126, and RR-00036. The authors would like to thank Mrs Pat Verplancke for her assistance in the preparation of this manuscript.

REFERENCES

1. C. LeGrimellec, P. Poujeol, and C. De Rouffignac, Pflug. Arch. 354:117 (1975).

2. S. F. Wen, R. L. Evanson, and J. H. Dirks, Am. J. Physiol. 219:570 (1970).

3. F. Morel, N. Roinel, and C. LeGrimellec, Nephron 6:350 (1969).

4. G. A. Quamme and J. H. Dirks, Am. J. Physiol. 238:F187 (1980).

5. M. Brunette and M. Aras, Am. J. Physiol. 221:1441 (1971).

6. C. De Rouffignac, F. Morel, N. Moss, and N. Roinel, Pflüg. Arch. 344:309 (1973).

7. J. H. Dirks and G. A. Quamme, in":"Homeostasis of Phosphate and Other Minerals", S. G. Massry, E. Ritz, and A. Rapado, eds., Plenum, New York (1978).

8. M. G. Brunette, N. Vigneault, and S. Carriere, Am. J. Physiol. 227:891 (1974).

9. H. H. Bengele, E. A. Alexander, and C. P. Lechene, Am. J. Physiol. 239:F24 (1980).

10. M. G. Brunette, N. Vigneault, and S. Carriere, Pflüg. Arch. 373:229 (1978).

11. M. Burnatowska, C. A. Harris, R. A. L. Sutton, and J. H. Dirks, Am. J. Physiol. 233:514 (1977).

12. S. Carney and L. Thompson, Am. J. Physiol. 240:F12 (1981).

13. G. A. Quamme, Am. J. Physiol. 238:E573 (1982).

14. K. J. Pederson, Trans. Faraday Soc. 35:277 (1939).

15. E. E. Schneeberger and A. B. Morrison, Lab. Invest. 14:674 (1965).

16. P. C. Hallson, G. A. Rose, and S. Sulaiman, Clin. Sci. 62:17 (1982).

17. G. Johansson, U. Backman, B. G. Danielson, B. Fellström, S. Ljunghall, and B. Wikström, J. Urol. 124:770 (1980).

18. I. Melnick, R. R. Landes, A. A. Hoffman, and J. F. Burch, J. Urol. 105:119 (1971).

19. J. W. Hamilton, F. W. Spierto, R. R. MacGregor, and D. V. Cohn, J. Biol. Chem. 246:3224 (1971).

20. J. F. Habener and J. T. Potts, Endocrinology 98:197 (1976).

21. C. A. Anast. J. L. Winnocker, L. R. Forte, and T. W. Burns, J.Clin. Endocrinol. Metab. 42:707 (1976).

22. T. B. P. Connor, J. Toskes, L. G. Mahaffey, L. Martin, J. Williams, and M. Walser, Johns Hopk. Med. J. 131:100 (1972).

23. J. Freitag, K. Martin, M. Conrades, E. Bellorin-Font, S. Teitelbaum, S. Klahr, and E. Slatopolsky, J. Clin. Invest. 64:1238 (1979).

24. E. T. Littledike and C. D. Arnaud, Proc. Soc. Expt. Biol. Med. 136:1000 (1971).

25. J. H. Dirks and G. A. Quamme, in:"Phosphate and Minerals in Health and Disease", S. G. Massry, E. Ritz, and H. Jahn, eds., Plenum, New York (1980).

26. E. Slatopolsky, E. Rosenbaum, P. Mennes, and S. Klahr, in:"Homeostasis of Phosphate and Other Minerals", S. G. Massry, E. Ritz, and A. Rapado, eds., Plenum, New York (1978).

INFLUENCE OF BICARBONATE ON THE RENAL HANDLING

OF MAGNESIUM

N. L. M. Wong, G. A. Quamme, and J. H. Dirks

Dept. of Medicine, Health Sciences Centre Hospital
University of British Columbia, Vancouver, Canada

INTRODUCTION

Metabolic acidosis has been shown to increase the urinary excretion of calcium, but the effects of acidosis on renal magnesium excretion are variable. Increases in urinary magnesium have been demonstrated in some[1,3] but not all studies of experimental metabolic acidosis in humans[4,5]. The reason for these contrasting results is not apparent. On the other hand, acute administration of acid in experimental animals failed to increase urinary magnesium[6].

The effect of metabolic alkalosis on altering magnesium excretion is more consistent than that seen in metabolic acidosis. During acute infusion of sodium bicarbonate, the fractional excretion of calcium and magnesium falls[6,7]. This reduction in calcium excretion is mainly due to enhanced reabsorption in the distal nephron[7]. The present experiments were performed in order to examine the effect of acid-base changes on magnesium excretion.

METHODS

Clearance and micropuncture experiments were carried out on 116 acutely thyroparathyroidectomized (TPTX) mongrel dogs of both sexes. The animals were divided into 5 groups:

Group 1: Normal control (n=29). Dogs were given intravenously 3% body weight of Ringer's solution prior to micropuncture in order to match the excretion of sodium in groups 2 and 3.

Group 2: Acute metabolic acidosis (n=19). Dogs were infused intravenously with 150 mM of NH_4Cl until blood pH fell to a level similar to that seen in the chronic acidotic group.

Group 3: Chronic metabolic acidosis (n=21). The dogs were fed 10 g/day of ammonium chloride for 3 days prior to study.

Group 4: Volume expansion normal control (n=22). These dogs received 7% body weight of Ringer's prior to experimentation, to increase sodium excretion to a level similar to that of Group 5.

Group 5: Acute metabolic alkalosis (n=25). In this group, the dogs were infused with a Ringer's solution containing 90 mM $NaHCO_3$.

The micropuncture and analytical methods were as previously described from this laboratory[8,9]. Tubule fluid bicarbonate was measured, using the picapnotherm method of Vurek[10].

RESULTS

The mean clearance data from these 5 groups of animals are presented in Table 1. Following acute NH_4Cl infusion, the fractional excretion of magnesium was similar to that of Group 1;

Table 1. Mean Clearance Data

	Group 1 Normal n=29	Group 2 Acute Acidosis n=19	Group 3 Chronic Acidosis n=21	Group 4 Vol.Exp. Normal n=22	Group 5 Alkalosis n=25
GFR (ml/min)	23.4+1.2	16.0+1.6*	20.8+1.8	24.0+1.8	22.6+1.3
P_{HCO3} (mM)	21.1+0.5	13.3+0.4	12.9+0.6*	16.6+0.6	30.6+0.5•
P_{Na} (mM)	148+1	142+1*	152+1	149+1	151+1
UF_{Mg} (mM)	0.49+0.01	0.50+0.01	0.49+0.01	0.49+0.01	0.50+0.01
FE_{HCO3} (%)	2.7+0.3	2.9+0.5	0.9+0.1*	6.1+0.6	22.8+1.8*•
FED_{Na} (%)	4.3+0.5	4.3+1.0	4.8+0.9	10.4+1.5	9.2+1.1
FE_{Mg} (%)	16.4+1.3	15.2+1.0	20.4+1.6*	29.7+2.2	21.9+1.8•

P = plasma concentration; UF = ultrafilterable;
FE = fractional excretion; *P<0.01 compared to Group 1;
• P<0.01 compared to Group 4.

Table 2. Mean Micropuncture Data

	Group 1 Normal n=29	Group 2 Acute Acidosis n=19	Group 3 Chronic Acidosis n=21	Group 4 Vol.Exp. Normal n=22	Group 5 Alkalosis n=25
Proximal					
RF_{Na} (%)	66+1	66+2	64+1	64+2	66+1
RF_{Mg} (%)	78+1	76+2	78+3	83+2	80+3
RF_{HCO_3} (%)	53+2	42+3*	24+2*	55+2	61+2•
Distal					
RF_{Na} (%)	6.1+0.6	6.2+0.5	7.2+0.7	16.4+1.6	15.3+1.3
RF_{Mg} (%)	17.9+1.1	17.9+1.7	23.6+1.5*	33.5+2.7	26.8+1.4•
RF_{HCO_3} (%)	10.6+0.9	8.4+1.6	4.3+0.8*	13.2+1.3	26.9+1.5•

RF = rejected fraction; *$p < 0.01$ compared to Group 1; • $p < 0.01$ compared to Group 4.

however, when animals were fed NH_4Cl for a period of 3 days, the fractional excretion of magnesium rose to 20%, which was significantly higher than that seen in Group 1. These data indicate that acute acidosis has no effect on fractional excretion of magnesium whereas chronic metabolic acidosis augments magnesium excretion.

Group 4 serves as a control group for Group 5. During acute infusion of $NaHCO_3$ (Group 5), despite similar rates of Na excretion in Groups 4 and 5, the fractional excretion of magnesium was significantly lower in Group 5 than that seen in Group 4. These data indicate that acute metabolic alkalosis reduces the fractional excretion of magnesium.

The micropuncture data are shown in Table 2. These indicate that acute and chronic acidosis and metabolic alkalosis have no effect on the proximal reabsorption of magnesium. The fraction of magnesium remaining in the distal tubule was the same during acute acidosis and control, but rose significantly during chronic acidosis. These data indicate that chronic acidosis reduced magnesium reabsorption at the site beyond the late proximal tubule. During metabolic alkalosis, the fraction of magnesium remaining in the distal tubule fell following alkali infusion. Accompanying this reduction in magnesium excretion the fraction of filtered bicarbonate remaining in the distal tubule increased. It appears that the reabsorption of magnesium in the distal tubule is related to the delivery of bicarbonate.

DISCUSSION

In the present experiment, acute metabolic alkalosis increased, whereas chronic metabolic acidosis decreased magnesium reabsorption in the distal tubule. The precise site within the nephron where acid-base changes affect magnesium transport is still unclear. This report clearly indicates that such changes occur between the late proximal tubule and the distal sampling site; this is compatible with the notion that the thick ascending limb is the site of alteration on magnesium transport under acid-base changes. Our present experiments indicate that chronic metabolic acidosis reduces and acute metabolic alkalosis enhances magnesium transport at a site beyond the proximal tubule. It is of interest that the amount of magnesium reabsorbed by the distal tubule is strongly correlated with the bicarbonate delivery. Whether bicarbonate has a direct or indirect effect on magnesium transport remains to be elucidated.

ACKNOWLEDGEMENTS

This study was supported by grants from the Medical Research Council of Canada to Drs J. H. Dirks and N. L. M. Wong (MT1915).

REFERENCES

1. F. K. Jabir, S. D. Roberts and R. A. Somersley, Clin. Sci. 16:119 (1957).
2. A. G. Hills, D. W. Parsons, G. O. Webster, Jr., O. Rosenthal, and H. Conover, J. Clin. Endocrinol. 19:1192 (1959).
3. H. E. Martin and R. Jones, Am. Heart J. 62:206 (1961).
4. E. J. Lennon and W. F. Piering, J. Clin. Invest. 49:1458 (1970).
5. R. J. McCollister, A. S. Prasad, R. P. Doe, and E. B. Flink, J.Lab. Clin. Med. 57:928 (1958).
6. D. R. Roy, L. K. Blouch, and R. L. Jamison, Am. J. Physiol. 243:F197 (1982).
7. R. A. L. Sutton, N. L. M. Wong, and J. H. Dirks, Kidney Int. 15:520 (1971).
8. J. H. Dirks, W. J. Cirksema, and R. W. Berliner, J. Clin. Invest. 44:1160 (1965).
9. N. L. M. Wong, G. A. Quamme, R. A. L. Sutton, and J. H. Dirks, J. Lab. Clin. Med. 94:683 (1979).
10. G. G. Vurek, D. G. Warnock, and R. Coisey, Analyt. Chem. 47:765 (1975).

URINARY EXCRETION OF CITRATE - INFLUENCE OF METABOLISM

AND ACID-BASE CONDITIONS

S. Adler

Montefiore Hospital and University of Pittsburgh
School of Medicine, Pittsburgh, PA 15213, U.S.A.

INTRODUCTION

Citrate, a known inhibitor of calculus formation, is important
in the field of urolithiasis, since a reduced citrate excretion has
been reported in some idiopathic calcium stone formers[1]. This
presentation reviews the urinary excretion of citrate with special
emphasis on the influence of acid-base effects.

BODY CITRATE METABOLISM

The major sources of blood citrate are the gastrointestinal
tract and bone with a lesser contribution from skeletal muscle.
Hypocitratemia develops in G.I. malabsorption[2]; hypocitratemia due
to decreased bone resorption and bone remodeling is not well
defined. The major organs utilizing blood citrate are the liver and
the kidney. Renal utilization differs from that of liver as some
citrate is excreted in the urine while some is metabolized.

RENAL HANDLING OF CITRATE

The features of renal citrate handling are shown in Fig. 1.
More than 90% of blood citrate is ultrafilterable passing readily
through the glomerulus. Small differences in binding exist from
patient to patient but are relatively small and clinically
insignificant. In man, 5 to 30% of filtered citrate is excreted.
Whereas in rats and dogs it is much smaller, averaging 3 to 7% in
rats. The proximal tubule reabsorbs between 70 to 95% of filtered
citrate and returns it to the blood or metabolizes it.

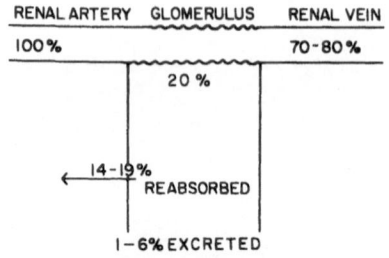

RENAL ARTERY GLOMERULUS   RENAL VEIN

100%   70-80%

20%

14-19% REABSORBED

1-6% EXCRETED

PHYSIOLOGIC FEATURES

1) 90-95% BLOOD CITRATE ULTRAFILTERABLE
2) 5- 30% FILTERED LOAD EXCRETED ($C_{cit} < C_{cr}$)
3) PROXIMAL TUBULE REABSORPTIVE SITE
4) PROXIMAL TUBULE UTILIZES LUMINAL AND
   PERITUBULAR CITRATE
5) NET UTILIZATION OF CITRATE

Fig. 1. Handling of citrate by the human renal kidney.

Table 1. Causes of Altered Citrate Excretion.

1. Acid-base changes
2. Blood bicarbonate concentration
3. Potassium depletion
4. Volume expansion
5. Acetazolamide
6. Starvation
7. Organic acids
8. Metabolic inhibitors
9. Magnesium
10. Vitamin D
11. ? PTH, calcium, estrogens

Table 2. Effects of Metabolic Acidosis and Alkalosis on Renal
Cortex and Plasma Concentrations of Citrate.

Condition	pH	Blood Total CO_2 (mM)	Citrate (mM)	Renal Cortex Citrate (μmol/g)
Acidosis	7.18	9.3	0.087	0.154
Control	7.44	20.5	0.141	0.351
Alkalosis	7.54	30.6	0.147	0.881

RENAL CITRATE UTILIZATION

The fate of citrate utilized by the kidney is uncertain. A large proportion is converted to CO_2 and H_2O. It is not well appreciated that in the isolated perfused kidney addition of citrate to glucose, pyruvate or lactate in the perfusate causes a reduction in fractional sodium excretion[3]. This decrease is associated with enhanced calcium reabsorption and decreased excretion. In general, citrate excretion, not utilization is measured. No systematic studies have been performed examining citrate utilization in stone formation.

Active transporters of citrate have been identified on proximal tubule basolateral and luminal membranes[4]. Although unanswered questions exist, most investigators feel the basolateral transporter is electroneutral while the luminal surface transporter is electrogenic. Citrate transport into the proximal cell may be rate limiting since cell entry precedes metabolism. Extracellular acid-base conditions affect both transporters[5]. Inside the cell the citrate enters the mitochondrion where it is metabolized[5].

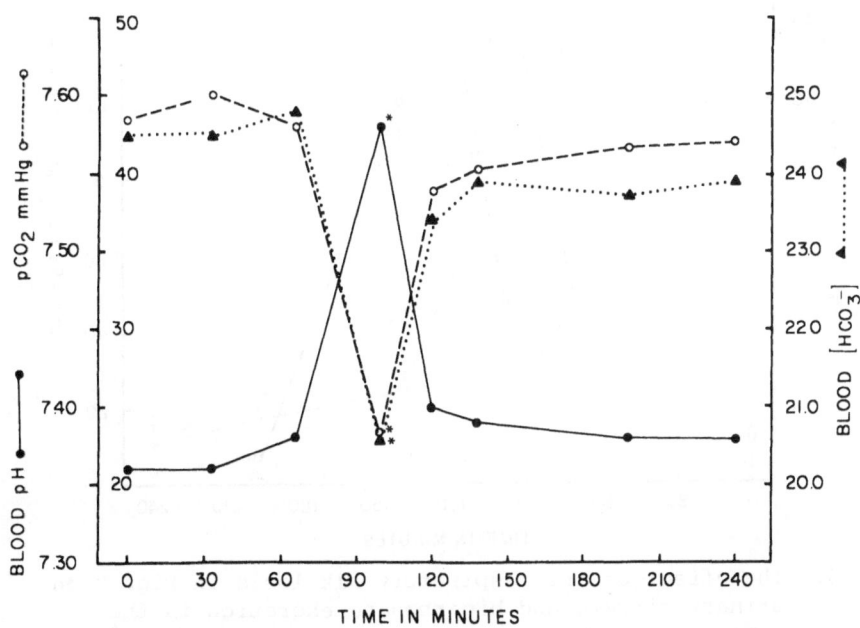

Fig. 2. Blood acid-base parameters during respiratory alkalosis induced in 6 normal subjects by voluntary hyperventilation (* differ from control P < 0.01).

CAUSES OF ALTERED CITRATE EXCRETION

Table 1 lists the factors altering citrate excretion. Table 2 shows data obtained on the effect of acid-base balance on rat renal cortical citrate content[6].   Acidosis lowered citrate content while alkalosis raised it.   These changes appear to be due to altered tubular cell utilization.   Thus, when rat renal cortical slices are incubated at different levels of bicarbonate or different levels of CO_2 tension, citrate decarboxylation is altered.   Acidosis increases decarboxylation while alkalosis decreases it.   Published data show that acidic media increase brush border citrate transport. Recently, it has also been reported that brush border vesicles obtained from chronically acidotic animals show increased citrate transport in vitro even when medium pH is unaltered[7].   Citrate movement into the cell from the peritubular side is also enhanced by acidosis.   Thus, acidosis increases citrate entry into the cell. If this were unaccompanied by increased utilization, cell citrate content would increase.   Yet, renal cortical citrate content falls in acidosis owing to increased cellular citrate metabolism.

Unpublished data from our laboratory demonstrate how rapidly acid-base changes may affect citrate excretion.   Six normal men

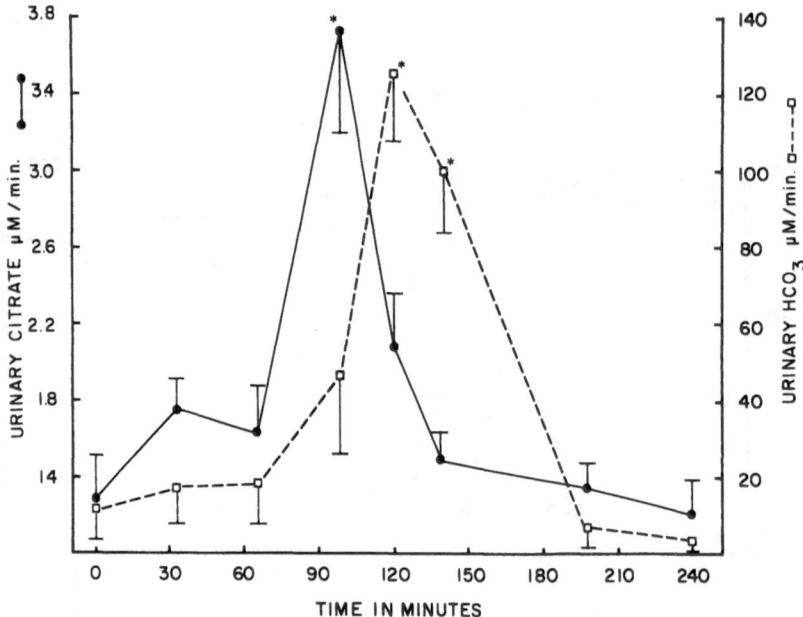

Fig. 3. The effect of the respiratory alkalosis in Fig. 2 on urinary citrate and bicarbonate excretion in the 6 subjects. Each bar indicates the mean ± SEM (*differ from control P < 0.01).

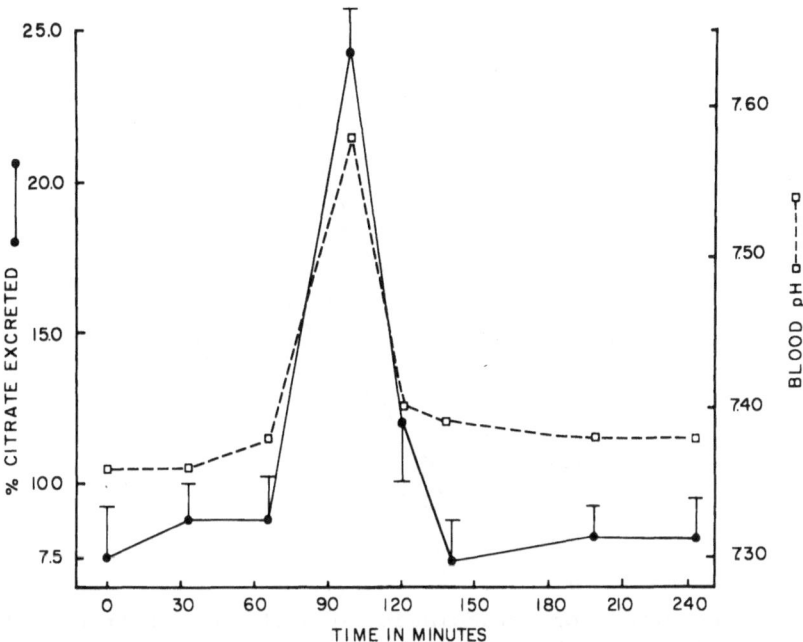

Fig. 4. The correlation between changes in blood pH and urinary
citrate excretion during respiratory alkalosis in the
6 subjects. Each bar indicates the mean ± SEM.

were studied in the resting state, then during 15 min of voluntary
hyperventilation followed by a recovery period.   Fig. 2 shows the
respiratory alkalosis induced during the hyperventilation period and
the rapid return of blood acid-base parameters during recovery.
Fig. 3 shows that both urinary citrate and bicarbonate rose during
respiratory alkalosis.   The increase in citrate excretion preceded
that of bicarbonate and returned to baseline before bicarbonate.
Fig. 4 shows the correlation between changes in blood pH and urinary
citrate. This phenomenon could be important in physiologic states
such as sleep during which a respiratory acidosis occurs.

Is pH the only blood acid-base parameter that affects citrate
excretion?   No. The second through fifth causes shown in Table 1
are examples of conditions in which acid-base changes affect citrate
excretion.   Potassium depletion, for example, reduces citrate
excretion despite concomitant metabolic alkalosis, possibly due to
accompanying renal intracellular acidosis.   When we isohydrically
raised or lowered the blood bicarbonate concentration in rats with
differing potassium states, citrate excretion rose when bicarbonate
was elevated and decreased when it was lowered despite constancy of
blood pH in all animals[8].   Similarly, when rats were volume
expanded[9] with mannitol or saline, which lowered the blood

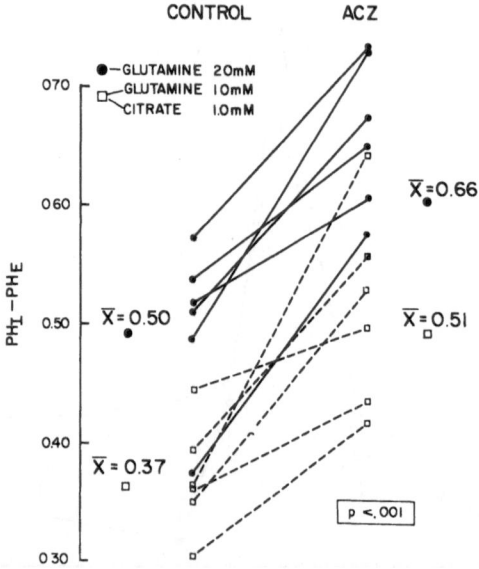

Fig. 5. The effect of actazolamide (0.5 mM) on the transcellular pH
gradient in isolated rat renal tubular cells. Cell pH was
determined from the distribution of ^{14}C-DMO.

bicarbonate concentration at a constant blood pH, citrate excretion
decreased despite an increased filtered load. This decrease in
citrate excretion was not caused by the expansion per se. When
rats were expanded with a saline-bicarbonate solution to prevent a
reduction in blood bicarbonate concentration, urinary citrate
excretion was increased not decreased. Blood pH remained constant.
Similarly, in acidotic rats where volume expansion did not lower the
bicarbonate concentration or change pH, citrate excretion was
increased. These data show that bicarbonate, independent of blood
pH alters citrate excretion; decreasing it when bicarbonate is
reduced.

Acetazolamide reduces citrate excretion in humans. Although
most investigators have assumed that the accompanying metabolic
acidosis is responsible, it has been suggested that acetazolamide
may directly lower tubular cell pH[5]. To investigate this problem,
we incubated isolated rat renal tubules in the presence or absence
of acetazolamide. As shown in Fig. 5, acetazolamide increased cell
pH. Fig. 6 shows citrate utilization was simultaneously decreased
suggesting that intracellular alkalosis reduced citrate utilization.
Other metabolic parameters were measured in these tubules and the
rise in cell pH caused changes in glutamine, glutamate, and ammonia
metabolism consistent with the effect of cellular alkalosis[10]. As
reductions in citrate utilization should increase citrate excretion

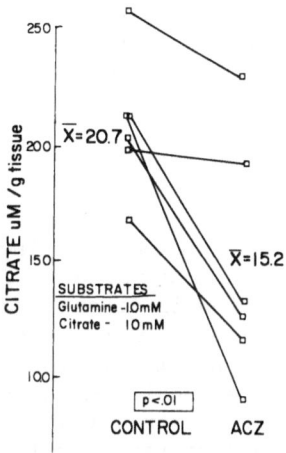

Fig. 6. Effect of acetazolamide on the utilization of medium
citrate by isolated rat renal tubular cells incubated with
1.0 mM glutamine and 1.0 mM citrate as substrates.

we conclude that the reduction in citrate excretion in patients
taking acetazolamide is not due to the effect of the drug on cell
pH. The data suggest that decreased citrate excretion in patients
taking acetazolamide is due to the systemic metabolic acidosis.
Our experiments in vitro were acute, so chronic experiments give a
different result. Although various models have been proposed, the
precise mechanism by which cell pH regulates citrate metabolism is
unknown. The most commonly accepted model, proposed by Simpson,
suggests that the major rate limiting step in the proximal tubular
citrate utilization is the pH gradient across the renal
mitochondrial membrane[5]. Our results support his conclusion,
particularly recent data obtained using isolated rabbit renal
tubules showing that lowering extracellular pH increased the
transmitochondrial pH gradient[11].

Table 1 shows other causes of altered citrate excretion.
Organic acids, metabolic inhibitors and vitamin D, all affect
citrate excretion[5]. The relationship to renal stone disease
remains uncertain. There are data suggesting citrate excretion is
higher in women than men and that this difference may be related to
estrogens[12,13]. During the estrogen portion of the menstrual cycle
citrate excretion appears to increase. There is a suggestion that
low estrogen states are associated with reduced citrate excretion.
In parathyroid disease correlations are difficult to ascertain. In
primary hyperparathyroidism both normal and decreased citrate
excretion have been reported in patients with renal calculi[14].
However, only citrate excretion has been measured, not citrate
utilization, and the latter may be important for regulating the
excretion of calcium or other substances. The effect of starvation

and G.I. malabsorption on citrate have been carefully studied. Both blood and urinary citrate fall in patients with these disorders[2]. Urinary citrate excretion returns to normal when magnesium and citrate are given, but eithr given alone does not restore normal urinary excretion. These observations may explain, at least partially, the high incidence of stones found in patients with malabsorption.

In conclusion, much is known regarding urinary citrate excretion. In humans it varies markedly from individual to individual and its regulation is determined largely by proximal tubular cell transport and metabolism. Active citrate transport occurs on both the luminal and basolateral sides of the proximal cell and cellular acid-base conditions help regulate citrate utilization. Many factors alter citrate excretion, particularly acid-base conditions, blood citrate levels, gastrointestinal citrate absorption, magnesium and hormones. In at least one instance the change in citrate excretion occurs within minutes. Each of the factors enumerated may be important for the pathogenesis of renal stone disease.

REFERENCES

1. D. Rudman, M. H. Kutner, S. C. Redd, II, W. C. Waters, G. G. Gerron, and J. Bleier, J. Clin. Endocrinol. Metab. 55:1052 (1982).
2. D. Rudman, J. L. Dedonis, M. T. Fountain, J. B. Chandler, G. G. Gerron, G. R. Fleming, and M. H. Kutner, New Engl. J. Med. 303:657 (1982).
3. W. H. Waugh and T. Kubo, Am. J. Physiol. 217:277 (1969).
4. K. E. Jorgensen, U. Krasgh-Hensen, H. Roigaard-Peterson, and M. I. Sheikh, Am. J. Physiol. 244:F686 (1983).
5. D. P. Simpson, Am. J. Physiol. 244:F223 (1983).
6. S. Adler, B. Anderson, and L. Zemotel, Am. J. Physiol. 220:989 (1971).
7. A. D. Jenkins, T. P. Dousa, and L. H. Smith, Kidney Int. 25:266 (1984).
8. D. S. Fraley and S. Adler, Proc. Soc. Exp. Biol. Med. 157:393 (1978).
9. S. Adler, D. S. Fraley, and B. Zett, Kidney Int. 20:475 (1981).
10. V. B. Delaney and S Adler, Kidney Int. 25:274 (1984).
11. S. Adler, E. Shoubridge, and G. K. Radda, Clin. Res. 31:514A (1983).
12. S. G. Welshman and M. G. McGeown, Br. J. Urol. 48:7 (1976).
13. M. Menon and C. J. Mahle, J. Urol. 129:1158 (1983).
14. P. O. Schwille, D. Scholz, M. Paulus, W. Engelhardt, and A. Sigel, Invest. Urol. 16:457 (1979).

THE RENAL HANDLING OF CITRATE

P. Deetjen

Institute of Physiology, 6010 Innsbruck, Austria

Second-year medical students already know that citric acid is
an especially valuable substance.   They learn that of the metabolic
processes in the body, the "citric acid cycle" is of utmost
importance: not only is this the final metabolic pathway of glucose
but also it is the pathway for many other substrates.   Thus, nobody
will doubt that citrate is a valuable metabolic substrate.
However, against all expectations the kidney seems to handle this
substance rather carelessly. Examination of the total urinary
output shows a daily loss of more than 3 mmol which is 5 times the
amount contained in plasma or approximately the entire pool in the
total extracellular fluid.   But we also know that Mother Nature is
not wasteful. All other substrates and fuels in our metabolism are
preserved most carefully and only traces of glucose, amino acids,
fatty acids, and the like appear in urine.

A urologist will not hesitate to give a reasonable explanation
for this peculiar behavior of citrate.   Citrate is a potent
chelator of calcium. Thus, citrate in the tubular fluid reduces the
concentration of ionized calcium and decreases the risk of
precipitation of calcium concrements in tubular fluid and in urine.
However, this is the teleologic view of a well-informed urologist.
But, how does the kidney know about these connections?

Citric acid has a simple chemical structure. It is a
tricarboxylic acid of which at physiological pH more than 90% is
completely ionized. This means that it appears mainly as a
trivalent anion (Fig. 1). Organic anions are handled in a rather
complex manner in the kidney. They often show a certain degree of
protein-binding, particularly to albumen. This also has been
claimed to be true for citrate. However, these studies were

181

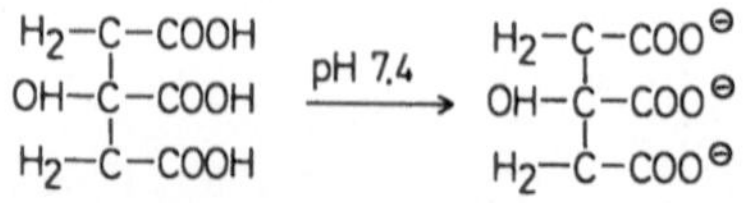

Fig. 1. pH-dependent dissociation of citric acid.

performed in vitro at room temperature[1]. It was not taken into account that plasma protein-binding decreases with increasing temperature. Measured at $37^{\circ}C$, citrate concentration in the glomerular ultrafiltrate approaches that of plasma water, thus, the triple-charged citrate ion circulates in blood unbound to larger molecules and is freely filtered at the glomerulus.

Also, many weak organic acids are extracted from the peritubular blood and are accumulated in the tubular fluid along the proximal tubule. The classical standard substance to study the secretion process is p-amino hippurate (PAH). Twenty years ago we introduced the method of continuous micro-perfusion of single nephron segments in vivo to determine quantitatively the kinetic constants of PAH secretion[2]. With increasing plasma concentrations, the proximal tubular fluid concentration increases proportionally to an approximately 5 times higher concentration (Fig. 2). If this maximum is reached, a further increase in plasma concentration apparently leads to depression of the secretory mechanism and does not augment tubular fluid concentration further.

At about the same time stop-flow experiments in dogs showed that proximal citrate secretion was detectable when ^{14}C-labelled precursors of citrate were infused[3]. However, it also was noted that simultaneous reabsorption of citrate took place in the proximal tubule and that this reabsorption was more effective than secretion[3,4]. Such a bidirectional transport of organic anions along the proximal tubule is not an unusual feature. A well studied example is urate. This also has drawn considerable attention from urologists since it belongs to the concrement-forming substances. Some years ago we performed continuous microperfusion experiments in rats to measure the bidirectional fluxes of urate[5]. Fig. 2 summarizes the findings and shows how urate is filtered and reabsorbed, but also secreted, along the proximal tubule.

Similar experiments to study the kinetic properties of the bidirectional movement of citrate were jeopardized by some uncontrolled factors. The proximal tubular cells were not only able to synthetize but also to degrade citrate[6,7]. Thus, transport studies at the tubular level did not help to clarify the underlying mechanisms. In this situation we received help from studies using the technique of membrane vesicles and the new techniques of ion-sensitive electrodes that allow measurements of intracellular ion activities.

182

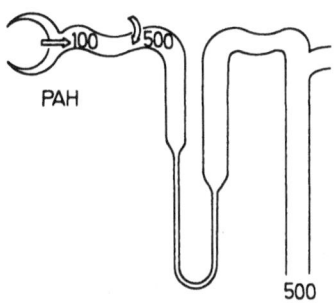

PAH

500

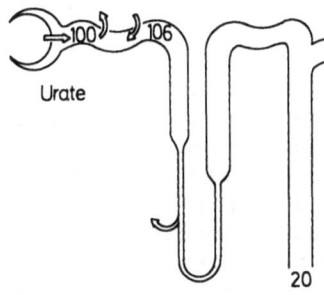

Urate

20

Fig. 2.   Renal handling and balance of organic anions. Top: p-amino
          hippurate (PAH) as an example of a substance which is
          filtered and secreted. Bottom:Urate as an example of a
          substance which is filtered and secreted but also undergoes
          reabsorption along the proximal tubule and in Henle's loop.

     In the vesicle technique either brushborder or basolateral
membranes are isolated from isotonic homogenates of rat kidneys by
differential centrifugation.   The membrane fractions
spontaneously form vesicles.   The composition of the intra- and
extravesicular spaces can be manipulated, allowing analysis of the
driving forces for transport.   The method offers the advantage not
only of studying the transport properties of the brush border or the
basolateral membrane separately but also of studying it free of
metabolic reactions.

     In a series of elegant studies Wright et al[8-11] have elaborated
the transport characteristics of the brush border membrane for
citric acid cycle substrates.   They were able to demonstrate that
the major tricarboxylic acid cycle intermediates, including citrate,
are transported from the renal tubular filtrate into the cell via a
common Na^+-dependent system.   Among these intermediates, succinate
had the greatest affinity.   The transport of both succinate, a
dicarboxylic acid, and of citrate, a tricarboxylic acid, depolarized

183

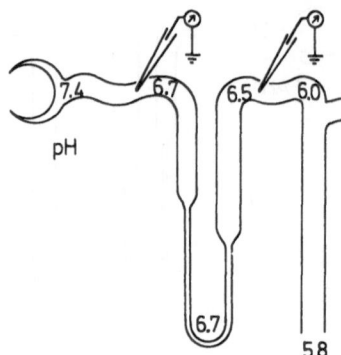

Fig. 3. pH values in tubular fluid along the nephron[12].

the brush border membrane. Thus, the transport of these ions
caused a positive charge to be translocated. However, both
substances are polyvalent anions and, if transported as such,
hyperpolarization of the membrane would be expected. This apparent
contradiction was solved by the finding that 3 Na^+ ions were
transported per substrate molecule. But even with this
stoichiometry only the transport of the divalent succinate is
electrogenic while that of the trivalent citrate would be
electroneutral. The solution of this inconsistency came from the
observation that citrate transport is largely dependent on tubular
fluid pH. Lowering the pH from 7.5 to 5.5 increases the transport
rate 10-fold, while this manoeeuver has almost no effect on
succinate uptake. At a neutral pH of 7.4, citrate is almost
completely ionized. Since the pK_a values are 3.1, 4.8 and 6.4,
respectively, the concentration of divalent citrate will increase
considerably when the pH of tubular fluid is reduced.

We have measured the profile of tubular pH under free-flow
conditions using pH-sensitive glass electrodes[12]. As Fig. 3
demonstrates, there is already in the proximal convolution a
significant drop to pH 6.7. Applying the Henderson-Hasselbalch
equation to citrate dissociation, it can be calculated that by
reducing pH from 7.4 to 6.7, the dissociation of trivalent citrate
is reduced from 93% to 67%. This results in a 5-fold increase in
divalent citrate which apparently is accepted by the succinate
transporter (Fig. 4). Reabsorption of divalent citrate will
immediately lead to new transformation of tri- to divalent citrate
to maintain the 2:1 relation dictated by the tubular fluid pH. In
this way citrate is sufficiently reabsorbed, but never as
effectively and completely as succinate. On the other hand,
reabsorption is sensitive to all changes in tubular pH. This is in
good agreement with many reports in the literature that an increase
in tubular pH augments citrate excretion[13].

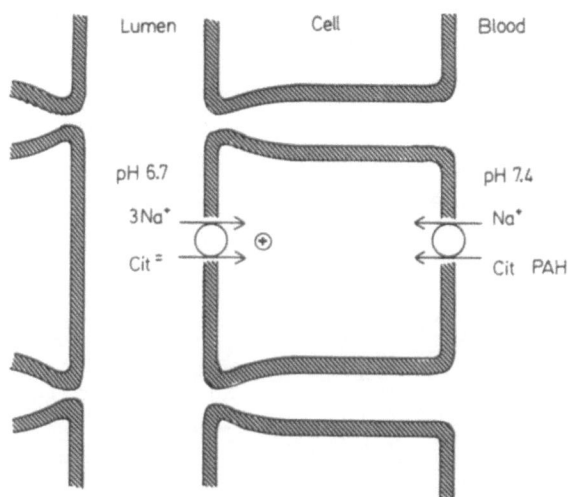

Fig. 4.   Citrate co-transport in the luminal and the basolateral
          membrane of proximal tubular cells.

     At the peritubular membrane of proximal tubular cells a similar
system seems to operate[14,15].   It also transports tricarboxylic
acid cycle intermediates into the cell (Fig. 4).   It is driven by an
Na^+ gradient and is electrogenic, carrying a positive charge.
However, it has a different pH sensitivity.   Transport is maximally
accelerated between pH 7.4 and 8.2.   In contrast to the luminal
membrane, maximal transport occurs against a proton gradient.
Furthermore the basolateral transport system exhibits competitive
inhibition with PAH and other organic anions while the luminal
system does not.   The intimate linkage of transmembranal citrate
movement to Na^+ fluxes gives some insight into the driving forces.

     The recent development of ion-sensitive microelectrodes by us
and others[16] has helped to enlarge our knowledge on the
intracellular activity of all major ions, their transmembranal
fluxes and their interdependence and coupling.   All transport
systems seem to be energized (Fig. 5) directly or indirectly by the
Na^+/K^+-ATPase localised at the basolateral membrane.   This Na^+-K^+-
exchange pump accumulates K^+ in the cell and is the main source of
the electrical polarization of the cell membrane.   The pump keeps
intracellular Na^+ on a low level which creates a Na^+ gradient and
establishes the driving force for all the Na^+ coupled transport
systems[17].   From the total net reabsorbed Na^+ ions, 2/3 are
channeled through the paracellular shunts and only 1/3 goes through
the cell itself and is actively extruded at the basolateral
membrane.   However, it is this fraction that creates the driving
force for the transmembranal movement of all other substances
including citrate.

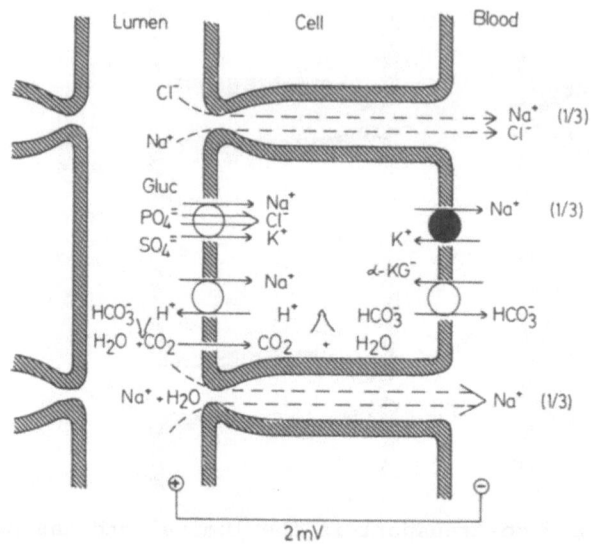

Fig. 5. Transmembranal ion fluxes and transport coupling in
proximal tubular cells.

A compilation of all data available at present allows the
formulation of a model for the tubular handling of citrate.
Citrate is almost freely filtered, with a net reabsorption occurring
in the proximal tubule (Fig. 6). Urinary excretion, therefore, is
restricted and the excretion rate is less than 1/3 of the filtered
load.   Due to the high filtration rate, however, renal citrate
excretion accumulates to a quantity which is equal to the amount
present in the total extracellular fluid volume. With increasing
tubular fluid pH there is an increase in urinary citrate excretion.

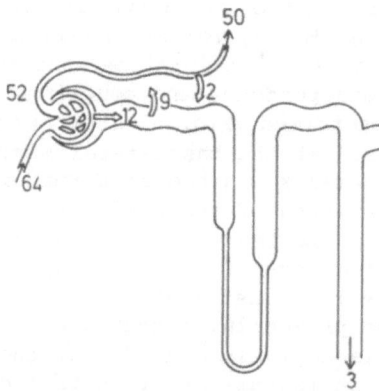

Fig. 6. Renal handling and balance of citrate (adapted from
reference 7).

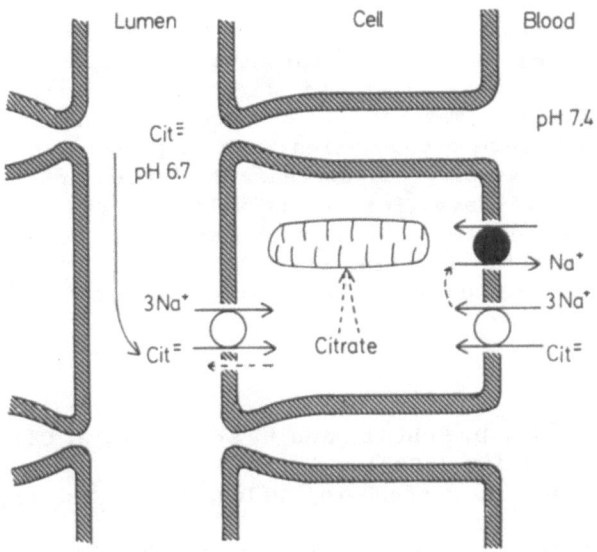

Fig. 7. Model of citrate handling in proximal tubular cells.

Unlike most other tissues the tubular cells are able to utilize
citrate as a substrate for their metabolic processes[7]. Together
with the liver, the kidney is the most important site for the
regulation of plasma citrate as well as of other tricarboxylic acid
cycle metabolites[18,19]. The proximal tubular cells ensure their
sufficient supply with these fuels by specific transport systems on
both the luminal and basolateral sides (Fig. 7). The transport is
coupled to Na^+ and dependent on active Na^+ transport. It receives
its driving force from the Na^+ gradient, directed from the
extracellular spaces into the cell. With 3 Na^+ ions, one molecule
of citrate is transported. For the luminal cell membrane it was
shown that citrate is transported as a bivalent anion. Transport,
therefore, is electrogenic and tends to depolarize the cell.
Citrate transport at the basolateral membrane operates in a similar
way but may exhibit some differences. It is still controversial
whether citrate along this membrane surface is transported in a tri-
or divalent form and, therefore, is electrogenic or not[14,20]. If
the latter is true, it is noteworthy that the concentration of
divalent citrate at neutral pH of 7.4 is only 1/5 of that at the
luminal side and that transport rates at both membranes differ
according to the same proportion. The metabolic utilization of
citrate within the cell seems to be the dominant reaction. Under
normal conditions it masks the potential ability of these cells to
extract citrate from the blood and to secrete it into the urine.
Such a capacity, however, can be demonstrated when poorly
metabolized analogs are used[14,15], or when the infusion of
precursors like succinate, fumarate or maleate increase

intracellular citrate syntheses[4,6,18]. Reduction of the basolateral citrate uptake by a possible competitive inhibition with other organic anions may also alter significantly the intracellular citrate equilibrium. The rate of citrate transport is limited by the fact that citrate dissociation is pH-dependent. Under control conditions, the physiological decrease of luminal pH is sufficient to render enough citrate from the trivalent to the bivalent form to enable bulk reabsorption. With increases in pH, however, citrate buffering becomes the limiting step and greater fractions of the filtered load remain unreabsorbed in the tubular fluid.

REFERENCES

1. P. O. Schwille, D. Scholz, and K. Schwille, J. Clin. Chem. Clin. Biochem. 2):169 (1982).
2. P. Deetjen and H. Sonnenberg, Pflüg. Arch. Ges. Physiol. 278:48 (1963).
3. Y. J. Kook and W. D. Lotspeich, Am. J. Physiol. 215:282 (1968).
4. A. P. Grollman, W. G. Walker, H. C. Harrison, and H. E. Harrison, Am. J. Physiol. 205:697 (1963).
5. R. Greger, F. Lang, and P. Deetjen, in:"International Review of Physiology", K. Thurau, ed., University Park Press, Baltimore (1973).
6. S. Baruch, R. L. Burich, and V. F. King, Am. J. Physiol. 225:388 (1973).
7. H. Nieth and P. Schollmeyer, Nature, 209:1244 (1966).
8. S. H. Wright, I. Kippen, J. R. Klinenberg, and E. M. Wright, J. Membr. Biol. 57:73 (1980).
9. S. H. Wright, S. Krasne, I. Kippen, and E. M. Wright, Biochim. Biophys. Acta 640:767 (1981).
10. S. H. Wright, I. Kippen, and E. M. Wright, Biochim. Biophys. Acta 684:287 (1982).
11. S. H. Wright, I. Kippen, and E. M. Wright, J. Biol. Chem. 257:1773 (1982).
12. F. Lang, S. Silbernagl, and P. Quehenberger, in:"Hydrogen Ion Transport in Epithelia", J. Schulz, ed., Biomedical Press, Elsevier, North-Holland (1980).
13. D. P. Simpson, Am. J. Physiol. 244:F223 (1983).
14. G. Burckhardt, Pflüg. Arch. Ges. Physiol. (in press).
15. K. J. Ullrich, H. Fasold, G. Rumrich, and S. Klöss, Pflüg. Arch. Ges. Physiol. (in press).
16. F. Lang, G. Messner, W. Wang, and H. Oberleithner, Klin. Wschr. 61:1029 (1983).
17. F. Lang, G. Messner, W. Wang, W. Paulmichl, H. Oberleithner, and P. Deetjen, Pflüg. Arch. Ges. Physiol. (in press).
18. M. A. Crawford, Biochem. J. 88:115 (1970).
19. B. H. Selleck and J. J. Cohen, Am. J. Physiol. 208:24 (1965).
20. K. E. Joergensen, K. Kragh-Hansen, H. Roigaard-Petersen, and M. J. Sheikh, Am. J. Physiol. 244:F686 (1983).

EFFECTS OF METABOLIC ACIDOSIS AND ALKALOSIS ON THE RENAL

BRUSH BORDER MEMBRANE TRANSPORT OF CITRATE

A. D. Jenkins, T. P. Dousa, and L. H. Smith

Nephrology Research Unit, Mayo Clinic, Rochester
Minnesota, U.S.A.

INTRODUCTION

The systemic acidosis in patients with distal renal tubular acidosis (RTA) may be responsible for the hypocitraturia[1]. The ability of renal mitochondria to metabolize citrate via the tricarboxylic acid cycle is thought to control the renal clearance of citrate. Metabolic acidosis increases the entry of citrate into the matrix space of mitochondria, cytoplasmic citrate levels fall, reabsorption of citrate from tubular fluid is enhanced, and less citrate appears in the final urine. Metabolic alkalosis has an opposite effect[1].

The influx of citrate from tubular fluid across the luminal membrane should influence cytoplasmic citrate levels. The luminal brush border membrane (BBM) of proximal tubular cells is equipped with a Na^+-gradient-dependent transport system for citrate[2]. In vitro lowering of the extravesicular pH increases citrate uptake into renal BBM vesicles[3]. The effects of in vivo metabolic acidosis or alkalosis on the BBM transport of citrate, however, have not been studied. Chronic exposure to the acidotic state may affect the BBM transport systems in a different way than pH status in vitro.

METHODS

Adult male Sprague-Dawley rats were allowed free access to a standard rat diet and were given distilled water from experimental Day 1 through experimental Day 6. Individual 24-h urine specimens (Initial) were collected from Day 5 to Day 6 for the measurement of

189

citrate excretion. The animals were then divided into 3 groups (3 to 4 rats/group) having similar mean citrate excretions. From Day 6 through Day 12, each group was maintained on drinking water containing 5% dextrose, and either 150 mM NH_4Cl (acidosis), 150 mM NaCl (control), or 150 mM $NaHCO_3$ (alkalosis). A final set of 24-h urine specimens were collected from Day 11 to Day 12. On Day 12, central venous blood samples were drawn, and the kidneys were removed for the preparation of BBM vesicles.

BBM vesicles for each group were prepared from renal cortex by the calcium precipitation method[4]. The uptake of citrate in the presence of a Na^+ gradient (outside inside) was measured by the rapid filtration technique[4]. The final concentration of citrate in the incubation medium was 0.1 mM. Uptake was measured in triplicate at each time point (20 s, 2.5 min, and 120 min), and the mean was entered as n=1. A total of 5 such experiments were performed. Multiple pairwise comparisons were made between the 3 experimental groups using Student's t-test.

RESULTS

Initial urinary citrate excretion was 41 ± 5 mg/24 h in each of the 3 groups (Table 1). Final citrate excretion was lower in the acidotic rats, unchanged in the control rats, and higher in the alkalotic rats. The changes in fractional citrate excretion (FE) were parallel to the changes in total citrate excretion.

Na^+-gradient-dependent uptake of citrate (pmol/mg protein/2.5 min; mean $\pm$ SEM) was greater in the acidotic group (411 ± 43) than that in the control group (204 ± 40, P<0.001, paired t-test) and that in the alkalotic group (164 ± 19, P<0.005, paired t-test). No significant difference was found between the alkalotic group and the control group.

Table 1. Effect of Metabolic Acid-Base Manipulation on Urinary Citrate Excretion (mean $\pm$ SEM).

Group	Initial (I) (mg/24 h)	Final* (F) (mg/24 h)	I vs. F (paired t-test)	FE (%) (Final)
Acidosis	41 ± 5	1.4 ± 0.4	<0.005	2.3
Control	41 ± 5	40 ± 2	ns	44
Alkalosis	41 ± 5	128 ± 7	<0.001	114

*P < 0.001 for acidosis vs control; acidosis vs alkalosis; or control vs alkalosis

DISCUSSION

Metabolic alkalosis raises urinary citrate excretion, while metabolic acidosis lowers it[5]. These effects are accompanied by changes in renal cortical citrate levels and are due to an alteration of intrarenal citrate handling, since plasma citrate levels and the glomerular filtration rate do not change appreciably[1,5].

In the present study, the induction of a mild metabolic acidosis with NH_4Cl resulted in a dramatic fall in citrate excretion and FE. Metabolic alkalosis induced with $NaHCO_3$ had an opposite effect: citrate excretion and FE tripled.

The most striking effect of metabolic acidosis was on the Na^+-gradient-dependent transport of citrate into BBM vesicles. Na^+-dependent citrate uptake at 2.5 min by BBM vesicles from acidotic rats was double that by BBM vesicles from control or alkalotic rats. Metabolic alkalosis did not significantly depress Na^+-dependent citrate uptake by BBM vesicles. Therefore, increased Na^+-dependent transport of citrate by renal BBM may, in part, be responsible for the increased proximal tubular reabsorption of citrate seen during metabolic acidosis. In contrast, decreased transport of citrate by renal BBM does not appear to be a major factor in the augmentation of the clearance of citrate induced by metabolic alkalosis. Inhibition of intracellular renal citrate metabolism is probably more important in this instance.

REFERENCES

1. D. P. Simpson, Am. J. Physiol. 244:F223 (1982).
2. I. Kippen, B. Hirayama, J. R. Klinenberg, and E. M. Wright, Proc. Natl. Acad. Sci. USA 76:3397 (1979).
3. S. H. Wright, I. Kippen, and E. M. Wright, Biochem. Biophys. Acta 684:287 (1982).
4. L. Cheng and B. Sactor, J. Biol. Chem. 256:1556 (1981).
5. M. A. Crawford, M. D. Milne, and B. H. Scribner, J. Physiol. 149:413 (1959).

RENAL HANDLING OF OXALATE

R. Hautmann and H. Osswald

Depts. of Urology and Pharmacology of the Medical
Faculty Rheinisch-Westfälische Technische Hochschule
Aachen, F.R.G.

INTRODUCTION

At the 3rd International Symposium on Urolithiasis and Related
Clinical Research, Knox stated that research on the renal handling
of oxalate did not match the importance of this substance in
urolithiasis.   Indeed, he noted that the Handbook of Renal
Physiology did not even list oxalate in the index.   The inability
to measure urinary and, in particular, plasma oxalate precisely
undoubtedly accounts for this lack of data[1].

Today, there is general agreement that mild hyperoxaluria is
the major risk factor in the genesis of calcium oxalate stone
disease[2].   Therefore, it is important to know how the kidney
handles and excretes oxalate.   Renal elimination of substances
proceeds via the three mechanisms, glomerular filtration, tubular
secretion and diffusion. The different secretion mechanisms of
oxalate will be discussed based on studies in laboratory animals and
how these observations relate to findings in man.   Knowledge of the
renal handling of oxalate in man, although limited at present, is
important in the understanding of the contribution of oxalate to the
supersaturation of urine with calcium oxalate.

GLOMERULAR FILTRATION

Several studies show that plasma oxalate is filtered freely by
the glomerulus.   No protein binding of ^{14}C-oxalate has been
observed[3-5].   If oxalate exists in plasma as a doubly negatively
charged ion, one would predict from the Donnan potential that the
oxalate concentration in the ultrafiltrate would be slightly higher

than that in the plasma. Micropuncture data, however, have demonstrated an ultrafiltrate to plasma ratio of oxalate of 1.0. Therefore it appears to be valid to calculate the filtered load of oxalate from the measured plasma levels.

The filtered load of oxalate (F_{ox}) is the product of plasma oxalate (P_{ox}) and the rate of glomerular filtration (GFR). Since accurate measurement of plasma oxalate is difficult and conflicting data have been reported, one can use approximate estimations from the ^{14}C-oxalate pharmacokinetics, ^{14}C-oxalate clearance and urinary oxalate excretion to calculate plasma oxalate in man. The most reliable measurement amongst these is the oxalate concentration in urine. Therefore, to minimize the uncertainty of the assumptions, the calculation of plasma oxalate concentration should take into consideration the amount of oxalate excreted in the urine, since the concentration of oxalate in urine is high compared with that in plasma. F_{ox} also equals the ratio of the excreted amount of oxalate to the fractional excretion of oxalate. The fractional excretion of oxalate (FE_{ox}) is defined by the ratio of the clearance of ^{14}C-oxalate divided by GFR, where the renal clearance of oxalate (C_{ox}) is determined from the ^{14}C isotope concentration in plasma and urine and the GFR. Tracer clearance methods are extremely accurate. The renal clearance of the ^{14}C-labeled compound is identical to the clearance of the unlabeled compound since oxalate is not metabolized in mammals[6,7].

With a daily oxalate excretion of 0.3 mmol and a fractional excretion of oxalate of 1.4, the filtered load of oxalate is 0.21 mmol/24 h and the calculated plasma oxalate concentration is 1.2 μmol/l. Thus, the filtered load of oxalate contributes about 70% of urinary oxalate. The critical concentration of oxalate in the urinary tract, therefore, clearly depends on the plasma oxalate levels and the GFR.

PLASMA OXALATE

Using chemical methods, Akcay and Rose[8] found plasma oxalate levels of 2.26 μmol/l. Earlier reported plasma levels were between 15 to 100 μmol/l[4,9-12]. Since there is little evidence that filtered oxalate undergoes net tubular reabsorption to a significant extent, the true plasma oxalate concentration is in the range of 1 to 2 μmol/l[13] and the filtered load of oxalate between 0.17 and 0.35 mmol/24 h in normal man.

OXALATE PHARMACOKINETICS

The measurement of plasma oxalate after rapid intravenous administration of insulin and C^{14}-oxalate in man, resulted in a volume of distribution of oxalate of 32.5 litres. This value corresponds to approximately 65 to 70% of total body water, suggesting that oxalate is not freely diffusible into all body compartments. The volume of distribution of oxalate contains the oxalate pool, averaging 3.7 mg. The pool size is small and, because of the short half-life of elimination of 91.7 min, the turnover of the oxalate pool must be rapid. Inasmuch as 98% of the administered tracer is recovered unchanged in urine, the non-renal loss of oxalate is not appreciable[13,14].

TUBULAR HANDLING

Evidence For Tubular Secretion

The concentration of oxalate in tubular fluid has been studied by several investigators using micropuncture techniques in rats. When the endogenous filtrate was collected along the proximal convolution, most of the data showed higher oxalate concentrations in the tubular fluid compared to inulin, indicating net tubular secretion of oxalate. In isolated perfused tubules of the rabbit kidney, net tubular oxalate secretion was demonstrated[15]. The oxalate to inulin concentration ratios in the distal tubule and in the final urine were close to the values of the late proximal tubule indicating that there is no net secretion of oxalate beyond the proximal convolution. In these studies, the fractional excretion of oxalate into the final urine were close to the values of the late proximal tubule indicating that there is no net secretion of oxalate beyond the proximal convolution. In these studies, the fractional excretion of oxalate into the final urine was between 1.09 and 1.28. This means that only between 9 and 28% of urinary oxalate is derived from net tubular secretion under normal conditions. Table 1 summarizes the findings from rat micropuncture studies[5,16-19].

Table 1. Free-Flow Micropuncture Data. Fractional Oxalate Recovery along the Nephron in Rats (Means ± SEM).

Oxalate Recovery (% Filtered Load)			References
Proximal	Distal	Urine	
120 ± 4 early	121 ± 3	126 ± 3	Weinman et al
125 ± 6 late	-	-	
126 ± 4 late	-	128 ± 3	Knight et al
130 ± 3 late	-	127 ± 2	
109 ± 2	111 ± 3	109 ± 2	Greger et al
86 ± 5	81 ± 3	120 ± 10	Hautmann and Osswald

Table 2. The Renal Clearance of Oxalate (Adapted from Greger[29]).

Substance	Dose (mmol/kg)	C_{Ox}/GFR	Reference
Caronamide	0.1	0.65	Cattell et al
Chlorothiazide	0.06	1.05	Knight et al
Furosemide	0.06	1.05	Knight et al
Hydrochlorothiazide	0.03	1.00	Greger et al
Indanyl-oxyacetic acid	0.2[a]	1.09	Knight et al
Para-aminohippurate	1.45	0.91	Greger et al
Para-aminohippurate	0.5-2.5	1.14	Knight et al
Piretanide	0.04	0.88	Greger et al
Probenecid	0.7	1.11	Hautmann and Osswald
Probenecid	0.35	0.90	Greger et al
Urate	0.48[a]	0.90	Greger et al
Urate	0.25[a]	1.04	Knight et al

a: No accurate value since prime was followed by constant infusion. (Caronamide was tested in dogs, all other data were obtained in rats.)

The mechanism by which oxalate is secreted by the epithelium of the proximal tubule seems to be somewhat different from the known organic anion secretion pathway. As shown in Table 2, many substances known to be secreted by the organic anion transport mechanism in the proximal tubule interfere with oxalate secretion. It is apparent that all of these substances decrease fractional oxalate clearance. Values below 1 indicate tubular reabsorption. However, probenecid has only a small effect on oxalate excretion, although this substance is a potent blocker of p-aminohippurate secretion. Also the location of probenecid-sensitive anion secretion is different from that of oxalate secretion, which is highest in S_1, the early proximal tubule, and lowest in S_3, the straight part of the proximal tubule segment. This is the opposite of the situation for PAH transport[15].

Tubular oxalate secretion in man was studied using the Chinard method, where oxalate was injected together with inulin into the renal artery, and followed by urine collection at 30 sec intervals. It was found that urinary oxalate excretion exceeded that of inulin by a factor of 2.3. This was interpreted as being indicative of net tubular secretion of oxalate, since it was found using the same technique in dogs that probenecid and PAH reduced oxalate recovery in the urine[20]. Thus there is good evidence that the proximal tubular secretion of oxalate is dependent on active transport and can be inhibited by a variety of substances also secreted into the proximal tubule. However, the exact mechanism of transtubular oxalate transport awaits elucidation.

Evidence for Tubular Rebsorption

When the proximal tubule is perfused with saline containing
[14]-C oxalate, net tubular outflux of oxalate was demonstrated[7].
The outflux of ^{14}C oxalate seemed to be unsaturable and independent
of the chemical concentration of oxalate[19].

In a different series[20], the tubular outflux of oxalate was
enhanced by intravenous infusion of sodium citrate. The effects of
calcium chloride and sodium citrate infusion on oxalate delivery
into the proximal tubule and final urine were compared in
parathyroidectomised Sprague Dawley rats[21]. Sodium citrate
chelates with calcium ions in the tubular fluid and leaves a larger
fraction of oxalate in its ionized form. Ionized oxalate is known
to diffuse readily through biological membranes. It should be
pointed out, that the infused sodium citrate lowered the free
calcium concentration to such an extent that tetanic convulsions
developed after 120 min. Although such low calcium concentrations
in blood and such high citrate loading of the kidney do not occur
under normal conditions, it shows that there is a reported extensive
tubular reabsorption of oxalate in man[22]. However, they are
derived from calculations of clearance data and fractional excretion
of oxalate using erroneously high plasma oxalate levels. Since the
urinary oxalate excretions in these earlier studies compared well
with recent data, the assumption of net tubular reabsorption of
oxalate appears to be a calculation artefact.

To summarize the present knowledge of the tubular handling of
oxalate (Fig. 1); oxalate is freely filtrable at the glomerulus,
there is net tubular secretion of oxalate in the proximal tubule and
only small amounts of oxalate undergo tubular reabsorption under
physiological conditions.

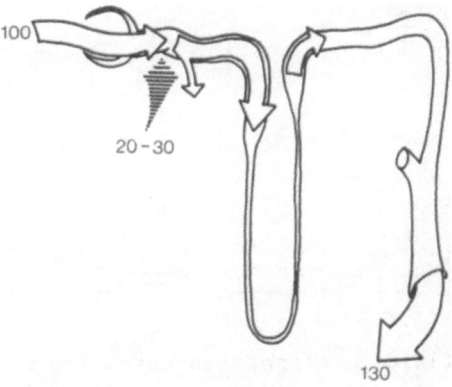

100

20-30

130

Fig. 1. Oxalate transport along the nephron.

Concentration Profiles of Oxalate along the Nephron

To understand calcium oxalate stone formation it is important to know the oxalate concentration at any point of the nephron. Based on the above data on the tubular handling of oxalate, the concentration profile of oxalate can be calculated along the nephron. Fig. 2 shows the tubular fluid to plasma concentration ratio from the Bowman space to the final urine[23]. Note that the concentration ratios at the ordinate are given in a logarithmic scale. It is obvious, that there is a continuous rise in the tubular oxalate concentration reaching its highest value at the duct of Bellini. In terms of concentration gradients, the oxalate concentration in the distal nephron segments exceeds the plasma oxalate concentration by a factor of 300. It is unlikely that supersaturation takes place at the bend of the loop of Henle since the oxalate concentration is only 2- to 3-fold higher than the plasma

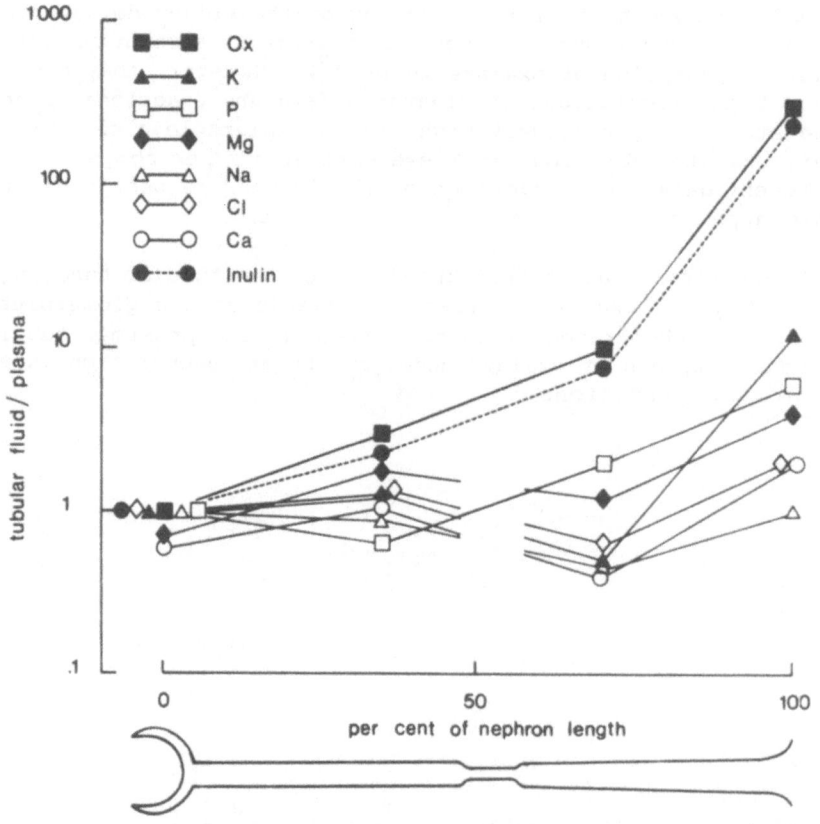

Fig. 2. Tubular fluid to plasma concentration ratio from the Bowman space to the final urine. The absolute concentrations of these substances are given in the Table.

concentration. The most variable concentration of oxalate occurs in the collecting ducts, where there are different rates of water reabsorption, depending on the fluid balance of the body.

Other ions which contribute to crystallization are Mg, P, K, Na, Cl. However, there are not enough data on the tubular concentrations of these ions at the bend of Henle's loop, where Na, K, Cl, Ca, and Mg concentrations can probably increase several-fold over their respective plasma concentrations. Only oxalate undergoes considerable concentration along the nephron compared to inulin. The concentrations of the other solutes, particularly that of calcium, are not much different from their plasma values. Urinary oxalate concentration can also be influenced by diuretic state. If urinary oxalate concentration (U_{ox}) is plotted against the apparent urinary flow rate (Uv)[23], the resulting curve is defined by $U_{ox} = 1/Uv \times GFR \times FE_{ox} \times P_{ox}$. The exponential increase in urinary oxalate concentration during antidiuresis coincides with the increased risk of stone formation in that situation.

OTHER FACTORS THAT INFLUENCE URINARY EXCRETION OF OXALATE IN MAN

Zarembski and Hodgkinson[24] showed the relationship between the daily excretion of calcium and oxalate in normals and in patients with a low and high urinary excretion of calcium, and a direct effect of urinary flow rate on the excretion of oxalate as well as diurnal and daily variations in the urinary excretion of oxalate.

CONCLUSIONS

Our current knowledge on the renal handling of oxalate cannot explain calcium oxalate stone formation, but it predicts that (i) an increase in plasma oxalate leads to an increase in oxalate excretion; (ii) a low urinary flow rate increases urinary oxalate concentration; and (iii) the contribution of other solutes critical to urinary supersaturation of calcium oxalate can now be better assessed from the known tubular oxalate concentrations. From the calculated oxalate concentration profile the primary nucleation site is unlikely to be intranephronic[23]. As we have hypothesized earlier, accumulation of oxalate in the papillary interstititium might be of critical importance in stone formation[25-27].

REFERENCES

1. F. G. Know, R. F. Greger, F. C. Lang, and G. R. Marchand, in:"Urolithiasis Research", H. Fleisch, W. G. Robertson, L. H. Smith and W. Vahlensieck, eds., Plenum, New York (1976).
2. W. G. Robertson, M. Peacock, D. D. Ouimet, P. J. Heyburn, and

A. Rutherford, in:"Urolithiasis: Clinical and Basic Research", L. H. Smith, W. G. Robertson and B. Finlayson, eds., Plenum, New York (1981).

3. W. R. Cattell, A. G. Spencer, G. W. Taylor, and R. W. E. Watts, Clin. Sci. 22:43 (1962).

4. H. E. Williams, G. A. Johnson, and L. H. Smith, Clin. Sci. 41:213 (1978).

5. E. J. Weinmann, S. J. Frankfurt, A. Ince, and S. Samsons, J. Clin. Invest. 61:801 (1978).

6. T. D. Elder, and J. B. Wyngaarden, J. Clin. Invest. 39: 1337 (1960).

7. R. Greger, F. Lang, H. Oberleithner, and P. Deetjen, Pflüger's Arch, 374:243 (1978).

8. T. Akcay and G. A. Rose, Clin. Chim. Acta 101:305 (1980).

9. P. M. Zarembski and A. Hodgkinson, Biochem. J. 96:717 (1965).

10. P. Nuret and M. Offner, Clin. Chim. Acta 82:9 (1978).

11. V. V. S. E. Dutt and H. A. Mottola, Biochem. Med. 9:148 (1974).

12. A. Hodgkinson and R. Wilkinson, Clin. Sci. Mol. Med. 46:61 (1974).

13. R. Hautmann and H. Osswald, Invest. Urol. 16:195 (1979).

14. H. Osswald and R. Hautmann, Urol. Int. 34:440 (1979).

15. H. O. Senekjian and E. J. Weinman, Am. J. Physiol. 243:F271 (1982).

16. T. F. Knight, H. O. Senkjian, and E. J. Weinman, Kidney Int. 15:38 (1979).

17. R. Greger, F. Lang, H. Oberleithner, and H. Sporer, Renal Physiol. 2:57 (1979/80).

18. R. Hautmann and H. Osswald, Fortschr. Urol. Nephrol. 9:7 (1977).

19. R. Hautmann and H. Osswald, Arch. Pharmakol. 304:277 (1978).

20. R. Hautmann, H. Osswald, and W. Lutzeyer, in:"Urolithiasis Research", H. Fleisch, W. G. Robertson, L. H. Smith and W. Vahlensieck, eds., Plenum, New York (1976).

21. H. Osswald, J. A. Haas, R. M. Meyer-Hentschel, and R. Hautmann, in:"Urolithiasis:Clinical and Basic Research", L. H. Smith, W. G. Robertson and B. Finlayson, eds., Plenum, New York (1981).

22. P. M. Zarembski and A. Hodgkinson, Invest. Urol. 1:87 (1963).

23. R. Hautmann and H. Osswald, J. Urol. 129:433 (1983).

24. P. M. Zarembski and A. Hodgkinson, Clin. Chim. Acta 25:1 (1969).

25. R. Hautmann, A. Lehmann, and S. Komor, J. Urol. 123:317 (1980).

26. R. Hautmann, A. Lehmann, and S. Komor, Eur. J. Clin. Invest. 10:173 (1980).

27. R. E. Hautmann, A. Lehmann, and H. Osswald, in:"Urolithiasis:Clinical and Basic Research", L. H. Smith, W. G. Robertson and B. Finlayson, Plenum, New York (1981).

28. T. F. Knight, H. O. Senekjian, K. Taylor, D. A. Steplock, and E. J. Weinman, Kidney Int. 16:572 (1979).

29. R. Greger, in:"Renal Transport of Organic Substances", R. Greger, F. Lang, and S. Silbernagel, eds., Springer Verlag, Berlin (1981).

200

RELATION OF SEVERITY OF RENAL IMPAIRMENT TO TISSUE CALCIUM CONCENTRATION IN THE HUMAN KIDNEY

L. Gimenez, K. Solez, and W. G. Walker

Depts. of Medicine and Pathology, John Hopkins
University School of Medicine and the John Hopkins
Hospital, Baltimore, Maryland, U.S.A.

INTRODUCTION

Ibels et al[1] recently reported that calcium in kidneys from patients with end-stage renal disease is 8-fold greater than in normal kidneys. We have extended these observations by examining the calcium content of renal tissue obtained at biopsy and representing a wide range of severity of renal impairment. This preliminary report focuses upon two questions: (i) Can a correlation be demonstrated between the concentration of calcium within the kidney and the degree of functional impairment? (ii) Does phosphate play a significant role as a determinant of renal calcification in human renal disease?

MATERIALS AND METHODS

Kidney tissue was obtained from 71 patients with a variety of renal diseases who underwent renal biopsy for diagnostic purposes at The Johns Hopkins Hospital between 1976-1977. All the samples (mean weight 1.3 ± 0.5 mg) were frozen in O.C.T. (a commercial mixture containing: distilled water; Carbowax; and dimethyl-benzol-ammonium chloride), to prevent dehydration. Tissues for controls were obtained from autopsied patients who at the time of death had a normal serum creatinine, without macro- or microscopic evidence of diseased kidneys or past history of renal disease. All samples were digested without 0.1 ml of 12 N HCl with heat until totally dissolved. Calcium was measured by atomic absorption spectrophotometry[2] and expressed as mg Ca/100 g of wet tissue. Serum creatinine (SCr), which provided an index of renal function, serum calcium (SCa) and phosphate (SPO4) were

measured in the clinical chemistry laboratory. Statistical analyses
were carried out using Student's t-test for unpaired data,
Wilcoxon's Rank Sum test for unpaired data, Pearson's product-moment
correlation coefficient and Spearman's rank correlation coefficient.

RESULTS

Renal tissue from 71 patients comprised the study sample; 56
were from patients with glomerular disease, 5 from patients with
essential hematuria, 4 with vascular disease and 6 with additional
miscellaneous disorders. Because of the small numbers in all
subsets but glomerular disease, all data were analysed together to
define the relation between renal Ca deposition and the severity of
renal functional impairment. The complete data set was analysed by
testing for correlations between renal tissue Ca, SCr, SPO4 and SCa
and the serum CaxP product. Age represents a potentially
confounding variable in the group with more severely impaired renal
function evident in older patients and hence was included in the
variables examined.

Table 1 presents the correlations between the variables of
interest and the probability that the observed correlation could
have arisen due to chance. Significant correlations were

Table 1. Relationships between Serum Creatinine, Serum Calcium,
Serum Phosphate and Renal Tissue Calcium in Patients
with Renal Disease.

	SCr	Tissue Ca	SCa	SPO4	CaxP	Age
SCr	–	0.047^b	0.17^b	0.001^b	0.005^b	0.001
Tissue Ca	0.24^a	–	0.37^b	0.012^b	0.027^b	0.385
SCa	-0.20^a	-0.13^a	–	0.038^b	0.51^b	0.654
SPO4	0.47^a	0.37^a	-0.31^a	–	0.001^b	0.336
CaxP	0.41^a	0.33^a	0.10^a	0.92^a	–	0.250
Age	0.40	0.10	0.06	0.15	0.17	–

a Correlation coefficient (r) between indicated variables.
b Probability that observed correlation coefficient could have
  arisen by chance. Values for correlation coefficient that are
  significantly different from 0 and their corresponding
  significance levels are underlined.

demonstrated between tissue Ca and SCr, between tissue Ca and the plasma CaxP product and between serum creatinine and plasma CaxP product. Levels of significance are also included in Table 1. Age correlated significantly with SCr levels but when the above correlations were recalculated as partial correlation coefficients, the values shown in Table 1 were unchanged and the significance levels remained the same. Among the significant correlations in Table 1, the variables which appear to be the most important determinants of renal tissue calcium are serum phosphate and creatinine. The strong association between the degree of impairment in renal function, elevation in serum phosphate, CaxP product and the amount of calcium in renal tissue indicate that the increase in phosphate associated with decreasing renal function may be the primary event in the pathophysiological sequence that leads to calcium deposition, interstitial inflammation and acceleration of renal failure. Comparison of data from these biopsies from patients with normal renal function (serum creatinine < 1.5 mg/dl) with data from impaired renal function (Table 2) yields additional support for this view. Serum phosphate is significantly greater in the group of patients with renal impairment, as is the CaxP product. The progressive elevation of the CaxP product is attributable almost exclusively to the rising phosphate since the values for serum calcium exhibited only a small and non-significant difference. Values for tissue Ca in the normal kidneys were less than that for either group of patients with renal disease.

DISCUSSION

These data indicate that progressive accumulation of calcium occurs in the kidney in human renal disease as renal function declines and that this is probably determined by the increased concentration of serum inorganic phosphate that results from the progressive decrease in renal function. The associated increase in CaxP product may well be the proximate cause of this increased Ca deposition but the increased product is almost entirely attributable to the elevation in serum inorganic phosphate.

There is strong evidence indicating that the increased calcium deposition and the accompanying interstitial inflammation accelerate the loss of renal function in experimental models of uremia[3,4] and that rigid restriction of phosphate preserves renal function with increased survival. Similarly, the use of agents that inhibit nephrocalcinosis are also effective in preserving renal function in these models of experimental uremia[5]. That this mechanism may also be operative in patients with end-stage renal disease has been suggested by the observation of Collier and colleagues[6-8] and, more recently, by Maschio et al[9].

Table 2. Comparison of Data from Biopsy Material in Patients with
Normal and Impaired Renal Function (mean $\pm$ SEM).

	Group 1 (SCr$<$1.5 mg/dl)	t-test (t/P)	Group 2 (SCr$>$1.5 mg/dl)
SCr (mg/dl)	1.02 $\pm$ 0.06 (n=41)		4.88 $\pm$ 0.67 (n=30)
SCa (mg/dl)	8.92 $\pm$ 0.15 (n=30)	1.1/0.27	8.59 $\pm$ 0.28 (n=18)
SPO4 (mg/dl)	3.80 $\pm$ 0.16 (n=28)	-3.2/0.003	4.89 $\pm$ 0.30 (n=18)
CaxP (mg/dl)^2	33.6 $\pm$ 1.4 (n=28)	-3.1/0.003	41.6 $\pm$ 2.4 (n=18)

The present study, which identified a correlation between
serum creatinine and renal Ca content for all biopsy material
studied, provides preliminary evidence that calcium deposition
may begin much earlier in the course of diffuse disease.   In
view of the demonstration that phosphate restriction preserves renal
function in experimental uremia, it is important to ask whether or
not phosphate restriction relatively early in diffuse renal disease
may not retard the rate of loss of renal function, thereby
permitting the patient to survive for a longer period before
dialysis becomes necessary.

REFERENCES

1. L. Ibels, A. Alfrey, W. Huffer, P. Craswell, and R. Weil, Am. J. Med. 71:33 (1981).
2. W. Tew, C. Malis, and W. G. Walker, Analyt. Biochem. 112:346 (1981).
3. L. Ibels, A. Alfrey, L. Haut, and W. Huffer, New Engl. J. Med. 298:122 (1978).
4. L. Haut, A. Alfrey, S. Guggenheim, B. Buddington, and N. Schrier, Kidney Int. 17:722 (1980).
5. L. Gimenez, W. G. Walker, W. Tew, and J. Hermann, Kidney Int. 22:36 (1982).
6. V. Collier, W. Mitch, and M. Walser, Clin. Res. 26:564A (1978).
7. M. Walser, W. Mitch, and V. Collier, Clin. Nephrol. 11:66 (1979).
8. M. Walser, W. Mitch, and V. Collier, in:"Contributions to Nephrology", G. Berlyne, ed., S. Karger, Basel (1980).
9. G. Maschio, L. Oldrizzi, N. Tessitore, A. D'Angelo, E. Valvo, A. Lupo, C. Loschiavo, A. Fabris, L. Gammaro, C. Rugiu, and G. Panzetta, Kidney Int. 22:371 (1982).

CALCIFICATION SITES IN HUMAN KIDNEYS - A REM STUDY

F. Hering, G. Lueoend, T. Briellmann, A. Guggenheim,
H. Seiler, and G. Rutishauser

Urologische Klinik, Abteilung Chirurgie, Kantonsspital
Basel, and Institut für Anorganische Chemie and
Geologie - Palaeontologie Institut der Universität
Basel, Switzerland

INTRODUCTION

In 1936 Randall and Melkin[1] reported that papillary tip calcification occurred more frequently in patients with stone disease than in non-stone formers. Since then many authors[2-7] have regarded so-called Randall's plaques as the first manifestation of urinary stones; yet, little is known about intrarenal crystallization[8,9]. The aim of this study was to attempt to detect primary sites of intrarenal crystallization and to describe any differences that there might be between stone formers and healthy persons[10,11].

METHOD

Immediately after nephrectomy or heminephrectomy (e.g. small tumors or stones) specimens were taken from cortex, medulla and papilla. One part was stored at 4°C in cacodylate buffer and prepared for scanning electron microscopy studies 12 h later, the other part was frozen for chemical analysis (content of calcium, magnesium, sodium, potassium, cadmium, lead, copper and zinc). Before surgery a 12-h urine sample was collected and analyzed for calcium, oxalate, phosphate, magnesium, urate, citrate, sodium and potassium. The relative supersaturation with respect to calcium oxalate was calculated by a Fortran IV computer program.

RESULTS AND DISCUSSION

Out of 5 stone-forming kidneys, 4 showed intratubular deposition of calcium-containing crystals lining the tubules like

205

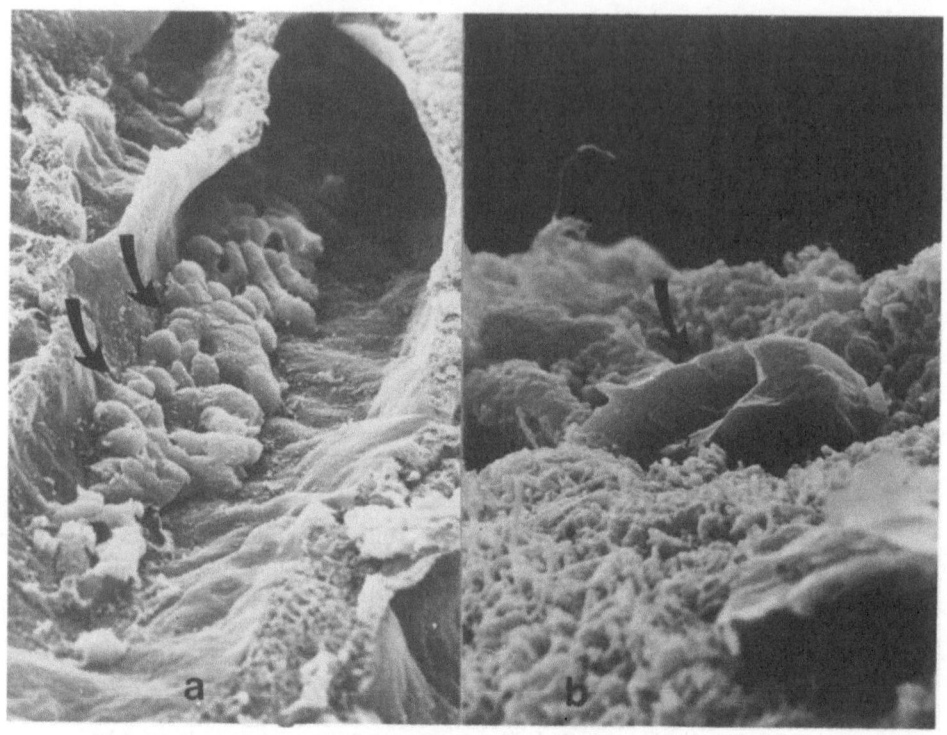

Fig. 1. (a) Calcium containing crystals (arrow) lining a collecting
duct of a recurrent CaOx stone former. Section is made near
the papillary tip. (b) Calcium concretion (arrow) on the
papillary tip of a stone former. Magnification, digital
600:1 and 5,500:1.

Table 1. Ion Content of Different Parts of Kidneys from Stone
Formers (n=5) and Non-Stone-Formers (n=10). (Mean ± SD in
ppm).

Ion	Stone-Formers			Non-Stone-Formers		
	Cortex	Medulla	Papilla	Cortex	Medulla	Papilla
Ca	485+50	875+296	1034+586	648+442	910+533	2450+2565
Mg	646+105	623+108	450+84	668+75	647+112	723+255
Cd	100+67	41+43	28+49	126+95	49+56	14+12

paving stones (Fig. 1a). Additionally 2 cases exhibited crystal
deposition on the papillary tip similar to Randall's plaques (Fig.
1b) and irregular, partially destroyed urothelium (Fig. 2a) in
comparison to a normal renal pelvis (Fig. 2b). Three of the 10
non-stone-forming kidneys exhibited intratubular calcification in

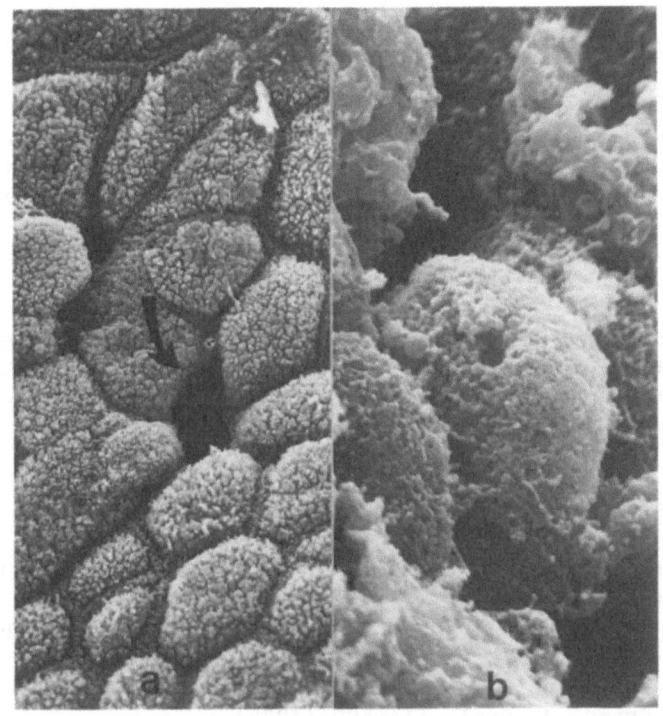

Fig. 2. Urothelium of (a) a stone bearing kidney and (b) a stone
free kidney near the papillary tip. Magnification,
(a) digital 6,000:1;(b) 2,400:1.

Table 2. Urinary Composition in Stone-Formers and Normals
(mean + SD).

Urine	Stone-Formers	Non-Stone-Formers
Calcium (mmol/l)	2.9 + 1.1	2.6 + 2.2
Oxalate (mmol/l)	0.15 + 0.22	0.06 + 0.07
Citrate (mmol/l)	0.22 + 0.19	0.6 + 0.45
Relative Supersaturation Ca Oxalate	8.2 + 8.1	2.1 + 3.1

the same manner as stone formers, while Randall's plaques were
absent. One non-stone-forming kidney demonstrated intertubular
tissue calcification.

No relation between crystal formation and calcium concentration
of the tissue investigated by EDAX analysis was found, but there was
evidence of a marked increase of calcium concentration from cortex
to papilla (Table 1). In contrast, the magnesium concentration of

the papillae was the lower in the stone-forming than in the non-stone-forming kidneys.

Of the heavy metals, the cadmium content of the papillary tip was higher in the stone-forming group (Table 1). Likewise 3 of 5 stone kidneys and only 1 papilla of the non-stone-bearing kidney contained lead normally not present in kidneys. Possibly heavy metals play a role in stone formation by destroying the epithelium of the collecting ducts. An altered tubular surface may induce heterogenous nucleation or retention of formed crystals.

There was no significant correlation between the urinary concentration of calcium and oxalate and crystal formation, but in general stone patients showed a much higher urinary supersaturation of calcium oxalate (Table 2).

REFERENCES

1. A. Randall and P. D. Melkin, Trans. Amer. Ass. Gen. Urin. Surg. 29:323 (1936).
2. C. W. Vermeulen, E. S. Lyon, J. E. Ellis, and T. A. Borden, J. Urol. 97:573 (1967).
3. R. S. Malek and W. H. Boyce, J. Urol. 109:551 (1973).
4. E. L. Prien, J. Urol. 114:500 (1975).
5. W. R. Jordan, B. Finlayson, and M. Luxenberg, Invest. Urol. 15:465 (1978).
6. C. K. Anderson, in:"Urinary Calculous Disease", J. E. A. Wickham, ed., Churchill Livingstone, Edinburgh (1979).
7. E. Hienzsch, A. Hesse, C. Bothor, W. Berg, and J. Roth, Urol. Res. 7:223 (1979).
8. B. Finlayson and F. Reid, Invest. Urol. 15:442 (1978).
9. H. G. Rushton and M. Spector, J. Urol. 127:598 (1982).
10. R. Hautmann, A. Lehmann, and H. Osswald, in:"Urolithiasis, Basic and Clinical Research", L. H. Smith, W. G. Robertson, and B. Finlayson, eds., Plenum, New York (1981).
11. R. S. Wright and A. Hodgkinson, Invest. Urol. 9:369 (1972).

THE INFLUENCE OF GLUCOSE AND INSULIN ON CALCIUM

EXCRETION IN THE URINE

R. G. Willis, R. Green, C. Gordon, and N. J. Blacklock

University Depts. of Physiology, Urology and Medicine
University of Manchester, U.K.

INTRODUCTION

Administration of refined carbohydrate or glucose to man increases calcium (Ca) excretion in the urine[1], but it is not known whether or not this is a direct effect. The normal increase in Ca excretion which occurs following the administration of glucose is exaggerated in stone forming patients[2,3], and such patients frequently show an abnormal plasma insulin response to a standard glucose tolerance test[4]. This paper investigates in the rat the causes of the increased Ca excretion provoked by glucose and the suggestion that hyperinsulinaemia per se may produce a similar increase in Ca excretion[5].

METHODS

Male Sprague-Dawley rats weighing 200 to 250 g were starved over-night but allowed free access to water. They were anaesthetised with Inactin (B.Y.K.) (120 mg/kg body weight i.p.) and placed on a heated table at 37°C. Catheters were inserted into a jugular vein for infusions, a carotid artery for measurement of blood pressure, and into the left ureter to collect urine. Saline (0.9% containing ^{3}H-inulin) was infused at 200 µl/min for 1 h and then at 150 µl/min for 2 h. During this time all animals reached a steady state as regards urine output and glomerular filtration rate (GFR), and control collections of urine and plasma were taken. Thereafter, animals were assigned to one of four groups which received the following infusions (at 150 µl/min) for a further 4 h, each infusate containing ^{3}H-inulin:(a) 0.9% saline was continued (control group n = 20); (b) 2.5% glucose in 0.9% saline

209

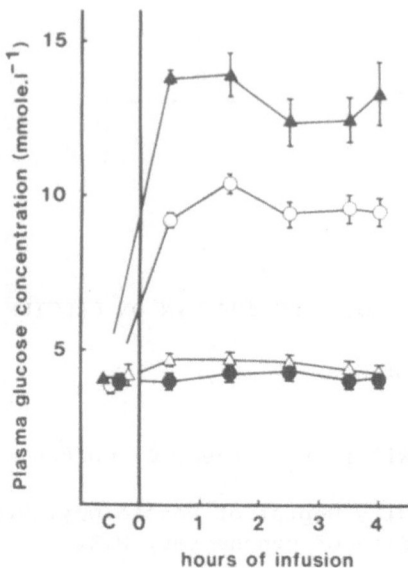

Fig. 1. Plasma glucose concentration in rats infused with saline
(●), 2.5% glucose in saline (O), 5% glucose in saline (▲)
and insulin with 2.5% glucose in saline (Δ). Prior to
time O, saline alone was infused (period C). (Mean ± SEM).

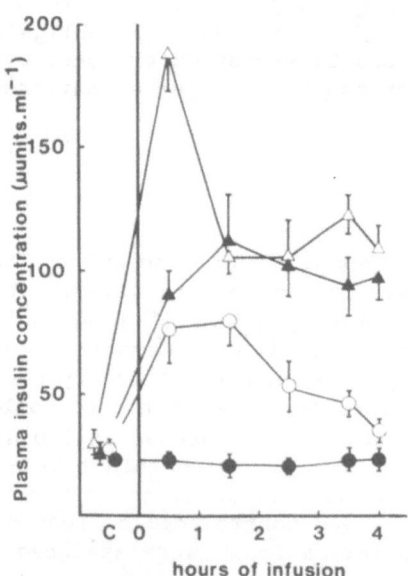

Fig. 2. Plasma insulin concentrations during glucose and insulin
infusions. For symbols, see Fig. 1. (Mean ± SEM).

210

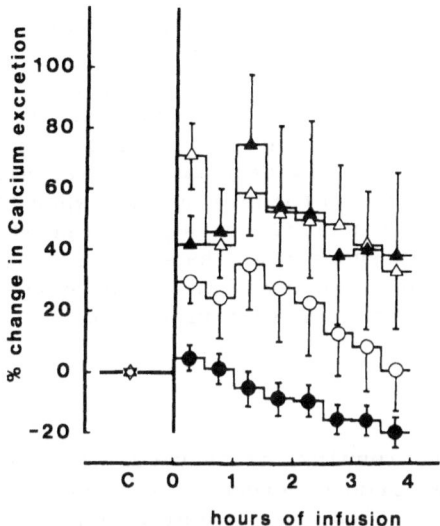

Fig. 3. Change in Ca excretion during glucose and insulin/glucose
infusions. For symbols, see Fig. 1. (Mean ± SEM).

(n = 10); (c) 5.0% glucose in 0.9% (n = 10); (d) 0.1 U Atrapid
insulin (Novo) was given as a bolus, followed by infusion of 2.5%
glucose on 0.9% saline, containing Actrapid insulin (0.1 U/h; n =
10). Urine was collected over 30 min periods, blood was sampled
every hour from the tail vein (0.2 ml) and at the end of the
experiment a large blood sample was obtained from the carotid
cannula. Urine and terminal plasma were analysed for Ca, Na, K,
Cl, glucose and osmolality. Glucose and insulin concentrations were
determined in the hourly plasma samples, the latter by a specially
scaled down radioimmunoassay technique. Aliquots of all urine and
plasma samples were counted in a liquid scintillation counter for
[3]H-inulin concentration to calculate GFR. Evaluation of the data
was made using one-way and two-way analysis of variance.

RESULTS

     As expected, infusion of glucose-containing solutions produced
a graded increase in plasma glucose which rapidly attained stable
levels (Fig. 1). The rise in plasma glucose was associated with an
increase in plasma insulin concentrations which remained stable with
the 5% glucose infusion, but fell after 2 h in the 2.5% glucose
group (Fig. 2). In both infusions, there was a significant rise in
Ca excretion (Fig. 3) but no significant change in either GFR or Na
excretion. Both infusions produced a small rise in urine flow rate
and a significant increase in urine Ca concentration; the 5%
glucose infusion gave significant glycosuria in some animals.

The infusion of insulin with glucose resulted in plasma glucose concentrations close to the control values (Fig. 1), but plasma insulin was elevated to levels comparable with those in animals receiving 5% glucose (Fig. 2). We have thus produced animals which are euglycaemic with high plasma insulin levels. Following the infusion of insulin, urinary Ca excretion was significantly increased, to a degree comparable to that when 5% glucose was given (Fig. 3). Urine Ca concentration was increased only in the first sample, however, and thereafter there was a significant rise in urine flow rate with no increase in Ca concentration. A small reduction in GFR together with a rise in Na excretion also occurred.

DISCUSSION

From the above results, it is clear that, in the rat, an increase in plasma glucose concentration results in an increase in both urinary Ca excretion and concentration. Since there was no associated changes in GFR or plasma Ca concentration, it is unlikely that this was due to changes in the filtered load of Ca, and therefore altered tubular reabsorption of Ca is the most probable explanation. The amount of Na excreted (a factor known to influence Ca excretion[6]) cannot be implicated since glucose infusion produced no significant alteration in Na excretion rate. Insulin infusion resulted in an increased excretion of Ca similar to that produced by an elevated plasma glucose concentration. Measurements of GFR and plasma Ca during insulin infusion again suggest that these changes are due to altered tubular handling of Ca, but since, in contrast to the experiments where glucose alone is infused, there is also a marked increase in urine flow rate and Na excretion (both of which may alter urinary Ca excretion), it is not possible to conclude that the same mechanisms are affected. Obviously, further investigation at the single nephron level is necessary to clarify the mechanisms underlying these changes and the site at which they occur.

REFERENCES

1. R. D. Lindeman, S. Adler, M. J. Yiengst, and E. S. Beard, J. Lab.Clin. Med. 70:236 (1967).
2. J. Lemann, W. F. Piering, and E. J. Lennon, New Engl. J. Med. 280:232 (1969).
3. D. E. Barilla, J. Townsend, and C. Y. C. Pak, Invest. Urol. 15: 486 (1978).
4. P. N. Rao, C. Gordon, D. Davies, and N. J. Blacklock, Br. J. Urol. 54:575 (1982).
5. R. A. DeFronzo, C. R. Cooke, R. Andres, G. R. Faloona, and P. J.Davis, J. Clin. Invest. 55:845 (1975).
6. M. Walser, Am. J. Physiol. 200:1099 (1961).

THE EFFECT OF INDOMETHACIN AND FLURBIPROFEN ON CALCIUM EXCRETION AND GLOMERULAR FILTRATION RATE IN THE ANAESTHETIZED RAT

S. L. Greenwood, R. Green, and N. J. Blacklock

Depts. of Physiology and Urology, University of Manchester, U.K.

INTRODUCTION

Calcium stone disease is commonly associated with hyper-calciuria which, if left untreated, can lead to a high incidence of recurrent stone formation[1,2]. It has been shown recently that the prostaglandin synthetase inhibitors, indomethacin and flurbiprofin, restore Ca excretion to normal in patients with idiopathic hyper-calciuria and it has been suggested that they may be useful in treating this disorder[3,4]. In conscious experimental animals indomethacin reduces Ca, Na and water excretion without associated changes in renal haemodynamics[5,6] implicating a role for prostaglandins in the regulation of Ca excretion by a direct action on the tubular transport processes. Prior to studying possible prostaglandin-Ca interaction in the nephron by micropuncture, we have investigated the effects of indomethacin and flurbiprofen on renal haemodynamics and Ca excretion in the anaesthetized rats.

METHODS

Male Sprague-Dawley rats were anaesthetized in Inactin (5-ethyl-5-(1'-methyl-propyl)-2-thiobarbiturate; 110 mg kg^{-1} body weight and catheters placed in the left jugular vein, right carotid artery and left ureter. Rats were infused with saline (140 mmol/l NaCl) containing ^{3}H-inulin (1.0 μCi/ml) and sodium PAH (5.8 mg/ml) at 100 μl/min for 8 h. Control animals received saline infusion throughout. After 5 h, experimental animals received indomethacin (10 mg/kg) in buffered saline or flurbiprofen (10 mg/kg) infused over a 15 min period. Urine and plasma samples were collected hourly beginning 2 and 2.5 h from the start of infusion

respectively and analyzed for ^{3}H-inulin and PAH. Glomerular
filtration rate (GFR) was measured as the clearance of ^{3}H-inulin and
effective renal plasma flow estimated as the clearance of PAH
(C_{PAH}). Urine flow rate was measured gravimetrically and Ca
concentration determined in urine and in a terminal plasma sample.

RESULTS

There were no significant differences in plasma Ca
concentration, measured in the terminal plasma sample, between
control and experimental groups (in mmol/l, control 1.29 $\pm$ 0.05,
indomethacin-treated 2.16 $\pm$ 0.04; flurbiprofen-treated 2.13 $\pm$
0.06). Rats achieved a stable urine flow rate in response to
saline after 2 to 3 h of infusion. Analysis of variance indicated
no significant effects of time on any of the variables measured and
the results have been analysed using a 't'-test to compare
corresponding collection periods in controls with drug treated rats.

Fig. 1a shows urine flow rate, Ca excretion and urinary Ca
concentration in the 5th and 7th hours of infusion i.e. 1 h prior to
(Control - C) and after (Experimental - E) drug administration.
Indomethacin significantly reduced urine flow rate and Ca excretion
($P<0.005$). The lowered Ca excretion with indomethacin was
associated with reduced urinary Ca concentration ($P<0.005$) in
addition to decreased urine flow. Flurbiprofen also lowered Ca
excretion ($P<0.005$) but failed to alter significantly urinary Ca
concentration. Thus the reduced Ca excretion reflected lowered
urine flow rate ($P<0.005$).

Fig. 1b shows the GFR and effective renal plasma flow measured
as the C_{PAH} in the 5th and 7th hours of infusion. In addition to
lowering Ca excretion, indomethacin and flurbiprofen significantly
reduced GFR ($P<0.005$), the lowered GFR with flurbiprofen being
associated with reduced renal plasma flow ($P<0.005$). Renal plasma
flow is not affected by indomethacin.

DISCUSSION

The results of this study in the anaesthetized rat confirm
previous observations that indomethacin reduces Ca excretion in the
rat[3]. Indomethacin and flurbiprofen have also been shown to reduce
Ca excretion in man[3,4] although a recent publication has suggested
that flurbiprofen may have no effect[7]. In conscious rats,
inhibition of prostaglandin synthetis results in reduced Ca
excretion without associated changes in renal haemodynamics implying
that inhibition of prostaglandin synthesis leads to a net increase
in Ca reabsorption by the tubules. In contrast, in the
anaesthetized rat both indomethacin and flurbiprofen reduce GFR and

214

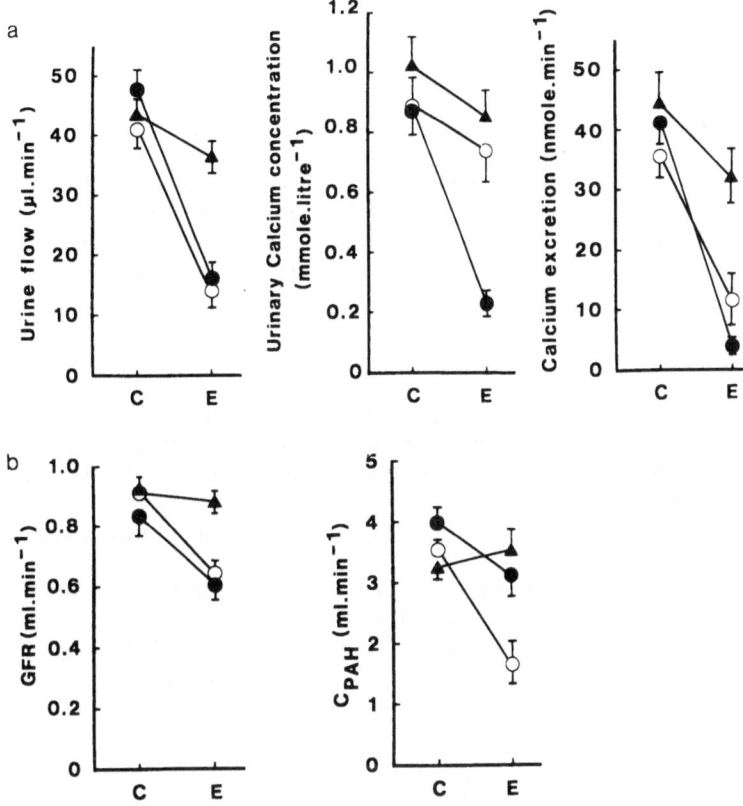

Fig. 1. Effect of indomethacin and flurbiprofen on (a) urinary flow
rate, Ca concentration and excretion and (b) renal
haemodynamics (▲———▲) Control (n = 12); ●———●
Indomethacin (n = 9); O———O Flurbiprofen (n = 8). Values
are means ± SEM in the 5th and 7th hours of infusion; i.e.
1 h before (Control - C) and 1 h after (Experimental - E)
drug administration.

the consequent reduction in filtered load of Ca may be sufficient to
account for its lowered excretion without involving altered tubular
Ca transport. However, indomethacin reduces urinary Ca
concentration which may implicate altered tubular Ca handling. The
latter may not be directly attributable to prostaglandin synthetase
inhibition, however, because flurbiprofen did not affect urinary Ca
concentration.

As well as altering Ca excretion by different mechanisms,
indomethacin and flurbiprofen have different effects on renal
haemodynamics. Flurbiprofen, but not indomethacin, reduces renal
plasma flow (estimated by C_{PAH}) although both drugs lower GFR.

215

Several possible explanations for the differences between the effects of these two cyclo-oxygenase inhibitors include (a) a difference in potency between the two drugs at 10 mg/kg, and (b) effects of either drug on renal function 'per se'. Further experiments would resolve these possibilities.

The results of this study imply that indomethacin may be more effective in reducing urinary Ca concentration than flurbiprofen. However, in anaesthetized animals it is not possible to conclude that either drug has a direct effect on renal tubular transport.

REFERENCES

1. R. E. Williams, Br. J. Urol. 50:459 (1963).
2. A. F. Stewart and A. E. Broadus, Ann. Rev. Med. 32:457 (1981)
3. A. C. Buck, C. J. Lote, and W. F. Sampson, J. Urol. 129:421 (1983).
4. P. N. Rao and N. J. Blacklock, J. Int. Med. Res. Suppl. 2:24 (1983).
5. A. C. Buck, W. F. Sampson, C. J. Lote, and N. J. Blacklock, Br.J. Urol. 53:485 (1981).
6. J. Haylor and C. J. Lote, J. Physiol. 298:371 (1980).
7. P. J. R. Shah and G. A. Rose, Br. J. Urol. 56:1 (1984).

IV. METABOLISM

STUDIES ON THE ENDOGENOUS PRODUCTION OF OXALATE IN MAN

B. Nordenvall, L. Backman, and L. Larsson

Dept. of Surgery, Karolinska Institute at Danderyd
Hospital and Dept. of Clinical Chemistry, University
Hospital, Linköping, Sweden

INTRODUCTION

Interest in oxalate metabolism has increased because of its
importance in urinary stone formation.   Oxalate is a metabolic end-
product in man and is excreted in the urine[1].   The two main
precursors of oxalate are glyoxylic acid[2] and ascorbic acid[3].
Serine is a minor precursor[4].   Glycine is thought to be the most
important precursor of glyoxylic acid[5].   Glycine and ascorbic acid
each contribute about 40% of the urinary excretion.   Intestinal
absorption is reported to be less than 10% of the ingested amount[6].

One purpose of this investigation was to study urinary oxalate
excretion as an indicator of endogenous oxalate production in a
model in which exogenous oxalate sources were excluded.   The other
purpose was to study the effect of a short-time parenteral load of
glycine and ascorbic acid on urinary oxalate excretion.

MATERIAL AND METHODS

We have studied 6 patients with malnutrition (considerable
weight loss and/or subnormal serum albumin and transferrin) who were
given total parenteral nutrition (TPN) in preparation for major
surgery.   The clinical data are given in Table 1.   None of the
patients had had kidney stones before the period of treatment.   The
infusion schedule and the composition of the TPN solutions are shown
in Table 2.   Parenteral nutrition was given through a central line.
No local or septic complications occurred during the study.   In one
patient (no. 1), urinary oxalate excretion was determined for 20
consecutive days during TPN.   In 5 patients (nos. 2 to 6) a study

Table 1. Clinical Data on 6 Patients Treated with Total Parenteral
Nutrition before Major Surgery.

Patient	Sex	Body weight	Age (years)	Notes
1	M	54	54	Recurrent gastric ulcer for 10 years. Gastric retention. Weight loss 11 kg/4 weeks
2	M	39	74	Pancreatic malignancy. Weight loss 18 kg/9 months
3	M	62	74	Colon malignancy. Weight loss 8 kg/6 weeks
4	F	39	46	Recurrent pancreatitis for 10 years. Weight loss 15 kg/9 months
5	F	49	76	Gastric malignancy. Gastric retention. Weight loss 15 kg/3 months
6	F	69	67	Esophageal malignancy. Weight loss 10 kg/6 months

of the urinary oxalate excretion for 12 consecutive days of TPN was
planned. On days 4 and 5, glycine solutions, containing 10 and
20 g respectively, were added to the TPN between 08.00 and 16.00.
The study was stopped after 5 days in patient 6, as she decided not
to undergo radical surgery and was therefore no longer motivated to
accept TPN. In the other 4 patients, ascorbic acid was added to
the TPN solutions on days 8,9 and 10 (1.3 and 3 g respectively)
between 08.00 and 16.00.

The amino acids glycine and serine were analyzed by an Amino
Acid Analyzer (Kontron). Twenty-four-hour samples were collected
(08.00 to 08.00) in plastic bottles containing 90 mmol of
hydrochloric acid to maintain oxalate in solution. Oxalate was
determined by the method of Hodgkinson and Williams as modified by

Table 2. Infusion Schedule and Composition of the Total Parenteral
Nutrition Solutions per 24 h.

Amino acids (Vamin[R] with 10% glucose)	1000 ml	08.00 - 20.00
Fat emulsion (Intralipid[R] 20%)	1000 ml	08.00 - 20.00
Glucose (10%)	1000 ml	20.00 - 08.00
Energy content	12.8 MJ (3050 kcal)	
Content of calcium	9 mmol	
magnesium	3.3 mmol	
glycine	2.1 g	
serine	7.5 g	
oxalate	0	

Tiselius[7]. The upper reference limit[8] was 450 μmol/24 h. Oxalate excretion was expressed in relation to creatinine excretion to compensate for errors in urine collection[8]. The upper reference limit for oxalate was 30 mmol/mol creatinine[8]. Urinary calcium and magnesium were analyzed by atomic absorption and creatinine by AutoAnalyzer with alkaline picrate[9]. The reference range[12] was 9 to 22 mmol/24 h. Data are presented as means ± SEM.

RESULTS

In patient no. 1 the oxalate excretion was unchanged during a 3-week period of TPN with a mean excretion of 376 ± 14 μmol/24 h (35.8 ± 1.7 mmol/mol creatinine). The mean urinary excretion of oxalate was 326 ± 19 μmol/24 h and of creatinine 6.7 ± 1.2 mmol/24 h in 5 patients during the first 3 days of TPN. A glycine load given for 2 days did not change the oxalate excretion. The oxalate excretion increased during the ascorbic acid load and reverted to pre-load levels within 1 day (Fig. 1). The urinary excretions of calcium and magnesium were normal and unchanged throughout the investigation. The day-to-day variations of urinary volume and creatinine excretion were minimal during the study. The serum concentrations of glycine and serine increased during the glycine load.

DISCUSSION

The endogenous metabolism of oxalate in man has been studied using feeding experiments[3,6] and by radioisotopic techniques[5]. These studies imply influence of enterally given oxalate or oxalate precursors. We have therefore examined patients in whom exogenous

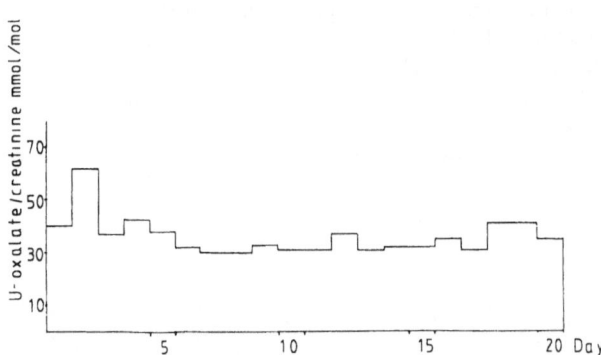

Fig. 1. Mean urinary oxalate/urine creatinine/24 h in 5 patients during total parenteral nutrition (one patient (no.6) was only studied for 5 days.

oxalate sources were excluded by means of TPN. The fecal loss of oxalate is small[10], and the urinary excretion of oxalate may therefore be considered equal to the endogenous synthesis of oxalate during TPN. It was in this study found to be about 325 umol/24 h. These patients had a high oxalate/creatinine quotient probably because of their low urinary excretion of creatinine. The study showed that the endogenous oxalate production was unchanged during TPN for 3 weeks. The long-term cyclic variations in daily excretion observed in one patient receiving enteral feeding[6] was not found in the patient examined during 20 days in our study.

The amino acid glycine has been shown to be the precursor of about 40% of the urinary oxalate[5]. In our study a parenteral glycine load resulted in increased serum concentrations of glycine and serine. In spite of this, oxalate excretion was unchanged, indicating that the production of oxalate is independent of short-term increases in serum concentrations of glycine and serine. Our study confirmed earlier findings of the importance of ascorbic acid as an oxalate precursor[5].

REFERENCES

1. H. E. Archer, A. E. Dormer, E. F. Scowen, and R. W. E. Watts, Clin. Sci. 16:405 (1957).
2. J. S. King and A. Wainer, Proc. Soc. Exp. Biol. Med. 128:1162 (1968).
3. K. Takenouchi, K. Aso, K. Kawase, H. Ichikawa, and T. Schimoni, J. Vitaminol. 12:49 (1966).
4. B. M. Dean, R. W. E. Watts, and W. J. Westwick, Clin. Sci. 35:325 (1968).
5. G. L. Atkins, B. M. Dean, W. J. Griffin, and R. W. E. Watts, J. Biol. Chem. 239:2975 (1964).
6. P. M. Zarembski and A. Hodgkinson, Clin. Chim. Acta 25:1 (1969).
7. H.-G. Tiselius, Invest. Urol. 15:5 (1977).
8. H.-G. Tiselius, L. E. Almgård, L. Larrson, and B. Sörbo, Eur. Urol. 4:241 (1978).
9. A. L. Chasson, H. J. Grady, and M. A. Stanley, Am. J. Clin. Path. 35:83 (1961).
10. A. Hodgkinson and R. Wilkinson, Clin. Sci. Mol. Med. 46:61 (1974).

RED BLOOD CELL TRANSMEMBRANE OXALATE FLUX IN IDIOPATHIC

CALCIUM OXALATE NEPHROLITHIASIS

A. Borsatti, G. Gambaro, F. Marchini, E. Cicerello, and B. Baggio

Institute of Internal Medicine, Postgraduate School of Nephrology, University Hospital, 35100 Padova, Italy

INTRODUCTION

The occurrence of mild hyperoxaluria "idiopathic" calcium-oxalate (CaOx) stone disease has been stressed recently[1,2]. It is thought to be due to a higher than normal intestinal absorption of oxalate[3,4], although abnormal renal handling of the ion cannot be ruled out. The underlying mechanism of both these abnormalities might involve a defect in the cellular transport of oxalate. To test this hypothesis, we have compared the rates of oxalate transport in red blood cells (RBC) in "idiopathic" CaOx stone forming patients and normal subjects. The results of this study are reported here.

PATIENTS AND METHODS

The study was carried out on 18 control subjects (12 males and 6 females) with no family history of renal stone disease, and 18 patients with "idiopathic" CaOx nephrolithiasis, selected as described previously[2] (15 males and 3 females). RBC oxalate exchange was assayed as follows[5]: 10 ml blood specimens were collected, washed three times in a solution containing 150 mM NaCl, 10 mM KCl, and 20 mM tris-HCl buffer (pH 7.4), resuspended to a hematocrit of 50% in the above solution supplemented with 10 mM sodium oxalate, and incubated at room temperature for 2 h. After centrifugation, the RBC were resuspended to a hematocrit of 20% in the same solution as above and subdivided into several aliquots to which a ^{14}C-oxalate tracer (8000-10,000 cpm) was added. At 10, 20, 30, 60, 90, 120 min and 24 h, aliquots were centrifuged and the ^{14}C-activity of the supernatant counted in a β-scintillation counter.

The flux rate was calculated according to the following expression: $(\ln(A_t-A_\infty)=\ln(A_0-A_\infty)-kt$, where t is time, k the flux constant, and A the quantity of labelled oxalate at time 0, t, and ∞.

RESULTS

The flux constant (K) was 0.25 ± 0.15 in controls, 1.30 ± 1.85 min^{-1} in "idiopathic" stone formers, the difference being statistically significant (t=2.40, P<0.025). Furthermore, 10 of the 18 stone forming patients showed K values greater than the normal range (mean + 2SD in controls) ($x^2 = 13.85$, P<0.0005).

DISCUSSION

Our data show that the majority of "idiopathic" CaOx stone formers have a faster than normal oxalate self-exchange in RBC. This observation strengthens the hypothesis that "idiopathic" CaOx nephrolithiasis may constitute a metabolic disease characterized by a cellular defect in oxalate transport. This may explain the increased intestinal absorption[3,4], the higher urinary excretion of oxalate[1,2], and also the high incidence of a family history of stones among patients with "idiopathic" CaOx nephrolithiasis[6,7]. A major criticism of our study lies in the use of RBC as a cellular model. However, RBC have been extensively used to study membrane transport systems[8], and many of the systems first identified in RBC have subsequently been found in other cell types. The existence of abnormal cellular transport of oxalate in stone-formers opens new prospectives in the understanding of the underlying mechanisms if CaOx stone disease. Furthermore, RBC could be used to assess the efficacy of the drugs most commonly prescribed to treat CaOx nephrolithiasis. Finally, the detection of a faster oxalate self-exchange in RBC might constitute a method for identifying individuals at risk of stone formation.

REFERENCES

1. W. G. Robertson and M. Peacock, Nephron 26:105 (1980).
2. B. Baggio, G. Gambaro, S. Favor, and A. Borsatti, Nephron 35:11 (1983).
3. A. Hodgkinson, Clin. Sci. 54:291 (1978).
4. M. Marangella, B. Fruttero, M. Bruno, and F. Linari, Clin. Sci. 63:381 (1982).
5. J. L. Cousin and R. Motais, J. Physiol. 256:61 (1976).
6. M. G. McGeown, Clin. Sci. 19:465 (1960).
7. S. Ljunghall, Br. J. Urol. 51:249 (1979).
8. P. R. Garey, G. Dagher, and P. Meyer, Clin. Sci. 59 (Suppl 6):1915 (1980).

THE EFFECT OF INGESTION OF MEGADOSES OF ASCORBIC ACID ON URINARY OXALATE EXCRETION IN NORMAL SUBJECTS AND STONE FORMERS

A. K. Pendse, A. K. Purchit, R. Ghosh, A. Goyal, and
P. P. Singh

Depts. of Biochemistry and Surgery, R. N. T. Medical
College, Udaipur-313001, Rajasthan, India

INTRODUCTION

In Western countries megadoses of ascorbic acid, ranging from 3 to 30 g, are being advocated as prophylactic and therapeutic measures against several diseases, notably the common cold and certain malignant conditions[1-6]. In India, it is common practice to use ascorbic acid in doses between 200 and 1000 mg/day during the post-operative period to achieve faster wound healing and to counter infection but there is an increased trend towards the use of megadoses of ascorbic acid.

The Udaipur region of India has a high prevalence of urolithiasis[7] and hyperoxaluria appears to be a significant etiologic factor[8]. It is thought that 35 to 50% of urinary oxalate derives from dietary ascorbic acid[2]. Oral ascorbic acid administration increases urinary oxalate, but there is a wide intra-individual as well as inter-individual response[2-9]. Megadoses of vitamin C may initiate calcium oxalate urolithiasis in some people and also may exacerbate stone formation in patients who have a history of the disorder[10]. Since it is not known whether or not stone-formers and normals repond differently to megadoses of ascorbic acid, we have studied the effect of such doses on urinary oxalate in these groups.

MATERIALS AND METHODS

Ten normal healthy males and 29 stone formers were included in the study. The normals were kept on a low oxalate diet during the period of study and for two days prior to it. The stone formers were placed on a standard, low oxalate, hospital diet for the same

225

duration. The first 24-h urine sample was collected before
ascorbic acid administration, then 6 g ascorbic acid (in 3 doses of
2 g) was given daily for 3 days. On the last day, a second 24-h
urine sample was collected and a third 48-h after discontinuation of
vitamin ingestion. Blood samples were also taken at the time of
collection of urine samples I and II. Serum and urinary ascorbic
acid[11], urinary oxalic acid[12] and calcium[13] were determined.

RESULTS AND DISCUSSION

We have found that, in normals as well as in stone formers,
oral administration of 6 mg day of ascorbic acid almost doubled the
mean 24-h urinary excretion of oxalic acid. There was no significant difference in the pattern between the two groups (Table 1).
That this increase is solely due to the ascorbic acid is shown by
the fact that urinary oxalate returned to the pre-loading level
after discontinuing the load. Lamden and Chrystowski[14] reported
that the amount of oxalic acid produced daily by ascorbic acid
supplements is proportional to the dose, such that 1 mg oxalic acid
is produced from 1 g ascorbic acid, 12 mg from 4 g, and 68 mg from
9 g. Schmidt et al[9], reported an increase in oxalic acid excretion
from 19 mg to 48 mg/day during the ingestion of 5 g of ascorbic acid
daily for 4 consecutive days in a healthy volunteer. They also
reported that on ingestion of 10 g of ascorbic acid daily, this
increase was in the range of 50 mg to 87 mg in 5 healthy volunteers.
Our values fall approximately within the same range.

Contrary to Schmidt et al[9] we also observed an increase in the
24-h excretion of calcium in the normals as well as in the stone
formers. This increase was significant, however, only in the stone
formers (P 0.01). This increase in calcium excretion, along with
that in oxalate, will further potentiate the risk of calcium oxalate
stone formation.

Normal serum and urinary ascorbic acid levels in both normals
and stone formers indicate that the ascorbic acid status of both
groups was normal. The administration of ascorbic acid resulted in
a predictable increase in these levels (mean $\pm$ SEM) from 0.89 $\pm$ 0.07
to 1.22 $\pm$ 0.14 mg/dl in normals and from 0.84 $\pm$ 0.06 to 1.55 $\pm$ 0.08
mg/dl in stone-formers.

Hoffer[1] has written, in relation to ascorbic acid administration, that "a discussion of toxicity that ignores efficacy is a
futile exercise". However, in this context we would like to add
further that conversely "the discussion of efficacy ignoring the
toxicity is not only a futile but may be a dangerous exercise".
because it has been clearly demonstrated that megadoses of ascorbic
acid cause hyperoxaluria[2-9] and may be instrumental in the formation
of calcium oxalate stones[10].

226

Table 1. The 24-h Urinary Excretion (Mean ± SEM) of Ascorbic Acid, Oxalic Acid and Calcium Before, During and 48-h After Ingestion of 6 g Ascorbic Acid by 10 Normal Men and 28 Stone-formers.

Period	Volume (ml)	Ascorbic Acid (mg)	Oxalic Acid (mg)	Calcium (mg)
Normals				
Pre-loaded (PL)	1996 ± 164	110.3 ± 12.2	20.6 ± 2.9	184.4 ± 18.6
Loaded (L)	2163 ± 213	1098.2 ± 145.1	43.6 ± 6.1	223.8 ± 12.2
Post-loaded (PTL)	2367 ± 281	153.7 ± 2.2	23.2 ± 2.2	197.4 ± 17.8
PL v L	ns	<0.001	<0.01	ns
L v PTL	ns	<0.001	<0.01	ns
PL v PTL	ns	ns	ns	ns
Stone-formers				
Pre-loaded (PL)	1563 ± 156	117.5 ± 17.1	29.3 ± 3.5	183.7 ± 20.3
Loaded (L)	1863 ± 140	1057.9 ± 148.2	54.7 ± 5.3	200.2 ± 20.3
Post-loaded (PTL)	1470 ± 142	138.0 ± 3.8	31.8 ± 3.8	133.8 ± 11.9
PL v L	<0.001	<0.001	<0.001	ns
L v PTL	ns	<0.001	<0.001	<0.01
PL v PTL	ns	ns	ns	<0.05

REFERENCES

1. A. Hoffer, New Engl. J. Med. 285:635 (1971).
2. A. Hodgkinson, "Oxalic Acid in Biology and Medicine", Academic Press, London (1977).
3. E. Cameron, L. Pauling, and B. Leibowitz, Rev. Canc. Res. 39:663 (1979).
4. E. Ginter, Adv. Lipid Res. 16:167 (1978).
5. C. W. M. Wilson and H. S. Loh, Lancet 1:638 (1973).
6. L. Pauling, Proc. Nat. Acad. Sci. 67:1643 (1970).
7. A. K. Pendse, A. K. Srivastava, J. L. Kumawat, H. S. Sharma, R. Ghosh, A. Goyal, and P. P. Singh, Int. Cell. Surg. Bull. 188: (1982).
8. P. P. Singh, A. K. Pendse, R. Ghosh, and A. Goyal, Asian Med. J. (in press).
9. K. H. Schmidt, V. Hagmaier, D. H. Horning, J. P. Vuilleumier, and G. Rutishauser, Am. J. Clin. Nutr. 34:305 (1981).
10. L. H. Smith, New Engl. J. Med. 298:856 (1978).
11. S. Natelson, "Techniques of Clinical Chemistry", Charles C. Thomas, Springfield (1971).
12. A. Hodgkinson and A. Williams, Clin. Chim. Acta 36:127 (1972).
13. H. Varley, A. H. Gowenlock and M. Bell, "Practical Clinical Biochemistry", Vol. I, Heinemann, London (1976).
14. M. P. Lamden and G. A. Chrystowski, Proc. Soc. Exp. Biol. Med. 85:190 (1954).

INTERACTIONS OF STEROID HORMONES AND PYRIDOXINE IN THE

REGULATION OF OXALATE METABOLISM IN RATS

S. K. Thind, V. Sharma, and R. Nath

Dept. of Biochemistry, Postgraduate Institute of
Medical Education and Research, Chandigarh, India

INTRODUCTION

Endogenous oxalate excretion in man and the rat is inversely
related to the amount of vitamin B_6 in diet. Pyridoxine-deficient
rats produce more oxalate from glycolic acid, ethylene glycol,
ethanolamine and xylitol. The effect of vitamin B_6 deficiency is
eliminated by hepatectomy, indicating that this effect is mediated
via the liver enzymes. The role of sex hormones in regulating
enzymes of oxalate biosynthesis[1] and a sex-related occurrence of
calcium oxalate calculi, with a higher prevalence in male rats fed a
vitamin B_6-deficient diet, have been reported[2]. The interaction of
pyridoxine deficiency and estradiol administration on the enzymes of
oxalate biosynthesis have been elucidated.

MATERIALS AND METHODS

Male Wister rats (100 to 120 g body weight) maintained on
specific dietary regimens and estradiol treatment (silastic implants
inserted Sc) were grouped in batches of 8 as follows:
SB - Pyridoxine deficient; SPF - Pyridoxine sufficient, pair-fed
with SB; (both groups were sham-operated and an empty implant
inserted); EB - Pyridoxine deficient + estradiol implant; and EPF -
Pyridoxine sufficient, pair-fed with EB + estradiol implant. After
one month, at sacrifice, blood, liver and kidneys were collected.
The pyridoxine status of the animals was ascertained by determining
the erythrocyte alanine transaminase (ALT) levels[3]. Glycolic acid
oxidase (GAO), glycolic acid dehydrogenase (GAD) and lactate
dehydrogenase (LDH) levels were assayed[1]. The specific activities
(U/mg protein) were converted to percentage, taking SPF as 100%.

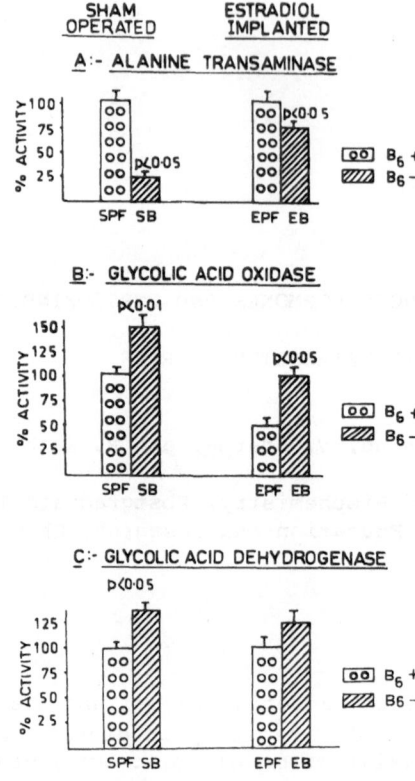

Fig. 1. Effect of vitamin B$_6$ deficiency and estradiol administration of ALT, GAO and GAD levels. SPF, SB, EPF and EB-treatment as given in text.

RESULTS

Feeding a pyridoxine-deficient diet for one month led to an 80% decrease in ALT levels in the case of sham-operated animals, and a 33% decrease in estradiol-treated animals (Fig. 1). Vitamin B$_6$ deficiency increased GAO levels by 45% in both sham-operated and estradiol-treated animals. Estradiol administration decreased GAO levels by 50%. GAO levels in SPF and EB were similar. A negative correlation (r = -0.557, P<0.01) was observed between ALT and GAO levels in these animals. Similarly, a negative correlation (r = -0.554, P<0.05) was observed between ALT and GAD levels, suggesting that pyridoxine status regulates these two major enzymes of oxalate biosynthesis. LDH levels of both liver and kidney were unaffected by either treatment.

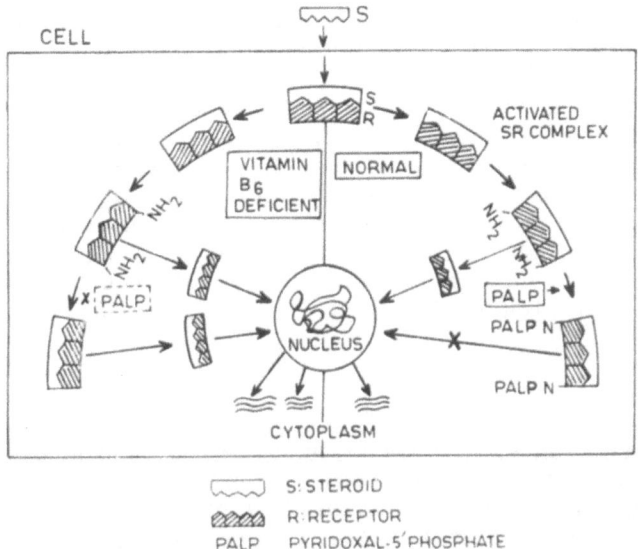

CELL

VITAMIN B₆ DEFICIENT

NORMAL

ACTIVATED SR COMPLEX

NUCLEUS

PALP

PALP

PALP N

PALP N

CYTOPLASM

S: STEROID
R: RECEPTOR
PALP   PYRIDOXAL-5'PHOSPHATE

Fig. 2. Role of pyridoxine in translocation of steroids to the nuclei.

DISCUSSION

The most accepted hypothesis, that the decrease in glyoxylate:glycine aminotransferase during pyridoxine deficiency leads to accumulation of glyoxylate thereby, producing hyperoxaluria, however, cannot explain why, during pyridoxine deficiency, glycolate is a better precursor of oxalate than glyoxylate. The increase in liver GAO and GAD levels seen in this study explains the hyperoxaluria observed during pyridoxine deficiency from glycolate and other compounds (viz. ethylene glycol, ethanolamine, xylitol) which are metabolized to oxalate via glycolate. It appears likely that the glyoxylate produced in the peroxisomes may have a different metabolism from that produced in the cytosol[4]. If it is assumed that the peroxisomal membrane does not allow the entry of glyoxylate[4], then the only enzyme remaining to convert it to oxalate in the cytosol is LDH, whose activity has been shown to be unaffected by pyridoxine deficiency. This explains the lack of hyperoxaluria from glyoxylate in pyridoxine-deficient animals. Recently, it has been shown also that at non-saturating levels of glyoxylate, complete hepatectomy has no effect on oxalate production from glyoxylate. Thus, liver may not play a major role in the conversion of glyoxylate to oxalate. As glyoxylate is highly toxic it would normally not attain saturating levels.

The interaction of pyridoxine with the steroid hormones has been recently proposed. PALP (pyridoxal-5'-phosphate), a coenzyme of pyridoxine, has been shown to regulate translocation of steroid hormones in liver by forming Schiff's base with ɛ-lysine residues exposed (on steroid-receptor complex) during activation, thereby preventing its nuclear translocation and binding[5] (Fig. 2). During pyridoxine deficiency this PALP modulation is lost, leading to increased translocation of the steroid-receptor complex to the nuclei[6]. Thus, an increased translocation of androgens to the nuclei may be a cause of increased enzyme levels observed during pyridoxine deficiency[7,8].

REFERENCES

1. V. Sharma, M. S. R. Murthy, S. K. Thind, and R. Nath, Biochem. Int. 3:507 (1981).
2. S. N. Gershoff, J. Nutr. 110:117 (1970).
3. H. Kishi and K. J. Folkares, J. Nutr. Sci. Vitaminol. 22:225 (1976).
4. A. M. Rofe and J. B. Edwards, Biochem. Med. 20:323 (1978).
5. Editorial, Nutr. Rev. 38:93 (1980).
6. J. Holley, D. A. Bender, W. E. Coulson, and F. K. Symes, J. Ster. Biochem. 18:161 (1983).
7. V. Sharma, S. K. Thind, and R. Nath, Biochem. Med. (1984) (in press).
8. V. Sharma, S. K. Thind, and R. Nath, Spec. Sci. Tech. (1984) (in press).

GLYOXYLATE OXIDATION AND ENZYMES OF OXALATE

BIOSYNTHESIS IN THIAMINE-DEFICIENT RATS

S. K. Thind, H. Sidhu, and R. Nath

Dept. of Biochemistry, Postgraduate Institute of Medical
Education and Research, Chandigarh-160012, India

INTRODUCTION

Glyoxylic acid (GA) is the major precursor of endogenous
oxalate and is mainly derived from glycine, glycolate and hydroxyproline. It can be either converted to CO_2 in liver and kidney
mitochondria by TPP-dependent α-ketoglutarate:GA carboligase[1] and
via the glyoxylate oxidation cycle[2], or it can be oxidized to
oxalate by glycolic acid oxidase (GAO) and lactate dehydrogenase
(LDH). Thiamine deficiency leads to excessive accumulation of GA
in tissues and its increased excretion in urine[3,4] and may result in
a greater incidence of renal calculi[5,6]. There are, however,
contradictory reports on the effect of thiamine deficiency on
oxalate excretion[7,8]. The present study tries to elucidate the
biochemical cause of the hyperoxaluria in thiamine deficiency.

MATERIALS AND METHODS

Male weanling Wistar rats (40-50 g body weight) were divided
into two groups: a thiamine-deficient group (TD) were fed a
thiamine-deficient diet ad libitum (n=8) and the second pair-fed
(PF) with the TD group but given 100 µg thiamine HCl/rat/day.

After four weeks when the TD rats showed symptoms of vitamin B_1
deficiency, they were sacrificed and blood collected in heparinized
vials. The vitamin B_1 and B_6 status was assessed by measuring the
specific activities of erythrocyte transketolase (ETK)[9] and
glutamate pyruvate transaminase (EGPT)[10], respectively. Liver and
kidney mitochondria were prepared in 0.25M sucrose buffered with
0.02M potassium phosphate buffer, pH 7.4, by differential

233

Table 1. Thiamine and Pyridoxine Status and the Mitochondrial Oxidation of U-^{14}C-Glyoxylate in Liver and Kidney of TD and PF Rats.

Group	Hemolysate		Liver Mitochondria		Kidney Mitochondria	
	ETK (U/mg protein)	EGPT x10^{-5} (U/mg protein)	U-^{14}C-GA oxidized to ^{14}C-CO$_2$ (nmol/min/mg/protein)	αKG:GA Carboligase (U/mg protein)	U-^{14}C-GA oxidized to ^{14}C-CO$_2$ (nmol/min/mg/protein)	αKG:GA Carboligase (U/mg protein)
Thiamine Deficient (n=8)	0.11+0.01***	4.36+0.30	0.93+0.09x10^{-3}	0.69+0.02	1.94+0.09x10^{-3}	0.78+0.06***
Pair-Fed Control (n=8)	0.33+0.17	4.80+0.17	2.31+0.08x10^{-3}	0.83+0.05	3.85+0.19x10^{-3}	2.89+0.11

***P<0.001 compared with the pair-fed controls.

centrifugation. The rate of oxidation of U-^{14}C-glyoxylate to ^{14}C-CO_2 was measured in tightly stoppered tubes containing 1.5 ml of 0.25M buffered sucrose, 10 μmol $MgSO_4$, 0.6 μmol ADP, 0.25 μmol pyruvate, 0.125 μmol of U-^{14}C-glyoxylate and 0.5 ml of mitochondrial preparation, in a final volume of 2.5 ml. ^{14}C-CO_2 was collected in small vials containing 0.2 ml of 10% KOH, and counted in a Packard scintillation counter. The α-KG:GA carboligase activity was measured in both liver and kidney mitochondria[11]. The activities of the oxalate-synthesising enzymes GAO, LDH and glycolic acid dehydrogenase (GAD), were measured in the liver supernatant but only LDH was measured in the kidney supernatant of TD and PF rats[12]. On two consecutive days before sacrifice, 24-h urine samples were collected from TD and PF rats and the urinary excretion of oxalate[13], citrate[14] and creatinine, determined.

RESULTS AND DISCUSSION

The growth rate of TD rats was normal for about 15 days after which they showed a decrease in food intake and cessation of growth. TD rats exhibited a significant decrease in ETK activity as compared to the PF controls (P 0.001) without affecting the EGPT levels indicating a normal pyridoxine status (Table 1). The mitochondrial oxidation of U-^{14}C-GA to ^{14}C-CO_2 was significantly decreased ($P < 0.001$) in both the liver and kidney mitochondria of TD rats (Table 1) as compared with PF controls, since thiamine deficiency leads to accumulation of glyoxylate, a potent inhibitor of γ-hydroxy-α-ketoglutarate aldolase[15] and α-KG-dehydrogenase[16]. The activity of α-KG:GA carboligase, a TPP-dependent enzyme was significantly decreased in kidney mitochondria ($P < 0.001$) and to a lesser extent (by 16%) in liver mitochondria of TD rats compared to the PF controls (Table 1). The αKG:GA carboligase activity resides

Table 2. Effect of Thiamine Deficiency on the Enzymes of Oxalate Biosynthesis in the Liver and Kidney Supernatant.

Group	Liver			Kidney
	GAO (U/mg protein)	GAD (U/mg protein)	LDH (U/mg protein)	LDH (U/mg protein)
Thiamine Deficient	5.59 ± 0.15***	0.31 ± 0.01	1.02 ± 0.07	2.58 ± 0.08
Pair-Fed Control	4.11 ± 0.19	0.31 ± 0.01	1.01 ± 0.07	2.33 ± 0.10

***$P < 0.001$ compared with pair-fed controls.

in the α-KG-dehydrogenase complex and a similar observation on the activity of α-KG-DH in TD rats has been reported[17]. Thus, in thiamine deficiency there is decreased conversion of GA to CO_2, which accumulates in blood and other tissues. This increased body pool of glyoxylate can be oxidized to oxalate[18]. A significant increase ($P<0.001$) in hepatic GAO activity and a lesser increase in the kidney LDH activity in TD rats was observed, while the liver GAD and LDH remain unaltered (Table 2). The increased synthesis of oxalate is also supported by the hyperoxaluria ($P<0.001$) in TD rats (0.41 ± 0.03 mg/day/100 g body weight) compared with PF (0.23 ± 0.02 mg/day/100 g). Glyoxylate is a potent inhibitor of key TCA cycle enzymes and competes with acetate for citrate bio-synthesis[19], leading to decreased ($P<0.001$) citrate excretion in urine (2.06 ± 0.24 mg/day 100 g in TD; 3.95 ± 0.23 mg/day 100 g in PF). Thus TD leads to hyperoxaluria, a decrease in urinary citrate excretion and a higher risk of calcum lithiasis.

REFERENCES

1. M. A. Schlossberg, R. J. Bloom, D. A. Richert, and W. W. Westerfield, Biochem. 9:1148 (1970).
2. E. E. Dekker and S. C. Gupta, Fed. Proc. 38:2339 (1979).
3. C. C. Liang, Biochem. J. 82:429 (1962).
4. R. M. Buckle, Clin. Sci. 25:207 (1963).
5. S. Davidson, A. P. Meiklejohn, and R. Passmore, "Human Nutrition and Dietetics", Williams & Wilkins, Baltimore (1959).
6. S. Dhanmitta, A. Valyasevi, and R. Van Reen, Nutr. Rep. Int. 2:87 (1970).
7. E. Takasaki, Invest. Urol. 7:150 (1969).
8. S. Hauschildt, R. Rudolph, and W. Feldheim, Int. J. Vitaminol. Nutr. Res. 42:457 (1972).
9. L. Boni, L. Kieckens, and A. Hendrikx, J. Nutr. Sci. Vitaminol. 26:507 (1980).
10. H. Kishi and K. Folkares, J. Nutr. Sci. Vitaminol. 22:225 (1976).
11. J. V. O'Fallon and R. W. Brosemer, Biochim. Biophys. Acta 499:321 (1977).
12. V. Sharma, M. S. R. Murthy, S. K. Thind, and R. Nath, Biochem. Int. 3:507 (1981).
13. A. Hodgkinson and A. Williams, Clin. Chim. Acta 36:127 (1972).
14. J. C. D. White and D. T. Davies, J. Dairy Res. 30:171 (1963).
15. R. G. Rosso and E. Adams, J. Biol. Chem. 23:5524 (1967).
16. A. Ruffo, E. Testa, A. Adinolfi, G. Pelizza, and R. Moratti, Biochem. J. 103:19 (1967).
17. C. J. Gubler, J. Biol. Chem. 236:312 (1961).
18. A. Weinhouse, in:"Symposium on Amino Acid Metabolism", W. D. McElroy and H. B. Glass, eds., John Hopkins Press, Baltimore (1955).
19. A. Ruffo, A. Adinolfi, G. Budillon, and G. Capobianco, Biochem.J. 85:593 (1962).

EFFECT OF PYRUVATE ON OXALATE-SYNTHESIZING ENZYMES IN LIVER

AND KIDNEY OF GLYCOLATE-FED RATS

M. S. R. Murthy, H. S. Talwar, S. K. Thind, and R. Nath

Dept. of Biochemistry, Postgraduate Institute of
Medical Education and Research, Chandigarh, India

INTRODUCTION

Oxalic acid, an end-product of metabolism, is known to cause
calcium oxalate stone formation when produced in large amounts in
the body both in animals and humans[1,2]. Glycolate is an important
precursor of oxalic acid[3] and its conversion to oxalate increases
several-fold in vitamin B_6 deficiency[4]. Chow et al[5] have reported
lowered oxalate excretion in glycolate-fed rats, when administered
alanine or pyruvate. But the mechanism of pyruvate action on
oxalate biosynthesis is still not clear. The present study was
undertaken to ascertain the biochemical mechanisms involved in the
inhibition of oxalate biosynthesis by feeding pyruvate to glycolate-
treated rats.

MATERIALS AND METHODS

A group of 24 male adult rats (4-months-old), were divided into
four sub-groups of 6 rats. Group I, orally fed with sodium
glycolate (50 mg/100 g body weight/day); Group II, orally fed with
sodium pyruvate (100 mg/100 g body weight/day); Group III, orally
fed both sodium glycolate and sodium pyruvate as in Groups I and II;
Group IV, normal controls. All the rats were fed stock diet
(Hindustan Lever) ad libitum. After 7 days of treatment, all the
rats were sacrificed and livers and kidneys removed for enzyme
analysis. Glycolate oxidase (GAO), glycolate dehydrogenase (GAD)
and lactate dehydrogenase (LDH) were assayed in liver homogenates;
in kidney homogenates only GAD and LDH were measured[6]. Protein in
all the samples was determined according to the method of Lowry et
al[7].

237

Table 1. Effect of Pyruvate Treatment on Oxalate-Synthesising Enzymes of Liver and Kidney in Glycolate-fed Rats.

	Normal	Glycolate	Pyruvate	Glycolate & Pyruvate
Liver				
LDH (U/mg protein)	1.79 $\pm$ 0.08	3.71 $\pm$ 0.30[c]	4.09 $\pm$ 0.30[c]	3.95 $\pm$ 0.35[c]
GAO (U/mg protein)	0.67 $\pm$ 0.18	1.33 $\pm$ 0.05[b,f]	0.99 $\pm$ 0.06	1.07 $\pm$ 0.09[g]
GAD (U/mg protein) x 10^{-2}	2.33 $\pm$ 0.08	1.86 $\pm$ 0.32	1.71 $\pm$ 0.42	1.59 $\pm$ 0.19[b]
Kidney				
LDH (U/mg protein)	2.55 $\pm$ 0.12	3.67 $\pm$ 0.18[c,d]	4.80 $\pm$ 0.34[c,g]	3.86 $\pm$ 0.15[c]
GAD (U/mg protein) x 10^{-2}	1.49 $\pm$ 0.07	0.18 $\pm$ 0.03[c]	0.23 $\pm$ 0.04[c]	0.15 $\pm$ 0.04[e]

1 U of LDH = enzyme required to produce ΔO.D.= 0.01/min at 340 nm at 25°C.
1 U of GAO = enyzme required to produce 1 nmol glyoxylate/min at 37°C.
1 U of GAD = enzyme required to produce 1 μmol oxalate/h at 37°C.
[a] $p<0.05$; [b] $p<0.01$; [c] $p<0.001$ as compared to normal group.
[d] $p<0.05$; [e] $p<0.01$; [f] $p<0.001$ as compared to pyruvate-fed group.
[g] $p<0.05$; [h] $p<0.01$; [i] $p<0.001$ as compared to pyruvate + glycolate-fed group.

RESULTS AND DISCUSSION

Rats fed glycolate or pyruvate for one week fhad no signs of
toxicity or change in growth pattern. Conversion of glycolate to
oxalate in the body is catalyzed by three main enzymes: GAO, GAD and
LDH[8]. Liver GAO acivity of glycolate-treated rats was
significantly increased ($P < 0.001$) as compared to normal controls
(Table 1). The enhanced GAO activity is probably due to substrate-
mediated induction as a result of proliferation of liver
peroxisomes[9,10]. Pyruvate feeding led to normalization of GAO.
This may be due to inhibition of GAO by lactate and acetate derived
from pyruvate[11], although pyruvate itself may not be inhibitory
(Fig. 1). The activity of liver GAD was reduced significantly in
the rats fed both glcolate and pyruvate as compared to the normal
controls ($P < 0.01$). There were no statistically significant changes
among the treated groups (Table 1). Liver LDH activity, although
the same among the treated groups, was significantly higher in each
of the treated groups ($P < 0.001$) as compared to the normal controls
(Table 1).

Kidney LDH also showed an increased activity in all treated
animals ($P < 0.001$) as compared to normal rats (Table 1). The enzyme
activity in pyruvate-fed rat kidneys was significantly higher than
in glycolate-fed rats ($P < 0.05$) and also in rats fed both glycolate
and pyruvate ($P < 0.05$). The increased LDH activity in liver and
kidney in glycolate-or pyruvate-fed groups as compared to the
normals could be due to excess substrate which may potentiate the
LDH enzyme protein, as both glycolate and pyruvate can act as
substrates for LDH. The GAD activity was significantly reduced

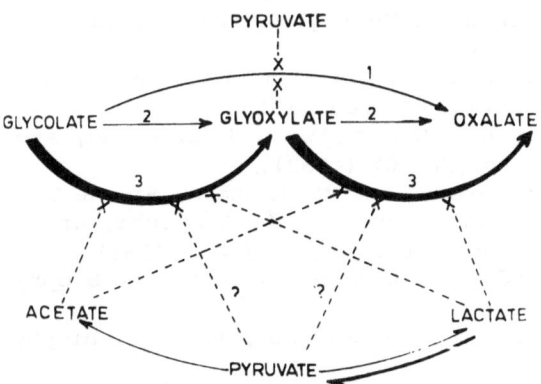

Fig. 1. Mechanism of the inhibition of oxalate biosynthesis by
pyruvate in glycolate-fed rats. (1 = GAD; 2 = LDH; 3 = GAO.
Bold arrows indicate increased enzyme activity due to
glycolate feeding; dotted lines indicate inhibition by
pyruvate or its metabolites.)

(P<0.001 in all cases) in kidneys of all treated rats as compared to the normal controls (Table 1).   The GAD activity is known to be significantly inhibited by glyoxylate[12].   Excess glycolate feeding can increase tissue glyoxylate levels by enhanced activities of LDH and GAO, and this increase in glyoxylate could inhibit the GAD of both liver and kidney. The decreased GAD activity by pyruvate feeding alone may be similar to GAD inhibition by glyoxylate as both pyruvate and glyoxylate are oxo acids.   Pyruvate feeding to glycolate treated rats further reduced the GAD activity in both liver and kidneys emphasizing the inhibitory effect of pyruvate on oxalate biosynthesis (Fig. 1).

CONCLUSION

     In glycolate induced hyperoxaluria GAO may play an important role in the endogenous synthesis of oxalate.   The present study reveals the importance of pyruvate in regulating the activities of oxalate-synthesizing enzymes in rat liver and kidney.

REFERENCES

 1. L. Hagler and R. H. Herman, Am. J. Clin. Nutr. 26:758 (1973).
 2. M. S. R. Murthy,. S. Talwar, S. Farooqui, S. K. Thind, and R. Nath, Int. J. Clin. Pharmacol. Ther. Toxicol. 20:434 (1982).
 3. K. S. Harris and K. E. Richardson, Invest. Urol. 18:106 (1980).
 4. T. J. Rundysan and S. N. Gershoff, J. Biol. Chem. 240:1889 (1965).
 5. F. H. C. Chow, D. W. Hamer, T. P. Boulay, and L. D. Lewis, Invest. Urol. 15:493 (1978).
 6. V. Sharma, M. S. R. Murthy, S. K. Hind, and R. Nath, Biochem. Int.3:507 (1981).
 7. O. H. Lowry, N. J. Rosebrough, A. L. Farr, and R. J. Randall, J. Biol. Chem. 193:265 (1951).
 8. M. S. R. Murthy, H. S. Talwar, S. K. Thind, and R. Nath, Ann. Nutr. Metab. 26:201 (1982).
 9. D. Crane, R. Holmes, and C. Masters, Biochem. Int. 1:133 (1980).
10. R. A. Harris, N. W. Cornell, C. Straight, and R. L. Veech, Arch. Biochem. Biophys. 213:414 (1982).
11. D. W. Fry and K. E. Richardson, Biochim. Biophys. Acta 568:135 (1979).
12. D. W. Fry and K. E. Richardson, Biochim. Biophys. Acta 567:482 (1979).

IS MAGNESIUM METABOLISM RELATED TO CALCIUM UROLITHIASIS?

G. W. Drach, J. Gaines, and J. Donovan

The Dept. of Surgery/Section of Urology, and Division of
Biostatistics, University of Arizona Health Sciences
Center, Tucson, Arizona 85724, U.S.A.

INTRODUCTION

Some investigators have demonstrated that the urinary ratio of
magnesium (Mg) to calcium (Ca) (usually expressed Mg/Ca x 100) is
significantly less in many stone formers than in normals. Based on
this observation physicians have administered magnesium as a means
of preventing new calcium stone formation, but success has been
inconclusive[1]. Other reports indicate that Mg/Ca ratios are not
relevant in stone former urines because urinary Ca is usually
elevated; Mg independently has minimal importance[2]. Furthermore,
there are no differences in the cellular metabolism of Mg between
stone formers and normals[3]. Most such studies have relied on long-
term observations (days or months) of serum and urinary (or even
cellular) Mg. These observations tend to average acute changes
which may occur when Ca and Mg are ingested and excreted
simultaneously[4]. If low urinary Mg is involved in the genesis of
calcium stone formation, then Mg administration should prevent
calcium stone formation. This is so[1].

We initially did <u>not</u> believe in the importance of magnesium,
but studies on out-patients in our metabolic unit defined a subgroup of patients who definitely had a low Mg/Ca ratio in urine,
which was related not to a high Ca excretion but to a low urinary
Mg. This observation stimulated the present study.

METHODS

The methodology has been described in full elsewhere[5]. It is
summarized in Table 1. The study group involved 93 Ca stone forming

241

patients and 11 normals who underwent an out-patient oral Ca/Mg loading test (Ca 1000 mg, Mg 53 mg, P 200 mg) modified from that of Pak[6]. Table 1 also records the observations made. Statistical analyses were performed by Anova and discriminant function tests.

Table 1. Design of Basic Study

Time	Test	Analyses
07.00 - 09.00	Fasting urine	Volume, Cr, Ca, Mg
09.00	Fasting blood	Ca, Mg, Cr
09.00	Oral Ca/Mg load	
09.00 - 13.00	Post-prandial urine	
13.00	Post-prandial blood	Ca, Mg

RESULTS

Table 2 summarizes the significant values for fasting and post-prandial observations in serum and urine. Most significant differences, however, were found in the ratios of Mg/Ca. We note that although the post-load serum ratios for Mg/Ca were not significantly different the urinary differences were maintained. Table 2 also shows the excretion rates of Ca and Mg and illustrates a significantly lower rate of post-load excretion of Mg in stone formers. The fractional excretion of the administered load of Mg (23% in normals and 16% in stone-formers) also differed between the two groups although that of calcium did not (2.4% and 2.0% respectively). Finally, discriminant analysis of all of the variables of Ca and Mg and their ratios revealed that the two criteria in Fig. 1 were most diagnostic.

Table 2. Blood and Urine Biochemistry Before and After Oral Ca/Mg Load in Normals (N) and Stone-Formers (SF) (mean $\pm$ SD).

Blood:				
Ca (mg/dl)	9.2 ± 0.3	9.4 ± 0.4	9.6 ± 0.3	9.9 ± 0.4*
Mg (mg/dl)	2.3 ± 0.2	2.2 ± 0.3	2.2 ± 0.3	2.2 ± 0.2
Mg/Ca	0.25± 0.02	0.23± 0.03*	0.23± 0.03	0.22± 0.03
Urine				
Ca (mg/dl)	2.8 ± 1.1	5.8 ± 4.2***	15.3 ± 6.5	18.4 ± 9.8
Ca (mg/h)	6.1 ± 2.3	10.8 ± 6.8***	12.1 ± 4.4	15.7 ± 5.9*
Mg (mg/dl)	1.9 ± 0.8	2.1 ± 1.9	9.6 ± 4.7	6.8 ± 4.1*
Mg (mg/h)	0.3 ± 0.1	0.3 ± 0.2	0.6 ± 0.2	0.5 ± 0.3*
Mg/Ca	0.69 ± 0.15	0.40 ± 0.27***	0.62 ± 0.15	0.40 ± 0.20**

*P<0.05; **P<0.01; ***P<0.001

242

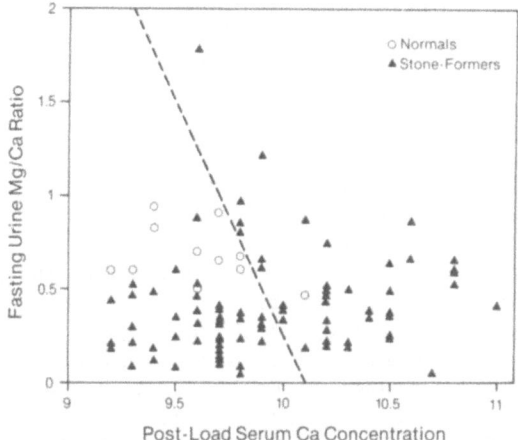

Fig. 1. Discrimination between stone-formers and normals on the
         basis of the Mg/Ca load test.

DISCUSSION

     It is known that Mg and Ca absorption tend to parallel each
other in a saturable, competitive transport mechanism probably
located in the small bowel. There is a second absorptive mechanism
for Mg, also in small bowel, which is believed to be ion-specific
diffusion-controlled and not saturable. Animal studies imply that
some competition between Ca and Mg transport exists in gut as well
as in renal tubules; hence, Ca absorption increases somewhat as Mg
absorption decreases. Perhaps this is also true of humans[7]. Fine
regulation of serum Mg is achieved, however, by renal excretion[8].

     It is important to note that irrespective of the post-prandial
changes in serum and urinary Mg created by oral Mg and Ca loading,
the fasting serum Mg of our stone formers was slightly lower and the
serum Ca slightly higher than that of our normals, such that the
serum Mg/Ca ratio in normals was significantly higher than that of
stone formers (Table 2).· This same relative deficiency of serum Mg
in Ca urolithiasis has been reported previously[9].

     Whatever the mechanism involved, our Ca urolithiasis patients
showed preferential Ca absorption and excretion over Mg absorption
and excretion when given orally amounts of both cations identical to
that given to a group of normal humans. This resulted in a
relative deficiency of urinary Mg (reflected by the Mg/Ca x 100
ratio) in 42% of our patients. Limitation to the requirement that
the ratio be less than 33 in both fasting and post-load states still
results in 34% of our patients with relative urinary Mg deficiency.
No normal person had this low ratio. Patients who fall into this
category are now usually placed on oral Mg therapy. Results of
such therapy will be reported in the future. These findings

hopefully will stimulate further investigation into the role of Mg metabolism in Ca urolithiasis.

REFERENCES

1. G. Johansson, Acta Med. Scand. (Suppl), 661:13 (1982).
2. C. D. Fetner, D. E. Barilla, J. Townsend, and C. Y. C. Pak, J. Urol. 120:399 (1978).
3. G. Johansson, U. Backman, B. G. Danielson, and B. Wikstrom, Invest. Urol. 18:93 (1980).
4. M. I. Resnick, D. Munday, and W. H. Boyce, Urology 20:385 (1982).
5. G. W. Drach, R. Perin, and S. Jacobs, J. Urol. 121:564 (1979).
6. C. Y. C. Pak, R. Kaplan, H. Bone, J. Townsend, and O. Waters, New Engl. J. Med. 292:497 (1975).
7. J. Aikawa, Wld. Rev. Nutr. Diet, 28:112 (1978).
8. J. H. Dirks and G. A. Quamme, Adv. Exp. Biol. Med. 103:51 (1978).
9. D. Scholz, P. O. Schwille, D. Ulbrich, W. M. Bausch, and A. Sigel, Urol. Res. 7:161 (1979).

LOW URINARY MAGNESIUM/CALCIUM RATIO DUE TO INCREASED URINARY CALCIUM EXCRETION IN ESSENTIAL HYPERTENSION

M. Cirillo, P. Strazzullo, A. Siani, P. L. Mattioli, R. Giannattasio, and V. Nunziata.

Clinica Medica II, 2nd Medical School, University of Naples, Naples, Italy

INTRODUCTION

A statistically significant association between blood pressure and frequency of kidney stone disease was reported many years ago[1]. More recently a mild degree of hypercalciuria has been described in patients with arterial hypertension[2,3]. Furthermore, a renal calcium leak as well as a high incidence of kidney stones has been found in the rat with genetic hypertension[4,5]. In the present paper we report on the urinary excretion of calcium and the urinary Mg/Ca ratio as potential risk factors for kidney stone disease[6] in patients with hypertension.

PATIENTS AND METHODS

A group of 60 patients with uncomplicated essential hypertension (30M and 30F; with a mean $\pm$ SEM age of 42 $\pm$ 3 years and a mean $\pm$ SEM body mass index 26.8 $\pm$ 0.6) and 60 comparable healthy volunteers (30M and 30F; 41 $\pm$ 2 years; body mass index 28.5 $\pm$ 0.5) were studied. No subject was on dietetic or pharmacological treatment. In all participants the 24-h urinary excretion of Ca, Mg and creatinine, the serum concentrations of total Ca, ionised Ca, Mg and creatinine were determined as previously described[3]. Parathyroid activity was assessed by the measurement of plasma PTH levels and urinary cAMP excretion. Student's t-test for unpaired observations was used for statistical analysis.

RESULTS

As shown in Table 1, hypertensive patients had significantly higher urinary Ca excretion with an appreciable reduction of the Mg/Ca ratio. Urinary Ca and Mg excretion were significantly interrelated in both groups of subjects, the correlation coefficients being 0.44 (P<0.01) in the hypertensive group and 0.40 (P<0.01) in the normotensive controls. The serum concentrations of total (2.42 $\pm$ 0.02 vs 2.54 $\pm$ 0.03 mmol/l) and ionised Ca (1.09 $\pm$ 0.01 vs 1.10 $\pm$ 0.01 mmol/l) were comparable in the two groups, while the mean level of serum Mg was slightly higher in the hypertensive group (0.88 $\pm$ 0.01 vs 0.81 $\pm$ 0.02 mmol/l, P<0.01). Both plasma PTH (2.79 $\pm$ 0.21 vs 2.21 $\pm$ 0.10 mUI/ml, P<0.05) and urinary cAMP (3.50 $\pm$ 0.14 vs 2.90 $\pm$ 0.11 nmol/100 ml GF, P<0.001) were increased in the hypertensive patients.

DISCUSSION

The present data confirm an increase in the urinary calcium excretion of untreated hypertensive patients, which seems to be due to a primary renal calcium leak[2,3]. The normal serum Ca levels and the mild degree of parathyroid overactivity also found in these patients are in keeping with the hypothesis of an altered renal calcium handling in hypertension.

Although Mg excretion was similar in patients and controls, the urinary Mg/Ca ratio was significantly reduced in the hypertensive group. This finding, together with the higher urinary calcium concentration, could account for the association between high blood pressure and urolithiasis previously reported[1]. The slight increase in the serum Mg levels of the hypertensives could be ascribed to the parathyroid overactivity[7] found in these patients.

Table 1. Data from Hypertensive (n=60) and Normotensive (n=60) Subjects (Mean $\pm$ SEM).

Urinary Variable	Normotensive	Hypertensive
Calcium (mmol/24 h)	3.54 $\pm$ 0.19	4.68 $\pm$ 0.25 **
Magnesium (mmol/24 h)	4.46 $\pm$ 0.19	4.94 $\pm$ 0.20
Mg/Ca ratio	1.23 $\pm$ 0.06	1.07 $\pm$ 0.05 *
Volume (ml/24 h)	1140 $\pm$ 60	1170 $\pm$ 70

* P<0.05; ** P<0.01

246

REFERENCES

1. S. Ljunghall and H. Hedstrand, Br. Med. J. 4:580 (1975).
2. D. A. McCarron, P. A. Pingree, R. J. Rubin, S. M. Gaucher, M. Molitch, and S. Krutzik, Hypertension 2:162 (1980).
3. P. Strazzullo, V. Nunziata, M. Cirillo, R. Giannattasio, L. A. Ferrara, P. L. Mattioli, and M. Mancini, Clin. Sci. 65:137 (1983).
4. D. A. McCarron, N. N. Yung, B. A. Ugoretz, and S. Krutzik, Hypertension 3:162 (1981).
5. B. C. Wexler and J. P. McMurtry, Br. J. Exp. Pathol. 62:369 (1981).
6. D. G. Oreopulos, M. A. O. Soyannwo, and M. G. McGeown, Lancet 2:420 (1968).
7. Z. S. Agus, A. Wasserstein, and S. Goldfarb, Am. J. Med. 72:473 (1982).

A STUDY OF FACTORS AFFECTING URINARY CITRATE LEVELS

A. K. Fraser, M. C. Gregory, G. A. Rose,
and C. T. Samuell

St. Peter's Hospitals and Institute of Urology
Endell Street, London WC2, U.K.

INTRODUCTION

Since citrate forms a soluble complex with calcium and has been
shown to reduce crystal formation in whole urine in vitro[1], hypocitraturia is regarded as a possible pathogenetic factor in calcium
urolithiasis. While gross hypocitraturia (in complete distal
renal tubular acidosis) is easily demonstrated, defining lesser
abnormalities may be more difficult because a number of physiological and pathological factors may affect urine citrate levels.
These include renal dysfunction, urine pH, sex and bacterial
infection. In this paper an attempt has been made to clarify the
role of these factors. The acute effect of oral citric acid
loading on urinary citrate has also been studied.

METHODS AND SUBJECTS

Urine citrate was assayed using citrate lyase. Plasma and
urine creatinine were measured by standard automated methods, and
urine pH by glass electrode. Specimens not analysed freshly were
stored at $-20^{\circ}C$. The following studies were carried out.

Renal Failure Study: Citrate, creatinine, and pH were measured
in timed 20-min urines collected from 50 patients (34 males, 16
females) with chronic renal failure (plasma creatinine > 0.2 mmol/l).
A simultaneous blood specimen was collected for creatinine
estimation. All patients had sterile urines and none was receiving
bicarbonate. Post-transplantation patients were excluded.

Urine pH Study: Seventeen normal volunteers were selected from the hospital staff 9 males ((24 to 39 years) and 8 females (19 to 32 years)). All had sterile urine and normal plasma creatinines. Urine citrate, creatinine, and pH were measured in timed 20-min specimens collected hourly during:forced urine pH changes induced across 8 h by sequential oral administration of sodium bicarbonate (1.8 g the previous evening and 2.4 g at the commencement of the period), and ammonium chloride (0.1 g/kg at the end of the third hour) and spontaneous urine pH changes throughout the waking day. Fifteen subjects took part in study (i) and 16 in study (ii).

Urine Infection Study: Urines from patients with known or suspected urinary tract infection, but normal plasma creatinine, were assayed fresh for citrate, and then reassayed after incubation at 37°C for 18 h. The type and concentration of any organism in the specimen were noted. Sterile urines were similarly incubated.

Citric Acid Loading Study: Seven normal males were given 10 mmol (2.1 g) or oral citric acid as a flavoured solution. Urines collected at 30 min intervals for 90 min pre- and 90 min post-load were assayed for citrate, creatinine, and pH.

RESULTS

In the renal failure study, the molar citrate:creatinine ratios (cit/creat) in relation to urine pH and simultaneous plasma creatinine are shown in Fig. 1. In the pH study, in terms of forced changes, the combined results for the group are shown in Fig. 2, indicating a significant correlation between urine cit/ creat and pH in both sexes. Individually, significant correlations ($r = 0.789 - 0.986$) were found in 14 of the 15 subjects. All subjects acidified their urine to pH 5.3 or less following ammonium chloride. In terms of spontaneous changes, the combined results again showed a significant correlation between urine pH and cit/creat in males ($r = 0.274$, $P = < 0.01$) and females ($r = 0.482$, $P = < 0.001$), albeit weaker than during the forced pH changes. Fifteen of the 16 subjects showed significant individual correlations, ($r = 0.521$ to 0.912). In the infection study, after 18 h incubation at 37° C the citrate level in urines infected with E. coli ($>10^6$ organisms/ml) was reduced to less than 0.1 mmol/l while no reduction was observed in sterile urines. In the citric acid loading study, no significant increases in cit/creat were seen post-loading either for the group as a whole, or for individuals, when changes in pH were allowed for.

DISCUSSION

Factors affecting urine citrate have been ignored in several studies on calcium stone formers, and there is a need to re-empha-

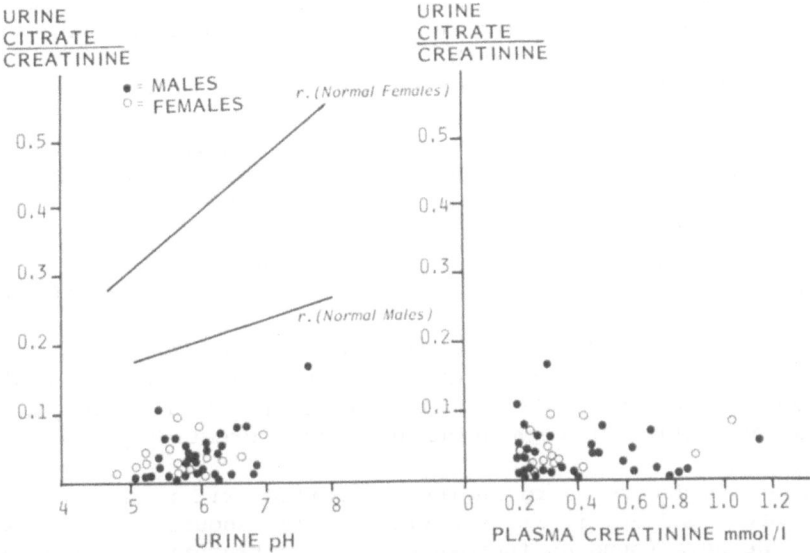

Fig. 1.   Urine citrate/creatinine ratios related to urine pH and
          plasma creatinine in chronic renal failure patients.
          The regression lines for normal subjects are shown.

sise their importance when interpreting patient results.   In this
study urine was found to be positively correlated with urine pH in
normal subjects of both sexes.   This was true both during periods
of forced and spontaneous pH changes, although the correlation was

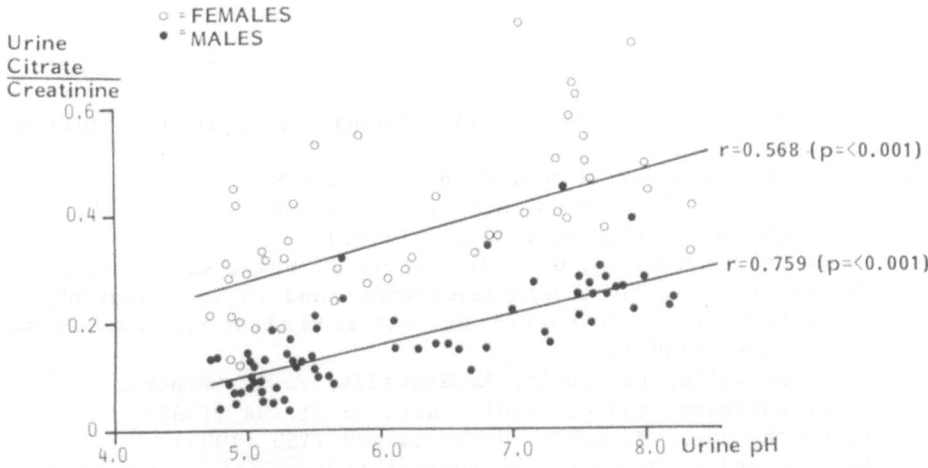

Fig. 2.   Effect of forced pH changes on urine citrate excretion in
          normal subjects.

stronger in the former case possibly due to more urines having pH values at the extremes of the range. This is in agreement with Dedmon and Wrong[2] but not with the findings of Nordin and Smith[3]. Although the correlation within any one subject is strong, there is a substantial between-subject variation leading to large scatter of values at any given pH. However, the above suggests that the relationship between citrate and pH in spot urines may be more revealing than daily citrate excretion. The finding that females had significantly higher citrate levels than males at all pH values confirms the findings of others[4-7] and emphasises the need for separate reference ranges, at least in the premenopausal years.

The hypocitraturia associated with established chronic renal failure[4,8] is clearly shown, ratios being depressed over the whole pH range in both sexes when plasma creatinine is >0.2 mmol/l. There was no correlation between urine and plasma creatinine.

There is debate as to whether hypocitraturia is seen in urinary tract infection[4] and if it is simply due to associated renal impairment. We have found an incidence of hypocitraturia in patients with E. coli infections but normal plasma creatine. On the basis of in vitro incubation studies bacterial consumption of citrate would seem to be responsible.

If hypocitraturia is important in calcium stone disease then raising levels might have therapeutic benefit. Oral citric acid is of little use, producing no significant change in urine when pH changes are allowed for, presumably due to rapid tissue uptake and catabolism. Urinary alkalinisation has been recommended for oxalate stone formers[9] and while bicarbonate clearly raises urine citrate in normals, its role in treatment needs further study.

REFERENCES

1. P. C. Hallson, G. A. Rose, and S. Sulaiman, Urol. Int. 38:179 (1983).
2. R. E. Dedman and O. Wrong. Clin. Sci. 22:19 (1962).
3. B. E. C. Nordin and D. A. Smith, Br. J. Urol. 35:438 (1968).
4. A. Hodgkinson, Clin. Sci. 23:203 (1962).
5. S. G. Welshman and H. G. McGeown, Br. J. Urol. 48:7 (1976).
6. H. Tiselius, in:"Urolithiasis:Clinical and Basic Research", L. H. Smith, W. G. Robertson, and B. Finlayson, eds., Plenum, New York (1981).
7. P. O. Schwille, D. Scholz, K. Schwille, R. Leutschaft, I. Goldberg, and A. Sigel. Nephron 31:194 (1982).
8. M. Menon and C. J. Mahle, J. Urol. 129:1155 (1983).
9. M. Butz and H. J. Dulce, in:"Urolithiasis:Clinical and Basic Research", L. H. Smith, W. G. Robertson, and B. Finlayson, eds., Plenum, New York (1981).

RELATION BETWEEN HYPERCALCIURIA AND VITAMIN D_3-STATUS

IN RENAL STONE FORMERS

T. Berlin, I. Björkhem, L. Collste, I. Holmberg,
and H. Wijkström

Dept. of Urology and Clinical Chemistry, Karolinska
Institute, Huddinge Hospital, Huddinge, Sweden

INTRODUCTION

An increased urinary excretion of calcium is common among
patients with recurrent urolithiasis. Another common abnormality
is a low-normal or subnormal serum phosphate level, the latter being
a stimulus for the renal conversion of 25-hydroxyvitamin D_3
(25-OH D_3) into the most active metabolite, 1,25-dihydroxyvitamin D_3
(1,25-$(OH)_2D_3$). Increased serum levels of 1,25-$(OH)_2$ D_3 have been
demonstrated in renal stone formers[1-3] and in patients with
hypercalciuria[4]. The major circulating form of vitamin D_3 is,
however, 25-(OH) D_3 and this metabolite is believed to reflect best
the endogenous synthesis and stores of vitamin D_3[5]. Previous
attempts to demonstrate increased concentrations of 25-(OH) D_3 in
serum from patients who form renal stones have failed[2,3]. Whether
or not the pool of 25-OH D_3 is increased in hypercalciuria is not
known. In order to study this possibility, we have determined
25-OH D_3 in stone forming patient with or without hypercalciuria.

METHODS

Seventy patients (50 males and 20 females) with (mainly
recurrent) urolithiasis participated in the study. The mean age of
the males was 43 years (range 15 to 71), and of the females 39 years
(range 17 to 67). They were all outpatients who consulted our
clinic between October and March. All patients with present or
previous hyperparathyroidism were excluded from the study. Blood
samples for calcium and phosphate measurement were taken on each of
3 consecutive days. A sample for determination of 25-OH D_3 was
taken on one of these days. A 24-h urine sample was collected for

each of the 3 days for determination of calcium. Serum 25-OH D$_3$ was determined by isotope dilution-mass spectrometry[6].

RESULTS

Serum 25-OH D$_3$ levels in relation to calciuria are summarized in Table 1. The male hypercalciuric stone formers (HCU) (calcium ≥ 8.1 mmol/24 h; n= 24) had significantly higher 25-OH D$_3$ levels (28.3 ± 2.3 ng/ml) than had the male normocalciuric (NCU) (calcium ≤ 6.0 mmol/24 h; n = 16) stone formers (17.6 ± 1.2 ng/ml; P<0.001). Male stone formers with an intermediate excretion of calcium (ICU) (≥6.1, ≤8.0 mmol/24 h; n = 10) had 25-OH D$_3$ levels between those of the other two groups (21.3 ± 1.2 ng/ml). The female stone formers with normocalciuria (n = 16) had a mean level of 25-OH D$_3$ (17.6 ± 1.3 ng/ml) identical with that of the male normocalciuric stone formers.

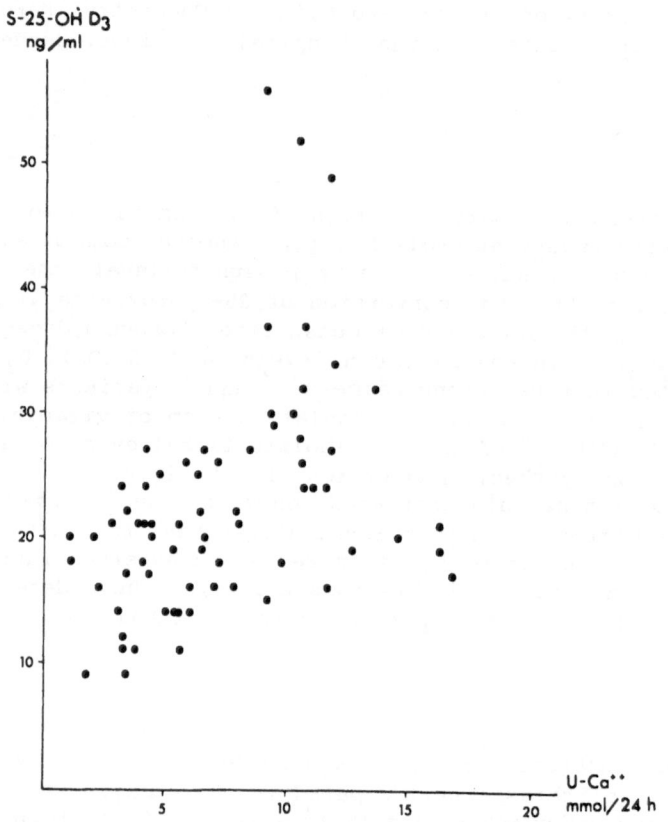

Fig. 1. Relation between serum level of 25-hydroxy vitamin D$_3$ and excretion of calcium in patients with urolithiasis. Individual values (r = 0.40).

Table 1. Serum levels of 25-Hydroxy Vitamin D_3, Calcium and Phosphate in the Different Groups of Patients. Mean $\pm$ SEM are given in the table.

	Males			Females		Males + females	
	NCU	ICU	HCU	NCU	ICU + HCU	NCU	ICU + HCU
	n=16	n=10	n=24	n=16	n=4	n=32	n=38
S-25-hydroxy vitamin D_3 (ng/ml)	17.6±1.2	21.3±1.2	28.3±2.3[a]	17.6±1.3	26±4	17.6±0.9	26.2±1.6[d]
S—Ca^{++} (mmol/l)	2.42±0.02	2.31±0.04	2.35±0.02[b]	2.35±0.02	2.43±0.05	2.39±0.02	2.34±0.02[e]
S—PO_4 (mmol/l)	0.96±0.06	0.90±0.10	0.85±0.04[c]	0.89±0.07	1.08±0.09	0.92±0.05	0.89±0.04[f]

[a] Significantly different from male NCU ($p < 0.001$).   [d] Significantly different from NCU ($p < 0.001$).

[b] Significantly different from male NCU ($p < 0.0025$).   [e] Significantly different from NCU ($p < 0.05$).

[c] Not significantly different from male NCU ($p > 0.05$).   [f] Not significantly different from NCU ($p > 0.05$).

The combined small group of female stone formers with a high and intermediate excretion of calcium (n = 4) had a mean 25-OH D_3 level (26 $\pm$ 4 ng/ml) significantly higher than that of the group of normocalciuric female stone formers. When the male and female stone formers with high and intermediate excretions of calcium were combined into one group (n = 38), the level of 25-OH D_3 was significantly higher (26.2 $\pm$ 1.6 ng/ml) than that of the corresponding group (n = 32) with a normal calcium excretion (17.6 $\pm$ 0.9 ng/ml; P<0.001). When the calcium excretion was plotted against the level of 25-OH D_3 for each individual patient, only a low correlation (r = 0.40) was obtained (Fig. 1). Serum calcium, while within the normal range, was slightly higher in the group of patients with a normal Ca excretion than in the group of patients with hypercalciuria (P<0.05; males + females). There was a tendency towards lower serum phosphate in patients with hypercalciuria, but this was not statistically significant. There was no correlation between serum 25-OH D_3 and either serum Ca (r = -0.06) or serum phosphate (r = 0.06).

DISCUSSION

The present assay of 25-OH D_3, based on isotope dilution-mass spectrometry, should be more specific than methods based on specific protein binding. The method is completely specific for the D_3-form of the vitamin and does not respond to 25-OH D_2. It should be pointed out that the relation between Ca excretion and serum 25-OH D_3 in the present work was evident only in a comparison between the two groups of patients. Within a given individual, there was only a weak correlation.

Since vitamin D_3 is the predominant form of vitamin D and 25-OH D_3 is its main circulating metabolite, it seems plausible that the values obtained reflect the total vitamin D status in the individuals. If $1,25\text{-}(OH)_2 D_3$ is the only important vitamin D metabolite, and the level of this metabolite is strictly regulated, it should not be important whether the vitamin D status is normal or high. It has been reported that $1,25\text{-}(OH)_2 D_3$ is at least 100-fold more effective than 25-OH D_3 in vivo with respect to intestinal absorption of calcium[7]. Thus 25-OH D_3 will act as a competitor of $1,25\text{-}(OH)_2 D_3$ for binding to intestinal receptors only when its concentration in the medium is about 900 times higher[8]. Since the concentration of 25-OH D_3 in serum is actually about 500 times higher than that of $1,25\text{-}(OH)_2 D_3$ it is evident that the level of 25-OH D_3 in serum might be of physiological importance. After completion of the present work two additional papers have appeared which support the contention that the level of 25-OH D_3 may be of importance for the development of hypercalciuria in renal stone formers[9,10].

ACKNOWLEDGMENT

This study has been described in detail earlier (Scand. J. Urol Nephrol 16:269-273, 1982) and is published here by courtesy of that journal.

REFERENCES

1. R. W. Gray, D. R. Wilz, A. E. Caldas, and J. Lemann, J. Clin. Endocrinol. Metab. 45:299 (1977).
2. A. E. Caldas, R. W. Gray, and J. Lemann, J. Lab. Clin. Med. 91:840 (1978).
3. H. Schmidt-Gayk, W. Tschöpe, B. Schellenberg, G. Scheierf, and S. Walch, Therapiewoche 29:2137 (1979).
4. F. H. Shen, D. J. Baylink, R. L. Nielsen, D. J. Sherrard, J. L. Ivey, and M. R. Haussler, J. Lab. Clin. Med. 90:955 (1977).
5. H. F. Deluca, "Monographs on Endocrinology", Springer, New York (1979).
6. I. Björkhem and I. Holmberg, Meth. Enzymol. 67:385 (1980).
7. J. Reeve, Br. Med. J. 2:888 (1979).
8. D. A. Procsal, W. H. Okamura, and A. W. Norman, J. Biol. Chem. 250:8382 (1975).
9. I. Eloma, S. L. Karonen, A. L. Kairento, and R. Pelkonen, Scand. J. Urol. Nephol. 16:155 (1982).
10. M. Johngen, "The Role of Vitamin D in the Pathogenesis of Urinary Calcium-Stone Disease", Ph.D Thesis, Amsterdam (1983).

V. CLINICAL UROLITHIASIS

INSTITUTION AND MANAGEMENT OF A STONE CLINIC

M. Peacock, W. G. Robertson, R. Norman, and P. L. Selby

MRC Mineral Metabolism Unit, The General Infirmary
Leeds LS1 3EX, U.K.

INTRODUCTION

The incidence of upper urinary stone disease has risen steadily throughout this century and renal colic is now one of the commonest causes of surgical admission to hospital. Spontaneous passage, removal, or dissolution of the stone does not, however, cure the underlying abnormalities responsible for stone formation and merely represents an episode in what is a recurrent disease. The high incidence and recurrence rates dictate that special facilities need to be provided for the management of patients if the disease is to be treated and prevented effectively. The facilities, their organisation, and the management of patients form the basis of this article. We have drawn heavily on experience gained in running a stone clinic in Leeds over the last 15 years, although each stone clinic is unique by virtue of its local environment and expertise.

PURPOSE AND OPERATION OF A STONE CLINIC

A stone clinic can be designed to serve a number of functions. It must provide a service for diagnosing the absence or presence of urinary stone disease. Having established that a patient is a genuine stone-former, it is essential for his, or her, further management that the clinic has the facilities to classify the stone disease into its various types; to identify the urinary and pre-urinary risk factors responsible for stone formation; to institute and monitor surgical and medical treatment, and finally, to train staff. In addition, the clinic should provide an environment in which research can be undertaken with the aim of improving management and eradicating the disease.

259

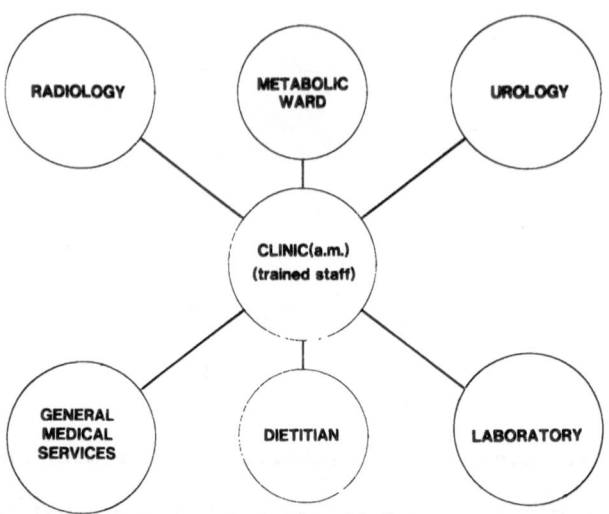

Fig. 1. Essential services associated with a stone clinic.

     To achieve its aim the clinic should be sited close to
essential services (Fig. 1).   The ideal site is within a general
hospital with access to the disciplines of urology, radiology and
clinical biochemistry.   Many other specialities, however, within
the general medical services will occasionally be required.   The
clinic, in addition, should have access to investigational beds,
staffed by skilled nurses and dietitians, in which metabolic studies
can be undertaken.   The clinic should be conducted by trained
physicians who appreciate the aims and limitations of management.
Since many of the biochemical variables to be measured are dietary
dependent, the clinic should be held in the morning so that blood
and urine can be collected from the patient after a standardised
overnight fast.   It is an advantage to have, within the clinic, a
room for the collection of specimens.

     The patient with stone should be handled like patients with any
other disease and the basic principles of clinical medicine
followed.   Failure to do so, or reliance on this being performed by
an outside department inevitably leads to misdiagnosis, wasteful
investigation and inappropriate treatment.   The essential
information gathered from the patient's history (such as age, sex,
occupation, previous surgery to the urinary and gastrointestinal
tract, urinary infection, stone recurrence rate, familial disease,
drug ingestion) and clinical examination (such as the presence and
absence of associated and non-associated disease) need to be
documented.   We have found that the documentation of the history
and clinical examination is most efficiently handled by providing a
unique set of patient case-notes for use only at the stone clinic.
The case-notes should contain space for the documentation of the

Table 1. Outline of an Instruction Sheet.

Instruction Sheet:	Name			Unit No.	
Appointment	X-ray	24-h Urine	Fasting Blood/Urine	Urine Culture	Stone Analysis
Date	Yes	Yes	Yes	No	Yes

results of biochemistry on fasting blood and urine and 24-h urine, of radiological procedures and of drug therapy. The average stone recurrence rate is such that the majority of patients need not be seen frequently at the clinic. It is essential, however, that when patients attend, the previous results are available and that any further investigations required have been arranged for that visit. To achieve the latter we have found it helpful to have an "Instruction sheet" (Table 1) which accompanies each patient and on which clear orders on the investigations required at the patient's attendance are given to secretarial, laboratory and other personnel. Computerised storage and retrieval of data can be extremely valuable both for patient management and for research but its cost effectiveness must be assessed by individual clinics.

MANAGEMENT OF PATIENTS

Diagnosis (Fig. 2)

A history of renal colic and/or passage of a stone combined with radiographic evidence of stone in the urinary tract are the essential requirements for establishing a diagnosis. Although the diagnosis is rarely a problem there are a number of pitfalls. Probably the commonest of these is the patient who has become addicted to analgesics. Such patients usually start off as genuine stone formers but their stone recurrence rate and symptoms are more severe than suggested by the radiography of the urinary tract or by the urinary biochemistry. 'Stones' are brought to the clinic or added to urine which on analysis reveals them to be of non-urinary origin. Some patients may add 'stones' or 'gravel' to the urine as a means of solving a psychological problem. In children there is often a family history of urinary stone disease and in adults the behaviour may be part of the Munchausen Syndrome.

Classification (Fig. 2)

Having diagnosed that a patient suffers from stone disease the next step is to the classification of the stone type. The most

261

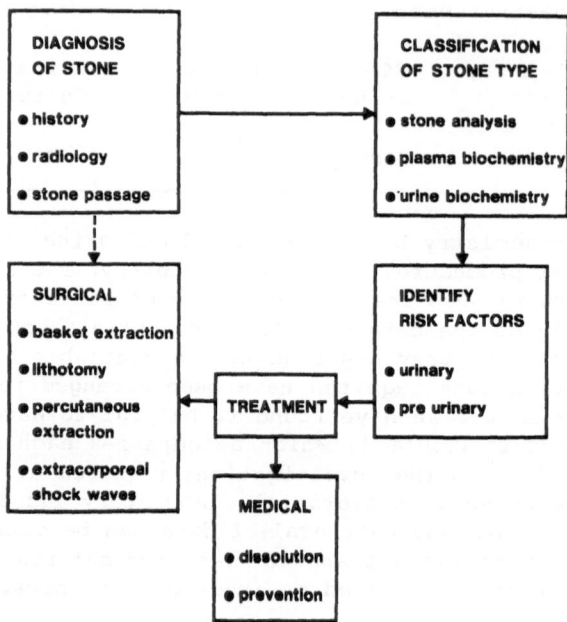

Fig. 2. Schematic outline of steps in the management of urinary
stone disease.

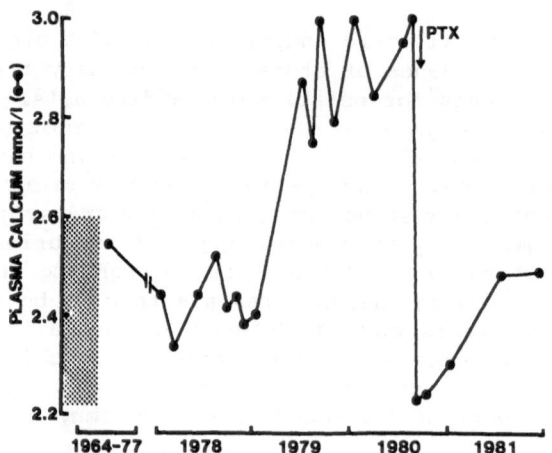

Fig. 3. Development of primary hyperparathyroidism in a patient
originally presenting with primary calcium stone disease.

important laboratory investigation for purposes of classification is the analysis of the stone itself. Where stones are unavailable, detailed analysis of plasma and urine biochemistry in conjunction with the information gathered from history, examination and radiography of the urinary tract are essential. The great majority of patients, even without analysis, can be classified into the four main types: calcium, infected, uric acid or cystine. These investigations also allow the patients with calcium stones to be classified further into those with primary or secondary disease.

Although most patients remain true to their initial stone classification, not all do so. Some may begin as primary calcium stone formers, but because of urinary obstruction, surgery or frequent instrumentation, become infected stone formers. Rarely, a patient with primary calcium stone disease may, with the passage of time, develop a secondary form of disease (Fig. 3).

Identification of Risk Factors (Fig. 2)

The risk factors responsible for stone formation can be considered to exist at two levels. Those in the urine (urinary risk factors) responsible for stone formation and its frequency and those outside the urine (metabolic and environmental risk factors) responsible for the urinary abnormalities and their severity.

Although there is general recognition of the particular risk factors which should be measured and of the most precise and accurate methodology for doing so, there is much less appreciation of the wide variation in the range of the risk factors in the normal population. All the urinary risk factors, to a greater or lesser extent, are dependent on age, sex and season and striking geographical and secular variations occur in their excretion. It is important, therefore, that the excretion of the urinary risk factors are assessed in relation to the ranges established in an appropriate normal population from which patients attending the stone clinic are drawn. All too often, normal ranges are inadequate because of lack of numbers or because the known determinants, outlined above, have been ignored. Few studies have aimed at establishing the optimal time at which to investigate patients in relation to the episode of stone passage. Ideally it should be at that time which separates stone formers from normals with respect to the urinary abnormalities. The period immediately following an episode of renal colic is not optimal. It takes about 2 months following colic for the abnormalities in the urinary excretion of the stone factors to become obvious again.

It is clear, from our own and published data, that the differences in the excretion of the urinary risk factors vary from clinic to clinic. These variations are due, in part, to the time

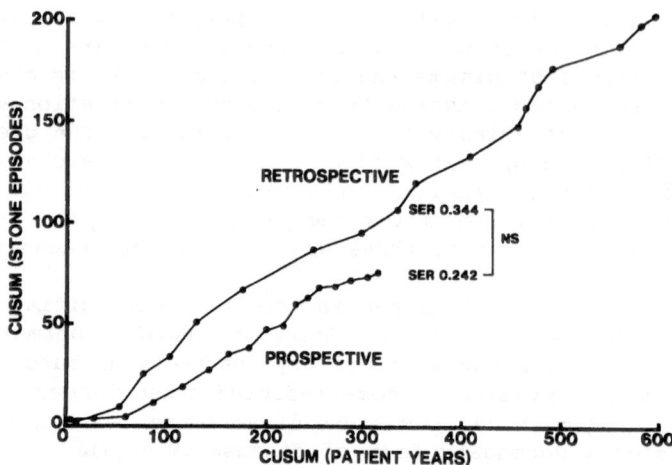

Fig. 4. A comparison of the retrospective and prospective stone
episode rates in a group of patients with primary calcium
stone disease.

Treatment

The quantitation of the response to preventive treatment
remains unsatisfactory. The majority of clinics rely on a decrease
in the stone recurrence rate as the sign of successful therapy.
Stones in situ are ignored since their quantification by
radiographic methods is unsatisfactory. Surgical removal of a
stone also poses a problem and it is a matter of opinion whether or
not it should be considered as an episode. Renal colic, despite its
classical features, is a symptom and if included as a criterion for
calculating the stone recurrence rate, can give misleadingly high
rates of stone recurrence.

The stone recurrence rate estimated retrospectively from
history assumes that the patient's memory is infallible - which is
rare - and that the recurrence rate is unaffected by regular
attendance at a stone clinic - which is not true (Fig. 4).

The evaluation of preventive therapy based on the stone
recurrence rate must take into account not only the "clinic effect"
but also the wide range in the episode rate between individuals.
In order to show that a particular treatment has a beneficial effect
in reducing the stone episode rate, it must be given for a
considerable length of time in a large number of patients before
statistically significant effects can be expected (Fig. 5).   To
show that a treatment has no effect on the episode rate i.e. to
prove the null hypothesis, takes much more time and many more

264

of investigation in relation to the stone episode and in part to subtle alterations in fluid and dietary intake as a result of advice from staff to patient, and from patient to patient.

Gross changes in bowel, bone and gut function are well known to affect the excretion of some of the urinary risk factors, particularly calcium, oxalate, pH, and citrate. Minor changes, difficult to diagnose, however, also alter their excretion. A small decrease in glomerular filtration rate, for example, often unappreciated by measuring plasma creatinine, decreases calcium absorption and excretion. Such small changes also affect the plasma biochemistry on which the classification of primary and secondary calcium stone type depends. A rise in plasma creatinine even within the normal range lowers plasma calcium and raises plasma phosphate and parathyroid hormone concentrations.

One of the most difficult problems in classification remains the diagnosis of calcium stone formers with idiopathic disease from those with mild primary hyperparathyroid disease. Accurate measurement of plasma calcium, total (corrected for plasma protein) and ionised, and plasma parathyroid hormone (C and N terminal fragments) are essential since several biochemical abnormalities are common to both conditions (Table 2).

Although a single set of biochemical variables obtained in blood and urine is of great value in classifying the stone type, follow-up biochemistry shows that using one set of variables gives an appreciable percentage of false positive and negative classifications. These mistakes can only be avoided by using mean data obtained from several clinic visits (Table 3).

Table 2. Biochemical Abnormalities which are Common to Idiopathic and Hyperparathyroid (HPT) Calcium Stone-formers.

	Plasma PO_4	PO_4 Reabsorption	Calcium Excretion	Calcium Absorption	Plasma $1,25(OH)_2D$
Idiopathic	↓	↓	↑	↑	↑
HPT	↓	↓	↑	↑	↑

Table 3. The % of False Positive and Negative Classifications Based on a Single Sample of Blood and Urine.

	'Calcium Leak'	Hypophos-phataemia	Hyper-calciuria	Hyper-oxaluria	Hyper-uricosuria
False positive	5%	15%	5%	10%	15%
False negative	5%	0%	5%	10%	5%

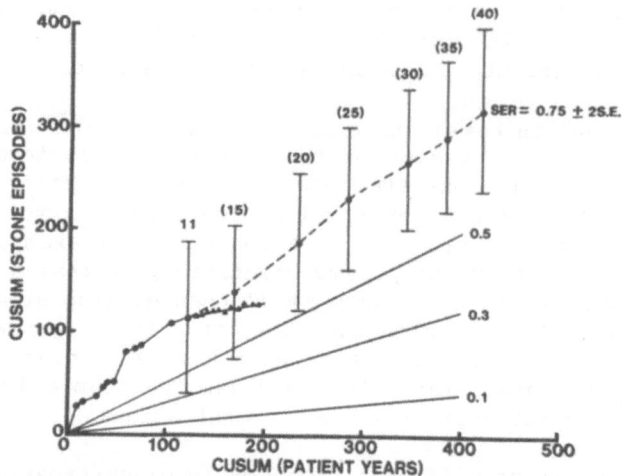

Fig. 5. The required reductions in stone episode rate in relation
to patient years to show significant effects of therapy.
SER = stone episode rate; ●-● before treatment;
---- extrapolated line; ▲-▲ on treatment.

patients. By and large, most published studies on treatment are
unsatisfactory because one or all of these variables have been
neglected and in only a few studies have an untreated group of
patients been included as a control.

CONCLUSIONS

A stone clinic probably provides the best environment for
managing patients effectively. To do so, it must be correctly
sited, be staffed with trained personnel, have access to a wide
variety of specialist expertise and have the facilities for
documentation of data essential for both clinical care and research.
More important than any of these, however, it must provide a
clinical service which encourages patients to attend and be followed
up over a number of years. Since the majority of patients are free
of symptoms between attacks of colic and are healthy men busy in
employment, the high degree of compliance necessary for
investigation and treatment can only be achieved by a clinic in
which patient care is the first priority.

TEMPORAL CHANGES IN URINARY RISK FACTORS FOLLOWING

RENAL COLIC

R. W. Norman, S. S. Bath, W. G. Robertson, and
M. Peacock

MRC Mineral Metabolism Unit, The General Infirmary
Leeds LS1 3EX, U.K.

INTRODUCTION

The optimal time for metabolic evaluation of a stone-former
following acute renal colic has not been established. Although
immediate in-patient studies are convenient, the results may be
biased by atypical diet, fluid intake, activity and renal function.
Early post-discharge assessment may reflect only temporary patient
compliance to advice on increasing fluid intake and decreasing
dietary excesses and therefore may not reveal the true risk of
recurrent stone formation[1].

To study this problem we followed several patients with
sequential 24-h urine collections following an episode of renal
colic and compared the results to those of a control group
collecting samples over the same period.

MATERIALS AND METHODS

Over a 3-month period, 13 consecutive males with acute renal
colic secondary to an obstructing radio-opaque ureteric calculus
were admitted from the casualty department. All had urine cultures
and plasma biochemical profiles performed on admission. They were
treated with fluids, antiemetics and analgesics as necessary.

Each agreed to provide 24-h urine samples, first in hospital,
and then at 1,2,3,8 and 12 weeks following discharge. These were
collected in plastic containers with hibitane preservative. The
volume and pH were measured immediately and aliquots were frozen
until all samples were available at the end of the three-month

period.   Those from each patient were analysed in a single batch
for calcium, uric acid, creatinine and alcian blue precipitable
polyanions (ABPP) as previously described[1].   Oxalate was measured
by ion-chromatography[2].   The individual risk factors of each 24-h
urine collection were combined to determine the relative probability
(P_{SF}) of forming stones[1].

In a separate, but otherwise identical, study beginning in
September, 10 normal male volunteers, aged 26 to 60 years (mean 40
years), provided 24-h urine collections at 0,1,2,3,4,8 and 12 weeks.

RESULTS

Eleven patients, aged 27-67 years (mean 41 years), completed
the protocol.   In 8 this was their first stone and in 3 it

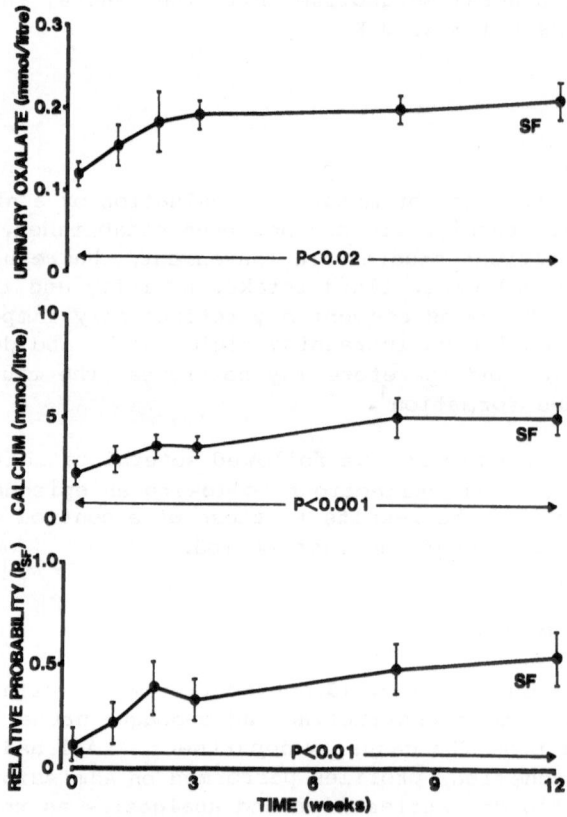

Fig. 1.   Changes in the 24-h urinary calcium and oxalate
concentration and P_{SF} in patients following acute
renal colic.

represented a recurrence. Two men underwent a ureterolithotomy during their admission. The others passed their stones during the follow-up period. All urine cultures were sterile. Plasma creatinine was 124 ± 13 μmol/l (mean ± SEM) at the time of admission compared to 93 ± 3 μmol/l after relief of the obstruction.

Patients produced a mean 24-h urine volume of 3.52 ± 0.46 litres in hospital but this fell progressively to 1.78 ± 0.21 litres by 12 weeks following discharge. The control group had a relatively constant volume varying from 1.41 ± 0.14 to 1.71 ± 0.18 litres throughout the study. Although the mean 24-h calcium excretion was consistently greater in the patient versus the control group, the largest differences were not apparent until the third month. The mean 24-h urinary calcium excretion in hospital was 6.24 ± 0.93 mmol but this increased to 9.07 ± 1.03 mmol at 12 weeks. The control values varied between 4.43 ± 0.58 mmol and 5.03 ± 0.64 mmol.

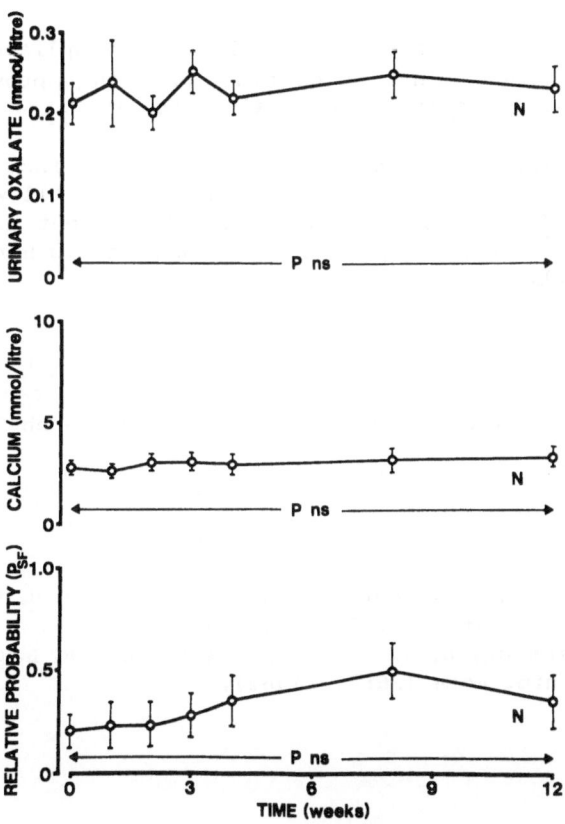

Fig. 2. Changes in the 24-h urinary calcium and oxalate concentration and P_{SF} in normal volunteers.

There were no major changes throughout the study period within the two groups in terms of the 24-h urinary pH and excretions of oxalate, uric acid, creatinine and ABPP.

A major effect of the decreasing urine volume was a progressive increase in the concentrations of oxalate and calcium in the patients compared to the controls (Figs. 1 and 2). A similar rise occurred in the P_{SF} (Figs. 1 and 2).

DISCUSSION

It is clear that 24-h urine studies of patients in hospital with acute renal colic yield an artificially low assessment of the risk of recurrent stone formation. Much of this effect is due to the high urinary outputs resulting from frequent encouragement to drink by the nursing staff. Also, the patients have low 24-h urinary excretions of calcium probably due to impaired dietary intake and renal function.

Following discharge, the initially good compliance with a high fluid intake decreases and, in combination with improved diet and renal function, there is a progressive rise in P_{SF}.

The accurate assessment of the urinary risk factors of CaOx stone disease requires at least a 3-month delay following acute renal colic. This usually will provide sufficient time for the stone to pass and for the patient to return to his normal dietary and fluid intake.

ACKNOWLEDGEMENT

R. W. Norman was funded by the Medical Research Council of Canada.

REFERENCES

1. W. G. Robertson, M. Peacock, P. J. Heyburn, D. H. Marshall, and P. B. Clark, Br. J. Urol. 50:449 (1978).
2. W. G. Robertson, D. S. Scurr, A. Smith, and R. L. Orwell, Clin. Chim. Acta 126:91 (1982).

ANATOMICAL LOCALIZATION OF URINARY RISK FACTORS

OF CALCIUM OXALATE STONE FORMATION

R. W. Norman, J. J. F. Somerville, M. Peacock, and
W. G. Robertson

MRC Mineral Metabolism Unit, The General Infirmary
Leeds LS1 3EX, U.K.

INTRODUCTION

A major limitation of urinary studies in calcium oxalate
(CaOx) stone disease is that the voided specimen represents the
final product of urine formation.   It is not known whether there
is a difference in the relative concentrations of the various risk
factors[1] between upper and lower urinary tract urine or between
one kidney and the other.   This could help to explain why stones
form most commonly in the upper tract and why some patients form
calculi only on one side.

The question is particularly significant with respect to the
glycosaminoglycans (GAGS) fraction of the alcian blue precipitable
polyanions (ABPP).   For example, if the mucosal GAGS lining the
urinary tract[2] were partially secreted, they would contribute to
the overall inhibitory activity of voided urine[3].   The effect
would be to make measurements on a 24-hour urine sample non-
representative of what is actually occurring in the upper tract.

To study this problem we collected and compared urine from
the renal pelvis and bladder in a group of volunteers.

MATERIALS AND METHODS

Twelve patients (4 males and 8 females, aged 18-76 years)
undergoing routine cystoscopy agreed to participate.   All had IVPs
in the previous three months.   Following induction of general
anaesthesia, standard preparation and draping, a cystoscope was
introduced into the bladder and a urine specimen was obtained in a

271

sterile glass bottle without preservative for bacterial culture
and risk factor analysis. The bladder was examined in the usual
fashion and emptied. A 4F or 5F ureteric catheter was passed up
one ureter until a steady drip of urine occurred. It was attached
to an upright sterile glass bottle and the patient was returned to
the recovery room. The ureteric catheter was removed after 10-15
ml of urine had been collected from the renal pelvis.

Each sample was analysed for calcium, magnesium, sodium,
phosphate, uric acid, creatinine and ABPP by methods previously
described[1]. Oxalate was measured by ion-chromatography[4] and the
GAGS were determined by the uronic acid content[5].

RESULTS

All patients had normal radiological, bacteriological and
cystoscopic examinations. There was no significant difference
between the upper and lower tract urine in terms of mean pH or
ratios of calcium, magnesium, sodium, phosphate, uric acid, and
oxalate to creatinine (Table 1). Analysis of the ABPP and its
constituent GAGS showed no difference between the bladder and the
renal pelvis (Fig. 1).

DISCUSSION

The data clearly show that there is no difference between
upper and lower tract urine in terms of the parameters measured.
In particular, the <u>free</u> urinary GAGS appear to originate in the

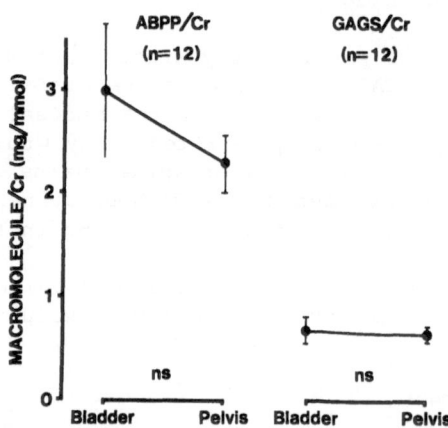

Fig. 1. Comparison of ABPP/creatinine and GAGS/creatinine
ratios in urine from the bladder and renal pelvis.

272

Table 1. Comparison of pH and Ion/Creatinine Ratios between Upper and Lower Tract Urine.

	Bladder mean ± SEM		Renal pelvis mean ± SEM		Significance
pH	6.0 ± 0.1		6.3 ± 0.01		ns
Ca/Cr (mmol/mmol)	0.32 ± 0.07		0.30 ± 0.04		ns
Mg/Cr (mmol/mmol)	0.32 ± 0.08		0.23 ± 0.03		ns
Na/Cr (mmol/mmol)	14.4 ± 3.1		12.7 ± 2.1		ns
PO_4/Cr (mmol/mmol)	1.4 ± 0.3		1.5 ± 0.2		ns
Urate/Cr (mmol/mmol)	0.39 ± 0.06		0.32 ± 0.04		ns
Ox/Cr (mmol/mmol)	0.020 ± 0.003		0.024 ± 0.005		ns

kidney and act on crystal agglomeration in solution[1]; the mucosal GAGS appear to originate in the urothelium and act on crystal nucleation at the urine-GAG interface[6]. Each has a distinct source and protective role in the pathogenesis of CaOx urolithiasis.

In conclusion, the normal collecting system provides a passive conduit for urine transport and makes no significant contribution to the 24-hour excretion of the risk factors of CaOx stone formation.

ACKNOWLEDGEMENT

R. W. Norman was funded by the Medical Research Council of Canada.

REFERENCES

1. W. G. Robertson, M. Peacock, D. H. Marshall, and P. B. Clark, Br. J. Urol.50:449 (1978).
2. B. Monis and H. D. Dorfman, J. Histochem. Cytochem.15:475 (1967).
3. K. A. Edyvane, R. L. Ryall, and V. R. Marshall, in:"Urinary Stone", R. Ryall, J. G. Brockis, V. Marshall, and B. Finlayson, eds., Churchill Livingstone, Melbourne (1984).
4. W. G. Robertson, D. S. Scurr, A. Smith, and R. L. Orwell, Clin. Chim. Acta 126:91 (1982).

5. N. Blumenkrantz and G. Asboe-Hansen, Anal. Biochem. 54:484
    (1973).
6. W. B. Gill, K. J. Ruggiero, and M. C. Frames, Invest. Urol.
    18:158 (1980).

AN AMBULATORY METABOLIC STUDY OF CALCIUM UROLITHIASIS IN

VENEZUELA

J. R. Weisinger, E. Bellorín-Font, V. Sylva,
J. Humpierres, and V. Paz Martínez

Division of Nephrology, Dept. of Medicine, Hospital
Universitario de Caracas and Centro Nacional de
Diálisis y Trasplante, Caracas, Venezuela

INTRODUCTION

Nephrolithiasis is an infrequent cause of death or end-stage renal disease[1]. Nevertheless, kidney stones in our country represent an important health problem because they may lead to urinary obstruction, infection, surgery and progressive loss of renal function. Venezuela is located in the stone belt of the Caribbean but epidemiological surveys in relation to the incidence of renal lithiasis are lacking. In one of our hospitals from 7,108 emergency room consultations during one year, 158 subjects (2.22%) presented with renal colic and in almost all of them a renal stone was demonstrated. A metabolic survey of patients with calcium stones has been conducted in our renal stone clinic in order to define the metabolic variables in our population and to plan a rational therapeutic approach directed to reduce the high recurrence of the problem.

METHODS

All patients with evidence of calcium urolithiasis were referred to our stone clinic at least one month after renal colic or surgical extraction of the stone. A clinical and dietary history was obtained and an ambulatory metabolic study, modified from that of Pak et al[2], was instituted for 2 weeks. In the first part, the patient ingested a regular diet, containing at least 1000 mg/day of calcium (with calcium supplements in the form of calcium carbonate, lactate and gluconate). Serum and 24-h urine samples were collected for calcium, phosphorus, uric acid and creatinine. A fasting blood sample was taken for determination of immunoreactive parathyroid

hormone (PTH).   A short acidification test using oral ammonium
chloride (100 mg/kg body weight) and a qualitative test for
cystinuria were performed.   The patients were then placed on a
calcium-restricted diet (<400 mg/day of calcium).   On day 8, after a
14-h fast, a 2-h urine sample was obtained for the fractional
excretion of calcium and cyclic AMP excretion.   This was followed
by an acute oral calcium load of 1000 mg (whole milk and calcium
gluconogalactogluconate).   Urine was then collected for 4 h with
measurements of fractional excretion of calcium and cyclic AMP
excretion.

Serum and urinary calcium were measured by atomic absorption
spectrophotometry.   Serum and urinary phosphorus by colorimetric
methods[3], serum and urinary creatinine by autoanalyzer[4].   PTH was
measured by radioimmunoassay using CH9 antisera, I[125]-labeled bPTH
(1-84) (kindly supplied by Drs. E. Slatopolsky and J. Morrisey,
Washington University, St. Louis, Mo) and pooled sera from patients
with renal failure as a standard.   This antibody reacts
predominantly with the carboxyl region of human PTH, and detects
both the intact hormone and its carboxyl terminus.   Cyclic AMP was
determined by radioimmunoassay[5].

RESULTS

A total of 174 subjects with calcium urolithiasis were studied
according to our protocol (93 males and 81 females).   The mean age
at the time of the study was 35.9 $\pm$ 9.2 years.   The mean number of

Table 1. Frequency of Abnormalities in 174 Patients with Calcium
         Urolithiasis.

	Number		Percent	
Hypercalciuria				
Reabsorptive	50		28.7	
Absorptive	27	82	15.5	47.1
Resorptive	5		2.9	
Hypercalciuria + Hyperuricosuria	21		12.1	
Hyperuricosuria	26		14.9	
Distal Renal Tubular Acidosis	4		2.3	
No Metabolic Abnormalities	41		23.6	

stones passed or surgically removed was 9.25 ± 28.6 per patient. The mean age at the time of the first stone was 30.1 ± 11.4 years and the mean number of operations performed was 5.83 per 100 stones.

Hypercalciuria was defined as urinary calcium excretion above 4 mg/kg/day of body weight in both sexes and, hyperuricosuria as a uric acid excretion >750 mg/day in males and >700 mg/day in females. Table 1 illustrates the results of the metabolic study. In 148 patients (76.4%), there was a definite metabolic abnormality, the most frequent being hypercalciuria which was noted in 82 patients (47.1%). These were further subdivided according to their fractional excretion of calcium and cyclic AMP excretion after a week on the calcium-restricted diet. Fifty had reabsorptive hypercalciuria with a fasting fractional excretion of calcium of 0.265 and a decrease in cyclic AMP excretion from 4.06 μmol/mg creatinine in the fasting period to 2.95 μmol/mg creatinine 2 h after the oral calcium load. Twenty-seven patients had absorptive hypercalciuria with a fractional excretion of calcium rising from 0.085 ± 0.004 in the fasting state to 0.36 ± 0.03 after the oral calcium load, and without significant change in the cyclic AMP excretion. Five patients had resorptive hypercalciuria with a high fractional excretion of calcium during the fasting state (0.22 ± 0.04) which increased to 0.57 ± 0.11 after the calcium load. The excretion of cyclic AMP was very high and was not modified by the oral calcium load. The mean serum PTH in these patients was 44.8 ± 26.9 μl Eq/ml (our normal range is 2 to 10 μl Eq/ml).

In 21 patients, hypercalciuria was associated with hyperuricosuria. Most of these patients had reabsorptive hypercalciuria. In 26 patients the only abnormality was hyperucosuria (mean uric acid excretion 839.1 ± 36.3 mg/24 h). Four patients had distal renal tubular acidosis; all of them had reabsorptive hypercalciuria. In the remaining 41 patients (23.6%) no metabolic abnormalities could be detected. These patients had a fractional excretion of calcium during the fasting state of 0.13 ± 0.01 increasing to 0.31 ± 0.02 after the oral calcium load. The excretion of cyclic AMP was unaltered.

DISCUSSION

In our group of patients with recurrent calcium urolithiasis, we were able to detect metabolic abnormalities that might be responsible for renal stones in 76.4% of the patients. Almost half of them were hypercalciuric, the majority with reabsorptive hyper-calciuria. This contrasts with other series, where absorptive hypercalciuria was the most common form of the disorder[6]. Another important finding is that all the hypercalciuric groups had some degree of hyperabsorption of calcium after the acute calcium load, especially the absorptive and resorptive hypercalciuric patients.

This is consistent with the observation of Coe et al[7], who have suggested that all idiopathic hypercalciuric patients belong to the same group. Therapy was instituted according to the specific abnormality as previously described[8].

ACKNOWLEDGMENTS

We acknowledge the helpful criticism and referral of patients from the Division of Nephrology and Urology at the Hospital Universitario de Caracas, the Policlinica Metropolitana and Instituto Medico La Floresta.

REFERENCES

1. W. C. Thomas, J. Urol. 113:423 (1975).
2. C. Y. C. Pak, R. A. Kaplan, H. Bone, J. Townsend, and O. Wales, New Engl. J. Med. 292:497 (1975).
3. C. H. Fiske and Y. Subbarow, J. Biol. Chem. 66:375 (1925).
4. O. Folin, J. Biol. Chem. 17:469 (1914).
5. A. L. Steiner, A. M. Kipnis, R. Utinger, and C. Parker, Proc. Natl. Acad. Sci. 64:367 (1967).
6. C. Y. C. Pak and R. A. Galosy, J. Clin. Endocrinol. Metab. 48:260 (1979).
7. F. L. Coe, M. Favus, T. Crockett, A. L. Strauss, J. H. Parks, A. Porat, C. L. Gantt, and M. Sherwood, Am. J. Med. 72:25 (1982).
8. C. Y. C. Pak, P. Peters, G. Hurt, M. Kadesky, M. Fine, A. Reisman, F. Splann, C. Caramela, A. Freeman, F. Britton, K. Sakhaee, and N. Breslau, Am. J. Med. 71:625 (1981).

HYPERURICOSURIC CALCIUM STONEFORMERS: EFFECT ON FASTING

AND CALCIUM HYPERABSORPTION

V. R. Walker and R. A. L. Sutton

Dept. of Medicine, University of British Columbia
Vancouver, B.C., Canada

INTRODUCTION

We have previously reported that serum urate, urinary urate and the fractional excretion of urate (FE_{urate}) do not differ between male idiopathic Ca stoneformers and normal subjects, following an overnight fast, and a similar non-linear negative correlation exists between FE_{urate} and serum urate levels in these two groups[1]. This latter observation demonstrates the role of the kidney in altering the distribution of urate between serum and urine. In 24-h non-fasting urine collections, Coe[2] has reported a 29% incidence of hyperuricosuria in Ca stoneformers. This value is similar to the 33% incidence we have found in male Ca stoneformers (urine urate > 800 mg/day). Coe and Kavalich[3] have suggested that excessive dietary purine may be a major factor contributing to hyperuricosuria in these patients. The present study examines other factors, apart from dietary purine, that may alter urinary urate excretion in idiopathic Ca stoneformers.

METHODS

A group of 40 male idiopathic Ca stoneformers, aged 43 ± 12 years (mean ± SD), comprised the patient population. Of this group, 13/40 demonstrated hyperuricosuria in a prior 24-h non-fasting urine collection while consuming their normal diets. Categorization of the hyperuricosuric (HU) and normouricosuric (NU) stoneformers into subgroups of Ca stoneformers according to their response to a standard 1 g oral Ca load is shown in Table 1 and is based on normal ranges described previously[4]. Sixteen normal healthy male subjects, aged 41 ± 12 years, comprised the control group.

279

Table 1. Categorization of HU (aged 40 ± 8 years) and NU (aged 44 ± 13 years) Stone-formers into Subgroups of Ca Stone-formers Based on their Response to a Ca Load Test[a] (Mean ± SD).

| | HU | | NU | |
	%	(n)	%	(n)
Normocalciuric	15	(2)	26	(7)
FNC[b] hyperabsorber	38	(5)	22	(6)
FHC[c]	8	(1)	30	(8)
FHC with hyperabsorption	38	(5)	22	(6)

[a]For normal ranges upon which subgrouping is based, see ref.4.
[b]Fasting normocalciuric.
[c]Fasting hypercalciuric.

All subjects were maintained on a restricted dietary Ca (<400 mg/day) and Na (<150 mEq/day) intake for one week prior to study. Following a 13-h overnight fast, 2-h urine collections were made and a blood sample taken at the midpoint of this collection. Subjects were given an oral purine-free 1-g Ca load as described previously[4], and a 4-h urine collection made immediately following the Ca load. Calcium, sodium, and creatinine were measured according to methods previously described[4], and serum and urinary urate were determined using the American Monitor uricase method (American Monitor Corp., Indianapolis, Indiana) using alkaline phosphotungstate with a uricase blank. Urinary electrolyte values are expressed as a ratio with urinary creatinine. Statistical analyses were performed with Student's 't'-test for paired or unpaired data.

RESULTS

No differences in fasting serum urate, Ca, Na, or creatinine were observed between HU and NU stoneformers or normal subjects. Following the fast, even though urinary Ca/Cr was higher in both HU (0.11 ± 0.02) and NU (0.11 ± 0.01) stoneformers than normal subjects (0.06 ± 0.01), urate/Cr, Na/Cr, volume excretion, and FE_{urate} did not differ. A similar positive non-linear correlation was observed between urinary Na and urate in the 2-h fasting urine collection in both the 40 stoneformers (r = 0.68, P 0.001) and 16 normal subjects (r = 0.79, P<0.001). A similar correlation between urine volume and urate excretion was also found in both stoneformers (r = 0.50, P< 0.001) and normal subjects (r = 0.77, P<0.001) and this correlation did not differ between the groups.

In response to the Ca load, no significant differences were found between HU and NU stoneformers in terms of increments of urate/Cr, Ca/Cr, Na/Cr, or volume excretion. However, differences were found

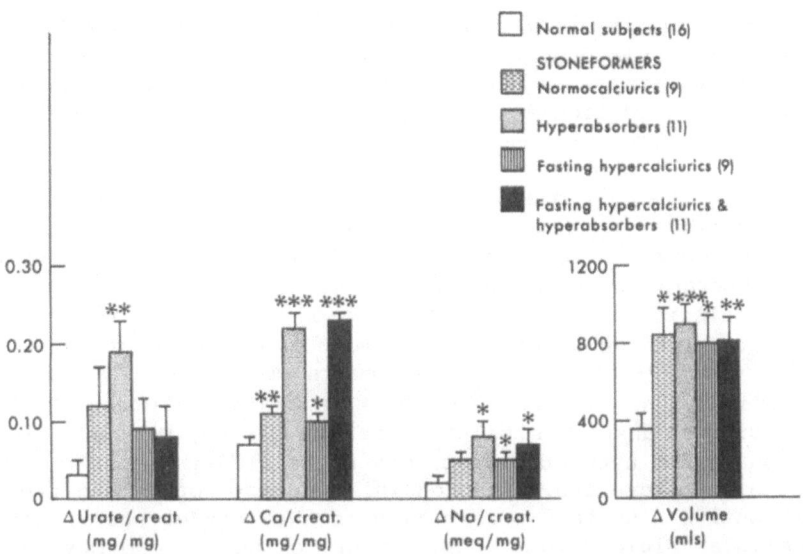

Fig. 1. Urinary changes in subgroups of Ca stoneformers following a
1g oral Ca load. These changes represent the difference
between a 2-h fasting urine values prior to the Ca load, and
4-h values post-load. Sub-grouping of the patients was
based on the values described previously[4].
*P<0.05; **P<0.01; ***P<0.001.

when compared with normal subjects, the stoneformers showing
significantly greater increments in all of these urinary factors.

To determine if urate excretion differed within the subgroups of
Ca stoneformers categorized according to their response to the Ca load
test, we divided the 40 stoneformers (13 HU and 27 NU) into their
respective subgroups and examined changes in urate excretion following
the Ca load, as shown in Fig. 1. No differences in fasting serum and
urinary urate, and Na excretion prior to the Ca load in these
subgroups were observed. However, in response to the Ca load, only
the fasting normocalciuric (FNC) hyperabsorbers of all the groups
including normal subjects demonstrated a significant increment in
urate excretion (paired 't'-test, P<0.001). This was not found in
fasting hypercalciuric (FHC) hyperabsorbers despite similar increments
in urinary Ca, Na, and volume in the two groups (FNC and FHC) of
hyperabsorbing stoneformers following the Ca load.

DISCUSSION

In the present study, hyperuricosuria (>800 mg/day) was
observed in 13 of 40 male idiopathic Ca stoneformers. Of these HU

stoneformers, 77% were Ca hyperabsorbers compared with 44% of the NU stoneformers. This observation suggested that Ca hyperabsorption in these HU stoneformers may be a factor contributing to their hyper-uricosuria, in addition to excessive purine intake as suggested by Coe and Kavalich[3]. The possible significance of this association between Ca hyperabsorption and hyperuricosuria was examined by categorizing the 40 stoneformers into subgroups and determining their increments in urate excretion in response to a Ca load (Fig. 1). When comparing pre- and post-load urinary urate values, only the FNC hyperabsorbers demonstrated a significant increment in urinary urate in association with that of Ca, Na, and volume excretion. This subgroup represented 38% of the HU stoneformers compared with 22% of the NU stoneformers (Table 1). The absence of a statistically significant increment in urate excretion in the FHC hyperabsorbers, despite similar increments in Ca, Na, and volume excretion to FNC hyperabsorbers, may be related to their antecedent fasting urate excretion, although this was not found to differ significantly. Another possibility is that differences in the extracellular fluid volume (ECFV) prior to the Ca load may have influenced the magnitude of urate excretion post loading. FHC hyperabsorbers lose more urinary Na along with Ca during fast, and may therefore have some contraction of ECFV. Steele[5] and Weinman et al[6] have observed a positive relationship between the ECFV and urinary urate excretion, and we have observed in the present study a positive non-linear correlation between urinary Na and urate during fast in both stoneformers and normal subjects. Thus, these studies following a fast indicate that the FNC hyperabsorbers are a subgroup of Ca stoneformers who exhibit enhanced excretion of urate as well as Ca following a Ca-rich meal, which may represent a particular hazard for initiation of further stone growth or formation.

ACKNOWLEDGMENT

This work was supported in part by the British Columbia Health Care Research Foundation.

REFERENCES

1. V. R. Walker and R. A. L. Sutton, Calc. Tiss. Int. 35 (Suppl.):A39 (1983).
2. F. L. Coe, in:"Nephrolithiasis, Pathogenesis and Treatment", F. L. Coe, ed., Year Book Medical Publishers, Chicago (1978).
3. F. L. Coe and A. G. Kavalich, New Engl. J. Med. 291:1344 (1974).
4. V. R. Walker and R. A. L. Sutton, Clin. Sci. 66:193 (1984).
5. T. H. Steele, J. Lab. Clin. Med. 74:288 (1969).
6. E. L. Weinman, G. Eknoyan, and W. N. Suki, J. Clin. Invest. 55:283 (1975).

CALCIUM OXALATE (CaOx) URINE SUPERSATURATION IN CALCIUM STONE

FORMERS (CSF): HYPERCALCIURIA VERSUS HYPEROXALURIA

A. Antonacci, G. Colussi, M. E. De Ferrari, G. Rombola, G. Pontoriero, M. Surian, F. Malberti, and L. Minetti

Renal Units E. O. Ca Granda Niguarda, Milano and Ospedale Maggiore, Lodi, Italy

INTRODUCTION

Calcium oxalate is the most frequent constituent of urinary calculi in idiopathic stone disease. Urinary excretion of both calcium (Ca) and oxalate (Ox) are recognised as risk factors[1]; however, there is still disagreement on the relative role played by each of the two in the genesis of urine supersaturation for CaOx. On the one hand, it has been shown that stone recurrence is related to oxalate excretion but not to calcium excretion[2]. On the other hand, it is widely recognized that reduction in Ca excretion (either by diet or with drugs) is highly effective in reducing the stone recurrence rate[3,4], even though Ox excretion may increase. This is because intestinal calcium absorption and Ca excretion are frequently increased in CSF and the decline in urinary calcium is typically more prominent than the modest increase in urinary oxalate[3]. The aim of our study was to evaluate CaOx urine supersaturation in relation to either Ca or Ox excretion in a large group of idiopathic CSF in an attempt to determine if either of the two has a more relevant clinical importance.

MATERIALS AND METHODS

Seventy-five consecutive idiopathic CSF (46 males and 29 females, aged 18 to 65 years) and 10 healthy volunteers (6 males and 4 females, aged 23 to 53 years) were studied. They were kept on a normal calcium (1 g/day) and oxalate (100 to 150 mg/day) diet; fluids, calories and salt were uncontrolled. After 10 days a 24-h urine was collected for Ca, Ox and creatinine, and a fasting blood for Ca and creatinine determination. CaOx urine supersaturation was

Table 1. Ca and Ox Excretions (UCaV and UOxV) and Urine Relative Supersaturation in 10 Controls (C) and 75 CSF patients.

	UCaV (mg/day)	UOxV (mg/day)	LogCaOxRS	Pts. with RS $>$1
C (10)	202 ± 74	31 ± 12	0.92 ± 0.2	3/10 (30%)
NC (34)	205 ± 60	37 ± 15	0.96 ± 0.15	16/34 (47%)
	$P < 0.001$	< 0.02	< 0.001	ns
IH (41)	388 ± 84	47.5 ± 19.5^{c}	1.13 ± 0.19^{c}	32/41 (78%)
NOx (52)	291 ± 129^{b}	33 ± 9	0.99 ± 0.13	26/52 (50%)
	$P < 0.05$	< 0.001	< 0.001	< 0.05
HOx (23)	362 ± 127^{d}	65.5 ± 12.7^{d}	1.23 ± 0.1^{d}	23/23 (100%)^{d}

P : b = 0.002; c = 0.01; d = 0.001, versus C

evaluated from a nomogram[5]; to avoid any effect of different urine volumes, all supersaturation data were normalized to a constant volume of 1.5 litre. Ca was measured by atomic absorption spectrophotometry and Ox by colorimetry[6]. Statistical analysis was performed by use of Student's t-test, x^2 evaluation and linear regression analysis.

RESULTS

Thirty-four of the patients were normocalciuric (UCaV<280 mg/day in females and <320 mg/day in males) and 41 of the patients were hypercalciuric (IH) (Table 1). Urine relative supersaturation (RS) was similar in NC and IH; oxalate excretion (UOxV) was also higher in IH than in NC and C. UCaV and UOxV were slightly correlated in all CSF (r = 0.26; P<0.05). Fifty-two patients had normal urinary oxalate excretions (UOxV<55 mg/day) and 23 had hyperoxaluria (HOx); HOx had higher RS, UCaV and percent of patients with urine supersaturation than NC and C. There was a progressive increase in RS values and frequency of supersaturation in different patient groups according to the presence or the absence of hypercalciuria and/or hyperoxaluria (Fig. 1). In all CSF, RS was better correlated with UOxV (r = 0.9; P<0.001) than with UCaV (r = 0.45; P<0.001).

DISCUSSION

From a physicochemical point of view, it is currently believed that both Ca and Ox play an equal role in determining CaOx urine supersaturation[3]. Previous reports that an increase in urinary Ca

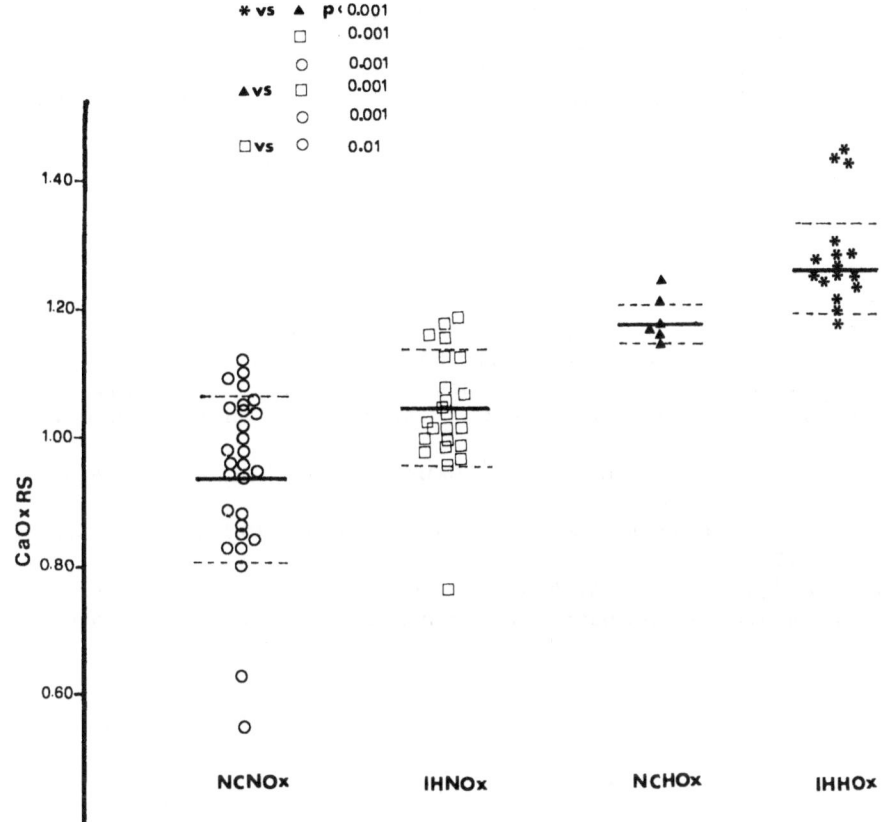

Fig. 1. Calcium oxalate relative supersaturation (CaOx RS, log
units) in the 4 CSF patient groups: normocalciuria-
normooxaluria (NC-NOx); hypercalciuria-normooxaluria (IH-
(NOx); normocalciuria-hyperoxaluria (Nc-HOx); and
hypercalciuria-hyperoxaluria (IH-HOx).

concentration caused only a modest increase in CaOx supersaturation
owing to the complexation of Ox have recently been revised after
correcting the stability constant for CaOx at physiological
temperature[3]. Thus the clinical importance of Ca or Ox
abnormalities as determinants of urine supersaturation would be
expected to depend upon their relative frequency. There are few
reports from which to evaluate the overall incidence of
hyperoxaluria in idiopathic CSF. Our data show that the incidence
of hyperoxaluria in unselected, idiopathic CSF, is somewhat lower
than previously reported in Italian patients[7]. While hyperoxaluria
per se is always associated with supersaturation of urine for CaOx,
neither hyperoxaluria nor hypercalciuria are necessary for urine
supersaturation to be present. However, the mean values of

relative supersaturation increase with an increase of Ca and Ox concentration. While hypercalciuria was more frequent than hyperoxaluria, the latter was more predictably associated with urine supersaturation. The higher values of urine RS were seen when the two disturbances occurred together. Thus it appears that, even though it occurs less frequently than hypercalciuria, hyperoxaluria is an important cause of supersaturation in CSF.

REFERENCES

1. W. G. Robertson, M. Peacock, P. J. Heyburn, D. M. Marshall, and P. B. Clark, Br. J. Urol. 50:449 (1978).
2. W. G. Robertson and M. Peacock, Nephron 26:105 (1980).
3. C. Y. C. Pak, M. Nicar, and C. Northcutt, Contr. Nephrol. 33:136 (1982).
4. A. L. Straus, F. L. Coe, L. Deutch, and J. H. Parks, Am. J. Med. 72:17 (1982).
5. R. W. Marshall and W. G. Robertson, Clin. Chim. Acta 72:253 (1976).
6. A. Hodgkinson and A. Williams, Clin. Chim. Acta 36:127 (1972).
7. B. Baggio, G. Gambaro, S. Favaro, and A. Borsatti, Nephron 35:11 (1983).

THE ORIGIN OF METABOLIC ABNORMALITIES IN PRIMARY CALCIUM STONE

DISEASE - NATURAL OR UNNATURAL SELECTION?

W. G. Robertson and M. Peacock

MRC Mineral Metabolism Unit, The General Infirmary
Leeds LS1 3EX, U.K.

INTRODUCTION

In the past, most papers on primary calcium stone disease have attempted to attribute this disorder to a single common pathological mechanism. This may take the form of the "abnormally" high excretion of some urinary constituent of stones, such as calcium or oxalate, or an excessively high urinary pH, or an "abnormally" low excretion of some protective factor which inhibits the rate of crystallization of calcium salts, or the occurrence of some "abnormal" promoter of crystallization or gluing agent which either sticks crystals together or anchors them to the wall of the urinary tract. In turn, these "abnormalities" have been attributed to some difference in diet or in metabolic activity or in genetic make-up between stone-formers and normals. Recently, however, it has become apparent that stone-formation is probably a multifactorial disorder and not attributable to any single pathological mechanism possessed by some discrete proportion of the population. In this paper, we have set out to study some of the biochemical and metabolic "abnormalities" described in stone-formers in relation to the values of these variables in the normal population. Only a few of the data can be included in this brief report.

METHODS

Twenty-four-hour urine calcium was measured in 60 male, primary calcium stone-formers and 60 age- and sex-matched controls. None had any disorder of calcium metabolism and all had good renal function. Calcium absorption, plasma $1,25-(OH)_2D_3$ and plasma phosphate were also measured. Twenty-four-hour urine calcium was measured before and after provocation with 40 μg of 25–OHD$_3$ given to 10 normal men and 10 primary calcium stone-formers.

RESULTS AND DISCUSSION

The top section of Fig. 1 shows the smoothed frequency distributions (expressed in %) of 24-h urinary calcium excretion in stone-formers and normals.   Although the mean ($\pm$ SEM) values (8.00 $\pm$ 0.38 and 5.95 $\pm$ 0.35 mmol/day respectively) are significantly different (P<0.001), there is a large overlap between the two groups.   Some investigators have inferred that the tail of skewed values in stone-formers represents a group of patients with abnormally high calcium excretions and they should be classed as "hypercalciuric".   However, this interpretation must be in doubt when the data are replotted allowing for a prevalence rate of stones

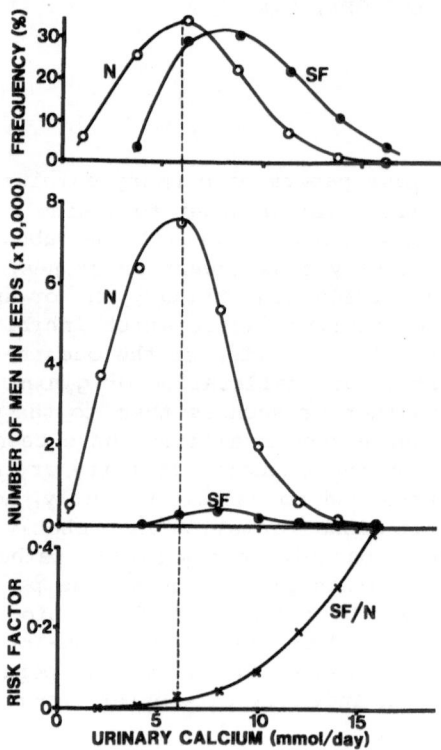

Fig. 1.   Frequency distributions of 24-h urinary calcium excretion
         in male, primary calcium stone-formers and controls,
         top: expressed as percentages; middle: expressed as true
         numbers in the male population in Leeds; bottom: expressed
         as a ratio of stone-formers to normals.

in men of 4%[1] (middle section of Fig. 1). Now all the stone-
formers actually lie within the distribution of urinary calcium
values in normal men, although most lie above the mean value in the
normal population. By dividing the number of stone-formers by the
number of normals at each level of urinary calcium, the relative
odds of being a stone-former (bottom section of Fig. 1) can be
calculated. This shows that, as urinary calcium increases, the risk
of being a stone-former rather than a normal also increases.
Similar distributions to those in Fig. 1 have been found for other
urinary risk factors of stone-formation, for calcium absorption, and
for plasma $1,25-(OH)_2D_3$ and phosphate concentrations. We conclude
that stone disease selects out those individuals who, although they
lie within the normal scale of metabolic activity, for some reason
are to be found at the high risk end of one or more of the risk
factor distributions. It is the combination of these separate
risks that determines the overall probability of stones in each
individual. It seems unlikely that this combination represents a
single common disease process.

But how do primary calcium stone-formers come to be in the high
risk half of one or more of the risk factors for stones? Are they

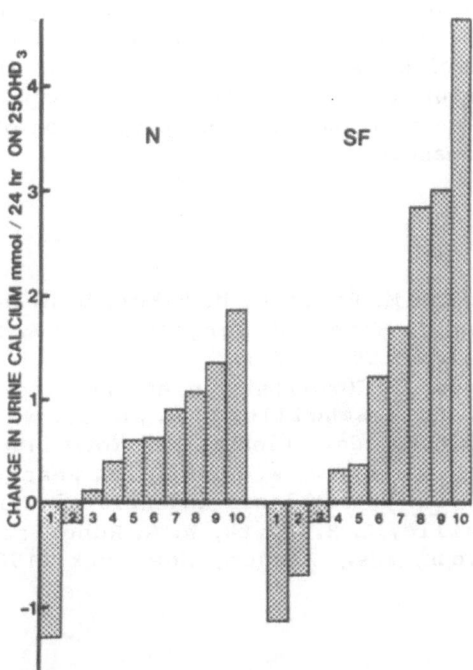

Fig. 2. The change in 24-h urinary calcium excretion in 10 male,
primary calcium stone-formers and their controls in
response to 40 μg 25-OHD$_3$.

more exposed to some stimulus, such as a diet overrich in protein, sugars, calcium and oxalate[2], or insufficient fluid intake, or a hot climate? Or are they a metabolically more active group of individuals who respond physiologically to a greater (or excessive) degree to even normal levels of stimulation from any of the above factors? Fig. 2 contains the results from a study to determine whether or not stone-formers are more sensitive to a stimulus from 40 g of $25-OHD_3$ given orally.   This shows the change in 24-h urinary calcium in 10 normal men and 10 stone-formers.   Although the mean ($\pm$ SEM) change in the stone-formers (1.2 ± 0.6 mmol/day) was not significantly different from that in normals (0.6 ± 0.3 mmol/day), there was a trend to higher values among the patients. A similar trend towards a higher response in stone-formers was noted[3] after an oral load of methionine (2.5 g/day).   Thus, as a group, stone-formers do not appear to be more sensitive than normals to the stimuli so far studied, although some individuals are clearly in the high risk half of the urinary calcium scale because they are more sensitive.   The effects of such stimuli extrapolated to the population as a whole markedly increase the number at risk of stones.

In conclusion, we suggest that there is no single cause of stone-formers being in the high risk range of a particular urinary risk factor; some are there because they are hypersensitive to some normal stimulus, others are there because they customarily receive some greater stimulus than normal.   Any factor which causes the distribution of a urinary risk factor in the population as a whole to move adversely, will increase the proportion of the population at risk of stone disease.

REFERENCES

1. W. G. Robertson, M. Peacock, M. Baker, D. H. Marshall,
     B.Pearlman, R. Speed, V. Sergeant, and A. Smith,
     Br. J. Urol. 55:595 (1983).
2. W. G. Robertson, in:"Urolithiasis and Related Clinical
     Research", P. O. Schwille, L. H. Smith, W. G. Robertson, and
     W. Vahlensieck, eds., Plenum, New York (1985).
3. B. Arora, P. L. Selby, R. W. Norman, M. Peacock, and W. G.
     Robertson, in:"Urolithiasis and Related Clinical Research",
     P. O. Schwille, L. H. Smith, W. G. Robertson, and
     W.Vahlensieck, eds., Plenum, New York (1985).

STUDIES ON URINE COMPOSITION IN PATIENTS WITH CALCIUM

OXALATE STONE DISEASE

H.-G. Tiselius and L. Larsson

Depts. of Urology and Clinical Chemistry
University Hospital, S-581 85 Linköping, Sweden

INTRODUCTION

The recurrent formation of calcium oxalate (CaOx) stones might be prevented by appropriate medical measures[1,2]. A number of urinary risk factors for stone formation have been identified, which are affected in different ways by the currently available forms of treatment. It appears reasonable to assume that the choice of medical treatment should be determined by the biochemical findings in the individual patient. For this reason it is necessary to have a routine programme for biochemical evaluation of stone-formers. In this paper we present the results from studies on urine composition in more than 700 patients with CaOx stone disese.

METHODS

Two 24-h urine samples from 483 male and 226 female CaOx stone-formers, and from 100 normal men and 40 normal women, were collected on an out-patient basis. Only patients with recurrent stone formation, with residual renal concrements, or who had been operated on to remove renal stones were investigated in this way.

Urine was analyzed for calcium, oxalate, magnesium, citrate, urate, creatinine (Cr), and inhibition of CaOx crystal growth rate in diluted urine (I_{GR}). The methodology has been described previously[3,4]. To compensate for errors in urine collection, and to enable comparison from one occasion to another, all urine variables were related to urinary creatinine.

RESULTS AND DISCUSSION

Urinary calcium was higher in both male and female stone formers (P<0.05), and the same was found for oxalate (P<0.05). On the other hand there were no significant differences in urate or magnesium excretion. A low excretion of citrate was observed in a large number of both male and female stone formers, and there was a pronounced similarity in the shape of the distribution curves of citrate.

Whereas stone-forming males had a slightly lower I_{GR} than normal subjects (P<0.05), female stone-formers had not. However, it should be emphasized that determination of I_{GR} was not possible in all women owing to frequent bacterial contamination of the samples.

In a previous study it was shown that calcium (Ca), oxalate (Ox), magnesium (Mg), citrate (Cit) and urine volume (V) were the most important determinants for the ion activity product of CaOx (AP_{CaOx})[6]. A CaOx risk index summarizes the effects of the different urine variables on the risk of forming a urine critically supersaturated with respect to CaOx:

$$((Ca/Cr)^{0.71} \times (Ox.Cr))/((Mg/Cr)^{0.14} \times (Cit/Cr)^{0.10})$$

This index approximately parallels AP_{CaOx} at the same urine volume. A volume factor is not included in it, because stone-formers appeared to increase their fluid intake during the collection period, thereby presenting larger urine volumes than they would normally. The frequency distribution curves of the CaOx-risk

Table 1. Normal range of Urine Variables and Proportion of Patients Outside the Normal Range.

Urine Variable	Normal Range		Stone Formers with Abnormal Values	
	Men	Women	Men(%)	Women(%)
Ca (mmol/mol Cr)	< 500	<600	40	42
Ox (mmol/mol Cr)	< 30	< 40	19	14
Cit (mmol/mol Cr)	>100	>125	32	32
Mg (mmol/mol Cr)	>200	>250	15	15
Ur (mmol/mol Cr)	< 300	<300	9	18
Volume (ml/24 h)	>1000	>1000	9	8
I_{GR}	>0.50	>0.40	36	8
CaOx risk index	< 550	<625	39	48

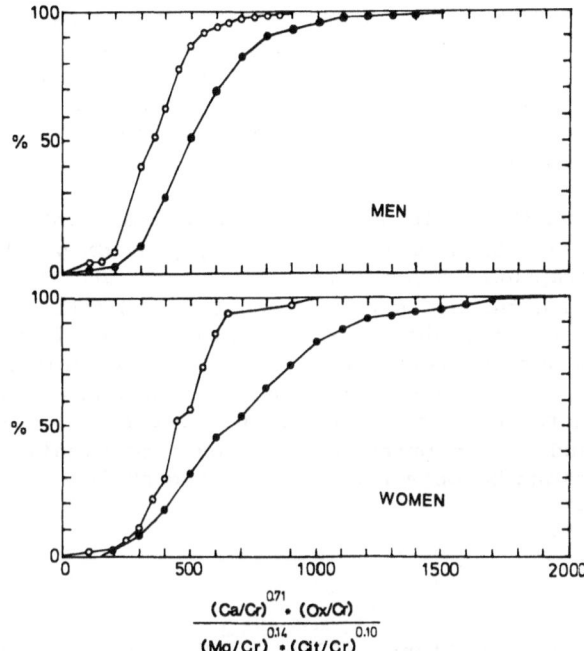

$$\frac{(Ca/Cr)^{0.71} \cdot (Ox/Cr)}{(Mg/Cr)^{0.14} \cdot (Cit/Cr)^{0.10}}$$

Fig. 1. Cumulative frequency distribution curves of the CaOx-risk index in normal subjects (O) and stone formers (●).

index is shown in Fig. 1. The difference between stone-formers and normal subjects is clear (P<0.001). Another simpler expression might also be useful:

$$(Ca/Cr)^{0.71} \times (Ox/Cr)$$

This product, previously shown to give an approximate estimate of CaOx supersaturation for a specific urine volume[7], resulted in a good separation of stone-formers and normal subjects. A more appropriate estimate of the supersaturation is the AP(CaOx)-index given by:

$$(3.8 \times Ca^{0.71} \times Ox)/(Mg^{0.14} \times Cit^{0.10} \times V^{1.2})$$

which includes urine volume. For a 24-h urine volume of 1500 ml, 28% of male and 15% of female stone-formers had an AP(CaOx)-index above 2.8, asumed to correspond to the formation product of CaOx (Robertson, personal communication). Normal limits of the urine variables and CaOx risk-index were chosen to include approximately 90% of normal subjects within the normal range (Table 1).

Classification of our stone-formers according to these criteria are shown in the same table. Combination of abnormalities were frequently encountered, and about 85% of the patients had one or several abnormalities in their urine composition. A completely normal urine composition was recorded in only 12% of male and 15% of female stone-formers.

We believe that this analytical programme might be useful in the routine evaluation of stone-formers, providing a basis for a selective therapeutic approach. Our results are thus much more encouraging than those recently presented by Ryall and Marshall[8]. The CaOx risk index might be particularly useful in the follow-up of stone-formers during treatment. Unfortunately this programme does not account for the inhibitory properties of whole urine, but a simple method for measuring this is not available. Neither are there any standardized principles for pH determination, but valuable information might be obtained by measuring pH in a fresh morning urine sample.

REFERENCES

1. E. R. Yendt., in:"Stones, Clinical Management of Urolithiasis", R. A. Roth and B. Finlayson, eds. Williams & Wilkins, Baltimore, London (1983).
2. C. Y. C. Pak, J. Urol. 128:1157 (1982).
3. H.-G. Tiselius, L. E. Almgård, L. Larsson, and B. Sörbo, Eur. Urol. 4:241 (1978).
4. H.-G. Tiselius and A.-M. Fornander, Clin. Chem. 27:565 (1981).
5. H.-G. Tiselius and L. Larsson, Eur. Urol. 6:90 (1980).
6. H.-G. Tiselius, Clin. Chim. Acta 122:409 (1982).
7. H.-G. Tiselius, Eur. Urol. 9:231 (1982).
8. R. L. Ryall and V. R. Marshall, Br. J. Urol. 55:1 (1983).

ALTERATIONS IN KIDNEY LOCATION WITH CHANGES IN PATIENT POSITION:

IMPLICATIONS FOR PERCUTANEOUS RENAL PROCEDURES

G. W. Drach, M. T. Yoshino, B. J. Hillman, and L. Creed

Depts. of Surgery and Radiology, University of Arizona
Health Science Center, Tucson, Arizona 85724, U.S.A.

INTRODUCTION

Accurate localization of the renal collecting system is
important for the safe and efficient performance of percutaneous
nephrostomy. That renal location changes with different body
positions is commonly accepted[1-3] but has not been systematically
studied. We employed computed tomography to demonstrate the extent
and unpredictability of in vivo renal mobility. Our results
demonstrate the importance of localizing the collecting system and
of continuous needle guidance during puncture.

METHODS

Ten patients believed to have no renal or perinephric disease
underwent abdominal CT scans. One cm thick scans at 1 cm intervals
(GE 8800 CT scanner) were performed in the upper abdomen during the
drip infusion of 150 ml of 60% meglumine iothalamate. The kidneys
were scanned with the patient in the supine, prone, right (RAO) and
left (LAO) anterior oblique positions.

Two of the authors (MTY and BJH) examined the scans for renal
disease, perirenal pathology, patient body habitus and liver and
spleen size and location. The slice representing the cephalocaudad
midpoint in each position was selected and the axial distance from
the xiphoid recorded. Projection-related alterations in renal
position were evaluated in the cephalocaudad direction. Measurement
of the vertical distance from the skin to the nearest aspect of the
collecting system, using the midpoint slice of each kidney in each
position, allowed us to assess anteroposterior renal motion.

Table 1. Alterations in Anteroposterior Location of the Renal Collecting Systems Relative to their Location in the Supine Position (Skin-Collecting System Distance in mm).

Patient	Prone		LAO	RAO
	Right	Left	Right	Left
1	+ 4	- 7	+26	+ 7
2	- 2	-11	+13	- 1
3	+10	+ 0	+13	+20
4	+29	+37	+ 9	+29
5	+ 8	+11	+11	+12
6	- 7	-16	+ 2	- 1
7	-10	- 8	+ 1	0
8	+37	0	+15	+33
9	- 7	- 7	+ 4	-11
10	- 4	+14	+18	+19

* Further from (+) or nearer to (-) the skin surface than when the patient was supine.

Table 2. Alterations in Cephalocaudad Location of the Renal Collecting Systems in the LAO and RAO Projections (Xyphoid-Collecting System Distance in mm).

Patient	Collecting System			
	Right		Left	
	LAO compared with:		RAO compared with:	
	Supine	Prone	Supine	Prone
1	+50	+20	+30	0
2	-50	0	-50	0
3	-50	0	-50	0
4	0	0	0	0
5	0	0	0	0
6	+80	+40	+40	0
7	-50	0	0	0
8	-50	0	-50	0
9	-50	+70	-20	+100
10	+70	0	+70	0

* Further from (+) or nearer to (-) the xyphoid than when the patient was supine or prone.

RESULTS

There was no consistent relationship between body habitus and position-induced change in either the anteroposterior or cephalo-caudad directions. Similarly, no significant renal, perirenal, splenic or hepatic pathology was observed. Measurements of antero-posterior alterations in the renal position in changing from supine to prone, RAO, and LAO positions are summarized in Table 1. Compared with the supine position, 9 kidneys were more anterior in the prone position, 10 more posterior and one maintained the same distance from the skin surface. When the right renal pelvic location in the LAO position is compared with its supine location, all were further from the skin, the increase varying between 1 and 26 mm. In the RAO projection, the left renal pelvis was further from the skin in 6 patients (range 7 to 33 mm), closer in 3 (range 1 to 11 mm), and one did not change in depth.

The cephalocaudad position of the kidneys in the prone position was closer to the feet 5 times, closer to the head 2 times, and unchanged 3 times relative to their location when the patients were supine. As shown in Table 2 there was considerable and variable alteration in the position of the right kidneys in the LAO projection relative to their locations in the supine and prone postures. In 9 of the 10 cases, the left kidney was at the same cephalocaudad level in both patient positions.

DISCUSSION

The results demonstrate the commonly accepted, but hitherto unproven, assertion that renal pelvic location varies with changes in patient position. Furthermore, it does so unpredictably in both antero-posterior and cephalocaudad axes. The left renal pelvis varies considerably in the cephalocaudad location when the RAO position is compared to the supine position. However, when this oblique position is compared to the prone position, only infrequent changes in cephalocaudad location were noted. This may be secondary to the tethering effects of the splenorenal ligament, which should be compressed when the patient is supine, but might be extended when the patient is prone.

Thus, the preferred clinical practice for nephrostomy placement should include localization with the patient in the position in which the procedure will be performed and continuous monitoring of renal pelvic position. To this end, collecting system location and depth should be determined in the nephrostomy position by sonography or by fluoroscopy following intravenous contrast material, or ideally, employing a combination of both modalities. This has not always been the case; even today, in many institutions, blind puncture is still employed. These older techniques are not acceptable. Sinner[4] has established that the morbidity of thoracic percutaneous procedures is directly related to the number of needle insertions. It seems reasonable to assume that a similar situation might exist for percutaneous renal procedures.

A second finding apparent from our scans, is that puncture in the opposite oblique position affords the longest course through the renal parenchyma. This observation is important because the longer needle tract afforded by oblique positioning stablizes the catheter once it has been placed in the pelvis. There also exists an advantage to an oblique approach as the expected needle trajectory is then aligned with the relatively hypovascular plane separating the anterior and posterior renal arterial distributions[1]. Finally, the oblique approach provides greater comfort and safety for the patient following the procedure, since it allows him to lie supine more easily without kinking or compressing the catheter[5]. The contralateral oblique is therefore the recommended patient position for performing percutaneous nephrostomy.

REFERENCES

1. W. H. Hollingshead, "Textbook of Anatomy", 3rd edn. Harper and Row, New York (1974).
2. C. Ney and R. M. Friendenberg, "Radiographic Atlas of the Genitourinary System", J. B. Lippincott, Philadelphia (1981).
3. P. Williams, R. Warwick, M. Dyson, and L. Bannister, "Grays Anatomy", 36th edn., W. B. Saunders, Philadelphia (1980).
4. W. N. Sinner, Acta. Radiol. 17:813 (1976).
5. D. G. Stables, N. J. Ginsberg, and M. L. Johnson, Am. J. Roentgenol. 130:75 (1978).

IN VITRO DETERMINATION OF OPTIMAL CONDITIONS FOR

COAGULUM PYELOLITHOTOMY

A. A. A. Lycklama à Nijeholt, E. Briët, and U. Jonas

University Hospital, Dept. of Urology, and Thrombosis
and Hemostasis Research Unit, Leiden, The Netherlands

INTRODUCTION

A clot, suitable for coagulum pyelolithotomy, must have the
following properties: (i) the formation must start after 1 min (for
optimal mixing and injection) but at the most within 5 min, (ii) the
clot must have a good elasticity, and (iii) the clot must be strong
(i.e. have good tensile strength).   The purpose of this study was
to determine the optimal conditions required for the formation of
suitable clots.   To this end we studied several combinations of
cyroprecipitate (cryo), platelet-rich plasma (p.r.p.), thrombin
(thromb) and calcium (Ca) under different conditions (temperature,
time, dilution) by means of thrombelastography and tensile strength
measurements.

METHODS AND RESULTS

A thrombelastograph was used to measure the reaction-time (R),
which corresponds with the clotting time, and the maximal amplitude
(MA), which correlates with the elasticity and the firmness of the
clot.   A specially constructed apparatus was used to measure the
tensile strength (F) which is the maximal stretching force endured
by the clot just before it breaks.

Preliminary experiments showed that the required properties and
conditions for good clot formation are: (a) $1 \text{ min} \leqslant R \leqslant 5 \text{ min}$,
(b) $MA \geqslant 50 \text{ mm}$ and (c) $F \geqslant 150 \text{ g/cm}^2$. Cryo with thrombin and p.r.p.
with Ca appeared to be unsuitable for the formation of a good clot.
Under these circumstances a good clot was obtained with cryo and Ca
with or without the addition of thrombin.

299

Table 1. Concentration Ranges of Ca and Thrombin Required for Optimal Clot Properties under Standard Conditions (Room Temperature and 15 min after Mixing).

Constants Factors	Variable components[*]	
	Ca	Thrombin
Cryo	10 to 33 mM	–
Cryo	–	**
Cryo + Ca optimal	–	0.2 to 0.8 U/ml
Cryo + Throm optimal	12 to 45 mM	–
P.r.p.	**	–

[*]Final concentrations; **Required properties not achieved.

The next step of the study was to determine the optimal conditions, using the optimal concentrations of cryo and Ca with or without the addition of thrombin. We studied the following conditions: (i) effect of pre-heating cryo for 15 min at 37°C compared with room temperature (22°C), (ii) the effect of measuring after an incubation time of 5, 10 and 15 min (= time after mixing), and (iii) the effect of dilution of the mixture with urine (at room temperature after 15 min).

Table 2. Effects of Varying Temperature and Incubation Time on Clot Properties at the Optimal Ca Concentrations (Cryo + Ca).

	Time (min)	Temperature	
		22°C	37°C
R (n = 82)	–	4 min 23 s ←— ns —→ 4 min 20 s	
A (mm) (n = 142)	5	18 ←— ns —→ 23	
		$p < 0.05$	$p < 0.05$
	10	68 ←— ns —→ 69	
F (g/cm^2) (n = 121)	5 to 7	66 ←— $p < 0.05$ —→ 326	
		$p < 0.05$	ns
	10 to 12	308 ←— ns —→ 369	

Table 2 shows that at room temperature an incubation time of 5 min is insufficient for obtaining a good clot. Pre-heating to $37^{\circ}C$ seems to improve the tensile strength after 5 min, but the amplitude (A) is still insufficient. If the mixture is incubated for 10 min, raising the temperature has no effect and under these conditions adequate clots are formed. A further increase of the incubation time (15 min) does not improve the clot properties.

Dilution of the mixture with urine at 10% does change the thrombelastogram results, while the tensile strength is only decreased significantly at a dilution of 30% or more.

Table 3. Effects of Varying Temperature and Incubation Time on Clot Properties at Optimal Ca and Thrombin Concentrations (Cryo+Ca+Throm).

	Time (min)	Temperature 22°	37°
A (mm)	5	49	
(n = 34)		↑ $P < 0.05$ ↓	
	0	58	
F (g/cm^2)	5 to 7	258 ← ns →	315
n = 135		↑ ns ↓	ns
	10 to 12	247	

Table 3 shows that when thrombin is added, a 5 min incubation time at room temperature is sufficient to obtain an adequate tensile strength. However, it appears that a longer incubation time is needed to obtain an amplitude A in excess of 50 mm. Further prolongation of the incubation time (15 min) has no effect.

Table 4. Summary of the Results (mean ± SD).

	Conditions	A (mm)	F (g/cm^2)
Cryo + Ca$_{optimal}$	Room temp, 10 min	68 ± 14	308 ± 35
Cryo + Ca$_{optimal}$	$37^{\circ}C$, 5 min	23 ± 30	326 + 53
Cryo + Ca$_{optimal}$ + thromb$_{optimal}$	Room temp, 5 min	49 ± 12.5	258 ± 51

Table 4 illustrates that the addition of thrombin to the mixture of cryo + Ca does not improve clot properties provided a waiting time of 10 min is acceptable.

DISCUSSION

The in vitro experiments described in this report show that good quality clots for coagulum pyelolithotomy can be produced by very simple methods, cryo precipitate and calcium ions. The quality of the clot is optimal after an incubation time of 10 min and pre-heating of the components is unnecessary. The addition of small quantities of urine has only minimal effects on the properties of the clot. Thrombin does acclerate the clotting process but does not improve clot properties. Since fatal emboli have been reported after its use in vivo we feel that thrombin should not be used. As a result of this sudy the method of our choice in vivo is as follows: (i) 30 volumes of cyroprecipitate (volume depending on size and distension of the pyelo-calyceal system), (ii) 2 volumes of calcium laevulate (10% sol, 325 mM) or 1 volume of calcium chloride (10% sol, 680 mM), (iii) mix the two components, inject the appropriate volume into the pyelum, using a butterfly needle, after occlusion of the ureter and aspiration of the urine. Wait   10 minutes for clotting to occur. Remove the clot and the entrapped stones.

A ONE DAY CELLULOSE PHOSPHATE (CP) TEST DISCRIMINATES

NON-ABSORPTIVE FROM ABSORPTIVE HYPERCALCIURIA

L. Knebel, W. Tschöpe, and E. Ritz

Dept. of Urology, Städtische Krankenanstalten
Mannheim, and Internal Medicine, University of
Heidelberg, F.R.G.

RATIONALE FOR DIAGNOSTIC WORKUP IN RECURRENT CALCIUM STONE FORMERS

Recurrent calcium urolithiasis is a major health problem in affluent societies. In view of the increasing cost of health services, there is strong pressure to use cost-effective procedures to identify patients in need of specific treatment. The value of thiazides for preventing recurrent calcium stone formation has not been established in placebo-controlled studies (indeed, one such study showed no benefit albeit with a large beta error[11]). Yet, strong circumstantial clinical evidence supports the validity of the original concept[2] that thiazides reduce the risk of stone recurrence, irrespective of whether the hypercalciuria is absorptive or non-absorptive in origin. Assuming that thiazides should first be tested in recurrent calcium stone formers in whom known secondary causes of hypercalciuria can be excluded, the aim of the present study to determine whether or not short-term administration of oral cellulose phosphate can identify individuals with resorptive hypercalciuria among recurrent calcium stone formers.

ONE-DAY CELLULOSE PHOSPHATE (CP) TEST

Forty-three healthy volunteers (20 females without hormonal contraception; 23 men; median age 35 years, range 20 to 55) were examined as outpatients on a free diet. A 24-h urine was collected in 2 litre PVC bottle containing 10 ml concentrated HCl, and a fasting 2-h urine collected between 08.00 and 10.00. On a subsequent day, patients took oral cellulose phosphate (Calcisorb[R], 5 g in the morning, 10 g at noon, 5 g in the evening). During that day, a 24-h urine was collected and the following morning a fasting

Table 1. Urinary Ca/Cr Ratio Before and After 24-h Oral Cellulose
Phosphate.

| Group | Urinary Ca/Cr (mmol/mmol) | | | |
| | Free diet | | Free diet + CP | |
	24 h	Fasting	24 h	Fasting
Controls (43)	0.32	0.22	0.17	0.12[*]
	(0.13-0.57)	(0.07-0.45)	(0.05-0.38)	(0.03-0.27)
Recurrent Stone Formers (80)	0.38	0.29	0.23	0.13[*]
	(0.12-0.96)	(0.03-0.91)	(0.05-0.5)	(0.03-0.27)
Recurrent Stone Formers with Skeletal Disease	0.51	0.55	0.43	0.42
	(0.22-0.78)	(0.19-0.90)	(0.15-0.73)	(0.28-0.90)

[*] $P < 0.01$

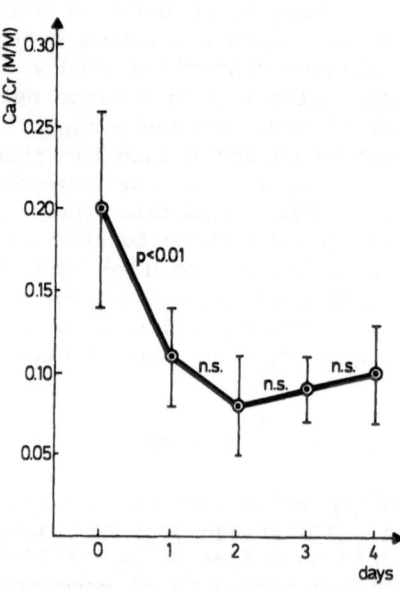

Fig. 1. Ca/Cr (fasting morning urines) in 8 normals after prolonged
administration of cellulose phosphate.

urine was obtained as described above.   Urinary calcium and
creatinine were determined by standard methods.

Daily urine collections were obtained from 8 healthy volunteers
prior to and during 4 days of oral cellulose phosphate.   Urinary
Ca/Cr which was 0.2 mmol/mmol prior to oral CP, decreased to 0.11 on
the 1st day of CP but failed to decrease further on subsequent days
(0.10 on the 4th day) (Fig. 1).   The normal ranges of the 24-h and
fasting morning urinary Ca/Cr ratio in healthy volunteers are given
in Table 1.

ONE DAY CP TEST IN RECURRENT STONE FORMERS

Whether or not the CP test could identify patients with
resorptive hypercalciuria was studied in 92 consecutive recurrent
calcium stone formers (51 male, 41 female; median age 37 years,
range 19 to 65).   All patients were excluded who presented with
hypercalcaemia or evidence of renal tubular acidosis, intestinal
problems or oxalosis.   As shown in Table 1, a decrease in the
fasting urinary Ca/Cr below the upper limit of the normal range
(0.27) was observed in 80 of the 92 patients.   Indeed, despite
hypercalciuria on an unrestricted diet, their fasting urine calcium
was identical with that of controls (Fig. 2).   In contrast, 12 of
the 92 patients failed to lower their fasting morning urine Ca/Cr
ratio below 0.27.   In 3, who had been normocalcemic on admission,

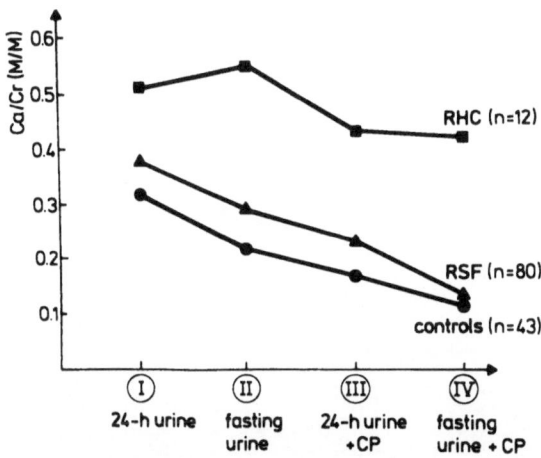

Fig. 2.   Effect of one-day administration of cellulose phosphate on
          urinary Ca/Cr ratios in controls, recurrent stone-formers
          (RSF) and in resorptive hypercalciuric (RHC) stone-formers.

primary hyperparathyroidism was established on the basis of urinary cAMP and intermittent hypercalcemia. The other 9 patients were postmenopausal women with no known skeletal disease and presumed to have postmenopausal osteoporosis.

PROPOSED EVALUATION OF RECURRENT STONE FORMERS

This study demonstrates that 24-h oral CP eliminates the contribution of intestinal absorption of Ca to the excretion of Ca in fasting morning urine samples, thus permitting discrimination between resorptive and other forms of hypercalciuria. In an effort, therefore, to provide cost-effective procedures to evaluate recurrent calcium stone formers, we propose to screen patients using serum calcium and the oral CP test. Normocalcemic patients who normalize their fasting urine calcium after CP administration for 24 h should be given thiazides. Patients who fail to lower their urinary calcium need further investigation of their increased skeletal resorption. The rare normocalcemic recurrent calcium stone former who suffers from primary hyperparathyroidism can be identified either from their urinary cAMP or from their serum iPTH.

REFERENCES

1. P. Brocks, C. Dahl, H. Wolf, and I. Transboel, Lancet ii:124 (1981).
2. E. R. Yendt and M. Cohanim, Kidney Int. 13:397 (1978).

SERUM PARATHORMONE AND URINARY AND NEPHROGENOUS CYCLIC AMP IN IDIOPATHIC HYPERCALCIURIA AND IN PRIMARY HYPERPARATHYROIDISM

V. Nunziata, G. di Giovanni, R. Giannattasio,
M. Riccio, A. Verrillo, and P. Strazzullo

Institute of Internal Medicine and Metabolic Diseases
Seconda Clinica Medica, 2° Facoltà di Medicina
via S. Pansini, Naples, Italy

INTRODUCTION

The mechanisms of idiopathic hypercalciuria (IH) in man are controversial. Primary hyperabsorption[1] or a renal tubular leak of calcium[2] have both been suggested. Reduced[3] or increased[4] parathyroid gland (PTG) activity has been described[5-7]. The purpose of this study was to evaluate PTG activity in hypercalciuric (HC) stone formers and to investigate the effect of various calcium intakes. In order to test the diagnostic validity of the adopted procedure, the results were compared with those obtained in a group of patients surgically proven to have primary hyperparathyroidism (HPT) with frank or intermittent hypercalcemia.

SUBJECTS AND METHODS

PTG activity was measured in 40 patients, 30 men and 10 women (mean age 39 years) with IH and stones, as well as in 20 age- and sex-matched normal controls. The HCs were diagnosed as absorptive (31) or renal (9) according to Pak et al[3]. In addition, 15 patients with surgically proven primary HPT, 10 frankly and 5 intermittently hypercalcemic, were investigated. All subjects were studied using an out-patient protocol of: (a) 24-h urine collections on days 5, 6 and 7 on a 400 mg Ca diet; (b) 2-h fasting urine collections between 09.00 and 11.00 and (c) 24-h urine collections on days 5, 6 and 7 on the same diet plus Ca supplementation up to 1000 mg Ca/day. Fasting blood samples were collected at the end of each diet and at the mid-point of the 2-h urine collection. Urines were analyzed for Ca, P, creatinine, and c-AMP; and plasma was analyzed for Ca, ionized Ca, P, creatinine, c-AMP[8,9] and PTH[10].

Table 1. Serum Biochemical Data (Mean ± SD).

| | Hypercalciuric | | Hyperparathyroid | | |
	Absorptive	Renal	Normo-calcemic	Hyper-calcemic	Normal
Total Ca (mmol/l)	2.29±0.19	2.35±0.07	2.52±0.09	2.95±0.25	2.33±0.15
Ionized Ca (mmol/l)	1.13±0.10	1.14±0.06	1.23±0.04	1.51±0.14	1.14±0.04
Phosphorus (mmol/l)	1.10±0.25	1.05±0.15	0.92±0.12	0.79±0.20	1.08±0.19
PTH (mIU/ml)	2.82±1.39	3.33±1.38	4.40±1.59	15.50±7.30	3.63±1.69
C-AMP (nmol/dl)	1.57±0.55	1.34±0.66	1.62±0.53	1.74±0.47	1.71±0.58

Table 2. Urine Biochemical Data (mean ± SD).

| | Hypercalciuric | | Hyperparathyroid | | |
	Absorptive	Renal	Normo-calcemic	Hyper-calcemic	Normal
Subjects	31	9	5	10	20
Calcium					
High Ca (mmol/day)	8.75±2.22	9.70±1.65	11.55±1.95	9.90±1.00	4.35±1.18
Low Ca (mmol/day)	6.40±1.04	7.95±1.35	8.35±1.40	7.95±1.10	3.35±0.20
Fasting (mg/dl GF)	0.08±0.03	0.14±0.02	0.11±0.04	0.22±0.04	0.06±0.03
Phosphorus					
High Ca (mmol/day)	22.68±7.51	23.26±5.43	22.31±1.90	21.31±4.06	18.76±4.93
Low Ca (mmol/day)	24.62±9.68	24.40±5.61	25.15±3.03	20.37±4.45	18.79±4.58
$TmPo_4$ (mmol/l GF)	1.27±0.39	1.11±0.18	1.03±0.16	0.75±0.34	1.23±0.21
Urinary c-AMP (nmol/dl GF)					
High Ca	2.60±1.00	2.80±0.60	2.50±0.75	6.26±1.30	2.89±0.71
Low Ca	3.26±1.03	3.50±0.75	2.76±1.00	7.57±1.67	3.30±0.83
Fasting	4.25±1.67	4.07±1.14	3.56±1.74	11.08±2.90	4.22±1.05
Nephrogenous c-AMP (nmol/dl GF)					
High Ca	1.05±1.00	1.29±0.60	1.10±0.65	4.55±1.30	1.32±0.61
Low Ca	1.74±0.89	2.20±0.99	1.34±1.00	5.88±1.50	1.62±0.81
Fasting	2.70±1.50	2.67±1.05	2.12±1.49	9.30±3.00	2.76±1.17

RESULTS AND DISCUSSION

The serum data from all subjects are shown in Table 1.
Compared to the normals, the total group of HCs, showed no
differences in serum Ca (either total or ionized), P, PTH or c-AMP.
As expected, the hypercalcemic HPT patients had a low serum P
(P < 0.001) and elevated PTH (P<0.001).   In the normocalcemic HPT
patients total and ionized Ca were borderline (P<0.001), serum P was
reduced (P<0.05) and PTH normal.

Table 2 contains the urine data from all subjects studied on
both Ca intakes and in the fasting state.   By definition, the renal
HCs had a high fasting urine Ca and this was also evident in the HPT
group (both hyper- and normocalcemic) (P<0.001).   Urinary P was
higher in the HCs compared to the controls on both Ca intakes
(P<0.05).   There was no difference in the tubular reabsorption of P
between HCs, normocalcemic HPT patients and normals.   Urinary and
nephrogenous c-AMP were the same at both Ca intakes in normals, HCs
and normocalcemic primary HPT patients.   Cyclic AMP was
significantly reduced by a high Ca diet in absorptive and renal HCs
and in normals (P<0.01).   A significant suppression of the
nucleotide between fasting and low Ca intake occurred in the
absorptive group and in the normals (P<0.01) but not in the group
with the renal leak.   It seems that the absorptive (P<0.01) and the
renal (P<0.05) groups recognized the different Ca diets, whereas the
normals did not.   A high dietary Ca also suppressed PTG function in
the primary HPT patients.   However, in the hypercalcemic HPT group,
nephrogenous c-AMP was significantly reduced on either a low or a
high Ca intake (P<0.05) whereas in normocalcemic HPT patients
dietary Ca appeared not to influence nucleotide excretion.

This study shows that in IH with stones, PTG activity is not
altered whether the fasting urine Ca is high or low.   The data do
not confirm previous reports of secondary HPT in renal HC[3-5] or
recent reports[11,12] showing some degree of PTG suppression.   In our
HCs, PTG activity appears to be the same as in normals on the basis
of serum PTH and urinary c-AMP excretion, and ionized Ca was not as
high as it should be when PTG function is inhibited[13,14].
Therefore the mechanism for HC must be the same in all patients
irrespective of the fasting urinary Ca.   Hyperabsorption of Ca, as
the predominant feature for HC[5], does not appear to be demonstrable
as the primary defect in our cases because of the lack of evidence
of significant PTG suppression.   The fact that, on a high Ca diet,
HC patients suppress their PTH normally indicates that some degree
of renal leak of Ca must occur.   On the other hand, if a renal leak
is present[12], a low Ca diet should not suppress the PTG, as happened
in our renal group on the 400 mg diet.   This significantly reduced
PTG activity only in normals and in absorptive HCs.   For these
reasons the predominant mechanism of HC seems to be a renal Ca leak.
Therefore the distinction between absorptive and renal HC appears of

no value[15] either on a pathophysiological or a therapeutic basis. Whether or not the determination of serum PTH and urinary and nephrogenous c-AMP represent valid diagnostic procedures for assessing small variations in PTG activity is debatable. In hypoparathyroidism, c-AMP has been found to be reduced but the data overlap those from normal people[16]. Similarly, in mild primary HPT we frequently have found a normal nucleotide excretion in contrast to Broadus et al[17]. From the above data it is concluded that PTG activity is normal in IH, whether primary hyperabsorption or a renal tubular leak of Ca is present. In agreement with Coe et al[12], the HC population seems homogenous in terms of Ca and P metabolism and the extent of a probable unique defect may cause HC with a high or low fasting Ca excretion.

REFERENCES

1. F. Albright, P. Hennemann, P. Benedict, and A. P. Forbes, Proc. Roy. Soc. Med. 46:1077 (1953).
2. P. H. Hennemann, P. H. Benedict, A. P. Forbes, and H. R. Dudley, New Engl. J. Med. 159:802 (1958).
3. C. Y. C. Pak, M. Ohata, E. C. Lawrence, and W. Snyder, J. Clin. Invest. 54:387 (1974).
4. F. L. Coe, J. M. Canterbury, J. J. Firpo, and E. Reiss, J. Clin. Invest. 52:134 (1973).
5. P. Bordier, A. Ryckewart, J. Gueris, and H. Rasmussen, Am. J. Med. 63:398 (1977).
6. A. E. Broadus, M. Dominguez, and F. C. Bartter, J. Clin. Endocrinol. Metab. 47:751 (1978).
7. C. Y. C. Pak and R. A. Galosy, J. Clin. Endocrinol. Metab. 48:260 (1979).
8. A. L. Steiner, C. W. Parker, and D. M. Kipnis, J. Biol. Chem. 247:1106 (1972).
9. J. F. Harper and G. Brooker, J. Cyc. Nucleotide Res. 1:207 (1975).
10. C. D. Arnaud, R. J. Goldsmith, P. J. Bordier, G. W. Sizemore, J. A. Larsen, and J. Gilkinson, Am. J. Med. 56:785 (1974).
11. F. P. Muldowney, R. Freaney, and J. G. Ryan, Quart. J. Med. 193:87 (1980).
12. F. L. Coe, M. J. Favus, T. Crockett, A. L. Strauss, J. H. Parks, A. Porat, C. L. Gantt, and L. M. Sherwood, Am. J. Med. 72:25 (1982).
13. P. Burckhardt and P. Jaeger, J. Clin. Endocrinol. Metab. 53:550 (1981).
14. R. A. L. Sutton and V. R. Walker, New Engl. J. Med. 302:709 (1980).
15. M. Peacock, Contrib. Nephrol. 33:152 (1982).
16. M. A. Weber, M. Klerekoper, I. R. Thornell, and G. S. Stokes, J.Clin. Endocrinol. Metab. 40:982 (1975).
17. A. E. Broadus, R. Lang, and A. S. Kliger, J. Clin. Endocrinol. Metab. 52:1085 (1981).

HYPERCALCIURIA IN PATIENTS WITH NORMOCALCEMIC HYPERPARATHYROIDISM AND STONE DISEASE

H. v. Lilienfeld-Toal, W. Koska, H. Franck, A. Hesse, and D. Bach

Depts. of Medicine and Urology, University of Bonn
Bonn, F.R.G.

INTRODUCTION

Normocalcemic primary hyperparathyroidism (pHpth) may be associated with renal stone disease[1-3]. In pHpth the renal tubular reabsorption of calcium (Ca) is increased. Therefore, relative to the serum Ca concentration, the urinary Ca excretion is low in pHpth[4]. Theoretically normocalcemic hypercalciuric stone formers should not have pHpth. In contrast, we present a group of stone formers who probably have pHpth with hypercalciuria despite normocalcemia.

PATIENTS AND METHODS

We identified 36 patients with recurrent stone disease and elevated immunoreactive parathyroid hormone (iPTH). It was measured with a C-terminal assay[5]. However, later cross-reaction studies showed that it is a mid-region assay[6]. A small group of patients was re-examined with two commercially available assays specific for the C-terminal region ("C-term h65-84 PTH")[7] and intact PTH ("h1-84PTH")[8]. Calcium was measured by atomic absorption, creatinine and phosphorus by AutoAnalyzer. Patients with elevated serum creatinine (above 1.1 mg/dl) were excluded.

RESULTS

Patients were grouped according to the 24-h urinary Ca on their individual diet and their serum Ca concentration (Table 1). Groups II and IV consisted of patients with elevated iPTH and hypercal-

Table 1. Patients with Elevated iPTH and Stone Disease (mean ±SD).

Group	SCa (mmol/l)	UCa (mmol/24h)	n	Diagnosis
I	Normal 2.45 ± 0.12	High 10.2 ± 3.6	11	?
II	High 3.11 ± 0.41	High 11.7 ± 5.2	9	pHpth
II	Normal 2.40 ± 0.16	Normal 2.8 ± 1.2	14	?
IV	High 3.08 ± 0.39	Normal 5.0 ± 0.8	2	pHpth

Table 2. Data from Patients in Group I (mean ± SD).

	iPTH (ngeq/ml)	SCa (mmol/l)	S Phosphate (mmol/l)	U Ca (mmol/24h)
Group I	67 ± 37	2.45 ± 0.12	0.79 ± 0.27	10.1 ± 3.6
Normal	7 - 27	2.25 - 2.55	0.8 - 1.6	below 6

Table 3. A Subgroup of 8 Patients of Group I After 2.5 Years Follow-up (mean ± SD).

	iPTH "c-term.h65-84" (ngeq/ml)	"h1-84" (ngeq/ml)	S Ca (mmol/l)	S Phosphate (mmol/l)
Patients	0.48 ± 0.49*	0.42 ± 0.07**	2.52 ± 0.18	0.95 ± 0.17
Controls	0.22 ± 0.09	0.17 ± 0.05	2.50 ± 0.10	1.30 ± 0.14

*$P < 0.03$; **$P < 0.001$

cemia; pHpth was confirmed in all of those who had surgery. Group I included patients whose data are given in Table 2. In 8 patients from Group I, the fasting Ca/creatinine excretion ratio was 0.047 ± 0.03 (mg/mg, normal below 0.11). After 2.5 years the 8 patients of Group I were reexamined (Table 3) on conservative therapy.

DISCUSSION

According to these data the combination of elevated iPTH and hypercalciuria in the presence of normal serum Ca is not a rare finding (Group I, Table 1).   Secondary hyperparathyroidism due to a renal leak - if it exists in idiopathic hypercalciuria[9,10] - can be excluded in the majority of these patients because they had a normal fasting Ca excretion. Re-examination of these patients after more than 2 years revealed a higher iPTH than in the controls and a relatively low serum phosphate but with a normal serum Ca.   This finding indicates that there is a persistent disorder of PTH secretion.   It is likely that this group of patients represents a subgroup of pHpth in whom the hypercalciuria results from hyperabsorption of dietary Ca[11].   It is conceivable that in these patients hypercalciuria prevents hypercalcemia.

REFERENCES

1. S. Ljunghall, R. Källsen, U. Backman, B. G. Danielson, L. Grimelius, H. Johansson, L. Thorén, and I. Werner, Acta Chir. Scand. 146:161 (1980).
2. L. Grimelius, H. Johansson, B. Lindquist, L. Thorén, and I. Werner, Acta Chir. Scand. 139:42 (1973).
3. G. Nichols and B. Flanagan, Trans. Assoc. Am. Physcns. 80:314 (1967).
4. B. E. C. Nordin, "Metabolic Bone and Stone Disease", Williams and Wilkins, Baltimore (1973).
5. H. v. Lilienfeld-Toal, I. Gerlach, H. U. Klehr, S. Issa, and E. Keck, Nephron 31:116 (1982).
6. H. v. Lilienfeld-Toal, unpublished results.
7. B. A. Roos, A. W. Lindall, D. C. Aron, J. W. Orf, M. Yoon, M. B. Huber, J. Pensky, J. Ells, and W. Lambert, J. Clin. Endocrinol. Metab. 53:709 (1981).
8. A. W. Lindall, J. Ells, J. Elting, and B. Roos, J. Clin. Endocrinol. Metab. 57:1007 (1983).
9. H. v. Lilienfeld-Toal, D. Bach, A. Hesse, H. Franck, and S. Issa, Urol. Res. 10:205 (1982).
10. P. Burckhardt and P. Jaeger, J. Clin. Endocrinol. Metab. 53:550 (1981).
11. A. E. Broadus, R. L. Horst, R. Lang, E. T. Littledike, and H. Rasmussen, New Engl. J. Med. 302:421 (1980).

VITAMIN D METABOLISM IN HYPERCALCIURIC PATIENTS

M. Schreiber, K.-H. Bichler, W. L. Strohmaier,
I. Gaiser, J. Krug, and H. J. Nelde

Dept. of Urology, University of Tübingen, D-7400
Tübingen, F.R.G.

INTRODUCTION

In many hypercalciuric patients it is impossible to determine the cause of the disorder by simple clinical procedures. Expensive and protracted investigations, such as the calcium-load test of Pak et al[1], are used but with these methods there are some diagnostic problems. In this study we measured 25-OH-D and $1,25(OH)_2$-D to see if they would be helpful in classifying the different types of hypercalciuria.

METHODS

Vitamin D metabolism was investigated in 33 patients with hypercalciuria. The serum levels of $1,25-(OH)_2$-D, 25-OH-D, calcium, phosphate, PTH and calcitonin were determined, along with the urinary excretions of calcium, phosphate and uric acid. Hypercalciuria was classified using the calcium-load test of Pak et al.[1]. Our 25-OH-D and $1,25(OH)_2$-D assays were based on the method of Mallon et al[2]. However, the serum extraction procedure was modified (Fig. 1). First, $1,25-(OH)_2$-D and 25-OH-D were extracted from serum with dichloromethane. Known quantities of ^{3}H-labeled $1,25-(OH)_2-D_3$ or $25-OH-D_3$ were added to calculate the recovery. The dichloromethane was completely evaporated on a rotary evaporator. The $1,25-(OH)_2$-D and 25-OH-D were resuspended and applied to and eluted from a Sephadex LH-20 column. After evaporation, the vitamin D metabolites were measured by separate competitive protein-binding assays. Calcium was determined by flame photometry, phosphate by a commercial test kit (Boehringer Mannheim, FRG), ionized calcium using an ion-selective electrode (Orion), and uric

315

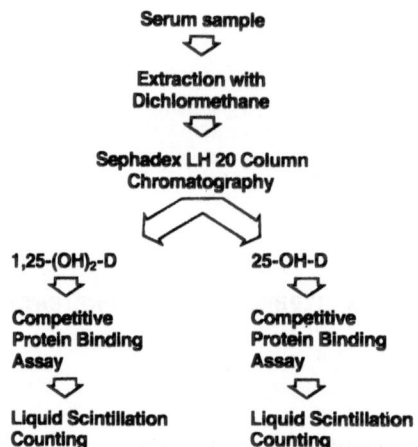

Fig. 1. Scheme for analysis of vitamin D metabolites.

acid by the Urica quant-test kit (Boehringer Mannheim, FRG). PTH
and calcitonin were measured by RIA (Byk-Mallinckrodt).

RESULTS

The mean ($\pm$ SD) 1,25-(OH)$_2$-D values found in our normals
compared well with the findings of Kaplan et al[3] (36 $\pm$ 9 and 34 $\pm$ 7
pg/ml respectively). The serum concentrations of 1,25-(OH)$_2$-D, 25-
OH-D, calcium, ionized calcium, PTH and calcitonin and the urinary
excretions of calcium, phosphate and uric acid in patients with the
different types of hypercalciuria are shown in Tables 1 to 4. In
renal and both types of absorptive hypercalciuria, we found a wide
range of 1,25-(OH)$_2$-D values from subnormal to high. Similar
results were found with 25-OH-D. Three of the 4 patients with

Table 1. Serum and Urine Data (mean $\pm$ SD) in 13 Patients with
Absorptive Hypercalciuria (Type 1).

Serum			Urine			
1,25(OH)$_2$-D	45.2 $\pm$ 14.1	pg/ml	Ca	9.20	$\pm$ 1.816	mmol/day
25-OH-D	21.3 $\pm$ 16.1	ng/ml	Pi	28.58	$\pm$ 10.94	mmol/day
Ca	2.41 $\pm$ 0.17	mmol/l	UA	3.39	$\pm$ 0.926	mmol/day
Ca^{2+}	1.14 $\pm$ 0.041	mmol/l				
Pi	0.96 $\pm$ 0.147	mmol/l				
PTH (AAS 44-68)	279 $\pm$ 134	pg/ml				
PTH (AAS 65-84)	258 $\pm$ 159	pg/ml				
Calcitonin	16 $\pm$ 5	pg/ml				

Table 2. Serum and Urine Data (mean ± SD) in 6 Patients with
Absorptive Hypercalciuria (Type 2).

Serum			Urine			
$1,25-(OH)_2-D$	43.2 ± 14.9	pg/ml	Ca	7.64 ± 1.49	mmol/day
25-OH-D	20.3 ± 9.2	ng/ml	Pi	32.77 ± 6.10	mmol/day
Ca	2.40 ± 0.091	mmol/l	UA	4.15 ± 0.80	mmol/day
Ca^{2+}	1.16 ± 0.029	mmol/l			
Pi	1.09 ± 0.159	mmol/l			
PTH (ASS 44-68)	255 ± 50	pg/ml			
PTH (ASS 65-84)	298 ± 181	pg/ml			
Calcitonin	29 ± 7	pg/ml			

Table 3. Serum and Urine Data (mean ± SD) in 10 Patients with
Renal Hypercalciuria.

Serum			Urine			
$1,25-(OH)_2-D$	42.7 ± 11.7	pg/ml	Ca	10.24 ± 3.04	mmol/day
25-OH-D	24.0 ± 8.6	ng/ml	Pi	31.17 ± 7.54	mmol/day
Ca	2.33 ± 0.144	mmol/l	UA	3.95 ± 1.07	mmol/day
Ca^{2+}	1.11 ± 0.030	mmol/l			
Pi	0.93 ± 0.194	mmol/l			
PTH (ASS 44-68)	281 ± 179	pg/ml			
PTH (ASS 65-84)	272 ± 191	pg/ml			
Calcitonin	21 ± 12	pg/ml			

resorptive hyperalciuria had increased serum concentrations of 1,25-
$(OH)_2-D$ and decreased 25-OH-D. PTH was increased, calcitonin was
normal.

DISCUSSION

The high concentrations of $1,25-(OH)_2-D$ in patients with
resorptive hypercalciuria can be explained by their primary
hyperparathyroidism[4,5] with high PTH and normal calcitonin levels.
In renal hypercalciuria, secondary hyperparathyroidism is said to be
present[1]. However, our results indicate a normal PTH in almost all
patients in this group. Also the $1,25-(OH)_2-D$ levels were
variable. In absorptive hypercalciuria, prolonged stimulation of
the intestinal mucosa by $1,25-(OH)_2-D$ is considered to cause the
increased absorption of calcium[3]. We found increased $1,25-(OH)_2-D$
in only 40% of these patients. Thus there must be other factors
causing intestinal hyperabsorption. There is a theory that
increased renal losses of phosphate result in enhanced synthesis of

Table 4. Serum and Urine Data (mean ± SD) in 6 Patients with Resorptive Hypercalciuria.

Serum			Urine			
$1,25\text{-}(OH)_2\text{-}D$	62.0 ± 28.4	pg/ml	Ca	8.57	$\pm$ 4.32	mmol/day
$25\text{-}OH\text{-}D$	11.8 ± 11.5	ng/ml	Pi	35.74	$\pm$14.07	mmol/day
Ca	2.84 ± 0.247	mmol/l	UA	3.50	$\pm$ 0.83	mmol/day
Ca^{2+}	1.49 ± 0.211	mmol/l				
Pi	0.70 ± 0.101	mmol/l				
PTH (AAS 44-68)	475 ± 115	pg/ml				
PTH (ASS 65-84)	375 ± 175	pg/ml				
Calcitonin	29 ± 16	pg/ml				

$1,25\text{-}(OH)_2\text{-}D$, independent of PTH[4,6,7]. However, hyperphosphaturia was not found in the present study. In absorptive hypercalciuria, calcitonin and PTH also were normal.

Our study demonstrates that only the group of patients with resorptive hypercalciuria were homogenous with respect to $1,25\text{-}(OH)_2\text{-}D$. The other types ranged from subnormal to increased values. PTH and calcitonin were normal. Absorptive and renal hypercalciuria could not be distinguished from the measurements made.

REFERENCES

1. C. Y. C. Pak, F. Britton, R. Peterson, D. Ward, C. Northcutt, N. A. Breslau, J. McGuire, K. Sakhaee, S. Bush, M. Nicar, D. A. Norman, and P. Peters, Am. J. Med. 69:19 (1980).
2. J. P. Mallon, J. G. Hamilton, C. Nauss-Karol, R. J. Karol, C. J. Ashley, D. S. Matuszewski, C. A. Tratnyek, G. F. Bryce, and O. N. Miller, Arch. Biochem. Biophys. 201:277 (1980).
3. R. A. Kaplan, M. R. Haussler, L. J. Deftos, H. Bone, and C. Y. C. Pak, J. Clin. Invest. 9:756 (1977).
4. W. Flury, Schweiz. Med. Wschr. 108:129 (1976).
5. M. R. Haussler, K. M. Bursac, H. Bone, and C. Y. C. Pak, Clin. Res. 23:322A (1975).
6. M. R. Hughes, P. F. Brumbaugh, M. R. Haussler, J. E. Wergedal, and D. J. Baylink, Science 190:578 (1975).
7. F. Shen, D. Baylin, R. Nielson, M. Hughes, and M. Haussler, Clin. Res. 23:423A (1975).

PROXIMAL TUBULE SODIUM HANDLING IN CALCIUM STONE FORMERS

G. Colussi, M. E. De Ferrari, P. Cosci, B. Corradi,
E. Benazzi, G. Pontoriero, G. Rombola, and L. Minetti

Renal Units, Ca' Granada Niguarda Hospital, Milan
and Ospedale Maggiore, Lodi, Italy

INTRODUCTION

It has been suggested that a high Na intake might be an etiological factor in idiopathic hypercalciuria (IH) and that in hypercalciuric Ca stone formers (CSF), Ca excretion (UCaV) can be normalized by reducing Na intake to less than 100 mEq/day without any change in Ca intake[1]. Moreover, in IH there might exist a proximal tubular "defect" in which there is reduced fractional reabsorption of Na, fluid, P, and possibly, Ca and Mg[2,3]. However, since the proximal tubule "defect" for Na is compensated at more distal sites of the tubule it cannot be the sole cause of the increased urinary Na excretion commonly seen in hypercalciuric patients[1,3]. We conclude that hypercalciuric patients must have an increased Na intake and have studied the relationship between Na intake, proximal tubular Na reabsorption and UCaV in healthy people and in a group of CSF to clarify the issue.

CASES AND METHODS

Fifteen healthy volunteers (C) and 32 idiopathic CSF were studied. Ten patients were normocalciuric (NC) (UCaV 320 mg/day in men, 280 mg/day in women on 1 g of Ca and a free Na diet); 22 had IH. After 7 to 10 days on a low Ca diet (approximately 400 mg/day) and a free intake of Na, calories and fluid, 24-h urines were collected and analysed for Ca, Na, P and creatinine. The maximum free water clearance was measured[3]. Eight C, 7 IH and 5 NC repeated the same protocol for 7 days after supplementation of the same diet with 6 g NaCl. The fractional delivery of filtered fluid to the distal tubule (ClDD) was evaluated from $ClDD = C_{H2O}2/GFR + C_{Cl}/GFR$.

Table 1. Plasma Values (PCa and PNa), Daily (UCaV and UNaV) and Fasting (CaE and NaE) Ca and Na Excretion, Renal Phosphate Threshold ($TmPO_4$/GFR) and Distal Chloride Delivery (ClDD) in Normal Subjects and Ca Stone Formers.

Group	PCa (mg/day)	PNa (mEq/1)	UCaV (mg/day)	CaE (mg/dl GFR)	UNaV (mEq/day)	NaE (mEq/1 GFR)	$TmPO_4$/GFR (mg/dl GFR)	ClDD (%)
C	9.4+0.5 (15)	138+3.4 (15)	132+47 (15)	0.03+0.03 (15)	150+51 (15)	1.07+0.87 (15)	3.8+0.6 (15)	10.6+4 (15)
IH	9.1+0.43 (22)	140+2.7 (22)	285+110[e] (22)	0.14+0.1[c] (22)	198+38[a] (10)	2.04+1.1[c] (22)	2.8+0.6[e] (22)	25.4+4.7[e] (22)
NC	9.2+0.3 (10)	138+4.5 (10)	153+63[i] (10)	0.08+0.05[c,m] (8)	196+69 (10)	2.2 +0.9[d] (10)	3.1+0.74[b] (10)	14.2+3.3[b]

P (vC) a = 0.05, b = 0. 02, c = 0.01, d = 0.001, e = 0.005, P (vIH) m = 0.05, i = 0.001.

Table 2. Effects of 6 g/day NaCl Supplementation in Normal Subjects (C), and in Idiopathic Hypercalciuric (IH) and Normocalciuric (NC) patients.

Group	Diet	UCaV (mg/day)	CaE (mg/dl GFR)	UNaV (mEq/day)	NaE (mEq/1 GFR)	TmPO$_4$/GFR (mg/dl GFR)	ClDD (%)
C (n=9)	Basal	135±55	0.03±0.02	135±35	0.73±0.6	3.99±0.5	9.6±2.8
	NaCl	146±76	0.04±0.03	230±46[d]	1.94±0.7[d]	3.62±0.7[a]	15.1±6.5[d]
IH (n=7)	Basal	310±95	0.17±0.12	201±43	2.66±1	2.9 ±0.45	16.8±4.4
	NaCl	356±144	0.21±0.14	308±56[d]	3.78±1.2[c]	2.6 ±0.62	21.5±5.2[b]
NC (n=5)	Basal	178±70	0.06±0.04	137±73	1.82±0.8	3.16±0.98	12.6±2.98
	NaCl	205±41[a]	0.07±0.04	239±53	2.35±1.2	3.1 ±0.8	13.4±4.3

P (NaCl v basal) a = 0.05, b = 0.02, c = 0.01, d = 0.001

RESULTS

The data on the low Ca + free Na diet are shown in Table 1. After NaCl supplementation, daily and fasting Na excretion and ClDD rose in 8 C to levels as high as in IH on the free Na diet (Table 2). Ca excretion remained unchanged and $TmPO_4/GFR$ slightly fell but remained higher than in the IH. ClDD and UNaV (basal and NaCl supplementation) were correlated in C ($r=0.58$, P 0.01) and in almost all the IH and NC the relationship fell within the 95% confidence limits observed in C. There were no significant correlations between $TmPO_4/GFR$ and ClDD and UNaV, nor between UCaV and ClDD and UNaV, either in C or in the patients. UCaV did not change after NaCl supplementation in IH and slightly increased in 5 NC. In the 12 CSF studied UCaV increased from 238 ± 125 to 293 ± 141 (P<0.05).

DISCUSSION

Our study confirms that IH have an increased distal delivery of glomerular filtrate and, as a consequence, have increased distal tubular reabsorption of Na and Cl, while the fractional reabsorption of their distal delivery remains unchanged[3]. In our patients, the reduction in proximal tubular fluid reabsorption was possibly related to their high Na intake. ClDD increased in C after NaCl loading to levels similar to those in IH, and the plots of ClDD v UNaV in almost every patient fell within the 95% confidence limits of the distribution in C. Thus, reduced proximal tubular Na reabsorption in Ca stone formers might not represent a tubular "defect" but be a physiological adaptation to a habitually high Na intake. In addition, there were no significant correlations between UCaV and either ClDD or $TmPO_4/GFR$ in C or in CSF. ClDD was as high in NC and in C after NaCl loading as in IH, but there was no hypercalciuria in the former group. Thus, it appears that hypercalciuria and proximal Na reabsorption are independent phenomena.

We have not observed any significant increase in Ca excretion in hypercalciuric CSF after NaCl supplementation in contrast to other studies[1]. However, our patients were only studied on a high Na diet and were not evaluated on lower Na diets.

REFERENCES

1. F. D. Muldowney, R. Freaney, and F. Maloney, Kidney Int. 22:292 (1982).
2. A. L. Sutton and V. R. Walker, New Engl. J. Med. 13:709 (1980).
3. Y. K. Lau, H. Wasserstein, G. R. Westbey, P. Bosanac, M. Gabrie, P. Mitnick, E. Slatopolsky, S. Goldfarb, and Z. S. Agus, Min. Electrol. Metab. 7:237 (1982).

EVIDENCE FOR MAGNESIUM DEPLETION IN IDIOPATHIC HYPERCALCIURIA

P. Bataille, A. Pruna, P. Leflon, I. Grégoire,
M. Finet, C. Galy, J. F. de Fremont, R. Makdassi,
and A. Fournier

Service de Néphrologie et Laboratoire de Biochemie
C.H.U., Hôpital Nord, 8000 Amiens, France

INTRODUCTION

Magnesium accounts for about 20% of the total inhibitory activity of urine with respect to calcium stone formation[1]. Magnesium depletion has been shown to cause calcification in the proximal tubule cells and in the tubular lumen in rats[2] and to be responsible for nephrocalcinosis in children. Based on these data, magnesium deficiency has been suspected as a factor in the pathogenesis of calcium stone formation although it has been observed only rarely[3]. Moreover, the data on magnesium excretion in stone formers are conflicting, and may even be normal[4] or increased[5]. These discrepancies may be explained by the fact that dietary calcium and calcium excretion were not taken into account, despite the fact that in normal individuals magnesium excretion is directly correlated with calcium excretion[6]. For these reasons it seemed interesting to us to study magnesium metabolism in various groups of idiopathic calcium stone-formers classified according to calcium excretion during a controlled calcium diet.

METHODS

Sixty controls and 82 patients with calcium urolithiasis were studied on an ambulatory protocol. They collected 24-h urines on a free diet and then after 4 days on a low calcium diet, containing no dairy products and providing approximately 400 mg of Ca per day. Creatinine, calcium, phosphate and sodium were measured in both urine collections. Magnesium was measured only in the urine collected after calcium restriction. Blood samples were drawn after the 4 days of calcium restriction for calcium, phosphate, magnesium, creatinine as well as alkaline phosphatase and parathyroid hormone in order to eliminate patients with specific causes of calcium stone-formation. Calcium, phosphate and creatinine were analysed colorimetrically using a Technicon AutoAnalyzer. Magnesium was determined in urine and plasma by the calmagite method.

RESULTS

Using the data of the controls, the patients were classified according to their urinary calcium excretion. Sixty were normocalciuric (NCa) on a free diet (calciuria < 0.1 mmol/kg/day); 17 patients who were hypercalciuric on a free diet, presented with diet-dependent hypercalciuria (DH), a diagnosis based on the return to normal of urinary calcium excretion after calcium restriction, when compared to controls on the same restricted diet (calciuria <0.07 mmol/kg/day). Idiopathic hypercalciuria (IH) was found in 29 patients who were hypercalciuric on a free diet and on a restricted diet (i.e. calciuria >0.1 mmol/kg/day on a free diet, calciuria 0.07 mmol/kg/day on calcium restricted diet).

Table 1 shows the values of the daily urinary excretion of calcium and magnesium in controls and in patients after 4 days on a low calcium diet. When compared to controls, both magnesium and calcium excretion were significantly higher ($P<0.01$) in patients with idiopathic hypercalciuria. Because of the possible role of magnesium in inhibiting calcium crystallisation urinary magnesium/ calcium ratios were calculated in both groups. The magnesium/ calcium ratios were significantly lower than normal only in those patients with IH. Serum magnesium was also found to be significantly lower ($P<0.05$) in this group than in the controls.

In each group there was a significant correlation between magnesium and calcium excretion (for controls: UMg = 1.53 + 0.37 UCa; $r = 0.37$; $P < 0.001$: for patients: UMg = 2.55 + 0.56 UCa; $r = 0.44$; $P< 0.001$). When the various subgroups of stone-formers were considered separately, positive correlations between calcium and magnesium excretions were found in normocalciuric patients ($r = 0.62$; $P<0.01$) and in those with diet-dependent hypercalciuria ($r = 0.45$; $P<0.05$), but not in patients with idiopathic hypercalciuria.

DISCUSSION

Our data, based on a short-term study, show that magnesium excretion on a low calcium diet is comparable in normocalciuric patients and in patients with diet-dependent hypercalciuria when compared to controls on the same Ca-restricted diet. On the other hand, the coexistence of a higher magnesium excretion and a lower plasma level of magnesium in stone-formers with idiopathic hyper-

Table 1. Daily Excretion of Magnesium and Calcium, Urinary Magnesium/Calcium Ratio and Plasma Levels of Magnesium and Calcium in Controls and Calcium Stone-formers on a Ca-Restricted Diet (Mean $\pm$ SEM).

	U Mg V (mmol/day)	U Ca V (mmol/day)	U Mg/U Ca	P Mg (mmol/l)	P Ca (mmol/l)
Controls n = 60	3.4 $\pm$ 0.6	2.02 $\pm$ 0.3	1.68 $\pm$ 0.15	0.84 $\pm$ 0.001	2.35 $\pm$ 0.06
N Ca n = 36	3.87 $\pm$ 0.17	2.84 $\pm$ 0.3	1.36 $\pm$ 0.08	0.2 $\pm$ 0.09	2.30 $\pm$ 0.07
DH n = 17	3.94 $\pm$ 0.30	3.78 $\pm$ 0.4	1.04 $\pm$ 0.13	0.85 $\pm$ 0.01	2.25 $\pm$ 0.08
IH n = 29	4.26 $\pm$ 0.28**	7.1 $\pm$ 0.4***	0.6 $\pm$ 0.04***	0.79 $\pm$ 0.01*	2.28 $\pm$ 0.07

Significance of the difference between controls and the stone-former group:

* P<0.05; ** P<0.01; *** P<0.001

N Ca = normocalciuric; DH = diet-dependent hypercalciuria; IH = idiopathic hypercalciuria.

calciuria suggests that there is a renal leak of magnesium leading to magnesium deficiency.

The following hypothesis may explain the higher magnesium excretion in idiopathic hypercalciuria. Since there is a well-known competition for tubular reabsorption between calcium and magnesium, an increased filtered load of calcium could increase magnesium excretion[6]. The following facts are not consistent with this hypothesis: (1) since there is no hypercalcemia in IH, there is no reason to postulate an increased filtered load; (2) there is ho correlation between calcium and magnesium excretion in IH.

A second hypothesis may be proposed. In most patients with IH there is relative hypoparathyroidism since the primary disorder is an increased intestinal absorption of calcium[7]. Since PTH stimulates magnesium reabsorption [8], relative hypoparathyroidism could explain the increase in magnesium excretion. This hypothesis is further supported by the lower plasma magnesium observed in patients with absorptive hypercalciuria [9].

The importance of magnesium in inhibiting the crystallization of calcium salts depends on the concentration of magnesium in relation to calcium rather than on the absolute amount of this ion. The urinary magnesium/calcium ratio represents an index of the propensity for stone-formation. This ratio is significantly decreased only in idiopathic hypercalciuric patients, although absolute magnesium is significantly higher in this group of patients. This suggests that magnesium supplements might be of particular therapeutic value in idiopathic hypercalciuria.

REFERENCES

1. S. Bisaz, B. Felix, F. Neuman, and H. Fleisch, Min. Electr. Metab. 1:74 (1978).
2. G. E. Bunce and G. A. King, Exp. Mol. Pathol. 28:322 (1978).
3. G. Johansson, U. Backman, B. G. Danielson, B. Fellström, S. Ljunghall, and B. Wikström, in:"Urolithiasis:Clinical and Basic Research", L. H. Smith, W. G. Robertson, and B.Finlayson, eds., Plenum, New York, (1981).
4. M. J. Nicar and C. Y. C. Pak, Min. Electr. Metab. 8:44 (1982).
5. F. L. Coe, M. J. Favus, T. Croukett, A. L. Strauss, J. H. Parks, A. Porat, L. Gant, and L. M. Sherwood, Am. J. Med. 72:25 (1982).
6. S. G. Massry and J. W. Coburn, Nephron 10:66 (1973).
7. F. P. Muldowney, B. Freaney, and J. G. Byan, Quart. J. Med. 49:87(1980).
8. G. Colussi, M. Sorian, G. Malberti, A. Aroldi, D. Rurale, and L.Minetti. Kidney Int., 22:96 (1982).
9. D. Scholz and P. Schwille, Min. Electr. Metab. 6:264 (1981).

MAGNESIUM EXCRETION IN RECURRENT CALCIUM UROLITHIASIS

R. Pfab, M. Hegemann, and W. Schütz

Dept. of Urology, The Technical University
8000 Munich 80, F.R.G.

INTRODUCTION

The rationale for using magnesium in the treatment of recurrent calcium stone formers is largely based on evidence from in vitro studies. Firstly, magnesium increases the solubility of calcium oxalate by forming a soluble complex with oxalate. Secondly, it inhibits the precipitation of calcium phosphate crystals[1], although it only has a limited inhibitory effect on the crystal growth of calcium oxalate[2]. The efficacy of magnesium treatment has been assessed in calcium stone formers[3,4]. Current opinion favours the view that magnesium significantly reduces stone recurrence in renal calcium stone formers but a few authors remain convinced that it has only a "placebo-effect" on patients with stones[5]. In search of the reason for the beneficial effect of magnesium therapy, we have measured magnesium excretion in patients with recurrent calcium urolithiasis to check for hypomagnesiuria.

MATERIALS AND METHODS

Magnesium excretion was measured in 122 recurrent calcium stone formers (83 males and 39 females, average age 41.2 ± 12.3 years) with no evidence of urinary tract infection and in 30 healthy subjects (19 males and 11 females; average age 35.3 ± 15.8 years). Each individual collected a 24-h urine sample on a free diet and fasting urine on the test day. Plasma and urinary biochemistry were measured using an SMA 12 Autoanalyzer and flame photometry. Urinary magnesium was determined by atomic absorption spectrometry and serum PTH by a C-terminal (65-84) radioimmunoassay. Results were compared using the Student one-tailed t-test.

RESULTS AND DISCUSSION

Low urinary magnesium concentrations in recurrent calcium stone formers have been reported[6]. Other investigators, however, have been unable to find significant differences in urinary magnesium excretion between healthy subjects and recurrent calcium stone formers[7]. Using a different approach, some authors have tried to quantitate the risk of calcium oxalate stone formation by calculating the urinary magnesium/calcium ratio. This ratio was found to be low in recurrent calcium stone formers[8]. However, increasing the magnesium/calcium ratio in urine does not necessarily reduce the relative supersaturation of calcium oxalate since any physiochemical effect of magnesium is related to its actual concentration in urine and not to the magnesium/calcium ratio[9].

Our findings indicate that magnesium deficiency does appear to be a significant pathogenetic factor in a subgroup of patients with recurrent calcium urolithiasis. This subgroup (M) consisted of 17 males and 10 females whose average age was 40.9 ± 18.4 years. Other obvious metabolic abnormalities were excluded, primary hyperparathyroidism (7), renal tubular acidosis (2), hypercalciuria (60), hyperuricosuria (19), hypocitraturia (4) and enteric hyperoxaluria (6). Magnesium deficiency in subgroup M was quantitated, as shown in Table 1 by determination of (i) the absolute concentration of

Table 1. Magnesium Excretion and Factors Influencing Renal Magnesium Transport (mean $\pm$ SD).

Variable		Subgroup M	Normocalciurics	Controls
24-h Urine:				
Mg	(mg/day)	83 ± 35.3**	103 ± 35.1	109 ± 47.66
Mg/Ca	(mg/mg)	0.47 ± 0.06*	0.52 ± 0.09	0.49 ± 0.12
		0.52 ± 1.10*	0.67 ± 0.07	0.54 ± 0.13
Mg/Cr	(mg/mg)	0.07 ± 0.03	0.67 ± 0.03	0.07 ± 0.04
Na	(mmol/day)	169 ± 83.7	179 ± 77.9	176 ± 71.6
Volume	(l/day)	2.09 ± 0.87	2.16 ± 0.96	1.56 ± 0.64
Fasting Urine:				
Mg/Ca	(mg/mg)	0.67 ± 0.03*	0.78 ± 0.13	0.72 ± 0.09
Mg/Cr	(mg/mg)	0.039 ± 0.010	0.042 ± 0.016	0.033 ± 0.015
Serum:				
Ca	(mg/dl)	9.27 ± 0.47	9.25 ± 0.39	9.51 ± 0.50
P	(mg/dl)	3.23 ± 0.55	3.06 ± 0.56	3.72 ± 0.65
PTH	(pmol/l)	60 ± 39	58 ± 31	56 ± 33

* $P < 0.01$ Subgroup M v Normocalciurics.
** $P < 0.01$ Subgroup M v Normocalciurics and Controls.

urinary magnesium and the magnesium/calcium ratio in a 24-h urine on a free diet, and (ii) the magnesium/calcium ratio in fasting urine. Such differences could not be detected using the magnesium/-creatinine ratio. Matched for sex and age, there was no significant difference between subgroup M and either the other nor mocalciuric patients or the control group.

Clinical studies suggest that magnesium is normally handled by a filtration-reabsorption process in the kidney[10]. The factors which influence renal magnesium transport are: (i) extracellular volume expansion, which produces a rapid urinary excretion of magnesium, (ii) hypercalcemia and hypophosphatemia, which result in marked hypermagnesiuria, and (iii) parathyroid hormone, which seems to enhance magnesium reabsorption in the loop of Henle. Our data on sodium excretion, 24-h urine volume, serum calcium, serum phosphate and serum PTH demonstrate that the significantly reduced urinary magnesium in subgroup M is not due to factors influencing the renal tubular reabsorption of magnesium (Table 1). We believe that the low urinary magnesium levels may be a pathogenetic factor in a metabolic subgroup of normocalciuric sterile calcium stone formers. In these patients oral magnesium supplements may be justified.

ACKNOWLEDGEMENTS

The authors wish to dedicate this paper to Prof. Dr. W. Mauermayer. The work was supported by grant 820181 of the Wilhelm-Sander-Stiftung.

REFERENCES

1. S. Bisaz, R. Felix, W. F. Neuman , and H. Fleisch, Min. Electrol. Metab. 1:74 (1978).
2. J. L. Meyer and L. H. Smith, Invest. Urol. 13:36 (1975).
3. P. Brundig, W. Berg, and H.-J. Schneider, Eur. Urol. 7:97 (1981).
4. G. Johansson, U. Backmann, B. G. Danielson, B. Fellström, S. Ljunghall, and B. Wikström, Magnesium Bull. 2:181 (1981).
5. M. I. Resnick, D. B. S. Munday, and W. H. Boyce, Urology, 4:385 (1982).
6. P. O. Schwille, I. Schlenk, N. M. Samberger, and C. Bornhof, Urol. Res. 4:33 (1976).
7. S. G. Welshman and M. G. McGeown, Br. J. Urol.. 47:237 (1975).
8. A. Hodgkinson, Clin. Sci. Mol. Med. 46:357 (1974).
9. C. D. Fetner, D. E. Barilla, J. Townsend, and C. Y. C. Pak, J. Urol. 120:399 (1978).
10. G. A. Quamme and J. H. Dirks, Rev. Physiol. Biochem. Pharmacol. 97 (1983).

THE DIAGNOSTIC VALUE OF RENAL TUBULAR REABSORPTION OF MAGNESIUM

CALCULATIONS IN CALCIUM-CONTAINING KIDNEY STONE FORMERS

V. Revúsová, J. Gratzlová, and V. Zvara

Medical Bionics Research Institute, Research Laboratory
of Metabolic Disorders in Renal Diseases, Dept. of
Urology, Bratislava, Czechoslovakia

INTRODUCTION

In our previous studies, a high incidence of hypomagnesemia was found among calcium-containing kidney stone formers. In the hypo-magnesemic patients, urinary magnesium excretion did not differ significantly from that of either healthy individuals or normo-magnesemic stone formers. However, oral and parenteral Mg supplementation caused a significant increment in urinary Mg excretion, suggesting that there was renal Mg wasting in these patients. To investigate this problem we have calculated TRMg% in a randomly selected group of calcium-containing kidney stone formers. The purpose of the study was to compare the diagnostic value of TRMg% and the urinary excretion of Mg as determinants of renal Mg wasting.

PATIENTS AND METHODS

Sixty-nine patients (53 males, 15 females, and one child aged 2 years) were investigated. Urinary magnesium, total serum Mg and plasma ultrafiltrable Mg prepared according to the method of Piemonte et al[1], were analyzed by atomic absorption spectrophometry.

RESULTS

The results in healthy subjects (group 1), in the complete group of patients (group 2), in the patients with impaired TRMg (group 3) and in the patients with hypomagnesemia (group 4) are summarized in Table 1. No significant differences in urinary Mg

Table 1. Laboratory Findings (mean+SD) in 17 Health Individuals
and in 69 Calcium-Containing Kidney Stone Formers.

Group	TRMg (%)	Serum Mg (mmol/l)	Urine Mg (mmol/day)
1	95.6 + 1.5	0.85 + 0.05	4.10 + 1.36
2	91.0 + 13.1	0.80 + 0.11	4.13 + 1.30
3	75.9 + 21.1	0.67 + 0.12	4.40 + 1.80
4	69.7 + 22.0	0.60 + 0.06	3.96 + 1.86
1:2	ns	ns	ns
1:3	P<0.02	P<0.001	ns
1:4	P<0.001	P<0.001	ns

excretion were found.   On the contrary, TRMg% was reduced in 10
patients indicating decreased renal Mg conservation.   The lowest
TRMg% values were found in 5 hypomagnesemic patients.

DISCUSSION

In our previous studies in calcium-containing kidney stone
formers, there was a great inter-individual variability in urinary
Mg excretion.   Urinary Mg values varied from the low-normal to
excessively high in comparison with the excretions in healthy
subjects.

A high incidence of hypomagnesemia in our patients suggested
that a renal leak of magnesium may have reduced serum Mg to
pathological levels.   However, the majority of hypomagnesemic
patients had a "normal" urinary excretion of Mg.   Although the
increment in urinary Mg following oral or parenteral Mg
supplementation suggested that there was impairment of renal Mg
conservation, measurement of urinary Mg alone was insufficient to
prove renal Mg wasting.

The results of this study have confirmed that calculation of
TRMg% is of greater value in detecting a renal leak of Mg than the
measurement of urinary Mg alone.   The lowest TRMg% values in
hypomagnesemic patients indicated a relationship between renal Mg
wasting and serum Mg depletion.   In addition, the decreased TRMg%
values in some normomagnesemic patients indicated that Mg deficiency
due to renal Mg wasting may have been present in some of the
patients with normal serum Mg values.

We have also found, that calculation of TRMg% is helpful in
Mg-loading and Mg-deprivation tests, where the interpretation of the
results may be incorrect in the patients with impaired renal Mg

conservation.   However, in the patients with renal insufficiency, TRMg% values decrease in proportion to renal impairment.   Thus in the calculation and interpretation of TRMg%, GFR must be taken into consideration.

REFERENCE

1. G. Piemonte, G. Luisetto, and N. Conte, Clin. Chim. Acta 45:261 (1973).

SOME STONE PROMOTING AND INHIBITING FACTORS IN FASTING AND
POSTPRANDIAL URINES OF STONE PATIENTS AND CONTROLS -
PRELIMINARY RESULTS

P. O. Schwille, G. Wölfel, I. Golberg, W. Bausch,
K. Bernreuther, G. Ruemenapf, and A. Sigel

Mineral Metabolism and Endocrine Research Laboratory
and Depts. of Surgery, Urology and Mineralogy
University of Erlangen, Erlangen, F.R.G.

INTRODUCTION

Little is known about the diurnal variation of urinary
supersaturation which might allow precipitation and crystalluria to
occur.   Previously, we found that urine voided after ingestion of
an oxalate-free calcium-rich test has a high degree of
supersaturation in terms of calcium oxalate[1]. The present work
describes the relative supersaturation of urine for brushite as well
as the associated crystalluria, before and after a test meal.   We
also measured several small molecular weight inhibitors.

PATIENTS AND METHODS

Healthy controls (n = 22; age   23-73, median 33 years;
M/F = 12/10) and patients with recurrent calcium urolithiasis
(RCU; n = 54) underwent our laboratory program to classify RCU, on
an out-patient basis, into those with normocalciuria (NC; n = 24;
age 20-69, median 41 years; M/F = 15/9), and those with idiopathic
hypercalciuria (I-HC; n = 30; age 24-68, median 44 years;
M/F = 21/0).   The study consisted of collecting a 2-h fasting
morning urine and a 3-h post-prandial urine, the latter following an
oxalate-free, synthetic liquid meal (Vavasorb, Pfrimmer; Erlangen,
FRG), supplemented with 2000 mg of calcium[2].   No urinary tract
infection or specific metabolic disorder was present in the
patients. At the time of examination 35% had stones present in
their kidneys.   The calcium/creatinine (Cr) ratio was measured in
the fasting and postprandial urine of all participants, but the
ratios with creatinine between cAMP inorganic phosphate, and the
stone inhibitors (magnesium, citrate, pyrophosphate) were obtained

335

in smaller groups.   These ions were analyzed by routine procedures, and the relative supersaturation product of brushite (RSP_{pi}) calculated from a nomogram[3].   Crystalluria was measured by a modification of a filter technique allowing the study of phosphate, but not oxalate, crystals.   Crystals were identified using polarisation microscopy and a crystalluria score calculated[4].

RESULTS

"Stone Promoters" (Table 1).   The calcium/creatinine ratio in N-C was normal during both the fasting and the postprandial period, whereas in I-HC it was elevated.   The phosphate/creatinine ratio during fasting was decreased in N-C, I-HC, contrasting with our own previous work[5].   After the meal urinary phosphate increased in only the stone patients, and tended to fall in the controls.   The median urinary pH in the stone groups was more alkaline, as found previously[5].   The RSP_{pi} was in the undersaturated range during fasting in all groups; it reached a peak in controls, while in stone patients there was considerably less undersaturation.   After a meal the RSP_{pi} in all groups rose into the metastable range of supersaturation, and in a few patients approached or exceeded the formation product of brushite.

"Stone Inhibitors" (Table 1).   Of the three small molecular weight inhibitors of crystal and stone forming processes, citrate appeared stable throughout, i.e. there is no citrate deficiency in stone formers, either in the fasting or postprandial urine[5]. Magnesium also was not decreased in stone disease under basal fasting conditions.   The postprandial magnesium in urine rose least in the N-C and most in the I-HC group.   Fasting pyrophosphate was markedly decreased in N-C, whereas post-prandial pyrophosphate neither differed from fasting values nor varied between the groups.

Crystalluria (Table 1).   Using a Millipore, instead of a Nucleopore filter[4], the predominant crystal phase in both fasting and postprandial urine of controls and stone patients was octacalcium phosphate (apatite) with an admixture of calcium oxalate in only a few patients.   As a rule, crystal size and the degree of aggregation did not grossly differ between the two groups.   Basal crystalluria in the fasting state was highest in N-C, not in I-HC, whereas postprandially the opposite was true.

Parathyroid gland function (Table 1).   The cAMP/creatinine ratio in fasting urine ws normal in N-C and I-HC.   Postprandially there was a fall of cAMP in all groups.   If one considers the three groups together pre- and post-prandially, then the fall in this indirect parameter of parathyroid gland function was highly significant (fasting - 0.41; post-prandially - 0.27; $P < 0.001$).

336

Table 1. Variables in Fasting and Postprandial Urine (Median (n)).

	Fasting Urine			Postprandial Urine		
	C	N-C	I-HC	C	N-C	I-HC
I. Stone Promoters						
Calcium/Cr (mM/mM)	0.17 (22)	0.20 (24)	0.34^c(30)	0.57 (22)	0.49 (24)	0.85^b(30)
Phosphate/Cr (mM/mM)	1.46 (17)	0.98^b(17)	1.09^b(17)	1.24 (17)	1.46 (17)	1.42 (17)
Urinary pH	6.4 (17)	6.5 (17)	6.5 (17)	6.0 (17)	6.2 (17)	6.3 (17)
RSP$_{pi}$	-0.60 (17)	-0.23^a(17)	-0.20 (17)	0.15*(17)	0.20 (17)	0.25*(17)
II. Stone Inhibitors						
Magnesium/Cr (mM/mM)	0.17 (17)	0.18 (17)	0.18 (17)	0.53 (17)	0.32^b(17)	0.60^a(17)
Citrate/Cr (mM/mM)	0.17 (17)	0.17 (17)	0.16 (17)	0.14 (17)	0.15 (17)	0.14 (17)
Pyrophosphate/ Cr (µM/mM)	0.94 (10)	0.10^a(10)	0.77 (10)	0.41 (10)	0.60 (10)	0.59 (10)
III. Crystalluria Score	0.50 (16)	1.0^a (16)	0.5 (10)	0.5 (5)	0.5 (16)	1.0^a (9)
IV. Parathyroid gland function						
cAMP/Cr (mM/mM)	0.42 (15)	0.39 (15)	0.48 (15)	0.24 (17)	0.25 (15)	0.33 (16)

a = P<0.05; b = P<0.01; c = P<0.001 versus C; * = P<0.05 versus corresponding value during fasting.

DISCUSSION

After a meal there was a marked increase in RSP_{pi} in urine into the metastable range of supersaturation. Thus, the theory of brushite being a possible nucleus for stone formation may well deserve further evaluation. A more detailed interpretation of crystalluria is difficult because of the small number of observations. We feel, however, that the existence of crystalluria in fasting urine is surprising, considering the rather low RSP_{pi}. Whereas in N-C the low pyrophosphate could explain their crystalluria, the underlying mechanisms in C and I-HC subjects are unknown. The fact that, in response to the meal, crystalluria in N-C is lower than it is basally probably does not detract from the usefulness of this kind of loading procedure. Support for the assumption comes from the postprandial increase in crystalluria in I-HC, which comprises about 40% of RCU patients, and I-HC most likely reflects a more severe state of stone disease. Also, crystalluria is determined by both the degree of supersaturation of the salt phase under study and the associated inhibitory activity. Thus, the failure of crystalluria to increase postprandially in N-C may be explained by a relative abundance of small molecular inhibitors as studied here, or of additional low and high molecular weight inhibitors[6]. Moreover, potential postprandial changes in crystalluria could have been masked in all groups by the suppressed parathyroid gland activity brought about by the oral calcium load. Significant crystalluria and a high RSP_{pi} are prominent features of primary hyperparathyroidism[4]. Finally, the calcium oxalate crystalluria which accompanies calcium phosphate crystalluria needs further evaluation in the groups studied.

ACKNOWLEDGEMENT

Support for this study was obtained from Deutsche Forschungsgemeinschaft (Sch 210/4-1).

REFERENCES

1. P. O. Schwille, E. Hanisch, and D. Scholz, (in press).
2. D. Scholz and P. O. Schwille, Dtsch. Med. Wschr. 106:999 (1981).
3. R. W. Marshall and W. G. Robertson, Clin. Chim. Acta 72:253 (1976).
4. P. G. Werness, J. H. Begert, and L. H. Smith, J. Cryst. Growth 53:166 (1981).
5. P. O. Schwille, D. Scholz, K. Schwille, R. Leutschaft, I.Goldberg, and A. Sigel, Nephron 31:194 (1982).
6. T. Kitamura, J. E. Zerwekh, and C. Y. C. Pak, Kidney Int. 21:379 (1982).

URINARY AND SERUM SULFATE IN IDIOPATHIC RECURRENT CALCIUM

UROLITHIASIS (RCU)

P. O. Schwille, A. Hamper, and A. Sigel

Mineral Metabolism and Endocrine Research Laboratory
and Depts. of Surgery and Urology, University of
Erlangen, F.R.G.

INTRODUCTION

Sulfate is present in considerable amounts in human urine and
serum[1], but little is known about sulfate in RCU. There are two
reasons for a possible relationship between sulfate and stone-
formation: (i) sulfate ions in tubular fluid or urine compete with
oxalate for complexing with calcium ions, and (ii) inorganic sulfate
under certain dietary conditions correlates directly with urinary
calcium[2], suggesting that idiopathic hypercalciuria (I-HC) may be
linked with either a high protein level in the diet, enhanced
intestinal absorption of dietary sulfate, increased hepatic sulfur
oxidation or altered renal sulfate handling. We report on the
sulfate in the 24-h and 2-h fasting urines, and in the serum of RCU
subjects and controls.

SUBJECTS AND METHODS

A total of 71 individuals (37 men and 34 women) with normal
kidney function took part in the study consisting of 19 healthy
controls (11 men and 8 women), 26 N-C (13 men and 13 women) and 26
I-HC (13 men and 12 women) stone patients, roughly matched for age.
All were examined in our outpatient stone clinic[3] and a 24-h urine,
a 2-h urine after a 12- to 15-h overnight fast, a 3-h postprandial
urine, and a fasting venous blood taken[4]. Sulfate was measured
colorimetrically in urine[5] before (inorganic sulfate) and after acid
hydrolysis (total sulfate), the difference being the esterified
sulfate, and also in serum[1]. Calcium, sodium and urea were measured
by routine methods.

339

Table 1. The Median Sulfate, Calcium and Sodium, in 24 h Urine (A:Excretion Rate; B:Excretion Related to Urinary Creatinine), and in 2-h Morning Fasting Urine (C:Excretion related to creatinine or creatinine clearance).

Analyte	Males			Females			Males + Females		
	C	N-C	I-HC	C	N-C	I-HC	C	N-C	I-HC
A.Sulfate (mmol)									
Total	32	24	35	28*	20	26	31	22^a	32
Inorganic	30	22^a	32	25*	18^a	25	29	20^b	30
Esterfied	2.5	2.3	0.9	3.4	1.4	2.4	2.9	1.9^b	2.3
Calcium (mmol)	5.4	4.4	8.2^a	3.3	3.3	7.5^c	4.3	3.9	8.1^c
B.Sulfate/Creatinine (mmol/mmol)									
Total	2.0	1.7^a	2.1	2.3	1.8	2.4	2.3	1.8	2.2
Inorganic	1.8	1.7	2.0	2.2	1.6	2.2	2.0	1.6^a	2.0
Esterfied	0.2	0.2	0.97	0.3	0.1	0.2	0.2	0.2	0.2
Sodium/Creatinine	12.4	14.1	12.8	9.8	12.4	14.6	11.6	13.3	13.8
C.Sulfate/Creatinine (mmol/mmol)									
Total	1.6	1.4	1.4	1.1	1.5	2.5	1.6	1.4	1.6
Inorganic	1.5	1.0^a	0.7^a	1.0	0.7	1.8^a	1.4	0.9	1.2
Esterfied	0.1	0.3	0.2	0.6	0.6	0.5	0.3	0.4	0.4
Ca/C$_{Cr}$ (µmol/dl)	1.9	2.0	3.0^c	1.3	1.3	2.4^b	1.4	1.5	2.8^c
Na/C$_{Cr}$ (µmol/dl)	85	82	131^a	48	81	121^a	52	82	127^b

*$P < 0.05$ vs males; $^a P < 0.05$, $^b 0.01$, $^c 0.001$ vs C.

Table 2. Correlation Coefficients from the Relationships between Urinary Calcium, Sulfate and Sodium.

	Calcium in fasting urine			Calcium in daily urine		
	C	N-C	I-HC	C	N-C	I-HC
Inorganic SO$_4$						
r	0.04	0.50	0.66	0.02	0.49	0.27
n	19	26	26	19	26	24
P	n.s	<0.01	<0.001	n.s	<0.01	n.s
Sodium						
r	0.26	0.39	0.43	0.30	0.18	0.57
n	17	26	25	19	26	24
P	n.s	<0.05	<0.05	n.s	n.s	<0.01

RESULTS

Total sulfate excretion was higher in males than in females
(P<0.01) but not in the 2-h fasting urine. Sulfate (total,
inorganic, esterified) was lower in N-C than in C, but unchanged in
I-HC (males + females). Urea excretion in (males + females) was
0.17 mol and 0.15 mol in C and N-C (P<0.05) and 0.15 mol in I-HC.
The median urine volumes were lower (but not significantly so) in C
than in N-C or I-HC subjects (Table 1). Division by creatinine
destroyed the significant differences seen with total and esterified
sulfate, but low inorganic sulfate persisted in N-C (males +
females). Sodium excretion in RCU (N-C, I-HC) was unchanged,
whereas the accompanying calcium was high.

In contrast to the 24-h urines there was a reduction in male
N-and I-HC, but an increase in female N-C patients in the sulfate/
creatinine ratio or sulfate/creatinine clearance ratios. The
difference disappeared when the two sexes were combined and no other
differences in fasting sulfate were detectable (males + females).
Calcium and sodium excretion were elevated in I-HC, but not in N-C
patients.

In the fasting urines of RCU there were significant
correlations between sulfate and calcium and sodium and calcium,
whereas in 24-h urines this was so only between sulfate and calcium
(N-C) and sodium and sulfate (I-HC) (Table 2).

The range of serum sulfate was 0.207 to 0.813 mM. Males did
not differ 'from females, nor did male or female patients differ from
the corresponding controls. After pooling the data sulfate was
decreased (P<0.05) in N-C (0.246 mM) compared with C (0.393 mM) but
was unchanged in I-HC (0.384 mM).

DISCUSSION

All fractions of urinary sulfate are higher in this study than
shown previously[6], while serum sulfate agrees with values obtained
by a more specific methodology[7]. We report that 24-h urinary
sulfate is low in normocalciuric (N-C) and normal in hypercalciuric
(I-HC) RCU, whereas in the fasting urine of RCU, sulfate is
statistically unchanged when considering male and female stone
patients together. The reasons for these conflicting observations
are unclear, but citrate, another multivalent anion, behaves
similarly in RCU[8].

In N-C, where inorganic sulfate in serum is decreased but is
only insignificantly lower in 2-h urine, net tubular sulfate
reabsorption may be reduced provided sulfate filterability is
unchanged. From normal sulfate and urea (another crude indicator

of protein consumption) we cannot support the "dietary protein excess theory" as leading to hypercalciuria through a greater endogenous "acid load" created by a surplus of sulfur-containing amino acids[9]. However, based on the correlations between urinary sulfate, calcium and sodium, it appears that the degree of hypercalciuria is in fact more related to renal sulfate rather than to sodium handling, at least during the more rigidly controlled 2-h urine period in the laboratory. Although hypercalciuria may be affected by dietary sodium[10] the nature of the sodium excess in the morning urines and the interrelations between sodium, sulfate and calcium deserve further study.

ACKNOWLEDGMENTS

This work was supported by Deutsche Forschungsgemeinschaft (SCHW 210/4-1) and Research Funds of the University Hospital, Erlangen (FRG).

REFERENCES

1. N. Weissman, and V. J. Pileggi, in:"Clinical Chemistry, Principles and Technics", R. J. Henry, D. C. Camion, J. W. Winkelman, eds., Harper & Row, Hagerstown, New York (1974).
2. S. A. Schuette, M. Hegsted, M. B. Zemel, and M. H. Linkswiler, J. Nutr. 111:210 (1981).
3. D. Scholz, and P. O. Schwille, Dtsch. Med. Wschr. 106:999 (1981).
4. G. Ploss, P. O. Schwille, and A. Siegel, in:"Urolithiasis and Related Clinical Research", P. O. Schwille, L. H. Smith, W. G. Robertson, W. Vahlensieck, eds., Plenum, New York (1985).
5. S. Swaarop, Clin. Chim. Acta 46:333 (1973).
6. L. Baldetorp and J. Martenson, Acta Med. SCand. 208:293 (1980).
7. D. E. C. Cole, and C. R. Scriver, J. Chrom. 225:539 (1981).
8. P. O. Schwille, D. Scholz, K. Schwille, R. Leutschaft, I. Goldbert, and A. Sigel, Nephron 31:194 (1982).
9. W. G. Robertson, P. J. Heyburn, M. Peacock, F. A. Hanes, and R. Swaminathan, Clin. Sci. 57:285 (1979).
10. F. P. Muldowney, R. Freaney, and M. F. Maloney, Kidney Int. 22:292 (1982).

URINE AND SERUM POTASSIUM IN PATIENTS WITH RECURRENT CALCIUM UROLITHIASIS (RCU) - RESULTS OF A PILOT STUDY

G. Ploss, P. O. Schwille, and A. Sigel

Mineral Metabolism and Endocrine Research Laboratory
Depts. of Surgery and Urology, University of Erlangen
Erlangen, F.R.G.

INTRODUCTION

Potassium metabolism in RCU has received little attention by stone researchers[1], despite the fact that potassium forms soluble complexes with oxalate[2], and is a key substance in renal acid-base and citrate regulation. In RCU, hypocitraturia and renal tubular acidosis-like hyperbicarbonateuria are well-documented[3,4] along with a tendency toward hypokalemia[3].

PATIENTS AND METHODS

All participants (n = 126) were studied on their unrestricted home diet. They underwent our laboratory examination program (collection of 24-h, 2-h fasting, and 3-h postprandial urines, with fasting blood drawn before the 2-h period), as adapted to an outpatient stone clinic[5]. RCU patients (n = 86) were subdivided into those with normocalciuria (in 24-h urine; and a calcium/creatinine ratio < 0.12 in 2-h fasting urine; n = 48, N-C), and with idiopathic hypercalciuria (in 24-h urine; and a calcium/creatinine ratio in 2-h fasting urine > 0.12, and/or in 3-h postprandial urine > 0.27, n = 38, I-HC). In about one third of RCU patients kidney stones were present at the time of examination, but no urinary tract infection or metabolic disorder was detectable. Healthy subjects with no metabolic disorder served as controls (n = 40, C). The male:female ratio was 68 (N-C 25, I-HC 19, C 24):58 (N-C 23, I-HC 19, C 16). The median ages were 40 for N-C, 43 for I-HC and 32 for C.

The following measurements were made: in serum (after a 12- to 15-h overnight fast) - creatinine and potassium; in capillary blood

Table 1. Potassium in 24-h Urine (A), in Fasting Serum (B), and in 2-h Fasting Urine (C).

	Males			Females			Males + Females		
	C	N-C	I-HC	C	N-C	I-HC	C	N-C	I-HC
A. Volume (ml)	1420	1850	1940[b]	1521	1570[*]	1850[a]	1465	1705[c]	1855[c]
Potassium (mmol/l)	40	30	28	43	36	28	40	31[a]	28[c]
Potassium (mmol)	56	53	53	51	48	58	55	52	56
B. Bicarbonate (mmol/l)	24	24	22	23	24	21 (5)	24	24	22[a]
Potassium (mmol/l)	4.4	4.3	4.2	4.3	4.3	4.1	4.3	4.3	4.2
C. Volume (ml)	233	140	350	198	370[b]	280	200	198	325[b]
Potassium (mmol/l)	42	65	26[c]	41	18[c]	24[c]	42	36	25[b]
Potassium (mmol)	8.1	8.6	8.6	8.2	6.1[**]	6.3[***]	8.2	7.0	7.6
Potassium C_{Cr}^{-1} .100 (µmol)	9.4	8.2	8.8	7.9	5.8[***]	5.7[***]	8.9	6.8[a]	6.7
Fe_K (%)	15	13	15	16	11	12[a][**]	15	12[a]	13
FE_{Kcorr} (%)	16	13	15	15	9.9[*]	11[a][***]	16	12[b]	12
C_K ml.min^{-1}	14	14	17	17	11	13[*]	15	13	14
pH	6.5	6.8	7.0	6.3	6.7	6.8	6.4	6.7	6.9

[*] P<0.05; [**] P<0.01; [***] P<0.001 vs males: a = P<0.05; b = P<0.01; c = P<0.001 vs C.

- bicarbonate (as a crude indicator of acid-base state); in urine (24-h, 2-h, 3-h collections) - creatinine, potassium, pH, all by routine methods. The percentage of potassium filtered and excreted (FE_K) was recalculated in order to detect inadequate distal tubular potassium secretion (FE_{Kcorr})[6].

RESULTS

Potassium in 24-h urine (Table 1): A clear influence of sex on potassium was not found in the C subjects, whereas in RCU this seemed to be the case in the 2-h fasting urine. The median potassium concentration was lower in RCU in both sexes, but was significantly reduced in the groups after pooling the data. However, the accompanying urine volume was also increased, and there was no diurnal variation in potassium excretion.

Bicarbonate and potassium in fasting blood (Table 1). On the basis of the small number of observations in each group, bicarbonate excretion tended to be lower in hypercalciuric (I-HC; males + females), but not normocalciuric, RCU. The median serum potassium concentration was lower in RCU (males, females), but the difference was not significant, contrasting with our previous report[3].

Potassium and pH in 2-h fasting urine (Table 1): Potassium concentration was lower in male (I-HC) and female (N-C, I-HC) RCU subjects, but was accompanied by a higher urine volume. However, potassium excretion rate was lower in females, compared with male NC and I-HC subjects. The same was true for potassium excretion normalized for creatinine clearance (as a measure of gomerular filtration rate) and, in female I-HC subjects, for the potassium clearance. Also FE_K in these females (I-HC) was decreased, as compared with the female N-C and the male I-HC subjects. Prior correction (FE_{Kcorr}), or pooling of data from both sexes (males + females), yield numerically similar values. One exception is that in so doing it appeared to restrict the enhanced net tubular potassium reabsorption, as reflected by the lower FE_K and FE_{Kcorr} values, to the N-C subgroup of RCU. However, the median values in I-HC were also lower than normal. There was a tendency toward higher urinary pH in RCU, approaching the level of significance ($P < 0.10$) in the pooled (males + females) N-C and I-HC groups. There were direct correlations between Fe_K and pH in all groups (males + females): for C, $r = 0.53$, $P < 0.001$, $n = 40$; for N-C, $r = 0.27$, $P < 0.10$, $n = 48$; and for I-HC, $r = 0.42$; $P < 0.01$, $n = 38$.

DISCUSSION

The lower potassium concentration in urine (24-h, 2-h) appears non-specifically mediated through the proportionately higher urine volume. Thus we cannot confirm decreased potassium excretion in the 24-h urine of male RCU patients[1]. However, we did find decreased potassium in the 2-h morning urine of the N-C subgroup, associated with rather stable serum potassium. The unaltered potassium clearance in the face of a low median potassium excretion and the virtually stable serum potassium suggests that the N-C group of RCU may be heterogeneous. For example, the female N-C sub-population might exhibit clear abnormalities, such as enhanced net reabsorption, while the male N-C may not have this abnormality. An increased intracellular potassium shift should be considered as one possibility. Should this assumption turn out to be correct, then the ensuing risk of hypokalemia may be circumvented by enhanced tubular potassium reabsorption thereby keeping serum potassium stable.

An altered potassium for hydrogen ion exchange process by the distal tubule possibly is reflected by the lack of a significant correlation between FE_K and pH in N-C subjects. However, as the correlation shown by the C subjects is the same in I-HC with signs of altered potassium metabolism especially in females and decreased blood bicarbonate, the nature and sequence of tubular events cannot be recognized.

We conclude that, first, the study of fasting urine samples may elicit potassium disturbances in RCU that are not detectable in 24-h urine; second, the linkage between stone forming processes, potassium and acid-base metabolism, are not well understood at present and deserve further investigation.

ACKNOWLEDGEMENT

This work was supported by Deutsche Forschungsgemeinschaft (Schw 210/4-1) and Research Funds of the University Hospital, Erlangen.

REFERENCES

1. S. G. Welshman and M. G. McGeown, Br. J. Urol. 47:237 (1975).
2. B. Finlayson, in:"Calcium Metabolism in Renal Failure and Nephrolithiasis", D. S. David ed., John Wiley, New York (1977).
3. P. O. Schwille, D. Scholz, K. Schwille, R. Leutschaft, I. Goldberg, and A. Sigel, Nephron 31:194 (1982).
4. U. Backman, B. G. Danielson, G. Johansson, S. Ljunghall, and B. Wikström, Nephron 25:96 (1980).
5. D. Scholz and P. O. Schwille, Dtsch. Med. Wschr. 106:999 (1981).
6. O. Schuck, Min. Electr. Metab. 7:54 (1982).

ACTIVITY OF ADENINE PHOSPHORIBOSYLTRANSFERASE (APRT) IN

PATIENTS WITH RENAL FAILURE AND UROLITHIASIS

A. Stenzel, P. Banholzer, W. Löffler, S. Reiter,
W. Gröbner, N. Zöllner, M. Hegemann, and R. Pfab

Medizinische Poliklinik der Universität München
and Urologische Klinik und Poliklinik der Technischen
Universität München, 8000 München, F.R.G.

INTRODUCTION

The common clinical manifestation of complete APRT-deficiency is 2,8-dihydroxyadenine (2,8-DHA) urolithiasis. Acute and chronic renal failure have also been reported[1]. On the other hand, homozygotes, either with late onset[2] or without symptoms[3], have been described. Heterozygous patients are usually symptom-free and only occasionally form stones[4]. It has been suggested that APRT-deficiency might not be a rare disease and is often overlooked in patients with renal failure or urolithiasis[1]. Thus, screening for APRT-deficiency in these patients seemed worthwhile.

METHODS

Three groups were studied: a control group (Group I) consisting of 524 unselected patients of the Medizinische Poliklinik; Group II consisted of 139 patients with chronic renal failure on hemodialysis. The underlying diseases represented the usual spectrum, but poorly unexplained cases of renal failure predominated. Care was taken to ensure that no patient had received blood transfusions during the last 6 months prior to measurement of APRT activity. The patients with urolithiasis (Group III, n=118) had passed stones at least once, or urolithiasis had been diagnosed unequivocally by ultrasound and/or X-ray. In 39 patients analysis of the stones was not available. In the others cystine (n=3), uric acid (n=16) and calcium oxalate (n=60; 3 of them mixed) were diagnosed by X-ray diffraction. In all of the 60 patients with calcium stones the metabolic classification[5] was known. Serum creatinine was normal in all stone patients.

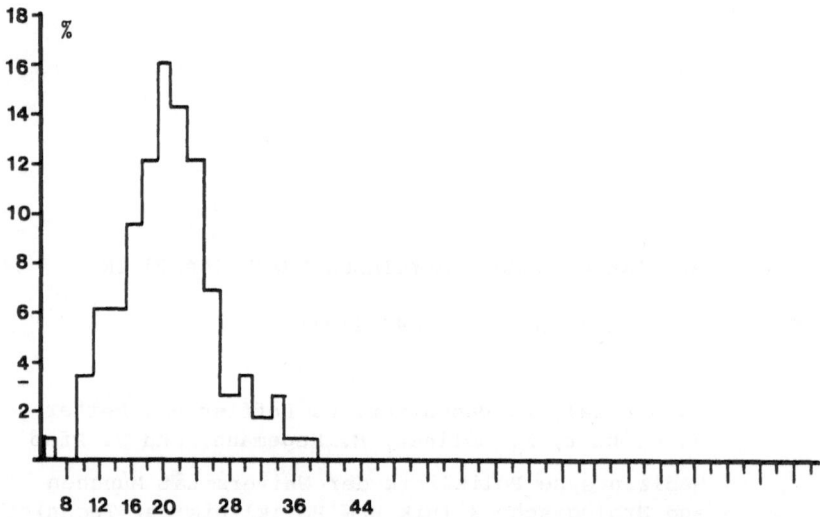

Fig. 1.   Distribution of APRT activity in hemolysate of unselected
           patients.   APRT activity is given on the abscissa in
           nmol/mg protein/h.   Class 4 covers activities from 3.1-4.9,
           class 6 from 5.1-6.9, etc.   The percentage of patients in
           each class is marked on the vertical line.

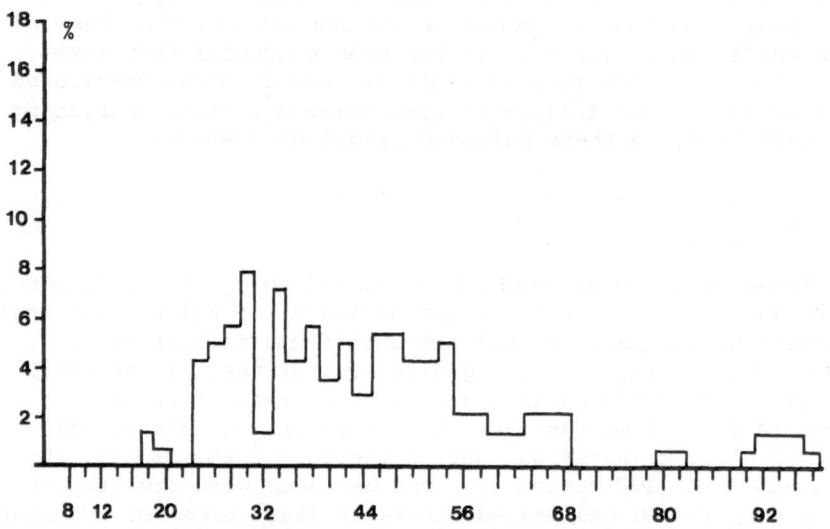

Fig. 2.   Distribution of APRT activity in hemolysate of patients
           with chronic renal failure on dialysis (Key as in Fig. 1).

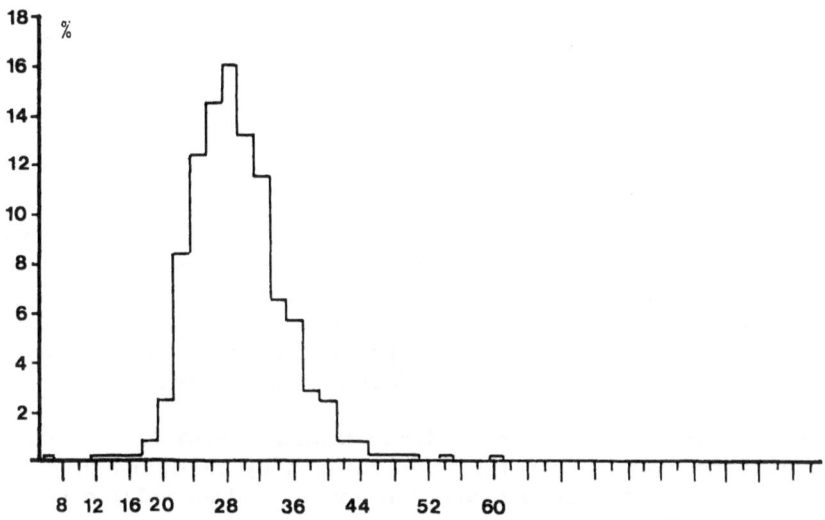

Fig. 3. Distribution of APRT activity in hemolysate of patients
with urolithiasis (Key as in Fig. 1).

APRT activity was measured micro-radiochemically in a
hemolysate[6,7].   One way analysis of variance and Duncan's multiple
range test were used to test the statistical significance of the
results.   Preconditions for the analysis were checked using the
Chi-suqare test (normal distribution) and the Bartlett test
(homogenity of variances).   If the latter condition was not
fulfilled, Welch's method[8] was used.

RESULTS AND DISCUSSION

APRT activity (mean ± SD) was 28.9 ± 5.7, 44.6 ± 17.1 and
20.8 ± 6.1 nmol/mg protein/h in control, dialysis and urolithiasis
patients, respectively.   The differences between groups were
significant (P<0.001).   APRT activities were distributed normally in
all groups of patients (Figs.1 to 3).   Within the distribution
particular to each group of patients, the number of patients with an
APRT activity below the 2 SD limit was 4 in the control group, none
in the renal failure group and 1 in the urolithiasis group.   Taking
the 2 SD limits of the control group as the limits of normal range,
APRT activity was lower than normal in 2 patients with renal failure
and in 31 patients with urolithiasis. Within the urolithiasis group
no significant differences in APRT activity could be demonstrated
between patients with different types of stones.   Although
occasional observations pointed in this direction, medications
(allopurinol, hydrochlorothiazide) were not found to influence APRT
activity significantly.

These results demonstrate that complete APRT-deficiency is not common even in patients with renal failure or urolithiasis. Presumably due to their younger erythrocyte population[9], patients on dialysis exhibit a considerably raised APRT activity and thus need their own standard. This finding is in contrast to previous investigations[10].

A lower APRT activity in stone patients has not been previously observed. In the present investigation this could not be traced to any (homo- or heterozygous) individuals nor to specific stone types. Although the difference between patients with urolithiasis and the control group is highly significant, there is considerable overlap between these groups. This is explained in part by the fact that the control group consisted of unselected patients.

We conclude from these findings that low APRT activity might be an unspecific risk factor for urolithiasis by allowing 2,8-DHA to be formed under certain dietary (and/or drug induced?) conditions, with 2,8-DHA crystals serving as a nucleus for a variety of stones.

REFERENCES

1. H. A. Simmonds and K. J. Van Acker, in:"The Metabolic Basis of Inherited Disease", J. B. Stanbury, J. B. Wyngaarden, D. S. Fredrickson, J. L. Goldstein, and M. S. Brown, eds., McGraw-Hill, New York (1983).
2. M. H. Gault, H. A. Simmonds, W. Snedden, D. Dow, D. N. Churchill, and H. Penney, New Engl. J. Med. 305:1570 (1981).
3. K. J. Van Acker, H. A. Simmonds, C. F. Potter, and J. S. Cameron, New Engl. J. Med. 297:127 (1977).
4. M. Kuroda, T. Miki, H. Kiyohara, M. Usami, T. Nakamura, T. Kotake, M. Takemoto, and T. Sonoda, Japan. J. Urol. 71:283 (1980).
5. D. Scholz, P. D. Schwille, and A. Sigel, Urologe A 19:202 (1980).
6. W. N. Kelley, F. M. Rosenbloom, J. F. Henderson, and J. E. Seegmiller, Proc. Natl. Acad. Sci. 57:1735 (1967).
7. P. Banholzer and W. Gröbner, Adenine phosphoribosyltransferase, in:"Methods of Enzymatic Analysis", Vol. III, H.U. Bermeyer, ed., Verlag Chemie, Weinheim (1983).
8. J. Pflanznagl, "Allgemeine Methodenlehre der Statistik", Vol. II, De Gruyter, Berlin (1962).
9. H. J. Becher, H. J. Weise, U. Volkermann, and P. Schollmeyer, Klin. Wschr. 58:1243 (1980).
10. M. A. Mansell, J. Allsop, M. E. North, R. J. Simmonds, R. A. Harkness, and R. W. E. Watts, Clin. Sci. 61:757 (1981).

THE SIGNIFICANCE OF HYPERURICEMIA AND HYPERURICOSURIA

IN CALCIUM OXALATE STONE FORMERS

R. Beeko, W. Schneeberger, A. Hesse, and
W. Vahlensieck

Rehabilitationskrankenhaus Bornheim-Merten, 5305
Bornheim-Merten, and Urologische Universitätsklinik
Bonn, 5300 Bonn-Venusberg, F.R.G.

INTRODUCTION

Calcium oxalate urolithiasis is frequently said to be a disease
of overnutrition. The formation of calcium oxalate stones depends
largely on urinary uric acid, calcium and oxalic acid. We have
determined the frequency of hyperuricemia, hyperuricosuria,
hypercalciuria and hyperoxaluria in recurrent calcium oxalate stone
formers on a free diet and after 5 days on a standard diet to study
the influence of nutrition on the risk factors for stone-formation.

METHODS

The patients studied consisted of 116 recurrent calcium oxalate
stone formers with an average age of 43.6 years (86 men, average age
44 years and 30 women, average age 42.5 years). Serum and urine
uric acid and the urinary excretion of calcium and oxalic acid were
measured. Normal serum uric acid was defined as < 5 mg/dl, latent
hyperuricemia between 5 and 6.4 mg/dl and hyperuricemia as > 6.5
mg/dl. Urinary excretion was considered normal when uric acid 3
mmol/24 h, calcium < 5 mmol/24 h and oxalic acid < 0.5 mmol/24 h. The
standard diet contained 2400 kcal/day (10050 Joules), 70 g protein
(80% animal), 250 g carbohydrates, 90 g fat, 800 mg calcium, 80 mg
oxalic acid, 2400 ml apple juice and fruit tea.

RESULTS

Serum uric acid decreased slightly on the standard diet. It
was 1 mg/dl higher in men than in women on both diets. On a free

Table 1. Serum Uric Acid of 116 Calcium Oxalate Stone Formers on the Free and Standard Diets (mean $\pm$ SD).

Group	Serum Uric Acid (mg/dl)	
	Free Diet	Standard Diet
Total	5.47 $\pm$ 1.28	5.39 $\pm$ 1.14
Men	5.71 $\pm$ 1.21	5.67 $\pm$ 1.06
Women	4.77 $\pm$ 1.24	4.61 $\pm$ 0.97

Table 2. Serum Uric Acid of 116 Calcium Oxalate Stone Formers on the Free and Standard Diets.

Diet	Serum Uric Acid (mg/dl)	Men (%)	Women (%)	Total (%)
Free	$\geq$6.5	17.2	2.6	19.8
	5.0 to 6.4	41.4	9.5	50.9
	<5.0	15.5	13.8	29.3
Standard	$\geq$6.5	13.8	1.7	15.0
	5.0 to 6.4	44.8	6.9	51.7
	<5.0	15.5	17.2	32.8

Table 3. Urinary Excretion of Uric Acid, Calcium, Oxalic Acid on the Free and Standard Diets in 116 Calcium Oxalate Stone Formers (mean $\pm$ SD).

Ion	Urinary Excretion (mmol/day)	
	Free Diet	Standard Diet
Uric acid	3.93 $\pm$ 1.54	2.90 $\pm$ 1.11
Calcium	5.94 $\pm$ 3.22	4.87 $\pm$ 2.72
Oxalic acid	0.53 $\pm$ 0.33	0.46 $\pm$ 0.28

diet, 71% of patients were hyperuricemic compared with 66% on the standard diet (Tables 1,2).

The stone formers had an increased excretion of uric acid, calcium and oxalic acid on the free diet, but after 5 days on the standard diet, their excretion rates were normal (Table 3).

The correlations between the various urinary factors were non-significant on each diet. The percentage of patients with an increased excretion of one or more factors was very high (Table 4).

352

Table 4. Recurrent Calcium Oxalate Stone Formers with an Increased
         Excretion of Uric Acid, Calcium, Oxalic Acid on the Free
         and Standard Diets.

Excretion Increased	% With Increased Excretion	
	Free Diet	Standard Diet
Uric Acid	67	34
Calcium	58	43
Oxalic Acid	35	20
Uric Acid + Calcium	44	14
Uric Acid + Oxalic Acid	29	6
Calcium + Oxalic Acid	27	11
Uric Acid + Calcium + Oxalic Acid	21	3
None Increased	17.2	30.2

DISCUSSION

The results of our study confirm that there is a high frequency
of hyperuricemia, hyperuricosuria, hypercalciuria, and hyperoxaluria
amongst recurrent calcium oxalate stone formers. It also confirms
the marked influence of nutrition, especially overnutrition, on the
risk of calcium oxalate urolithiasis. A decrease in serum uric
acid and in the excretions of uric acid, calcium and oxalic acid
could be seen on the standard diet, which is recommended by the
German Society of Nutrition as a fully balanced diet. It contains
less calories, proteins, etc than the average diet of individuals in
the industrialised countries. This means that by taking a balanced
diet alone, some patients' increased excretion of lithogenic
substances may be normalised and their risk of further stone
formation reduced.

URINARY EXCRETION PATTERN OF MAIN GLYCOSAMINOGLYCANS IN STONE FORMERS AND CONTROLS

A. Martelli, B. Marchesini, P. Buli, F. Lambertini, and R. Rusconi

Depts. of Clinical Pharmacology and Urology, University of Bologna, Italy

INTRODUCTION

Various inhibitors of calcium oxalate (CaOx) crystal growth and aggregation have been found in human urine. These findings led to the hypothesis that a deficiency of these substances may be involved in the generation of kidney stones. Among them, the urinary macromolecules, glycosaminoglycans (GAG), have been proved to be effective inhibitors of crystallization in vitro[1]. Several investigators have compared total GAG excretion of stone-forming subjects to that of normal controls but the results have been conflicting[2-4]. It should be emphasized that urinary GAGS are extremely heterogeneous with respect to molecular weight and charge density and the possibility exists that a selection of different GAG fractions has been obtained in different studies. We thus examined a GAG fraction characterized by less complete degradation in terms of both its uronic acid content and the relative distribution of its main components, chondroitin sulfate (ChS) and heparan sulfate (HS), in stone formers and normals.

PATIENTS AND METHODS

We studied 17 adult male subjects with recurrent CaOx nephrolithiasis without metabolic disturbances and 15 normal males. Both patients and subjects were on their usual diet, all had normal renal function, and none was taking drugs. The less degraded GAG fraction was extracted from 24-h urine using the isolation procedure described by Goldberg and Cotlier[5], and its uronic content measured by the conventional carbazole method[6]. Electrophoresis of urinary GAG on cellulose acetate membrane was carried out in EDTA/LiCl (pH

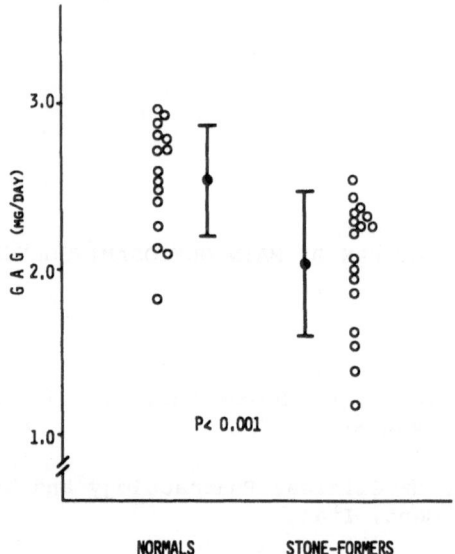

Fig. 1. The 24-h excretion of total GAG recovered as uronic acid
for stone-formers and normals.

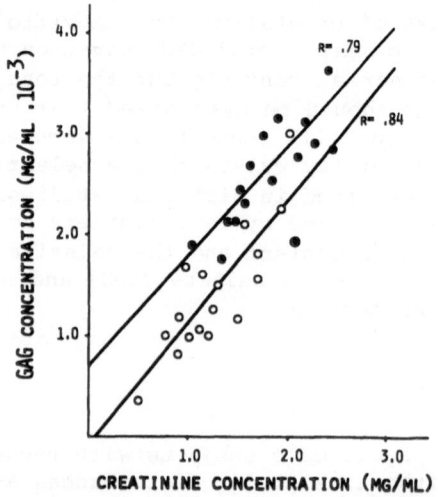

Fig. 2. GAG concentration plotted against creatinine concentration
for normal (●) and stone-forming (o) subjects.

8.4)[7]. The last procedure, which allows the separation of
connective tissue GAG, has never been applied to urinary GAG. To
identify individual GAG components, enzymatic treatment with
mucopolysaccharidases was performed on the extracted GAG. The
relative distribution of the main individual GAG components was
determined by densitometry after staining in alcian blue solution.
Mean values (+ SD) are shown, and differences between means assessed
by Student's t-test for unpaired data.

RESULTS AND DISCUSSION

    Fig. 1 shows that there is a decrease in the ratio of stone
formers to normals as the 24-h urinary excretion of GAG increases.
According to the statistical analysis, this difference is highly
significant ($P < 0.001$) and the dose-response relationship is
consistent with the hypothesis that low GAG excretion is a risk
factor in CaOx stone formation. Newton et al[8] have shown that ChS
and HS concentrations are strongly correlated with urinary
creatinine concentration and suggested that GAGS are filtered into
the urine. To gain further information about GAG excretion we
examined the relation between GAG and creatinine concentrations in
both populations. The two quantities were found highly correlated
in both normals ($r = 0.79$, $P < 0.001$) and stone formers ($r = 0.84$, $P < 0.001$) and two distinct regression lines describe the two groups.

    If, as probable, the mechanism of GAG excretion is similar in
stone formers and normals, our data suggest that unbound plasma GAG
concentration must be higher in normals than stone-formers. This
could be related to a higher amount of total GAG in plasma or to a

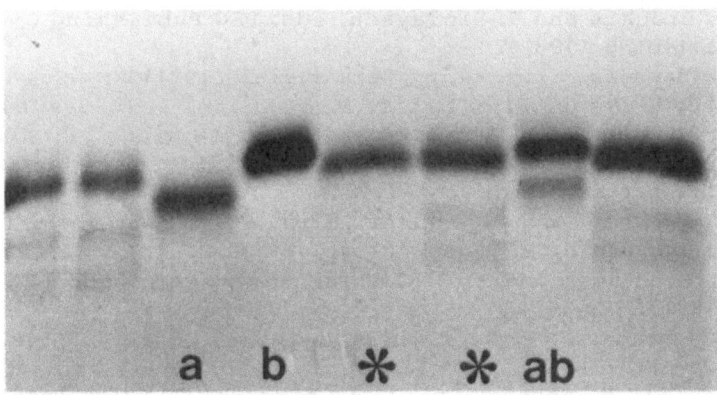

Fig. 3. Typical electrophoretic run of connective tissue (a=HS,
         b=Chs) and urinary GAGs from stone-formers and normals.

lower fraction bound. These results confirm previous findings in normals and will be the object of further studies on GAG clearance.

Three clear bands were obtained after electrophoresis of urinary GAG extracts (Fig. 3). Enzymatic digestion suggested that the first prominent band corresponds to isomeric ChS and the following two to HS(s). The possibility of obtaining two separable bands for HS has been reported[9], but the nature of the difference between the two forms has not, as yet, been determined. We have not observed significant differences between the two groups in either the migration rates of the individual GAG species or their suceptibility to enzymatic treatments. The relative ratio of ChS to HS in stone formers (3.31) and controls (3.01) was similar. Since no significant differences could be detected in terms of the excretion pattern of the main individual GAG components, the discrepancies of total GAG output reported in the literature cannot be ascribed to difference in the relative distribution of the main GAGS.

Among the possible explanations is the observation that small variations in the procedure can lead to considerable error in the total amount as well as the pattern of GAG excreted, and the possible presence of interfering non-GAG macromoleules. It can be concluded that the need remains for increased standardization in the isolation and characterization of these complex heterogeneous compounds when looking for differences that can be small between two populations.

REFERENCES

1. R. L. Ryall, R. M. Harnett, and V. R. Marshall, Clin. Chim. Acta 112:349 (1981).
2. K. Bichler, J. Sallis, and S. Broring, in:"Urinary Calculus", J. G. Brockis and B. Finlayson, eds. PSG Publishing Co., Littleton (1981).
3. C. T. Samuell, Clin. Chim. Acta 117:63 (1981).
4. W. G. Robertson, A. B. Latif, D. S. Scurr, A. M. Caswell, G. W. Drach, and A. D. Randolph, in:"Urinary Stone", R. Ryall, J. G. Brockis, V. Marshall, and B. Finlayson, eds., Churchill Livingstone, Melbourne (1984).
5. J. M. Goldberg and E. Cotlier, Clin. Chim. Acta 41:19 (1972).
6. T. Bitter and H. M. Muir, Analyt. Biochem. 4:330 (1962).
7. E. H. Schuchman and R. J. Desnik, Analyt. Biochem. 117:419 (1981).
8. D. J. Newton, J. E. Scott, and S. Amhad, Connect. Tiss. Res. 7:47 (1979).
9. G. Manley, M. Severn, and J. Hawksworth, J. Clin. Path. 21:339 (1968).

THE CONNECTION BETWEEN AMINO ACIDS, URINARY

ENZYMES AND STONE FORMATION

R. Azoury, S. Perlberg, N. Garti, Y. Wax, and
S. Sarig

The Casali Institute of Applied Chemistry
The Hebrew University of Jerusalem, Jerusalem, Israel

INTRODUCTION

About 30 enzymes have been identified in urine, none of whose activities is correlated with calcium oxalate (CaOx) kidney stone disease[1]. Recently, however, we reported[2] a significant difference in the activities of the urinary transaminase enzymes (GOT and GPT) between stone formers (SF) and normals. The average activity values of GOT and GPT in normal urines were found to be higher than those of SF by a factor of 3. GOT and GPT convert aspartic acid and alanine to glutamic acid. In vitro and in vivo studies[3,4] showed that glutamic acid is a potent inhibitor for CaOx precipitation. In this study the role of GOT and GPT activity in CaOx stone formation were studied along with evaluation of the effect of drug treatment on it.

MATERIALS AND METHODS

The inhibition test was carried out as follows. First morning voided urine specimens were collected from a group of healthy volunteers and SF, all of whom were on a free diet. The overall inhibitory potential of each urine was determined using the Discrimination Index (DI) described by Sarig et al[5]. Briefly, this is a precipitation test in which low DI values (<0.66) were associated with high inhibitory potential in the urine of normals. The urinary enzyme activities of GOT, GPT, LDH, AP and ɣ-GLU were measured in the first voided urine specimens using a Technicon SMAC Analyzer. Urine samples were analyzed for their amino acid content using an LKB 4400 Amino Acid Analyzer equipped with a gold column.

The Pearson correlation coefficient was used to assess the relation between the level of enzyme activity and the corresponding DI values among the SF and normal populations.

RESULTS AND DISCUSSION

The sum of GOT and GPT activity was found to be significantly higher (P<0.001) in the urines of 35 normals compared with 49 SFs (32:11 respectively). The correlation between the high GOT plus GPT activity and low DI values (which indicate high inhibitory potential) was -0.39 (Fig. 1). Thus, about 26% of the urinary inhibitory potential (reflected by low DI values) could be ascribed to GOT plus GPT activity. The activities of the other urinary enzymes (LDH, AP and γ-GLU), also show some differences between SF and normals. However, no significant correlation was observed between their activities and the urinary inhibitory potential.

Glutamic acid production is enhanced by GOT and GPT. McGeown[3] reported that the incidence of CaOx kidney stone formation was significantly reduced in rats fed glutamic acid. Recently, we have reported the involvement of glutamic acid in the crystallization of CaOx in vitro[2]. Also we have shown that incubation of SF urines with GOT or GPT increases the urinary inhibitory potential[4]. At the end of those incubations the ratio of $[glutamic\ acid]/([aspartic\ acid] + [alanine])$, denoted by AA_f, was significantly increased. In this study, AA_f values in the urines of SF and in the organic matrices of CaOx stones was found to be significantly lower (<0.57) than in urines of normals (>0.84).

This evidence leads us to examine the effect of drug treatment (phosphates, thiazides and allopurinol) on the urinary inhibitory potential and on the urinary GOT plus GPT activity. In the present study, 90% of SF have relatively low activity values (<18 I.U.) of GOT plus GPT in their urine before the start of medication.

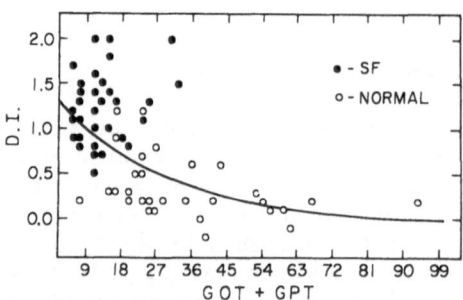

Fig. 1. The relationship between DI values and GOT plus GPT activity (I.U.).

Table 1. The Relative Changes in the Mean ($\pm$ S.D.) of GOT + GPT Activity (in IU) after Drug Treatment.

Treatment	(GOT + GPT) (I.U.)
Phosphate	14.5 ± 2.4
Thiazides	13.3 ± 3.1
Allopurinol	8.1 ± 6.3

Therefore an increase in the urinary activities of GOT and GPT to values above 18 I.U. was considered as being influenced by medication. A significant change ($P < 0.01$) in the mean values of GOT plus GPT activity was observed in the groups treated with phosphates or thiazides (Table 1), but there was no significant change in the group receiving allopurinol. On the other hand, treatment with allopurinol improved the urinary inhibitory potential, as reflected by the lower DI values, in the way the other groups did. The other urinary enzymes, which have been examined, did not show any significant change in their activity.

The present study reinforces the evidence concerning the involvement of glutamic acid, which is produced in situ by GOT and GPT in urine, in the crystallization of CaOx. The improvement in the inhibitory activity of urine during drug treatment may be explained in part by the change in GOT plus GPT activity. We may speculate that the basic deficiency of enzyme activity is due to (a) obstruction of excretion, (b) presence of specific blockers of enzyme activity, or (c) genetic deficiency. In each case, glutamic acid production in situ would be decreased, thereby reducing the inhibition of CaOx crystallization.

In conclusion, this study indicates that CaOx crystallization may be subject to biological control, by a mechanism involving the combined activities of GOT and GPT.

REFERENCES

1. H. Mattenheimer, in:"Methods of Enzymatic Analysis", H. U. Bergmeyer, ed., Verlag Chemie, Weinheim (1974).
2. R. Azoury, N. Garti, S. Perlberg, S. Sarig, Urol. Res., 10:185 (1982).
3. M. G. McGeown, Urology 78:381 (1957).
4. R. Azoury, S. Sarig, N. Garti, S. Perlberg, Urol. Res. 10:169 (1982).

5. S. Sarig, N. Garti, R. Azoury, Y. Wax, and S. Perlberg, J. Urol. 128:645 (1982).

URINARY ISOCITRATE EXCRETION IN NORMAL INDIVIDUALS AND

IN STONE PATIENTS

V. Graef, H. Schmidtmann, and K. Jarrar

Institute of Clinical Chemistry and Pathobiochemistry
and Dept. of Urology, University Giessen, F.R.G.

INTRODUCTION

It is well known that citrate forms a complex with Ca^{2+} ions.
The crystallization of calcium oxalate and the formation of calcium
oxalate stones are inhibited by the presence of citrate in urine.
However, there are other compounds in urine that form complexes.
We found that isocitrate possesses the same complex-forming ability.
Urinary isocitrate was determined in normal subjects and in stone
patients.

METHODS AND RESULTS

Isocitrate was measured as follows: To a 1 cm cuvette is added
2 ml of triethanolamine buffer (0.1 M, pH 7.5, containing 0.2 g
$MnCl_2/l$), 100 μl $NADP^+$ solution (5 mg/ml) and 100 μl urine.
Following addition of 20 μl isocitrate dehydrogenase (4 U/ml) (from
porcine heart; Boehringer Mannheim, F.R.G.) the increase in
absorbance is read in a spectrophotometer at 365 nm. Usually, the
reaction is finished after 5 min.

The specificity of the method was tested by use of other
organic acids instead of isocitrate. As shown in Table 1, the
method is highly specific. The acids tested gave absorbance that
were only 2 to 3% that of isocitrate. The acids were used in
concentrations of 500 mg/l, whereas urine contains these acids only
in a concentration of about 70 mg/l.

The preservatives sodium azide (3 g/l urine), thymol
(saturated), Merthiolate[R] (ethyl mercurithiosalicylate, 0.1 g/l) and

Table 1. Specificity of the Method for Isocitrate Determination.

Acid	Concentration (mg/l)	ΔE (365 nm)	"Isocitrate" (mg/l)
Isocitric acid	500	0.385	500
Citric acid	500	0	0
Glycolic acid	500	0.008	10.4
Pyruvic acid	500	0.008	10.4
Glutaric acid	500	0.009	11.7
Oxaloacetic acid	500	0.007	9.1
Lactic acid	500	0.010	13.0
Oxalosuccinic acid	500	0.011	14.3
Acetoacetic acid	500	0.008	10.4
Ascorbic acid	500	0.009	11.7

Table 2. Isocitrate in Urine of Normal Subjects and Stone Patients.

Subject	n	Sex	Isocitrate (mmol/l)	(mmol/24 h)
Normal	19	F	0.39 $\pm$ 0.19	0.60 $\pm$ 0.21
Normal	14	F	0.38 $\pm$ 0.17	0.55 $\pm$ 0.21
Normal	33	M+F	0.38 $\pm$ 0.18	0.58 $\pm$ 0.21
Oxalate stone	111	M+F	0.31 $\pm$ 0.13	0.60 $\pm$ 0.23
Urate stone	25	M+F	0.31 $\pm$ 0.12	0.70 $\pm$ 0.38
Phosphate stone	48	M+F	0.26 $\pm$ 0.12	0.61 $\pm$ 0.26

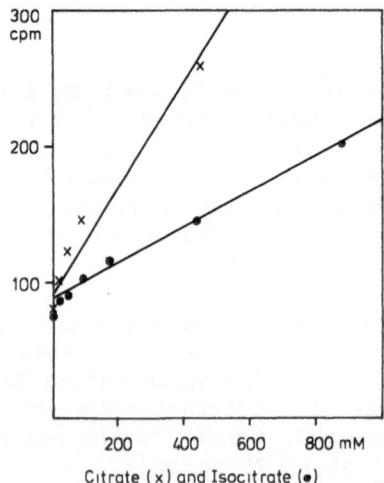

Fig. 1. Demonstration of the complex-forming effect of citrate and
isocitrate.

penicillin G/streptomycin sulfate (110 mg + 190 mg/l) did not inhibit the isocitrate dehydrogenase reaction. Therefore, these substances are suitable for the preservation of urines prior to isocitrate determination.

In order to determine if isocitrate in urine comes from citrate through the action of aconitase (if present in urine), 3 urines were filtered through a bacteria filter. Citric acid (500 mg/l) was added. The urines were (i) cooled at $0^{\circ}C$ and (ii) incubated at $37^{\circ}C$ for 12 h. After this time, isocitrate was determined. There was no difference in the mean isocitrate concentrations (78.8 mg/l and 75.4 mg/l respectively). This indicates that isocitrate in urine is not derived from urinary citrate.

In order to determine the complex-forming effect of citrate and isocitrate on Ca^{2+}, 10 ml of 4mM sodium oxalate solution, 50 μl ^{14}C-oxalate (0.05 μCi) and 500 μl potassium citrate (or isocitrate) solution of increasing concentration (0 to 870 mM) were mixed. Following the addition of 10 ml of 4 mM calcium acetate solution the reaction mixtures were allowed to stand at room temperature for 24 h. Aliquots of the clear supernatant (1 ml each) were added to 10 ml scintillation cocktail (Minisolve I, Koch-Light Lab.). The radioactivity was measured in all solutions. The results are shown in Fig. 1.

Isocitrate was determined in 24-h urines from healthy subjects and stone patients. To avoid bacterial destruction of isocitrate, the urines were collected over penicillin G/streptomycin sulfate (110 mg + 190 mg). As shown in Table 2, isocitrate excretion was not significantly different in urine from normal men and women. Patients with urate stones excreted a somewhat higher amount of isocitrate than healthy adults.

CONCLUSION

Because of the complex-forming effect of isocitrate, not only citrate but also isocitrate should be determined in the urines of stone formers.

URINARY CITRATE EXCRETION IN NORMALS AND PATIENTS

WITH IDIOPATHIC CALCIUM UROLITHIASIS

D. H. Hosking, J. W. L. Wilson, R. R. Liedke,
L. H. Smith, and D. M. Wilson

University of Manitoba, Winnipeg, Queens University
Kingston, Canada and Mayo Clinic, Rochester
Minnesota, U.S.A.

INTRODUCTION

In urine, citrate forms soluble complexes with calcium thereby decreasing the calcium ion activity and, secondarily, the relative supersaturation of both calcium oxalate and calcium phosphate[1]. In addition, citrate exerts an inhibitory effect on both hydroxy-apatite[2] and calcium oxalate crystal growth[3] although the contribution to the latter is minor. The mean urinary citrate excretion in patients with idiopathic calcium urolithiasis has been found to be significantly lower than in control groups[4-7] prompting the speculation that hypocitraturia may be an etiologic factor. There are few reports, however, on what constitutes an abnormally low urinary excretion of citrate[7,8].

To try and clarify the role of urinary citrate in idiopathic calcium urolithiasis we have conducted two studies. The first study was performed on healthy persons without urolithiasis to determine the urinary excretion of citrate in a normal population. The second consisted of a retrospective study to determine whether or not altered urinary citrate excretion is associated with stone growth or new stone formation in patients with urolithiasis.

MATERIALS AND METHODS

Control Urine Collections

The 24-h urinary excretion of citrate was measured in 43 normal women and 40 normal men, while following their usual diet and

367

activity.   Toluene was used as a preservative and the assay was performed using a citrate lyase technique.

Studies in Patients with Idiopathic Calcium Urolithiasis

The clinical courses of 132 consecutive patients with idiopathic calcium urolithiasis, all of whom had urine citrate determinations, were reviewed.   All had normal renal function, uninfected urine, and at the time of the urinary citrate determinations no patient was taking thiazides, orthophosphates, alkalis or acetazolamide.

In each patient, the stone formation rate prior to initial assessment was calculated as the sum of stones passed or removed prior to presentation plus the total number of stones visible on plain roentgenograms of the kidneys at the time of presentation divided by the duration of the disease in year.

During the follow-up, metabolic activity of the stone disease was determined according to the criteria outlined by Smith[9].

RESULTS

Studies on Normal Subjects

Regression lines for the urinary excretion of citrate versus age were calculated for both men and women.   No significant differences were observed.   A single regression line of urinary citrate excretion versus age was obtained for males and females combined.   A significant correlation was observed ($r^2 = 0.156$; P < 0.001; slope = 7.11 mg/year).   Using the line representing the 5th percentile as the lower limit of normal, a urinary excretion of citrate of 150 mg/24h at age 20 years was determined to be the lower limit of normal, increasing by 7.11 mg/24h per year after age 20. No persons in the control group were over the age of 70 years so the lower limit of normal for this age group could not be determined.

Studies in Patients with Idiopathic Calcium Urolithiasis

In 132 patients with idiopathic calcium urolithiasis, no correlation was detected between urinary excretion of citrate and age.   Comparison of the urinary citrate excretion in male and female stone formers revealed no significant differences.

Of 120 patients aged 29-70 years, 35 (29.2%) were found to have a level of urinary citrate excretion lower than the 5th percentile

of the control group.   These 35 patients constitute a
hypocitraturic group.

The age of onset of stone disease in the hypocitraturic group
was 39.8 $\pm$ 13.5 years (mean $\pm$ SD) which was not significantly
different from the age of onset of 36.9 $\pm$ 11.8 years (mean $\pm$ SD) in
patients with normal urine citrate excretion.   However, only 1 of
19 patients (5.3%) in the 30 to 39-year-old age group was
hypocitraturic.

The possibility that incomplete renal tubular acidosis, defined
as an inability to acidify the urine below pH 5.3[10], could account
for the presence of hypocitraturia was studied.   Twenty-four of the
35 hypocitraturic patients (68.8%) had at some time voided urine
with a pH of 5.3 or less suggesting that incomplete renal tubular
acidosis as defined above was not present in these 24 patients.

The severity of the stone disease prior to presentation was
determined by the stone formation rate.   The stone formation rate
in our patient population was 1.78 $\pm$ 2.84 stones per year (mean
$\pm$ SD) with a range of 0.03 to 13 stones per year.   There was no
correlation between the stone formation rate prior to presentation
and the 24-h urinary excretion of citrate (r^2 = 0.0064;P>0.05).

In those patients whose stone disease was initially treated
with fluid and dietary therapy only, the frequency of metabolic
activity[9] was determined for different levels of urinary citrate
excretion.   No variation in the frequency of metabolic activity was
identified with increasing levels of urinary citrate.   These
findings were unchanged even when patients with increased urinary
excretion of calcium and uric acid were excluded.

DISCUSSION

The urinary excretion of citrate in our normal population
increased with increasing age in both men and women.   It is
therefore necessary to take the age of the patient into account when
determining whether or not hypocitraturia is present.

Hypocitraturia was uncommon in the age range 30-39 years, the
age range including the mean age of onset of the stone disease in
our patient group.   This suggests that hypocitraturia may not be an
initiating factor in the stone disease of many patients with
idiopathic calcium urolithiasis.   No relationship was detected
between the urinary excretion of citrate and the stone formation
rate prior to presentation or the frequency of metabolic activity
during the follow-up period.

It is possible that hypocitraturia may reflect the presence of

an associated incomplete renal tubular acidosis.   In the majority
of our hypocitraturic patients an intact urine acidification
mechanism was demonstrated although it is possible that more
sophisticated acid load tests, such as described by Backman[11], might
reveal an abnormal renal handling of acid in these patients.

Normal values in the local population must be established
before hypocitraturia can be diagnosed in an individual.   Although
citrate in urine had important theoretical protective effects in
urolithiasis, we have been unable to demonstrate clinically any
association between urine citrate levels determined on urine
collected in an outpatient setting and the onset of stone disease in
patients with idiopathic calcium urolithiasis.

REFERENCES

1. A. B. Hastings, F. C. McLean, L. Eichelberger, J. L. Hall, and
   E. Da Costa, J. Biol. Chem. 107:351 (1934).
2. L. H. Smith, J. L. Meyer, and J. T. McCall, in:"Urinary Calculi",
   L. Cifuentes Delatte, A. Rapado, A. Hodgkinson, eds., Karger,
   Basel (1973).
3. J. L. Meyer and L. H. Smith, Invest. Urol. 13:36 (1975).
4. S. G. Welshman and M. G. McGeown, Br. J. Urol. 48:7 (1976).
5. P. O. Schwille, D. Scholz, M. Paulus, W. Engelhardt, and A.
   Sigel, Invest. Urol. 16:457 (1979).
6. D. Rudman, M. H. Kutner, S. C. Redd II, W. C. Waters IV, G. G.
   Gerron, and J. Bleier, J. Clin. Endocrinol. Metab. 55:1052
   (1982).
7. M. J. Nicar, C. Skurla, K. Sakhaee, and C. Y. C. Pak, Urology
   21:8 (1983).
8. A. Hodgkinson, Clin. Sci. 23:203 (1962).
9. L. H. Smith, Urol. Clin. N. Am. 1:241 (1974).
10. O. Wrong and H. E. F. Davies, Quart. J. Med. 28:259 (1959).
11. U. Backman, B. G. Danielson, G. Johansson, S. J. Ljunghall, and
    B. Wikström, Nephron 25:96 (1980).

DRUG NEPHROLITHIASIS: AN UNRECOGNIZED AND UNDERESTIMATED PATHOLOGY

M. Daudon and R. J. Reveillaud

Crystal Laboratory and Dept. of Internal Medicine and
Nephrology, Centre Hospitalier, Saint-Cloud, France

INTRODUCTION

The occurrence of drugs in urinary stones is a rare finding.
Apart from Ettinger's studies on triamterene[1], the only other papers
are confined to individual, isolated cases. When a stone is
present, the contribution of drugs to nucleation or growth should
always be considered.

In a series of 3,000 urinary stones, we have detected the
presence of mineral or organic compounds, probably of iatrogenic
origin, in 54 stones (1.8%). We have identified drugs in 33 cases
(1.1%).

MATERIALS AND METHODS

All stones were analyzed by microdissection and infrared
spectroscopy. The methods have been published elsewhere[2-4]. We
wish to emphasize the importance of macroscopic examination of the
calculi. The morphology is often sufficient to detect unusual
components either by the colour or by the texture of the layers.
When the presence of a drug is suspected further physical and
chemical studies are necessary either to identify the drug, if it is
not already known, or to establish the characteristics of its metabolites. The latter may be important[4], since the stones almost
always contain metabolites rather than the native drug itself. It is
essential that a complete drug history should be taken by the
physician in order to identify the drug(s) and dose(s) absorbed by
the patient during the months or years before the stone(s) was
recovered.

371

RESULTS

Our studies showed that 9 compounds were implicated:triamterene (11 cases), glafenine (10), phenazopyridine (4), piridoxilate (2), carbonates (2), sulfamethoxazole (1), sulfaguanidine (1), sulfadiazine (1) and flumequine (1).

Triamterene

In our experience only Cycloteriam, which contains 150 mg of triamterene and 3 mg of cyclothiazide, is actually responsible for stone formation. The drug is a complex mixture of triamterene and 7 metabolites, whose main component is always hydroxy-4'-triamterene ester sulfate[3]. Only one calculus was "pure", i.e. composed exclusively of triamterene derivatives and proteins. The patients had been taking Cycloteriam for periods varying from 4 months to 3 years, with a normal triamterene dose of 150 mg per day.

Glafenine

Glafenine was found in 10 stones in the form of three associated metabolites: glafenic acid, hydroxy-4'-glafenic acid and hydroxy-2-glafenic acid, the last-mentioned being unknown until we identified it in the stones[4]. Two out of 10 stones were "pure", another contained the drug in the nucleus. The taking of Glifanan was spread over periods from 6 weeks to 4 years with doses from 400 to 800 mg per day. All the stones were located in the renal pelvis and necessitated surgical removal.

Phenazopyridine hydrochloride

Four stones contained phenazopyridine metabolites adsorbed to pre-existing calculi. Chromatographic studies revealed the presence of one predominant metabolite accompanied by 5 others and traces of phenazopyridine. The main metabolite does not correspond to those previously described[5] and seems to be, as in the case of triamterene, an ester sulfate metabolite (unpublished).

Piridoxilate

Even though their morphology is a little special, piridoxilate-induced stones are made of pure or almost pure whewellite. The three peculiarities of these stones are: appearance during piridoxilate treatment in patients without previous stone disease, frequent recurrence (several stones/year) and progressive disappearance after stopping treatment.

Carbonates

Calcite was found in 0.8% of our 3000 stones, most often resulting from falsification with fine gravel or various exogenous stones. Calcite is sometimes detected in surgically-removed calculi. In two cases, we had the opportunity to correlate its presence in the stones with a regular absorption of carbonated drugs, mixture of calcium carbonate, magnesium carbonate, sodium bicarbonate and silicates. In one case, the patient eliminated numerous small stones made of "pure" calcite. The other one had a big stone in the renal pelvis, surgically removed, made of calcite (80%) and carbonated calcium phosphates.

Sulfamides

Each of the following, cotrimoxazole, sulfaguanidine and sulfadiazine respectively has been found in one stone under the form of N-acetylsulfamethoxazole[2], N-acetylsulfaguanidine[6], and N-acetylsulfadiazine. The last two metabolites induced "pure" stones after only few weeks of treatment.

Flumequine

Flumequine was found in a renal stone almost entirely formed of proteins[6]; the patient had chronic renal failure and received intermittent treatment with flumequine for several months.

DISCUSSION

We identified 9 drugs that may have a role in the genesis or growth of urinary stones; at least twenty drugs have been identified in the literature. In our series 1.1% of the stones contained identified drugs. There are probably more, perhaps 2 or 3%, if we include drugs like vitamin D, acetazolamide and uricosuric agents that increase the tendency for the formation of urinary calculi.

Several factors are involved in the precipitation of a drug in urine: a high renal excretion, low solubility of the drug and its metabolites in urine, a low urine volume, and prolonged treatment at a high drug dosage. Probably supersaturation is not the only factor involved in drug crystallization if we compare the low incidence of stones in regard to the very large consumption of some of these drugs. Also there may be a relationship between drug and urinary proteins or protein matrix or drugs may interfere with the urinary inhibitors of crystallization.

To our knowledge we report the first two cases of piridoxilate-induced stones. The mechanism may involve supersaturation of the mitochondrial oxidative potential due to the excess of glyoxylate despite the simultaneous intake of pyridoxine. Thus, the glyoxylate excess is converted to oxalate and excreted in the urine. These stones seem to be very rare but may have not been recognized since their morphology and composition are non-specific; they are characterisic of whewellite stones induced by hyperoxaluria[7].

As most of the drugs found in the stones are amphoteric or acidic, dissolution may be achieved in vivo by alkalinization of the urine. It may be possible to dissolve the drug, but the dissolution of the protein matrix will be more difficult. If it is retained in the kidney then secondary mineralization or infection may occur necessitating surgical treatment.

It seems essential that stone analysis should be improved so as to detect the presence of drugs. This would permit the interruption of the treatment by the drug involved, thus reducing the risk of aggravating the disorder and preventing stone recurrence. In patients with known calculus disease any previous use of these drugs should be established. For all of these patients such drugs should not be prescribed.

REFERENCES

1. B. Ettinger, N. O. Oldroyd, and F. Sorgel, J. Am. Med. Assoc. 244:2443 (1980).
2. M. Daudon, M. F. Protat, and R. J. Reveillaud, Ann. Biol. Clin. 36:475 (1978).
3. N. Daudon, M. F. Protat, and R. J. Reveillaud, Nephrol. 3:119 (1982).
4. M. Daudon, M. F. Protat, and R. J. Reveillaud, Ann. Biol. Clin. 41:105 (1983).
5. W. J. Johnson and A. Chartrand, Toxicol. Appl. Pharmacol. 37:371 (1976).
6. M. Daudon, M. F. Protat, and R. J. Reveillaud, Ann. Biol. Clin. 41:239 (1983).
7. M. Daudon and R. J. Reveillaud, Nephrol. (in press).

TRIAMTERENE SOLUBILITY AND METABOLISM ARE NOT CAUSATIVE

FACTORS OF TRIAMTERENE NEPHROLITHIASIS

F. Sörgel, B. Ettinger, L. Z. Benet, and P. O. Schwille

University of California, School of Pharmacy, and the
Kaiser Permanente Medical Center, San Francisco
U.S.A. and Chirurgische und Urologische Klinik
University of Erlangen, F.R.G.

INTRODUCTION

Although the risk of passing a kidney stone during triamterene
therapy is not yet fully understood[1,2] there is enough evidence to
suggest that deposition of triamterene and other drugs in kidney
stones is a frequent occurrence[3]. Since our initial report on the
presence of triamterene in kidney stones, only a few studies have
appeared on this topic and it still remains unclear as to why
triamterene is found in stones. We now report the true composition
of kidney stones passed during triamterene therapy, which may help
to explain why it is incorporated. Also, we will report the first
data on triamterene metabolism in patients passing these stones, as
well as in patients chronically using triamterene. Previously
published data will also be discussed in the light of our data.

RESULTS AND DISCUSSION

As shown in Fig. 1, many factors can influence the concentration of triamterene in urine, which is considered to be a critical
factor in the incorporation of triamterene into kidney stones.
From a recent study[4] it has also become evident that different drug
formulations considerably affect its absorption. Renal failure
considerably prolongs the half-life of triamterene and its
metabolites[5].

We studied a group of 103 patients taking Dyazide[R] regularly
for treatment of hypertension. In these patients we found a
pattern of metabolism very similar to that seen in healthy
volunteers, except for a tendency towards lower metabolic ratios in

375

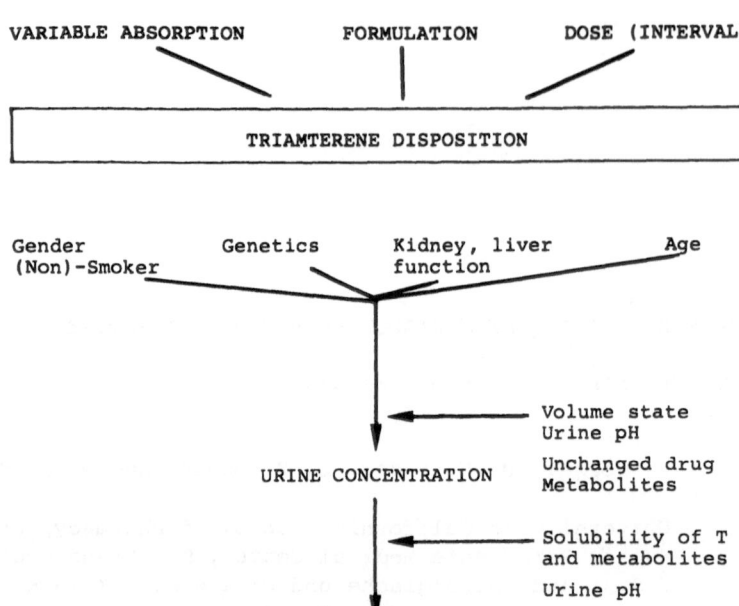

Fig. 1. Factors influencing the urinary concentration of
triamterene and its metabolites.

the patient group.   When patients who had passed kidney stones were
studied, it became evident that the metabolic handling of triamterene is not different from that of patients who take Dyazide
regularly.   The incorporation of triamterene into kidney stones is
a function of triamterene excretion and concentration, as well as
its solubility in urine.   Werness et al[6] reported solubility data
for triamterene and its metabolites in a 0.15 M NaCl buffer at 37°C.
They found a solubility of 6 to 7 µg/ml, which is considerably lower
than previously published by Pruitt et al[7] and Dittert et al[8].   We
found a solubility of triamterene in Sorensen buffer of about 30
µg/ml in the pH 4 to 6 range.   These discrepancies may be partly
due to the different buffer systems used.   The low solubility
reported by Werness et al[6] may have been caused by complex formation, as reported earlier[8].   We found that the solubility of triamterene in urine is lower than that measured in the 0.15 M NaCl
buffers used by Werness et al[6].   This would support their thesis
that chloride, the major anion of urine, reduces the solubility of
triamterene.   For hydroxytriamterenesulfate, the solubility is
higher in urine than in buffer.   Although there was a clear pH-
dependency of hydroxytriamterenesulfate solubility in buffer, there
was no correlation between urinary pH and the solubility in urine.
Werness et al[6], using a HPLC procedure, were able to measure and

determine the solubility of hydroxytriamterene in buffer. That compound revealed the lowest solubility of all compounds tested, but no concentrations of that metabolite were published. In our study in Dyazide[R] users, we found that the vast majority of patients, as well as the stone formers, approached or exceeded the apparent solubility of hydroxytriamterenesulfate in urine. For unchanged triamterene, however, the urinary concentrations were lower than the solubility in urine as determined by an equilibration method.

Werness et al[6] found high binding of triamterene and its meta-bolite to the stone matrix. This is an important finding, as it can be shown that triamterene stones have an unusually high matrix content. However, as our data on kidney stone analysis were not available to them, they erroneously concluded that the extent of matrix-binding correlates well with the amount of drug found in kidney stones. Our analysis of 66 kidney stones showed that 49% of the stones contained less than 5% of total triamterene-derived material. The average triamterene, hydroxytriamterene and hydroxy-triamterenesulfate content of the stones was 42.3%, 34% and 23%, respectively.

White and Nancollas[9] suggested that precipitation of triamterene and its metabolites may be a causative factor. They also found that the addition of triamterene or of its metabolites induces calcium oxalate crystal growth by heterogeneous nucleation.

Our data, however, do not support either hypothesis. The epidemiological data of Jick et al[2] suggest that "triamterene nephrolithiasis" may not be a problem complicating or prohibiting triamterene therapy. However, even for a rare side-effect selection of drug therapy has to consider the individual risk. That drug incorporation into stone material is not a unique event is shown by the report of Reveillaud and Daudon[3] (this conference). Therefore, in the future greater concern must be given to drug precipitation in kidney stones.

REFERENCES

1. B. Ettinger, N. O. Oldroyd, and F. Sorgel, in:"Urolithiasis: Clinical and Basic Research", L. H. Smith, W. G. Robertson, and B. Finlayson, eds., Plenum, New York (1981)
2. H. Jick, B. J. Dinan, and J. R. Hunter, J. Urol. 127::224 (1982).
3. R. J. Reveilland and M. Daudon, in:"Urolithiasis and Related Clinical Research", P. O. Schwille, L. H. Smith, W. G. Robertson, and W. Vahlensieck, eds., Plenum, New York (1985).
4. W. Stüber, E. Mutschler, and D. Steinbach, Arzneim.-Forsch. 30:1158 (1980).

5. B. Grebian, H. E. Geissler, and E. Mutschler, Arzneim.-Forsch.26:2125 (1976).

6. P. G. Werness, J. H. Bergert, and L. H. Smith, J. Lab. Clin. Invest. 99:254 (1982).

7. A. A. Pruitt, J. S. Winkel, and P. G. Dayton, Clin. Pharmacol. Ther. 21:610 (1977).

8. L. W. Dittert, T. Higuchi, and D. R. Reese, J. Pharm. Sci. 53:1325 (1964).

9. D. J. White and G. H. Nancollas, J. Urol. 127:593 (1982).

THE EFFECT OF A HIGH INTAKE OF TARTARIC ACID ON

URINARY AND PLASMA OXALATE

N. Fituri, N. Allawi, M. Bentley, and J. Costello

The Irish Stone Foundation, Meath Hospital, Dublin
Eire, and The Renal Research Laboratory, Allegheny
General Hospital, Pittsburgh, Pennsylvania, U.S.A.

INTRODUCTION

The metabolism of tartaric acid in man has not yet been fully elucidated. Finkle[1] concluded from his studies that parenteral tartrate appears unchanged in the urine. Studies by Chadwick et al[2] clearly demonstrated partial metabolism of sodium tartrate to CO_2 over 8 h after intravenous administration of ^{14}C-labelled DL-tartrate. Intestinal bacteria, they found, metabolized both D-and L-tartrate. After oral ingestion, as much as 46% of tartrate was converted to CO_2 and only 12% excreted unchanged in the urine. Other metabolites of tartrate in man have not yet been identified. Whether or not oxalic acid may be an end-product of tartrate catabolism was investigated by Chadwick et al[2]. They concluded that no significant formation of oxalate occurred. However, oxalate excretion in only one subject was studied. Kun and Hernandez[3] reported that the mitochondria of several animal tissues contain an enzyme system capable of oxidizing meso or D-tartrate. They proposed formation of glyoxylate from tartrate as follows:

$$D\ (-)\ or\ Meso\ Tartrate + NAD^+ \rightarrow Dihydroxyfumarate \xrightarrow{Mg^{2+}} Glyoxylate$$

Glyoxylate is readily converted to oxalate in vivo. Tartaric acid L(+), is present in many fruits and is widely used as a constituent of effervescent drinks. The Redoxon tablet preparation of ascorbic acid contains 800 mg of L(+) tartaric acid/g of ascorbic acid. A knowledge of the end-products of tartrate metabolism is therefore of considerable interest and in the present study its possible metabolism to oxalate was investigated.

MATERIALS AND METHODS

Tartaric acid L(+) (Analar grade) was obtained from BDH, England. Plasma and urinary oxalate, urinary urate, calcium, magnesium, citrate and the urinary inhibitory activity of calcium oxalate crystal growth were determined as previously described[4]. Tartaric acid was titrated to pH 5.2 with KOH before ingestion.

Four health subjects, 3 males and 1 female, ingested 8.0 g of L(+)tartrate (2 g x 4) daily for 5 days. Prior to ingestion 3 consecutive 24-h urines were collected and one blood sample obtained from each subject to determine control values. During ingestion of tartrate 24-h urines were collected daily for 5 days and blood samples taken on days 2 and 4. In addition, two 24-h collections were made one week post-ingestion.

Table 1. Urinary Oxalate Excretion Pre-, During and Post-Tartrate Ingestion (8 g/day) (Mean $\pm$ SD).

	Anhydrous Oxalic Acid (mg/24 h)		
Subjects	Control	During	Post
1	16.3 $\pm$ 2.4	20.2 $\pm$ 3.5	28.2 $\pm$ 4.4
2	24.1 $\pm$ 5.9	32.2 $\pm$ 10.9	47.2 $\pm$ 0.2
3	30.4 $\pm$ 4.9	37.9 $\pm$ 7.8	51.7 $\pm$ 6.6
4	24.1 $\pm$ 0.7	35.7 $\pm$ 13.0	33.7 $\pm$ 0.7
		ns	$P < 0.005$

Table 2. The Effect of Ingestion of Tartrate (8 g/day) on Plasma Oxalate, Urinary Urate, Calcium and Magnesium (Mean $\pm$ SD).

	Control	Tartrate	Post-Tartrate
Plasma Oxalate (μg/100 ml)	27.6 $\pm$ 8.8	38.6 $\pm$ 15.1	
Urinary Urate (mg/24 h)	398.1 $\pm$ 92.9	446.1 $\pm$ 96.3	399.0 $\pm$ 99.0
Urinary Calcium (mg/24 h)	161.6 $\pm$ 92.4	152.1 $\pm$ 92.6	170.0 $\pm$ 94.9
Urinary Magnesium (mg/24 h)	101.0 $\pm$ 27.6	106.0 $\pm$ 35.8	106.1 $\pm$ 31.8

RESULTS

All subjects showed an increase in urinary oxalate during ingestion which was not significant. One week post-ingestion, a highly significant increase (P<0.005) in urinary oxalate was observed over control values (Table 1). No significant change occurred in plasma oxalate, urinary urate, calcium or magnesium during or after tartaric acid ingestion (Table 2). Urinary citrate increased significantly on days 3, 4 and 5 of ingestion (P<0.025, <0,001, <0.01 respectively) and had returned to control values one week post-cessation of tartrate. The inhibitory activity of calcium oxalate crystal growth was not significantly altered during or after ingestion of tartrate.

DISCUSSION

The increase in urinary oxalate observed in 4 subjects during tartrate ingestion (Table 1) is supported by the findings of Sur et al[5] and are in contrast to those of Chadwick et al[2]. This increase, and more importantly the significant increase (P<0.005) in urinary oxalate one week post-tartrate ingestion, supports metabolism of this compound to oxalate in man. Whether this occurs by bacterial degradation in the gut or via tissue metabolism or a combination of both cannot be stated. Some ascorbic acid tablets contain large quantities of tartaric acid. Increases in urinary oxalate while ingesting these tablets[6], attributed to metabolism of ascorbate to oxalate, may have derived from the catabolism of tartrate.

The large increase in urinary oxalate after tartrate ingestion has ceased, suggests a possible alteration in the renal handling of oxalic acid during ingestion. This may be due to competition for renal excretory sites by oxalic and tartaric acids.

In man, oral tartrate ingestion increases bicarbonate production[2] and this in turn causes increased urinary citrate excretion[7,8]. The significant increases in urinary citrate during tartrate ingestion are in agreement with these findings. Despite the increase in urinary citrate no significant change in urinary inhibitory activity of calcium oxalate crystal growth was found, suggesting that citrate may not be a major factor in urinary inhibitory activity.

ACKNOWLEDGMENTS

We are grateful to Roche Pharmaceuticals Ltd., Hertfordshire, England, for supplying data on the Redoxon tablet.

REFERENCES

1. P. Finkle, J. Biol. Chem. 100:349 (1933).
2. V. S. Chadwick, A. Vince, M. Killingley, and O. M. Wrong, Clin. Sci. Mol. Med. 54:272 (1978).
3. E. Kun and M. G. Hernandez, J. Biol. Chem. 218:201 (1956).
4. N. Fituri, N. Allawi, M. Bentley, and J. Costello, Eur. Urol. 9:312 (1983).
5. B. K. Sur, H. N. Pandey, S. Deshpande, R. Pahwa, R. K. Singh, and Tarachandra, in:"Urolithiasis, Clinical and Basic Research", L. H. Smith, W. G. Robertson, and B. Finlayson, eds., Plenum, New York (1981).
6. M. Hatch, S. Mulgrew, E. Bourke, B. Keogh, and J. Costello, Eur. Urol. 6:166 (1980).
7. D. P. Simpson, Am. J. Physiol. 206:875 (1964).
8. M. Butz and H. J. Dulce, in:"Urolithiasis, Clinical and Basic Research", L. H. Smith, W. G. Robertson, and B. Finlayson, eds., Plenum, New York (1981).

ROLE OF FLUORIDE IN FORMATION OF CALCIUM OXALATE STONES

F. Hering, T. Briellmann, H. Seiler, and
G. Rutishauser

Urologische Klinik, Kantonsspital Basel, Institut für
Anorganische Chemie der Universität Basel, Switzerland

INTRODUCTION

Fluoridation of drinking water (an anticariogenic measure) leads
to a higher content of fluoride in urinary stones, especially
calcium oxalate stones[1,3,4,6-11,13]. The aim of this study was to
investigate the possible role of fluoride in the formation of
calcium oxalate stones.

METHODS

Male Wistar rats were treated with 0.8% ethylene glycol (v/v)
to induce calcium oxalate stone formation. In addition, one group
received 10 ppm fluoride in their drinking water. Urine samples
(collected while the rats were kept in metabolic cages), kidneys and
one femur were analyzed for calcium and fluoride contents.
Crystallization kinetics were studied in solutions mimicking normal
urine (pH 5.6, temperature 37°C, ionic strength 0.3 and ion
concentrations as in normal human urine). Sodium oxalate (39 μmol)
was added in the presence of various fluoride concentrations
(o,1,5,10 ppm). After 2 and 4 min the solutions were filtered
through glass filters of pore size 9 to 15 μm. The calcium oxalate
crystals retained were dissolved in hot acetic acid and the calcium
content measured by atomic absorption spectrometry.

RESULTS

Fluoride inhibited the ethylene glycol-induced calcium oxalate
stone formation or nephrocalcinosis in rats but increased the

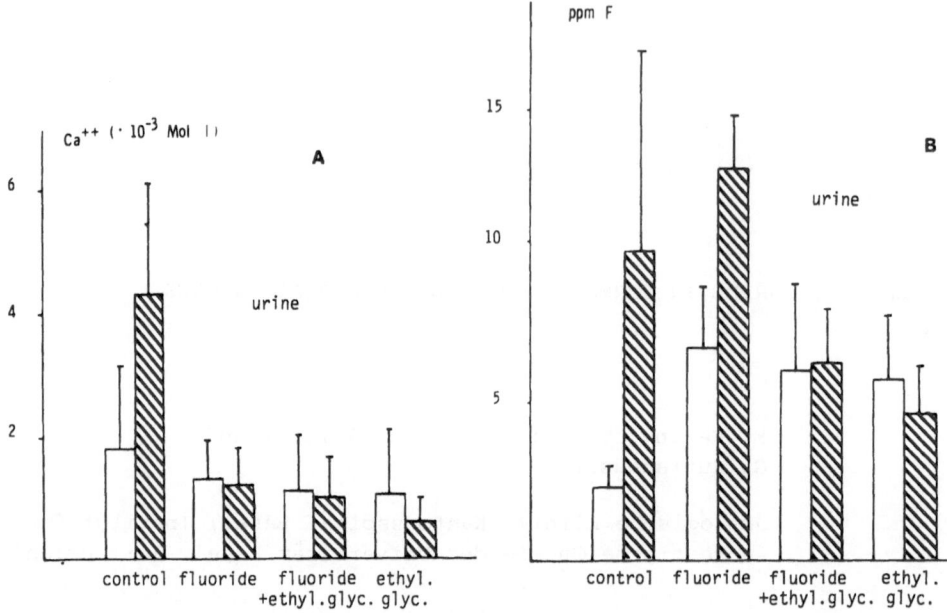

Fig. 1. (A) Urinary calcium excretion and (B) fluoride excretion;
control:drinking water without fluoride or ethyleneglycol,
fluoride:fluoride concentration in drinking water 10 ppm,
fluoride + ethyleneglycol:fluoride concentration in
drinking water 10 ppm, ethyleneglycol 0.8 Vol p.c.,
ethyleneglycol:only ethyleneglycol 0.8 Vol p.c. White
columns animals killed after 20 days, oblique shaded
columns animals killed after 60 days.

excretions of fluoride and calcium in urine (Fig. 1). Treatment
with ethylene glycol alone led to a much greater deposition of
calcium and fluoride in the kidneys (Fig. 2). No differences could
be detected in the fluoride content of the femur. Fluoride delayed
the dose-time-dependent initiation of calcium oxalate
crystallization, but promoted the formation of smaller crystals
(Fig. 3). Two min after adding oxalate to the solutions containing
10 ppm fluoride only 56% crystals were formed in comparison to a
control solution containing no fluoride. The values for the
solutions with 5 ppm and 1 ppm fluoride were 64% and 72%
respectively. After 4 min slight, but not statistically
significant, differences could be detected.

384

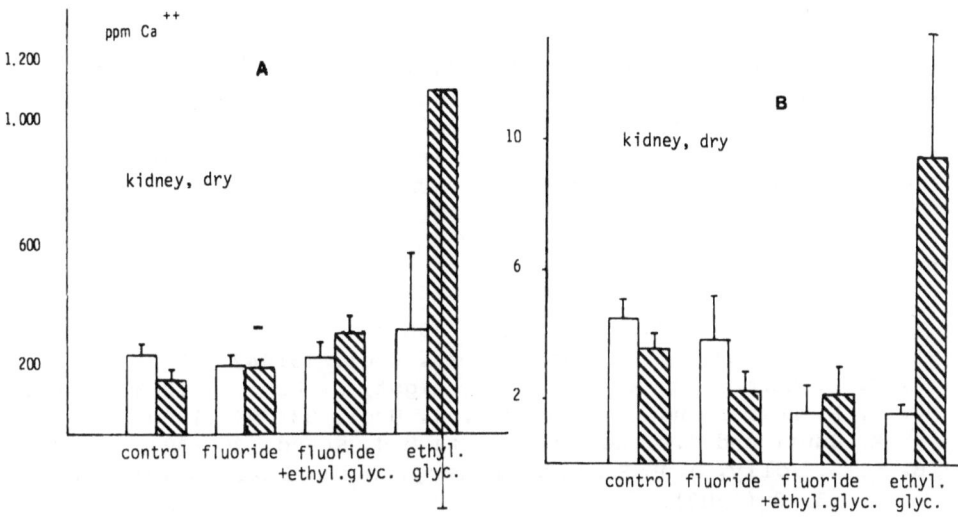

Fig. 2. (A)Calcium content and (B) fluoride content in rat kidneys, other conditions as in Fig. 1.

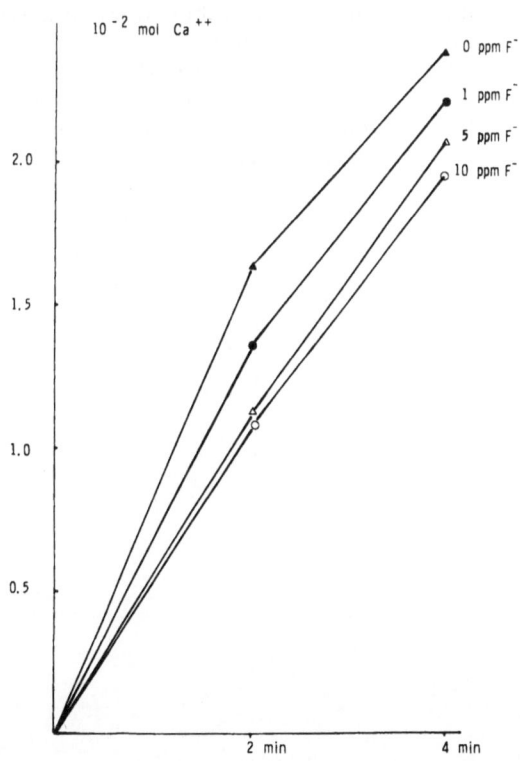

Fig. 3. Calcium content in retained crystals filtered 2 and 4 min after incubation with sodium oxalate in relation to fluoride concentration (0,1,5,10 ppm).

DISCUSSION

Since the intrarenal passage time[2] is about 3 to 4 min, the above data suggest that fluoride might delay intratubular calcium oxalate crystallization. If crystallisation does start, the crystals produced are smaller than in the absence of fluoride and more likely to be passed freely in the urine.

REFERENCES

1. A. Anasuya, J. Nutr. 112:1787 (1982).
2. B. Finlayson and F. Reid, Invest. Urol. 15:442 (1978).
3. J. R. Herman, B. Mason, and I. Light, J. Urol. 80:263 (1958).
4. J. R. Herman and L. Papadakis, J. Urol. 83:799 (1960).
5. M. Juuti and O.P. Heinonen, Acta Med. Scand. 206:397 (1979).
6. S. S. Jolly, O. P. Sharma, G. Garg, and R. Sharma, Fluoride 13:10 (1980).
7. S. Ljunghall, Br. Med. J. 18:439 (1978).
8. H. Luoma, T. Nuuja, Y. Collan, and P. Nummikoski, Calc. Tiss. Res. 20:291 (1976).
9. J. L. Meyer and G. H. Nancollas, J. Dent. Res. 51:1443 (1972).
10. R. Muller, A. Hesse, and H. J. Schneider, Jenaier Harnsteinsymposion, p.96, 1978.
11. L. Spira, Exp. Med. Surg. 14:72 (1956).
12. J. L. Summers and W. A. Keitzer, Ohio State Med. 71:25 (1975).
13. J. Zipkin, W. A. Lee and N. C. Leone, in:"Fluoride Drinking Waters", U.S.D.H.E.W., Washington (1962).

TRANSIENT HYPERCALCIURIA DURING ACUTE PYELONEPHRITIS

AND ACTIVE STONE FORMATION

F. Pizzarelli, C. Ciccarelli, and Q. Maggiore

Divisione Nefrologica, Centro Fisiologia Clinica
C.N.R., Reggio Calabria, Italy

INTRODUCTION

In 1939 Flocks[1] reported that "apparently a slight or intermittent obstruction...... in the urinary tract, such as the presence of a small stone in the kidney pelvis, was associated with a significantly higher calcium concentration in the urine from that kidney". Hennemann et al[2] suggested that urinary tract infection might cause hypercalciuria through an impairment of the tubular reabsorption of calcium. These hypotheses have never been tested and idiopathic hypercalciuria is currently regarded as being due to increased absorption of calcium from the gut and/or reduced tubular reabsorption of calcium of unknown cause[3]. This paper describes a patient who manifested transient renal hypercalciuria concomitantly with episodes of urinary tract infection and multiple stone formation. This association suggests that pyelonephritis and/or partial urinary obstruction due to stone growth may play a role in the genesis of hypercalciuria.

METHODS

Serum ionized calcium (Ca^{2+}) measurements were performed using the Orion specific electrode (Model SS20). Serum iPTH values were measured by radioimmunoassay using a C-terminal specific antiserum (Sorin, Saluggia, Italy). All other biochemical measurements were performed using standard methods. Fractional calcium excretion (FeCa%) was calculated from the serum Ca^{2+} and creatinine concentrations and simultaneous urinary creatinine and calcium excretions. The maximum tubular reabsorption of calcium (TmCa/GFR mmol/100 ml) was calculated as described by Marshall[4] and relative supersatura-

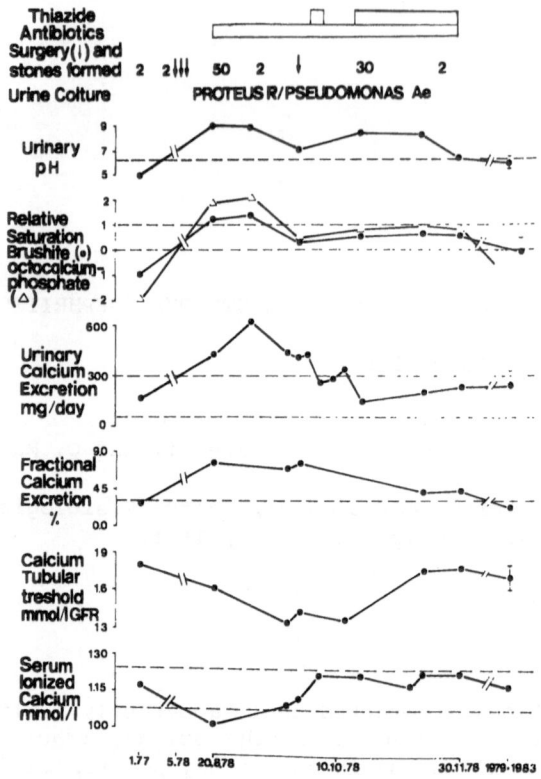

Fig. 1.   Biochemical data on patient (1977-1983).

tion (RS) for brushite and octocalcium phosphate (OCP) from the nomograms of Marshall and Robertson[5].

CASE REPORT (Fig. 1)

A 30-year-old man was referred to our Centre in January 1977, because he had recently passed two calcium oxalate calculi. At this time he was free from stones or urinary infection and his serum and urinary calcium, phosphate and urate concentrations were normal.
In May 1978, because of recurrent ureteral stones, he underwent bilateral ureterolithotomy at another hospital. A few days later another operation had to be performed because of urine leaking from the surgical wound. In August 1978, he came under our care with a vesico-cutaneous fistula and an indwelling vesical catheter. The pH of his urine was 9. Urine culture yielded colonies of Proteus Rettgeri and/or Pseudomonas Aeruginosa in excess of 10^6 colonies/ml. He was treated with antibiotics according to antibiotic sensitivity. As a result of the very high urinary pH, the relative supersatura-

Table 1. Biochemical Data

Analyte		Baseline (1977)	Acute phase[*] (1978)	Follow-up (1979-83)
Serum				
Phosphate	(mmol/l)	0.8	1.0	0.9
Uric acid	(mmol/l)	0.3	0.2	0.2
HCO_3[**]	(mmol/l)	-	26.0	23.0
iPTH	(mU/ml)	-	3.1	3.1
Urine				
Volume	(l/day)	2.2	2.2	1.8
Creatinine Clearance	(ml/min)	99.0	90.0	116.0
FENa	(%)	-	0.7	0.6
Phosphate	(mmol/day)	18.3	20.7	20.1
Uric acid	(mmol/day)	1.3	3.4	2.4

[*]Before HCT therapy; [**]Normal range:undetectable below 4.5 mU/ml

tions for brushite and OCP were both above the formation products of these salts. Accordingly he passed several small stones composed of calcium phosphate and struvite. At this time his daily urinary calcium excretion and FeCa% reached a peak value of 640 mg/day and 7.8% respectively. His Ca^{2+} (1.02 mmol/l) and TmCa/GFR (1.34 mmol/l) were both low. In September 1978, he underwent a left ureterolithotomy for recurrence of obstructing ureteral stones. Two small stones remained in the right kidney. Because his hypercalciuria persisted, hydrochlorothiazide (HCT 100 mg/day) was administered, which promptly reduced his urinary calcium to within the normal range and his serum Ca^{2+} to high-normal values.

By November 1978 signs of the infection had subsided and antibiotics and HCT were discontinued. In the following 5 years, his urinary pH was below 6 on 12 out of 15 occasions and his urine was undersaturated or within the metastable zone with respect to brushite and OCP. Urine cultures were negative in all but three determinations. Urinary calcium excretion remained within the normal range throughout the follow-up period after discontinuation of HCT therapy. In December 1981 the patient underwent a right pyelolithotomy because the 2 residual stones had increased in size.

DISCUSSION

This patient was investigated during a period of active stone formation due to infection of the urinary tract. Hypercalciuria appeared as a concomitant risk factor but subsided after HCT treatment and, once the drug had been withdrawn, did not recur as long as the urine remained sterile. The hypercalciuria was due to a renal leak as shown by the increased FeCa% and the low levels of Ca^{2+} and TmCa. Otherwise there was no evidence of other tubular disfunction or parathyroid hyperactivity (Table 1). Immobilization can be ruled out as the cause of hypercalciuria in this patient because his filtered load of calcium was reduced, rather than enhanced, as in paraplegic patients[6] nor can a defect in the tubular resorption of sodium account for the hyperalciuria, because, at its peak, the fractional Na excretion was normal (Table 1). The presence in the 24-h urine collections of clusters of calcium phosphate crystals, which dissolved following acidification of the urine prior to estimation of calcium, might explain the increased excretion of calcium. But, if this were so, one would also expect an increase in phosphate excretion. On the contrary, the 24-h phosphate excretion was normal (Table 1).

It is well known that urinary infection may cause tubular damage as shown by impairment of the concentrating ability of the kidney[7] and by interference with the mechanisms of urinary acidification[8]. Our observation suggests that acute pyelonephritis, and possibly stone growth by partially obstructing urinary flow, may have impaired the tubular reabsorption of calcium in this patient. Whether or not this mechanism operates in other patients with pyelonephritis and stones, remains to be identified.

REFERENCES

1. R. H. Flocks, J. Am. Med. Assoc. 113:1466 (1939).
2. P. H. Hennemann, P. H. Benedict, A. P. Forbes, and H. R. Dudley, New Engl. J. Med. 259:802 (1958).
3. F. L. Coe and M. J. Favus, in:"The Kidney", B. M. Brenner, and F. C. Rector, eds., Saunders, Philadelphia (1981).
4. D. H. Marshall, in"Calcium, Phosphate and Magnesium Metabolism", B. E. C. Nordin, ed., Churchill Livingstone, Edinburgh (1976).
5. R. W. Marshall and W. G. Robertson, Clin. Chim. Acta 72:253 (1976).
6. A. F. Stewart, M. Adler, C. M. Byers, G. V. Segre, and A. E. Broadus, New Engl. J. Med. 306:1136 (1982).
7. T. A. Stamey, "Urinary Infections", William & Wilkins, Baltimore (1972).
8. M. Cochran, M. Peacock, D. A. Smith and B. E. C. Nordin, Br. Med. J. 2:721 (1968).

UREAPLASMA UREALYTICUM AND RENAL STONES

H. Hedelin, J.-E. Brorson, L. Grenabo, and
S. Pettersson

Depts. of Urology and Microbiology, Sahlgrenska
Sjukhuset, Göteborg, Sweden

INTRODUCTION

Urease-producing bacteria, such as Proteus mirabilis, can be
detected in the urinary tract of most patients with infection
stones (struvite and carbonate apatite stones). Bacteria,
however, can not always be demonstrated in the urine samples of
the stones from these patients. Ureaplasma urealyticum is a
small urease-producing microorganism that differs from bacteria by
the lack of a cell wall. It is not recovered by ordinary
bacterial culture techniques and special methods are required for
its isolation and identification. U. urealyticum is cultured from
the urethra in about half of all sexually active adults[1,2]. It
has also been isolated, with a much lower frequency, from urine
obtained by suprapubic bladder punctures but not at all from the
upper urinary tract[3,4]. It is one of the causes of non-
gonococcal urethritis and it may induce chronic cystitis in
patients with a hypogammaglobulinaemia. It has not yet been
connected, however, to any upper urinary tract disease. U.
urealyticum does not synthesize folic acid and it is thus
resistant to penicillins, cephalosporins and sulphonamides as
well as other antimicrobial agents which act by interfering with
cell wall formation or folic acid synthesis. U. urealyticum has
been shown to produce bladder stones in rats[5,6] and to promote
crystallization of struvite and calcium phosphate in synthetic
urine[7]. In a preliminary study, its role has been demonstrated in
the development of urinary tract concrements in humans[8]. To
elucidate further this question, we have performed an extended
clinical study.

MATERIAL AND METHODS

Fifty patients, 26 males and 24 females, with a mean age of 52 years (range 23-73 years) consecutively operated on for renal stones were studied during a 10-month period in 1982-1983. The stones were removed by conventional surgical techniques, pyelolithotomy or nephrolithotomy, via a loin incision, in 48 patients and in 2 patients the stones were extracted percutaneously. In 9 patients the stone-bearing kidney had been subjected to previous stone surgery and in another 8 patients the contralateral kidney had been subjected to previous stone surgery. Antibiotics were given immediately before the operation and peroperatively to 16 patients. Only 1 patient received an antibiotic (doxycycline) which is known to be effective against U. urealyticum. Five patients had a single calyceal stone and 45 a pelvic stone with or without concomitant calyceal stones.

The day before operation a midstream voided urine specimen was obtained. When the renal pelvis was visualized at surgery it was punctured and urine aspirated. After removel the stones were divided and one half sent for chemical analysis and the other for culture according to the method of Nemoy and Stamey[9]. All samples were cultured for U. urealyticum, and bacteria under both aerobic and anaerobic conditions. The stones were analysed by conventional chemical methods.

RESULTS

Twenty-six patients had stones of metabolic origin (calcium oxalate, mixture of calcium oxalate and calcium phosphate or uric acid) and 24 had infection stones (magnesium ammonium phosphate and/or carbonate apatite).

Bacteria were cultured from the upper urinary tract in 3 (11.5%) of the 26 patients with non-infection stones (Table 1). In one patient U. urealyticum was cultured in a low concentration from the stone.

Bacteria were detected in the upper urinary tract in 18 of the 24 patients with infection stones. Sixteen of these patients had growth of urease-producing bacteria. U. urealyticum was cultured from the upper urinary tract in 7 of the 24 patients. In two of them U. urealyticum was the only microorganism detected in the pelvic urine or the stone. In another two, it was concomitant with non-urease-producing bacteria. Three patients had growth of urease- producing bacteria and U. urealyticum.

Previous renal stone surgery had been performed in half of the patients with infection stones and in 5 of the 26 patients

Table 1. Growth of Bacteria and U. Urealyticum in the Upper
         Urinary Tract of 50 Patients Operated on for Renal
         Stones.

| | U. Urealyticum | Bacteria | |
		Urease-producing	Total
Patients with non-infection concrements (n=26)	1	0	3
Patients with infection concrements (n=24)	7	16	18

with metabolic concrements. Five of the 7 patients with infection
concrements and growth of U. urealyticum in the upper urinary
tract had undergone previous renal stone surgery. In all 7
patients, in whom U. urealyticum was detected in the upper urinary
tract, it was cultured also from the stone, and in 3 it was
cultured from pelvic urine. This contrasts with the findings in
the 28 patients who had bacteria in the upper urinary tract. In
20 of them, the bacteria were detected from the pelvic urine and
in 17 patients the same species was also cultured from the stone.
In only one patient were bacteria cultured from the stone but not
from the pelvic urine.

DISCUSSION

    U. urealyticum was detected in the upper urinary tract in 7
of the 24 patients with infection stones, compared with 1 of the
26 patients with non-infection concrements. In 4 of the patients
with infection stones no other urease-producing microorganism
could be detected. Five of the 7 patients with growth of U.
urealyticum in the upper urinary tract had been subjected to
previous stone surgery. A spread to the upper urinary tract from
the known reservoirs of U. urealyticum in the lower urinary tract,
especially the urethra, may have occurred following the operation.
The fact that U. urealyticum was found more often in the stone
than in pelvic urine may be explained by the fact that it is more
easily detected there than in urine or that it persists in the
stone more readily than in urine. These findings emphasize the
importance of obtaining cultures not only from urine but also from
the stone.

    The recurrence rate of infection stones after surgery
remained high even after the introduction of antibiotics. The

presence of U. urealyticum in the upper urinary tract could be one of the explanations for this high recurrence rate.

The findings in this study appear to link the presence of U. urealyticum in the upper urinary tract with infection stones. We therefore suggest that cultures from pelvic urine and the stone should be performed not only with conventional bacterial culture techniques but also with techniques specific for U. urealyticum, This would allow appropriate therapy (doxycyclines) to be instituted to avoid unnecessary stone recurrence.

REFERENCES

1. W. R. Bowie, S. P. Wang, E. R. Alexander, J. Floyd, P. S. Forsyth, H. M. Pollock, J. S. Lin, T. M. Buchanan, and K. K. Holmes, J. Clin. Invest. 59:735 (1977).
2. P. A. Mårdh, L. Weström, and S. Colleen, in:"Proceedings of the Symposium on Genital Infections and their Complications", D. Danielsson, L. Juhlin, and P. A. Mardh, eds., Almqvist and Wiksell, Stockholm (1975).
3. P. A. Mårdh, A. Lohi, and H. Fritz, Acta. Med. Scand. 191:91 (1972).
4. A. C. Thomsen, J. Clin. Microbiol. 8:84 (1978).
5. A. M. Friedländer and A. I. Braude, Nature 247:67 (1974).
6. L. Grenabo, J. E. Brorson, H. Hedelin, and S. Pettersson, Submitted for publ in Urol. Res.
7. L. Grenabo, J. E. Brorson, H. Hedelin, and S. Pettersson, Submitted for publ. in J. Urol.
8. S. Pettersson, J. E. Brorson, L. Grenabo, and H. Hedlin, Lancet 1:526 (1983).
9. N. J. Nemoy and T. A. Stamey, J. Am. Med. Ass. 215:1470 (1971).

INFECTION CONCREMENTS INDUCED BY UREAPLASMA UREALYTICUM

L. Grenabo, J.-E. Brorson, H. Hedelin, and S. Pettersson

Depts. of Urology and Microbiology, Sahlgrenska
Sjukhuset, S-413 45 Göteborg, Sweden

INTRODUCTION

Infection with urease-producing bacteria as Proteus, Klebsiella, Pseudomonas or Staphylococcus has so far been considered a prerequisite for the formation of infection concrements, i.e. concrements composed of struvite and/or carbonate-apatite. Urease splits urea into ammonia and carbon dioxide and in the alkaline urine so formed, the formation products of struvite and carbonate-apatite are exceeded. In a recent clinical study a relationship between Ureaplasma urealyticum and infection concrements in the upper urinary tract was demonstrated[1]. U. urealyticum is a urease-producing microorganism commonly occurring in the lower urinary tract of adults but not ordinarily in the upper urinary tract. The ureaplasmas are not detected with conventional bacterial culture techniques, which may explain why infection concrements have not previously been associated with the organism.

The aim of this study was to investigate the crystallization caused by U. urealyticum (a) in vitro and (b) the concrement-forming capacity in vivo in rats. The results were to be compared with those of urease- and non-urease-producing bacteria.

MATERIAL AND METHODS

(a) In vitro crystallization was studied by encrustation on solid glass rods suspended in a glass reactor, perfused with synthetic urine, at 37°C for 20 h according to Griffith et al.[2]. After inoculation with U. urealyticum, Proteus mirabilis or urease-negative Escherichia coli, the amounts of encrusted calcium, magnesium and phosphate on the glass rods were analysed and the pH followed. To certain reactors acetohydroxamic acid (AHA), a potent urease inhibitor, was added. As controls, reactors with synthetic urine only or synthetic urine plus ureaplasma broth without microorganisms were used. All precipitated magnesium was assumed to be a constituent of struvite. The phosphate not present as struvite was assumed to be a constituent of calcium phosphates such as brushite, hydroxyapatite and carbonate-apatite. From the molecular weights of the various calcium phosphates and the ratio between phosphate (not present as struvite) and calcium, it was possible to calculate the type of calcium phosphate formed. The pH was measured with a surface pH electrode.

(b) In the animal experiments U. urealyticum was inoculated into the bladder of adult male rats. Rats inoculated with ureaplasma broth without microorganisms, heat-inactivated U. urealyticum, P. mirabilis, urease-negative Myoplasma hominis or E. coli were used as controls. After 2, 4 and 6 weeks the animals were killed and the incidence of concrement formation was recorded. The composition of the stones was analyzed chemically. Cultures for U. urealyticum and bacteria in bladder urine were performed before inoculation and at sacrifice[3].

RESULTS

(a) Inoculation of synthetic urine with U. urealyticum or P. mirabilis resulted in encrustation of calcium, magnesium and phosphate on the glass rods and in alkalinization of the urine (Table 1). The mean amount of encrusted struvite on each glass rod was 231 μg in the ureaplasma reactors and 899 ug in the Proteus reactors. The calcium phosphates were calculated to be brushite in the Ureaplasma reactors and hydroxy- and carbonate-apatite in the Proteus reactors. AHA prevented the alkalinization and crystallization caused by U. urealyticum and P. mirabilis. Inoculation with M. hominis, E. coli, synthetic urine only or synthetic urine plus ureaplasma broth caused no crystallization and the pH remained constant.

(b) Rats inoculated with U. urealyticum or P. mirabilis developed bladder concrements with a high frequency (Table 2). Rats inoculated with ureaplasma broth without microorganisms, with heat inactivated U. urealyticum with M. hominis or E. coli developed bladder concrements only in a few cases. All stones were composed of pure struvite. Urine cultures for U. urealyticum and bacteria were negative before inoculation in all rats and contaminating microorganisms were never found at sacrifice. U. urealyticum was never recovered at sacrifice in any rat inoculated with it, although 31 rats in this group developed bladder stones. Of the 3 E. coli-inoculated rats with stones, 1 had a positive culture.

396

Table 1. Maximum pH in Synthetic Urine and Encrustation on Glass Rods after Inoculation with Different Microorganisms (mean $\pm$ SEM).

Inoculate	Initial count of microorg.	pH	Encrustation (μg/rod)		
			Calcium	Magnesium	Phosphate
U. urealyticum	10^4	8.1 ± 0.1	8.7 ± 23.8	23.1 ± 10.4	294.8 ± 66.3
U. urealyticum + AHA	10^4	5.9 ± 0.1	0.9 ± 0.2	1.4 ± 0.1	38.5 ± 3.4
P. mirabilis	10^8	9.3 ± 0.1	389.6 ± 51.3	89.9 ± 14.1	898.0 ± 66.8
P. mirabilis + AHA	10^8	6.0 ± 0.1	0.5 ± 0.1	1.2 ± 0.1	33.6 ± 5.1
E. Coli	10^8	6.2 ± 0.0	0.9 ± 0.4	1.5 ± 0.1	36.3 ± 3.0
Synthetic urine only	-	5.7 ± 0.0	0.8 ± 0.2	1.3 ± 0.1	39.9 ± 7.5
Synthetic urine + ureaplasma broth	-	5.8 ± 0.0	1.0 ± 0.1	1.5 ± 0.1	45.1 ± 5.4

Table 2. Development of Bladder Concrements in Rats after
Inoculation with Different Microoroganisms.

Inoculate	No. of rats	Stone frequency after various times			
		2 weeks	4 weeks	6 weeks	Total
U. urealyticum	37	6/9	9/10	16/18	31/37
U. urealytcum (killed)	19	-	0/10	0/9	0/19
Ureaplasma broth only	22	0/8	1/8	0/6	1/22
P. mirabilis	51	6/17	10/15	15/19	31/51
M. hominis	27	0/9	0/9	1/9	1/27
E. Coli	22	1/9	1/7	1/6	3/22

DISCUSSION

Inoculation of synthetic urine in vitro with U. urealyticum or
P. mirabilis caused crystallization of struvite and calcium phosphates. The alkalinization caused by U. urealyticum was less
pronounced than that caused by P. mirabilis. The phosphate not
present as struvite consisted of brushite in the Ureaplasma experiments and hydroxy- and carbonate-apatite in the Proteus experiments.
This is explained by the fact that the formation product of brushite
is exceeded at a lower pH than that of the apatites[4]. The alkalinization and crystallization was due to the urease activity of the
microorganisms as AHA prevented these effects and they were not seen
after inoculation with urease-negative E. coli either. Inoculation
of U. urealyticum or P. mirabilis into the bladder of rats caused
the develpoment of bladder concrements composed of struvite with a
high frequency. Despite the fact that U. urealyticum was not
recultured at sacrifice living ureaplasmas were a prerequisite for
the formation of bladder concrements in this study. These results
and previous clinical data[1] suggest that U. urealyticum is
associated with the formation of struvite and/or calcium phosphate
stones and that the microorganism should be sought in patients with
infection stones.

REFERENCES

1. S. Pettersson, J. E. Brorson, L. Grenabo, and H. Hedelin, Lancet
   1:526 (1983).
2. D. P. Griffith, D. M. Musher, and C. Itin, Invest. Urol. 13:346
   (1976).
3. M. C. Shepard, and C. D. Lunceford, Appl. Microbiol. 20:539
   (1970).
4. J. S. Elliot, W. L. Quaide, R. F. Sharp, and L. Lewis, J. Urol.
   80:269 (1958).

STONE ANALYSIS AND URINARY TRACT INFECTION IN RENAL

STONE PATIENTS

K. Holmgren, B. Fellström, B. G. Danielson,
S. Ljunghall,and F. Niklasson

Depts. of Urology, Internal Medicine and Clinical
Chemistry, University Hospital, S-751 85 Uppsala
Sweden

INTRODUCTION

The influence of bacterial urease in the calculogenesis of struvite and apatite calculi is well known[1-4]. The significance of urinary tract infection (UTI) among other stone formers and its relationship to the types of stones is less clear. The aim of the present study was to investigate the frequency of UTI in patients that had been admitted to the clinic for renal stone disease. Stone analysis, frequency and level of surgery for stones in relation to infection were also included in the survey.

METHODS

Throughout the years 1975-1981, 1325 patients were hospitalized at the University Hospital in Uppsala for stone disease and 374 (28%) had experienced UTI with at least one positive urine culture (midstream urine). There were 1919 positive urinary cultures performed. A total of 780 patients were operated on for stone, including transuretheral procedures. From the operated patients, 619 stone analyses were performed using infrared spectrophotometry. The localization of the stones in the urinary tract in relation to infection and stone content was also studied.

RESULTS

E. coli was the most common microorganism among the hospitalized stone formers and was found in 60% of the cases. Other organisms included Staphylococcus albus 33%, Enterococci 28%,

Table 1. The Distribution (%) of Stone Analyses in Infected and
        Non-Infected Stone Formers.

Organism	Oxalate-containing Calculi	Calcium phosphate Calculi	MAP Calculi
E. Coli	65	19	16
Staph. albus	59	30	11
Enterococci	59	30	11
Proteus	22	50	28
Klebsiella	53	24	23
Non-infected patients	86	13	1

Proteus 20% and Klebsiella 17%. Some patients had more than one
microorganism. In 81% of the cases with E. coli the infection was
found during or after the patient were admitted to the clinic, while
56% of the cases with Proteus infection was found prior to admission
to the clinic. Calcium-containing calculi were found in more than
90% of the analyzed calculi and magnesium ammonium phosphate (MAP)
in 6%. The most common finding in this series was mixed calcium
oxalate/calcium phosphate stones (44%). The oxalate-containing
calculi were found in 86% of the analyzed calculi in the non-
infected patients and the MAP in only 1%. Among the patients with
UTI the MAP calculi represented 11 to 28% of the analyses with the
highest value in cases with Proteus. The frequency of oxalate-
containing stones was between 22 and 65%, with the lowest value from
patients with Proteus infections (Table 1).

In patients without infection, 37% had been operated in the
kidney and 63% in the ureter. The infected patients, on the other
hand, were more often operated in the kidney, especially in cases
infected with Proteus (Table 2). In 33% of the pure oxalate-
containing calculi the stones were located in the kidney at
operation while the pure calcium phosphate calculi were equally
located in the ureter and the kidney. The MAP calculi were most
often (79%) found in the kidney at operation.

DISCUSSION

In another investigation[5] the consecutive distribution of
microorganisms in stone formers was studied. The Enterococci were
absent and Pyocyaneus much more common than in the present study.
The reason why the results did not correspond so well might be
explained by geographical differences. The stone content was comparable with that found in another investigation[6]. In the present
study, all of the analyzed stones had been removed by surgery and
one might have expected a higher frequency of MAP calculi. On the

Table 2. Frequency (%) of Kidney and Ureteral Operations or Manipulations for Stones in Infected and Non-Infected Patients.

	Kidney operations	Ureteral operations or manipulations
Non-infected	37	63
Total infected	51	49
E. coli	56	44
Staphylococcus albus	45	55
Enterococci	50	50
Proteus	68	32
Klebsiella	49	51

other hand, the frequency of pure phosphate calculi was high compared with that found by other investigators.

There was a distinct difference in the pattern of stone composition between infected and non-infected patients, especially with respect to oxalate-containing calculi. The non-infected patients had a higher frequency of oxalate-containing stones compared with the infected patients (Table 1). Oxalate calculi are usually formed in non-infected urine. Of course, some of the patients with oxalate calculi will be secondarily infected but some authors believe that all infection stones result from metabolic stones that have been secondarily infected[7].

Only patients with Proteus infections had a different pattern of stones despite the fact that both Staphylococcus albus and Klebsiella often produce urease. There was a difference in stone composition between the non-infected patients and patients infected with non-urease producing microorganisms, such as E. coli and Enterococci.

Most of the oxalate-containing calculi were located in the ureter at operation. Phosphate calculi and especially stones containing MAP are often larger and heavier than oxalate stones[8], which may explain why phosphate calculi more often were located in the kidney and apparently not so easily passed down the ureter.

REFERENCES

1. D. P. Griffith, Kidney Int. 13:372 (1978).
2. D. M. Musher and D. P. Griffith, J. Infect. Dis. 131:177 (1975).
3. D. P. Griffith, B. M. Musher, and C. Itin, Invest. Urol. 13:346 (1976).

4. J. B. Hellström, Br. J. Urol. 10:348 (1938).

5. J. Simon, M. Fuss, and E. Yomassowski, Eur. Urol. 6:129 (1980).

6. B. Otnes, Scand. J. Urol. Nephrol 17:85 (1983).

7. L. H. Smith, in:"Renal Calculi: A Guide to Management", W. C. Thomas, ed., Springfield, Illinois (1976).

8. B. Otnes, Scand. J. Urol. 17:191 (1983).

VESICAL CALCULI IN PATIENTS WITH NEUROGENIC URINARY

BLADDER DYSFUNCTION

B. Suryaprakash, M. S. Rao, S. K. Thind,
S. Faidyanathan, and A. K. Goel

Depts. of Urology and Biochemistry, Postgraduate
Institute of Medical Education and Research
Chandigarh-160012, India

INTRODUCTION

Vesical calculi occur in 28% of adult paraplegics[1] and are associated with hypercalciuria, urinary stasis and infection involving urea-splitting bacteria. The incidence of urolithiasis is higher in children than in adults following spinal injury[1].

PATIENTS AND METHODS

Thirteen cases of neurogenic bladder with vesical calculi (12 male and 1 female aged 18 to 50 years) were referred to this Institute during the last 5 years. The nature of the underlying neurological disease, which resulted in bladder dysfunction and the level and duration of neurological lesion were noted. The initial urological management prior to referral was recorded. The patients were given a physical examination and a urine culture made. Serum creatinine was measured and intravenous urography, retrograde urethrography, and cystography carried out. Subsequent urological management was tailored to the needs of the individual patient.

RESULTS

The clinical data on the patients are shown in Tables 1 to 4. Serum creatinine was <1 mg/dl in 2 patients and between 1 and 3 mg/dl in the remaining 11. Urine culture yielded Proteus Rettgeri in one, Proteus Mirabilis in another and mixed bacterial flora in 11. KUB revealed a co-existent staghorn calculus in one case. IVP showed undilated upper tracts in 9 patients and bilateral hydro-

Table 1.   Nature of Neurological Lesion

Spinal Cord Injury	8
Transverse Myelitis	2
Prolapsed Intervertebral Disc	1
Lymphoma with Spinal Cord Compression	1
Recurrent Spinal Cord Tumour (Neurolipoma)	1

Table 2.   Level of Spinal Lesion

	No. of Cases	
	Complete	Incomplete
C-4/5	1	1
T-12	0	1
L-1	1	6
L-3	0	2
L-4	0	1

Table 3.   Duration of Neurological Lesion

Time (months)	No. of Cases
0-12	1
12-24	8
24-36	3
48-60	1

Table 4.   Initial Urological Management

Management	No. of Cases.
In-dwelling Urethral Catheter Drainage	7
Crede Manoeuvre	2
Suprapubic Cystostomy	1
Involuntary Urine	2
Condom	1

nephrosis in 4. The cystograms showed grade IV vesicoureteral reflux in one. A retrograde urethrogram in one patient showed a urethral diverticulum containing a stone. Suprapubic cystolithotomy was performed in 12 cases. In a 19-year-old female, the stone was removed transurethrally after dilating the urethra up to No. 28F. Increased autonomic activity which responded to i.v. administration of 10 mg phentolamine, was observed in a tetraplegic patient. The patient with renal stones subsequently underwent pyelolithotomy uneventfully. In the other case, a urethral diverticulum was excised along with the stone and urethroplasty performed. The subrapubic wound healed well in all 12 cases and urine leakage did not occur after removal of the urethral catheter. Stone analysis revealed various combinations of calcium, oxalate, phosphate, uric acid, magnesium and carbonate. After removal of the vesical calculi, phenoxybenzamine (10 mg/6 h) was prescribed to one tetraplegic patient to produce satisfactory vesical emptying; another patient was prescribed clonidine (2 mg/8 h). Clean atraumatic intermittent catheterization is being practised by the remaining patients. Follow-up IVPs showed resolution of hydronephrosis in all 4 cases. Vesical calculi did not recur in any case for up to 2 years.

DISCUSSION

Prolonged in-dwelling catheters with infection was the major cause of bladder stones in 8 patients and in 5, complete vesical emptying was not achieved either without treatment or when they employed Crede's manoeuvre. In contrast, none of the patients (>100) who have practised intermittent catheterisation at this Institute as a first line of management after injury, have developed vesical calculi, the follow-up being between 1 and 13 years. Clean autraumatic intermittent catheterization performed every 4 h from the day of injury ensures complete vesical emptying. It reduces the urinary infection rate and ischemia from repeated over-distension of the urinary bladder wall[2]. Local damage to the bladder and urethra from the presence of an indwelling catheter is prevented thereby reducing the risk of stone formation. Urinary calculi were found in 45% of children with spinal cord injury who had an indwelling Foley catheter[1]. Of these stones, 85% were in the bladder. In contrast, only 4% of patients treated by intermittent catheterization developed calculi; 25% of which were vesical calculi. Calcium oxalate was present in all calculi. Burr[3] showed that in 'early' calculi (removed up to 30 months from the onset of the cord lesion), the calcium to magnesium ratio was significantly higher than in later stones. Similarly, samples taken from sites nearer to the centres of calculi contained more calcium and less magnesium than did those from more peripheral sites. The ratio was independent of the level of the cord lesion, the sex of the patient, or the anatomical site of the stone.

405

The incidence of stone disease in patients with poor bladder function was 22% in World War II paraplegics and 18% in Korean War paraplegics. In contrast, in those with good bladder function the incidence of stone disease was markedly reduced, being 2.5% and 4.5% respectively[4]. Current management of vesical calculi in patients with neurogenic bladder dysfunction may be classified into preventive and therapeutic. The former include general measures such as hydration and early ambulation. Intermittent catheterization should be practised from the very onset of illness. Subsequently, satisfactory vesical emptying can be achieved by external urethral sphincterotomy[5] or pharmacotherapy in cases of detrusosphincter dyssynergia and by continued intermittent catheter-ization or pharmacotherapy (phenoxybenzamine, indoramin[6]) in cases of hyporeflexic bladders. The therapeutic aspects of vesico-lithiasis include cystolithotomy, transurethral ultrasonic litho-lapaxy, treatment of urinary infection and management of underlying vesical dysfunction as well as patho-anatomical lesions such as urethral stricture. The physician taking care of spinal cord injury patients should adopt a holistic approach[7] and involve a urologist, microbiologist and clinical biochemist besides a neurosurgeon, orthopedic surgeon, clinical psychologist and rehabilitation nurse. With improved investment in spinal cord injury research[8], and establishment of specialized centres for civilian traumatic paraplegic and tetraplegic patients, it is possible that vesical calculi will no longer be encountered by 1990.

ACKNOWLEDGEMENT

Our gratitude to the Indian Council of Medical Research.

REFERENCES

1. J. A. Tori and L. S. Kewalramani, Paraplegia 16:357 (1978-79)
2. J. Lapides, A. C. Diokno, B. S. Lowe, and M. D. Kalish, J. Urol. 111:184 (1974).
3. R. G. Burr, Paraplegia 10:56 (1972).
4. J. Connelly, R. H. Hackler, and R. C. Bunts, J. Urol. 108:558 (1972).
5. M. S. Rao, B. C. Bapna, S. Vaidyanathan, V. N. Bhat, C. L. Gupta, M. J. Reddy, and K. M. K. Rao, Indian J. Surg. 40:201 (1978).
6. S. Vaidyanathan, M. S. Rao, P. L. Sharma, K. S. N. Chary, and R. P. Swamy, J. Urol. 129:96 (1983).
7. H. S. Talbot, Paraplegia 17:32 (1979).
8. S. Vaidyanathan and M. S. Rao, in:"Emergency and Disaster Medicine", N. P. Singh, ed., National Association for Critical Care Medicine, New Delhi (1981).

406

BIOCHEMICAL STUDIES IN PARAPLEGIC RENAL STONE PATIENTS

R. G. Burr, I. Nuseibeh, and C. D. Abiaka

The Ludwig Guttmann Institute of Spinal Injuries
Stoke Mandeville Hospital, Aylesbury, Buckinghamshire
HP21 8AL, U.K.

INTRODUCTION

Paraplegics have a higher than normal incidence of renal calculi[1]. Hypercalciuria is common in the early months following the onset of a spinal cord lesion, but calculi from such patients are almost invariably associated with chronic urinary infection and the majority consist principally of calcium phosphate and magnesium ammonium phosphate (MAP)[1].

This paper reports the results of a series of studies of biochemical factors related to stone formation in patients with spinal cord lesions.

MATERIAL AND METHODS

Three groups of subjects were studied; paraplegics with no history of urinary stones, but hospitalized for a variety of reasons, paraplegics with stones and chronic urinary infection, and apparently healthy non-paraplegic control subjects. All were male and the duration of paraplegia was more than 1 year.

Serum Ca, P_i, albumin, total protein and urate were determined by Technicon SMA II, plasma Na, K, Cl and HCO_3^- by Tecnicon 660, urinary citrate and urate enzymtically[2,3], and inorganic pyrophosphate (PP_i) by a modification of the method of Russell and Hodgkinson[4].

Urinary pH, Na, K, NH_4, Ca, Mg and P_i were determined and relative saturation (RS) with brushite, octacalcium phosphate

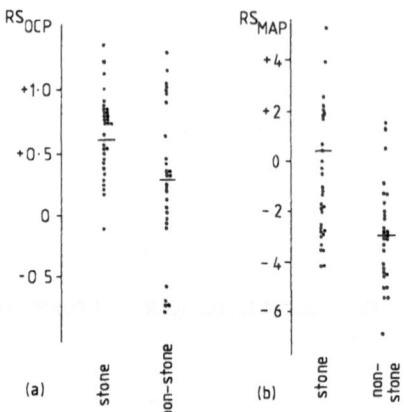

Fig. 1. Maximum values of calculated relative saturation (RS) for
(a) OCP and (b) MAP observed during a 48-h period in
paraplegic patients with and without renal stone.

(OCP) and MAP obtained as detailed elsewhere[5]. Urine pH was
measured immediately or preserved with hibitane[5]. Urine for urate
analysis was kept for up to 5 days at $4^{O}C$, for PP at $-20^{O}C$.
Citrate was determined on the day of completion of collection, the
sample being kept in ice during collection.

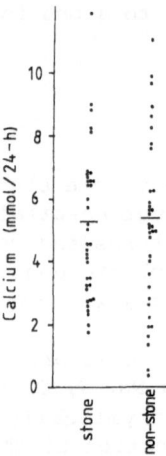

Fig. 2. Urinary Ca excretion in paraplegic patients with and
without renal stone, duration of cord lesion 1 year.

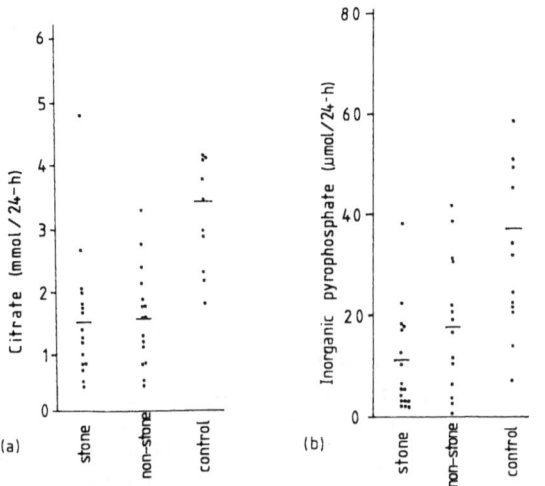

Fig. 3.   Urinary excretion of (a) citrate and (b) PP_i in stone-
forming paraplegics, paraplegics with no history of urinary
stone and healthy controls.

RESULTS

The results of interest are given in the Figs.1-4.   Each point
is the mean result for one patient. Urinary pH, NH_4, 24-h urate
excretion and RS of urine with OCP and MAP were significantly higher
in the stone-formers than in the paraplegics without stones ($P < 0.01$).

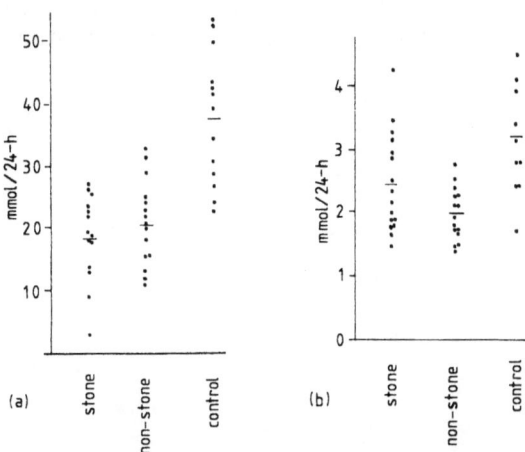

Fig. 4.   Urinary excretion of (a) P_i and (b) urate in stone- and
non-stone-forming paraplegics and in healthy controls.

All stone-formers' urines were oversaturated with brushite or OCP for part of each day; 38% (10/26) had urine that was oversaturated with MAP for part of each day. The excretions of citrate, P_i, PP_i, urate and creatinine and 24-h creatinine clearance were lower in the paraplegics than in the control subjects (P<0.01). Serum Ca, P_i, and HCO_3^- were within normal limits but 17% (13/75) of all patients had hypercalciuria and 30% (16/54) had hyperuricaemia.

DISCUSSION

The low excretions of P_i and urate we attribute to the effects of diet. The patients were hospitalized and had a low level of muscular activity and, presumably, poor appetite. By contrast many of the control subjects were highly active young men, whose ages were not significantly different from those of the patients. The low PP_i excretion was probably secondary to the low excretion of P_i [4]. The low urinary citrate is partly explained by urinary infection.

There is a need for further study of the excretion of citrate by paraplegics and of the possible roles of citrate, PP_i and urate in stone-formation in paraplegia. Oversaturation with MAP is possibly a spasmodic or localized phenomenon in some stone-formers.

REFERENCES

1. R. G. Burr, Int. Rehabil. Med., 3:162 (1981).
2. S. G. Welshman and H. McCambridge, Clin. Chim. Acta 46:243 (1973)
3. Urica Color, The Boehringer Corporation, Lewes.
4. R. G. Russell and A. Hodgkinson, Clin. Sci. 31:51 (1966).
5. R. G. Burr and I. Nuseibeh, Br. J. Urol. 55:162 (1983).

THE EFFECTIVENESS OF HEMODIALYSIS AND CONTINUOUS AMBULATORY PERITONEAL DIALYSIS (CAPD) IN CONTROLLING PLASMA OXALATE CONCENTRATIONS

N. Fituri, B. Keogh, and J. Costello

The Irish Stone Foundation, Meath Hospital, Dublin Eire, and The Renal Research Laboratory, Allegheny General Hospital, Pittsburgh, Pennsylvania, U.S.A.

INTRODUCTION

Oxalosis or calcium oxalate deposition in the tissues has been reported not only in cases of primary hyperoxaluria[1] but in several patients with chronic renal failure of long duration[2]. In these patients, crystal deposition has also been found to occur in the kidney and in extrarenal tissue including the myocardium. Previous studies[3] have suggested that peritoneal dialysis is less successful than hemodialysis in the treatment of primary hyper-oxaluria. Salyer and Keren[2] concluded from their studies on patients in chronic renal failure that hemodialysis was more effective in lowering plasma oxalate levels than peritoneal dialysis. This study was undertaken to compare the effectiveness of hemodialysis and CAPD in controlling plasma oxalate concentrations in a number of patients in chronic renal failure.

METHODS

The patients, consisting of 8 on hemodialysis and 7 on CAPD, had been on dialysis for similar periods of time, with a minimum of two years. Plasma oxalate was determined by a modification of the method of Hatch et al[4] as previously described[5]. Oxalate in the dialysate was assayed by the same method[5] using 30 ml of dialysis fluid. The oxalate removed in one patient on CAPD over a period of 18.5 h was determined. Urinary oxalate excretion was assayed as described by Costello et al[6].

Table 1. Plasma Oxalate Concentrations Pre- and Post-Hemodialysis.

Subjects	Pre-Dialysis	Post-Dialysis	% Decrease
1	852	476	44.1
2	560	250	55.4
3	620	360	41.9
4	828	455	45.0
5	710	436	38.6
6	971	522	46.2
7	495	270	45.5
8	490	230	53.0
Mean $\pm$ SD			46.2 $\pm$ 5.5

Each value represents the mean of triplicate determinations

Table 2. Plasma Oxalate Concentrations in Continuous Ambulatory Peritoneal Dialysis Patients (CAPD).

Subjects	Anhydrous Oxalic Acid (μg/100 ml)
1	490
2	450
3	470
4	410
5	380
6	290
7	490

Each value represents the mean of triplicate determinations

Table 3. Oxalate Removed in One Patient on CAPD Over 18.5 Hours.

Period of Dialysis		Plasma	Post-Dialysis Fluid	Oxalate Removed
Start	Finish	(Oxalate μg/100 ml)		(μg)
23.30	07.45	551.8	305.3	6,106
08.00	13.00	-	405.1	8,102
13.15	18.00	528.1	322.9	6,458
			Total Oxalate Removed	20.66 mg

Samples for analysis were taken at the end of each period of dialysis. Each value is a mean of quadruplicate determination.

RESULTS

Plasma oxalate concentrations in patients on hemodialysis were significantly higher pre-dialysis, than in patients on CAPD (P<0.005) (Tables 1 and 2). The decrease in plasma oxalate on hemodialysis treatment (mean $\pm$ SD) was 46.2 $\pm$ 5.5% (Table 1), while plasma values stayed relatively constant in the CAPD patients (Tables 2 and 3). The total oxalate removed in one patient on CAPD over 18.5 h was 20.7 mg, equivalent to 26.8 mg/24 h. Hemodialysis patients excreted markedly more oxalate in their urine (23.7 $\pm$ 11.6 mg/24 h) than did the CAPD patients (4.9 $\pm$ 2.9 mg/24 h).

DISCUSSION

The decrease in plasma oxalate during hemodialysis of 46.2% is considerably less than the 81 to 85 % observed by Zarembski and Hodgkinson[7]. The improved assay procedure for plasma oxalate of the present study[5] (normal range 27.3 $\pm$ 6.8 µg/100 ml; n= 19) may have given more reliable values. Plasma oxalate levels in the 8 patients on hemodialysis were significantly higher (P<0.005) than in the patients on CAPD, increasing the risk of oxalosis in these patients. This finding is somewhat surprising since treatment on hemodialysis was more efficient in reducing plasma oxalate concentrations than was CAPD (Tables 1 and 3). Furthermore, patients on hemodialysis excreted more oxalate in their urine than patients on CAPD. On CAPD, plasma oxalate values remained fairly stable, the amount of oxalate removed in one patient, 26.8 mg/24 h, being close to that believed to be synthesized endogenously in man[8]. As all these dialysis patients were on a low oxalate intake, the dietary oxalate contribution was minimal. On hemodialysis, the quantity of oxalate removed in the dialysate was not determined and consequently a direct comparison with the efficiency of CAPD in removing oxalate from the body cannot be made. However, CAPD was more effective in maintaining relatively constant plasma oxalate concentrations. Oxalate is known to inhibit several enzymes[9] and it is tempting to speculate that the higher plasma levels reached in the intervals between hemodialysis treatment may inhibit other enzyme reactions, resulting in increased oxalate synthesis in patients on hemodialysis. Experimental evidence to support this hypothesis is lacking.

While hemodialysis treatment has been shown to be more beneficial in cases of primary hyperoxaluria than peritoneal dialysis, the value of CAPD in treating patients in chronic renal failure deserves further study. These investigations are continuing in our laboratory.

REFERENCES

1. J. Walls, A. R. Morley, and D. N. S. Kerr, Br. J. Urol. 41:546 (1969).
2. W. R. Salyer and D. Kerens, Kidney Int. 4:61 (1973).
3. P. M. Zarembski, S. M. Rosen, and A. Hodgkinson, Br. J. Urol. 41:530 (1969).
4. M. Hatch, E. Bourke, and J. Costello, Clin. Chem. 23:76 (1977).
5. M. Maguire, N. Fituri, B. Keogh, and J. Costello, in:"Urolithiasis, Clinical and Basic Research", L. H. Smith, W. G. Robertson, and B. Finlayson, eds., Plenum, New York (1981).
6. J. Costello, M. Hatch, and E. Bourke, J. Lab. Clin. Med. 87:903 (1976).
7. P. M. Zarembski and A. Hodgkinson, Nature 212:511 (1969).
8. H. E. Williams and L. H. Smith, in:"The Metabolic Basis of Inherited Disease", J. B. Stanbury, J. B. Wyngaarden, and D. S. Fredrickson, eds., McGraw-Hill, New York (1972).
9. A. Hodgkinson, in:"Oxalic Acid in Biology and Medicine", Academic Press, London (1977).

ROUND TABLE DISCUSSION ON SECONDARY LITHIASIS

D. P. Griffith

Baylor College of Medicine, Houston, Texas, U.S.A.

DR GRIFFITH: Our Round Table will focus on secondary stone
formation.   DR WERNESS (ROCHESTER, Ma. USA) has presented an
overview of triamterene stones.   Now our discussion will target
upon infection stones.   There seems to be a general consensus that
the bacterial enzyme urease is primarily responsible for struvite
and carbonate apatite stones in humans.

DR BICHLER (TUBINGEN, FRG): We have special interest in infection
stones in children.   The plain abdominal radiographs and the
urinary chemistries describe an infection stone in a 12-year-old
boy.   This patient had a urea-splitting Proteus infection and no
obstructive uropathy.   He was successfully treated with surgical
stone removal and elimination of infection with antimicrobial
agents.   Infection-induced calculogenesis results in a vicious
cycle: Infection with urea-splitting organisms $\longrightarrow$ Over-production of
urease $\longrightarrow$ Degradation of urea $\longrightarrow$ Hyperammoniuria and alkaline
urinary pH $\longrightarrow$ Increased supersaturation of urine with struvite $\longrightarrow$
Precipitation of struvite and "nucleus" formation $\longrightarrow$ Rapid growth of
staghorn calculi $\longrightarrow$ Obstruction of urinary tract $\longrightarrow$ Re-infection.
Successful treatment can be achieved only by surgical removal of
stones thereby interrupting these events.

DR ROSENSTEIN (LONDON, UK): The recurrence rate in these stones can
be quite high, owing to residual microcalculi containing viable
urea-splitting bacteria.   We have been studying ureases and their
inhibition. I_{50} indicates the concentration of inhibitor that
inhibits 50% of the urease.   With this assay and a P. mirabilis
urease, 'Benurestat' (2-P. chlorobenamide acetohydroxamic acid) was
a much more effective inhibitor (I_{50} = 0.065 μg/ml) than
acetohydroxamic acid (AHA) (I_{50} = 2 μg/ml).   Urease from strains of

P. morgani is more resistant to urease inhibitors than all other bacterial species tested (mean I_{50} of AHA using four strains of P. morgani is 8.6×10^{-2}M and that of Benurestat is 3.4×10^{-3}M compared with a mean I_{50} of 2×10^{-3}M AHA and 3×10^{-5}M Benurestat using other species of Proteus. The P. morgani urease, in addition to being more resistant to inhibitors, is non-inducible, has a lower Km and different electrophoretic mobility. Vegetable ureases were more resistant to urease inhibitors than sonicated extracts of urease from P. vulgaris, P. mirabilis and P. rettgeri but more sensitive than urease from P. morgani. Because a permeability barrier exists at the cell wall to inhibitors (shown by the increase in I_{50} when using whole cells) anti-urease compounds should be tested using whole bacterial cells. The type of inhibition produced by the anti-urease compound is important. A non-competitive inhibitor such as AHA is useful therapeutically, since its effect will not be reduced by large amounts of substrate (urea) in the urine. A competitive inhibitor such as hydroxyurea, which has also been used therapeutically, will not be as successful because competitive inhibition is reversed in the presence of excess substrate.

We have found that the presence of AHA (2 mg/ml) can potentiate the antimicrobial activity of some antibiotics; it is itself slightly antibacterial (MIC 4 mg/ml). In some cases the combination of urease inhibitor and antimicrobial agent is synergistic, i.e. the effect of the two drugs in combination is greater than the total effects of the drugs measured separately. The potentiation effect is inconsistent; not all combinations of antimicrobial agent and urease inhibitor are synergistic with the same strains, not all strains showed the synergistic effect with the same combination of antibiotic and urease inhibitor. The potentiation effect is unrelated to urease production as it occurs using urease-negative mutants of Proteus and naturally occurring urease-negative bacteria. Our work has led us to believe that a synergistic combination of an antimicrobial agent and a urease inhibitor could be valuable in the postoperative management of patients with infected urinary calculi. Induction studies indicate that urease inhibitors may not be able to dissolve pre-formed stones, but may be able to act as prophylactic agents in preventing recurrence after surgery.

DR MARTELLI (BOLOGNA, Italy): We have been interested in the pharmacological potential of propionohydroxamic acid (PHA), a urease inhibitors. This is a summary of some of our experimental and clinical investigations. The original manuscripts should be consulted for specific methodological details.

Urease Activity

PHA has a urease inhibitory activity only slightly less than that of AHA. As PHA concentration increases from 15 to 100 uM, urease is progressively inhibited. Experimental models showed a reduction in calculogenesis in the presence of PHA.

Animal Toxicity

Rats and beagle dogs tolerated PHA at doses of 5 to 30 mg/kg/day for up to 26 weeks; no changes in behavior, growth, food consumption or hematological data were noted.

Mutagenicity

Mutagenicity was studied utilizing four strains of Salmonella typhimurium in the Ames Test. Three strains showed no evidence of mutations, while in the TA 98 strain, a slight retromutation appeared at PHA concentrations of 2,000 ug/plate.

Teratogenicity

Studies in pregnant rats and rabbits with orally administered PHA showed no statistically significant teratogenic effects in the offspring, although the fetuses did show a few more anomalies than controls. The incidence of anomalies seemed to parallel the dose of administered PHA; thus, the potential for embryofetotoxic effects has not been completely eliminated.

Pharmacokinetics

The half-life $(T_{1/2})$ in humans of PHA is about 20 h. We have used daily doses of 250 to 375 mg for the human clinical trials.

Clinical Trials

PHA has been administered to 48 patients; each had a chronic urea-splitting urinary infection and had residual or recurrent urinary stones. Dosages varied between 250 and 375 mg/day. Treatment was discontinued in 5 patients because of side-effects consisting of gastrointestinal disturbances, headache, loss of hair and mild anemia. The other 31 tolerated the medication for up to 32 consecutive months. Urinary ammonia and alkalinity were reduced in all patients.

In conclusion, we believe that PHA will be a useful pharmacologic agent in the patient with chronic urea-splitting bacteriuria who is at risk of urease-induced calculogenesis.

Table 1. Side-effects in Those Patients in Whom Treatment was not Terminated, Though Treatment might have been Temporarily Interrupted. More than One Side-Effect may have been Reported by a Given Patient.

	AHA (45)		Placebo (49)		Total (94)	
	No.	%	No.	%	No.	%
Side-Effects						
None	10	22.2	25	51.0	35	37.2
Tolerable	25	55.6	22	44.9	47	50.0
(Mild)	(22)	(48.9)	(19)	(38.8)	(41)	(43.62)
(Moderate)	(3)	(6.7)	(3)	(6.1)	(6)	(6.38)
Intolerable	10	22.2	2	4.1	12	12.77
Types of Tolerable Side-Effects						
Alopecia	1	2.2	2	4.1	3	3.2
Anorexia	2	4.4	2	4.1	4	4.3
Chest pain	2	4.4	1	2.0	3	3.2
Diarrhea	3	6.7	8	16.3	11	11.7
Faintness	0	0.0	1	2.0	1	1.1
Headache	8	17.8	12	24.5	20	21.3
Leg pain	1	2.2	0	0.0	1	1.1
Malaise	5	11.1	1	2.0	6	6.4
Muscle ache	2	4.4	0	0.0	2	2.1
Nausea	3	6.7	6	12.2	9	9.6
Nervousness	5	11.1	0	0.0	5	5.3
Rash with alcohol	2	4.4	1	2.0	3	3.2
Rash without alcohol	1	2.2	3	6.1	4	4.3
Shortness of breath	3	6.7	0	0.0	3	3.2
Swelling of legs	4	8.9	0	0.0	4	4.3
Tremulousness	4	8.9	0	0.0	4	4.3
Vertigo	3	6.7	2	4.1	5	5.3
Vomiting	2	4.4	4	8.2	6	6.4
Weakness	1	2.2	2	4.1	3	3.2
Other	20	44.4	13	26.5	33	35.1

DR GRIFFITH: Like Dr Martelli, we have been interested in the use of a hydroxamate - i.e., acetohydroxamic acid (AHA) for the palliative treatment of chronic urea-splitting urinary infection. We have previously reported experimental, pharmacokinetic and preliminary clinical investigations. Herewith, we report results from a double-blind clinical trial involving Lithostat[TH1] acetohydroxamic acid (AHA) and a placebo (mannitol). Efficacious treatment was defined as reduction of calculogenesis, as determined on sequential plain abdominal radiographs. Stone growth occurred in 8 out of 45 (17%) of the AHA group and in 23 out of 49 (46%) of the placebo group (x^2 = 9.02, P < 0.005). In those patients who were stone-free upon entry, stones occurred in none out of 3 (0%) of the AHA group and in 2 out of 7 (28%) of the placebo group. These sample sizes were too small to be statistically significant. In those patients who had stones in one or both kidneys upon entry,

Table 2. Patient Complaints (Both Tolerable and Intolerable) by Organ System. A Given Patient Commonly had more than One Complaint so that the Number of Symptoms Exceeds the Number of Patients.

	AHA (n = 45)		Placebo (n = 49)	
	Tol	Intol	Tol	Intol
Psychoneurologic Symptoms				
(No. of patients)	14	6	13	2
Headache	8	4	12	2
Malaise	5	2	1	2
Nervousness	5	1	0	0
Tremulousness	4	3	0	1
Gastrointestinal Symptoms				
(No. of patients)	6	3	12	1
Anorexia	2	1	2	0
Diarrhea	3	2	8	0
Nausea	3	1	6	1
Vomiting	2	0	4	1
Dermatologic/Muscular Symptoms				
(No. of patients)	9	7	6	2
Alopecia	1	4	2	1
Leg pain	1	0	0	1
Muscle ache	2	3	0	2
Rash	3	1	4	0
Swelling of legs	4	0	0	1

stone growth for the AHA group was 8 out of 42 (19%) and 21 out of 42 (51%) in the placebo group (x^2 = 8.9, P<0.005).

Tolerable symptoms (Table 1) and intolerable symptoms of a similar type but greater magnitude were more prevalent in the treatment group. Patients in the placebo group had a statistically greater probability of having no symptoms (25/49 = 52%) as compared to the treatment group (10/45 = 22%), (x^2 = 8.32; P<0.01). Patients in the treatment group were also more likely to have treatment discontinued because of side-effects (10/45 = 22.2%) as compared to the placebo group (2/49 = 4.1%, (x^2 = 6.93;P<0.01). Analysis of symptoms by organ system (Table 2) indicates that the treatment group had significantly more psychoneurologic and musculo/integumentary side-effects than the placebo group. No other organ system manifested significant side-effects. We concluded from this study that urease inhibitors in general and that Lithostat[TH] (AHA) in particular retard infection-induced calculogenesis. Long-term treatment is likely to be beneficial in those patients who do not develop intolerable side-effects.

DR RODMAN (NEW YORK, USA): Surgical extirpation of the stone is probably the only therapeutic modality which can cure a patient with staghorn stone disease induced by infection with a urea-splitting organism. For this reason, in an otherwise healthy patient, operative intervention is the treatment of choice for the first occurrence of this disease. Unfortunately, even when the surgeon believes that he has removed all the stone fragments in the operating room, the recurrence rate without adjunctive therapy is at least 30% in 6 years. The development of adjunctive therapies to surgical removal of struvite stones offers hope of improved palliative management. However, each of the adjunctive therapies is associated with significant toxicity. Because infection-induced stones are such a virulent medical problem, the use of these adjunctive modalities is justified, but only if the diagnosis of struvite stone disease is secure.

Hemiacidrin Irrigation

The use of acidic irrigation of the urinary tract was first suggested by Suby in the 1940s. He found that addition of magnesium to a citric acid/citrate buffer reduced irritation of the uroepithelium by a pH 4.0 solution. The magnesium was not added to hasten dissolution of stone material. Even with magnesium present, solutions of pH 4.0 are still quite irritating to the uroepithelium. Suby's original experiments used irrigation of the rabbit bladder to assess toxicity. We repeated his studies with urethral catheters and infusion of various test solutions from above through the ureter which had been exposed by a flank incision. With such a model, overnight irrigations of the urinary tract with saline produced no histological changes in the ureteral or bladder mucosa. By contrast, severe desquamation, submucosal hemorrhage and acute inflammation were produced by both hemiacidrin and a pH 4.0 buffer of 0.1MN citric acid/citrate. When evaluated in blind fashion, the severity of changes was worse without magnesium in the irrigations. However, even the hemiacidrin solution induced dramatic mucosal loss and focal hemorrhage. Since clinical use of hemiacidrin has been associated with radiographic changes, irrigation with this formulation must be reserved for those patients who are likely to benefit from them. They should not be used until a presumptive diagnosis of struvite stone disease is established.

Acetohydroxamic Acid (AHA)

We also have used AHA as a palliative agent and agree that it is effective in reducing the prevalence of infection stone recurrence. We have even seen a case of stone dissolution on AHA and antimicrobial agents. However, the clinical usefulness of AHA may be limited by its toxicities. In addition to the side-effects described earlier, we have encountered several cases of phlebothrombosis - all of which responded to medical treatment.

420

Shorr Regimen/Low-Protein Diet

Uncontrolled clinical studies of phosphate depletion (Shorr Regimen) and canine studies of protein restriction (to reduce urinary urea) have both been reported to retard calculogenesis of infection stones. Osborne has predictably achieved dissolution of struvite stones in dogs using various combinations of dietary protein depletion, urease inhibition and antimicrobial agents. Controlled clinical conformation of these approaches would be meritorious. Unfortunately, all chronic therapy is at risk of poor patient compliance.

VI. TREATMENT
DIETARY THERAPY

THE EFFECT OF "HIGH FIBRE BISCUITS" ON URINARY RISK FACTORS

FOR STONE FORMATION

P. N. Rao, I. L. Jenkins, W. G. Robertson, M. Peacock,
and N. J. Blacklock

Depts. of Urology, University Hospital of South
Manchester, Manchester, and Royal Naval Hospital
Haslar and MRC Mineral Metabolism Unit, The General
Infirmary, Leeds, U.K.

INTRODUCTION

Idiopathic hypercalciuria is a common finding in stone
formers[1-3]. Conversely, a reduction in urinary calcium decreases
the recurrence rate of stone formation[4]. Excessive absorption of
calcium from the intestine is the major cause of hypercalciuria[5]
but an increased consumption of fibre may reduce urinary calcium[3,6]
by binding calcium in the gut. If this is the mechanism by which
fibre reduces urinary calcium, however, there is the risk that more
oxalate might become available for passive absorption. This may
produce marginal hyperoxaluria, as in the case of other calcium-
binding agents, such as cellulose phosphate[7]. The most common form
of fibre supplement is cereal bran which contains a variable
quantity of oxalate. It is not known if this oxalate is "available"
for absorption.

The purposes of this study were to determine the oxalate
content of various types of bran and to measure the intestinal
absorption of calcium and the urinary excretion of calcium and
oxalate following dietary supplementation of soya bran produced from
hulls of soya beans.

PATIENTS AND METHODS

The oxalate contents of soya, rice, wheat and corn brans were
determined after de-fatting and acid extraction[8]. Eight healthy
male volunteers with no history of stone disease and 22 patients
with proven urolithiasis were included in a study to examine the
effect of specially formulated soya bran biscuits containing

4 to 4.5 g fibre, 7 g carbohydrate, 2.6 g fat and 1.3 g protein per biscuit. The biscuits were manufactured by Welfare Foods, Stockport, U.K. and Anglo-Dietetics Ltd., Wilton, U.S.A.

In 20 patients intestinal absorption of [47]Ca was measured by an external isotope counting method[9]. The investigation was repeated 2 to 4 weeks later, when 2 soya bran biscuits were ingested 15 min prior to the oral dose of [47]Ca.

Eleven stone formers with known hypercalciuria (9 of whom participated in the above study) and the 8 healthy subjects were studied as follows. On 3 consecutive days 24-h specimens of urine were collected. All subjects were given soya bran in the form of 2 biscuits to be taken before the 3 main meals of the day for 7 days. During the last 3 days of the regime, 24-h specimens of urine were again collected. The subjects were asked to keep other dietary factors constant as far as possible throughout the trial. After noting the volume, the urines were analysed for creatinine, calcium, magnesium, phosphate, oxalate and uric acid.

RESULTS

The oxalate contents of the brans (mg/100 g) were soya 17, wheat 240, rice 123, and corn 7.

In the normal subjects there was no significant difference in the urinary excretion of any of the parameters measured before and while taking the biscuits (Table 1). In the patients the intestinal absorption of [47]Ca was elevated before treatment in each patient, ranging from 36 to 98% (mean 64%) (normal range 25 to 35%). This was reduced in all the patients while taking soya bran to 6 to 59% (mean 29%) ($P < 0.001$). In 13 patients, calcium absorption returned to normal (Fig. 1).

The mean daily urinary calcium excretion of the 11 patients was 7.76 to 14.5 mmol/day (mean 9.7 $\pm$ 1.97) before treatment. This was

Table 1. Urinary Biochemical Profile of Health Subjects Before and While Taking Soya Bran Biscuits (Mean $\pm$ SD).

Urinary Excretion	Before (mmol/day)	After (mmol/day)
Calcium	4.5 $\pm$ 1.9	4.4 $\pm$ 2.1
Magnesium	5.4 $\pm$ 1.8	5.8 $\pm$ 2.0
Inorganic Phosphate	29.9 $\pm$ 7.4	31.1 $\pm$ 5.2
Uric acid	4.3 $\pm$ 0.8	4.24 $\pm$ 0.9
Oxalate	0.42 $\pm$ 0.06	0.40 $\pm$ 0.06

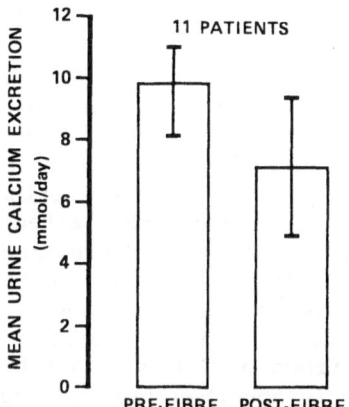

Fig. 1. ^{47}Calcium absorption before and while taking soya bran biscuits.

reduced to 3.62 to 11.36 mmol/day (mean 7.29 ± 2.09) while taking the biscuits. Calcium excretion was reduced in all the cases except one (P<0.01) (Fig. 2). Urinary oxalate did not increase in the 2 patients in whom it was measured.

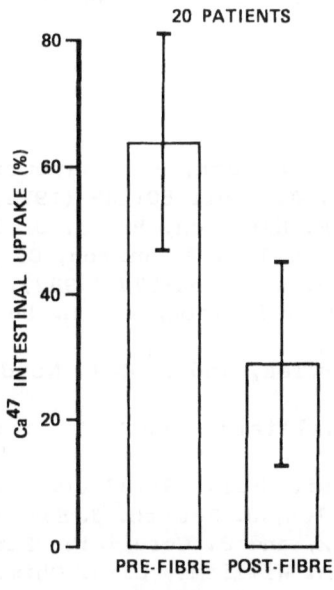

INTESTINAL ABSORPTION
OF CALCIUM

Fig. 2. Urinary calcium excretion (mmol/day) before and while taking soya bran biscuits.

427

DISCUSSION

Hyperabsorption of calcium has been shown to be the most common cause of hypercalciuria[8]. Calcium-binding agents have been successfully used to treat this type of hypercalciuria. Dietary supplements, such as fibre, either alone or along with other dietary measures have also been shown to reduce urinary calcium[3,6]. The mechanism by which fibre produces this effect is not known. It has been suggested that the phytate in fibre binds with calcium in the intestine and prevents its absorption. Alternatively, fibre may reduce the time available for calcium absorption by reducing intestinal transit time[6]. Another possible mechanism is the "nutrient dilution" effect of fibre. A fibre-rich diet reduces the rate at which glucose is absorbed from the gut[11] and this reduces the glucose-mediated insulin response shown to be abnormally high in stone-formers[12]. This mechanism certainly could explain why, in the present study, soya bran biscuits failed to reduce the calcium excretion in the normal subjects.

Whatever the mechanism involved, this study confirms that addition of soya bran fibre to the diet reduces the urinary excretion of calcium in hypercalciuric stone formers. It also appears that soya bran fibre consumption does not increase the excretion of oxalate in the urine. Since the biscuits used in this study are very palatable, they can be expected to encourage compliance by patients.

REFERENCES

1. W. G. Robertson, M. Peacock, P. J. Heyburn, D. H. Marshall, and P. B. Clark, Br. J. Urol. 50:449 (1978).
2. G. A. Rose and A. R. Harrison, Br. J. Urol. 46:261 (1974).
3. P. N. Rao, V. Prendiville, A. Buxton, D. G. Moss, and N. J. Blacklock, Br. J. Urol. 54:578 (1982).
4. P. J. Heyburn, W. G. Robertson, and M. Peacock, Nephron 32:314 (1982).
5. M. Peacock, F. Knowles, and B. E. C. Nordin, Br. Med. J. 2:729 (1968).
6. P. J. R. Shah, G. Williams, and N. A. Green, Br. J. Urol. 52:426 (1980).
7. C. Y. C. Pak, Invest. Urol. 19:187 (1981).
8. M. Fuss, D. Verbeelen, J. Geurts, J. Simon, A. Bergans, M. DeBacker, R. Six, and J. Coruilain, Eur. Urol. 4:324 (1978).
9. A. Hodgkinson and A. Williams, Clin. Chim. Acta 36:127 (1972).
10. M. MacLeod, J. Roy. Nav. Med. Ser. 57:88 (1971).
11. G. B. Haber, K. W. Heaton, and D. Murphy, Lancet 2:679 (1977).
12. P. N. Rao, C. Gordon, D. Davies, and N. J. Blacklock, Br. J.Urol. 54:575 (1982).

IS SALT RESTRICTION NECESSARY TO REDUCE THE RISK

OF STONE FORMATION?

P. N. Rao, E. B. Faraghar, A. Buxton,
V. Prendiville, and N. J. Blacklock

University Hospital of South Manchester
Manchester M20 8LR, U.K.

INTRODUCTION

Several studies have demonstrated a close association between idiopathic hypercalciuria and upper urinary tract stone disease. The cause of the hypercalciuria is not totally understood, but it is well known that the tubular reabsorption of sodium and calcium are closely related[1]. Studies in animals and man suggest that dietary and urinary sodium may influence urinary calcium excretion[2,3]. Except for a few isolated reports, however, there is little information on the role of dietary sodium in idiopathic hypercalciuria. We have examined the relationship between urinary sodium and calcium in a group of stone formers and investigated the effect of dietary sodium restriction in those who were hypercalciuric.

PATIENTS AND METHODS

The urinary data from 363 calcium oxalate stone formers were reviewed retrospectively. All patients supplied three 24-h specimens of urine whilst on a free diet at home and without medication. The mean urinary sodium and calcium excretions of each patient were calculated and the data analysed statistically. In a separate prospective study, 7 male stone formers (aged 43 to 63; mean = 53 years) with idiopathic hypercalciuria were investigated. Prior to the study they were interviewed by a dietitian who assessed their dietary intake of factors known to influence urinary calcium excretion and gave advice on how to keep these constant during the 12-day period of the trial. Twenty-four-hour urines were collected on 3 consecutive days after which they were prescribed a low sodium diet (Na < 100 mmol/day) by the same dietitian. This is the "no

added salt " diet frequently used in hospitals. They were allowed
to establish themselves on this diet for 5 days and 24-h urines
collected on 3 subsequent days.

RESULTS

There is a weak but statistically significant correlation
between urinary sodium and calcium (Spearman's r = 0.361; P<0.001;
Fig. 1). The correlation did not change when normocalciurics were
excluded.   The mean (+ SD) calcium value was 5.1 + 0.3 mmol/day
(normal < 7 mmol/day) and that for sodium was 175 + 58 mmol/day
(normal < 200 mmol/day).   Urinary calcium and sodium were normal in
215 (59%) patients, 88 (25%) were hypercalciuric and 101 (28%) had
hypernatriuria.   Forty-seven percent of hypercalciuric patients had
hypernatriuria whereas only 21% of normocalciurics excreted
excessive amounts of sodium (χ^2 = 19.16; P<0.001).

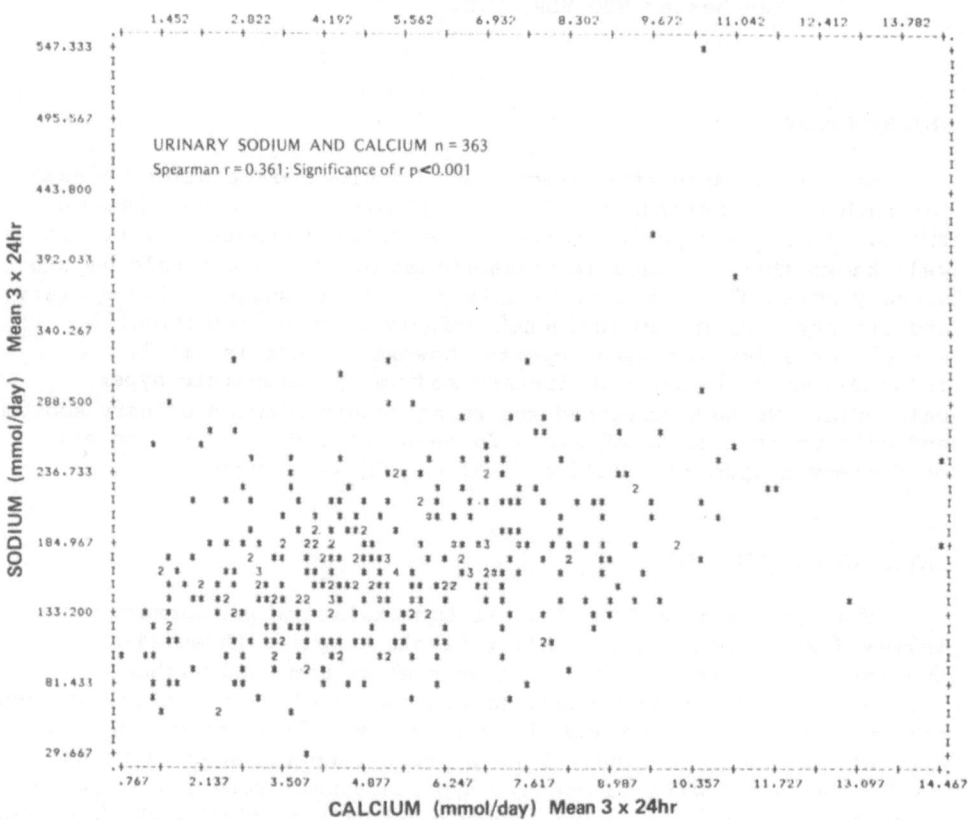

Fig. 1. Correlation between urinary sodium and calcium excretion
in stone-formers.

430

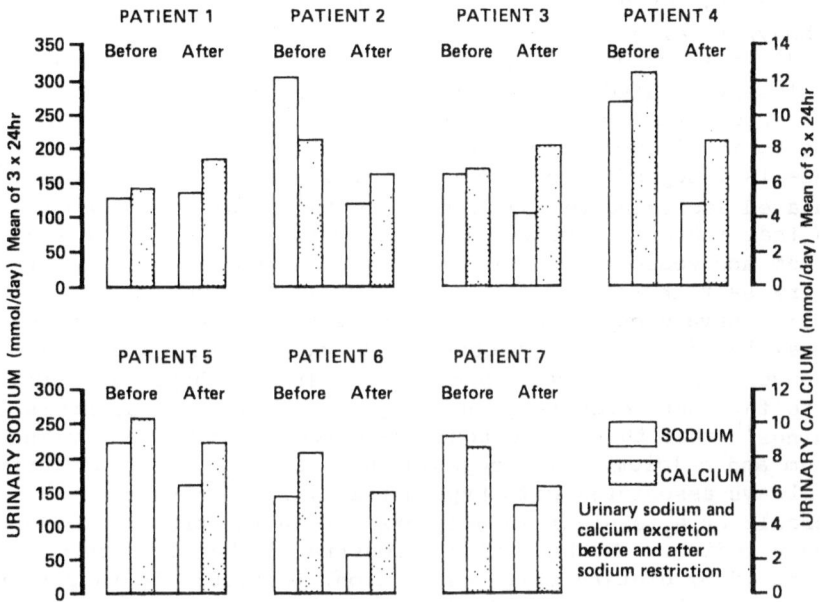

Fig. 2. Urinary sodium and calcium excretion (mean of 3 x 24-h
values) before and after dietary sodium restriction.

In the second study, urinary sodium exceeded 200 mmol/day in 4
patients. Urinary calcium dropped appreciably in all 4 following
sodium restriction. In one patient, it was reduced even although
the urinary sodium was only 147 mmol/day prior to advice. This
patient, however, managed to curtail his sodium intake quite
significantly as his urinary sodium was reduced to 53 mmol/day
after dietary advice. In the other two patients with normal sodium
excretion, calcium excretion, if anything, increased after salt
restriction. One of these may not have adhered to the advice as
his urinary sodium did not change after dietary advice (Fig. 2).

DISCUSSION

Flocks[4] was the first to recognize an association between
hypercalciuria and upper urinary tract stone. A few years later
Albright et al[5] described a group of stone-formers with
hypercalciuria, normal serum calcium and hypophosphataemia. Since
a cause for this was not identifiable, the term "idiopathic"
hypercalciuria was used. This is widely in use now although
several dietary and metabolic causes for hypercalciuria have since
been identified[6-8]. There is, however, a sub-group of patients in
whom the cause is unknown and their hypercalciuria is often
resistant to common methods of treatment.

Sodium, which plays an essential role in cellular functions of the body, is also a prominent constituent of the modern diet. It is well known that the renal tubular transport of sodium and calcium are closely related. About 80% of filtered calcium is reabsorbed in the proximal tubule and the thick ascending loop where calcium reabsorption is sodium-dependent. Reabsorption in the distal tubule is independent of sodium and here calcium excretion is regulated according to body requirements[1]. Walser[3] demonstrated in dogs that there is a direct relation between the renal clearances of calcium and sodium. Studies on humans demonstrated that increasing dietary salt increases urinary calcium excretion[2,9]. Sutton and Walker[10] have shown a positive correlation between urinary sodium and calcium in normal subjects and stone formers. In spite of this evidence, the role played by dietary sodium in hypercalciuria has not so far been adequately investigated. This study confirms the findings[10] that there is a positive correlation between urinary sodium and calcium. It suggests that although hypercalciuria is not always associated with hypernatriuria, the risk of hypercalciuria is significantly greater in the presence of a high urinary sodium. We have also demonstrated that urinary calcium can be reduced by dietary salt restriction, particularly in patients with concomitant hypernatriuria. We suggest that urinary sodium should be measured routinely in idiopathic calcium stone formers. Salt restriction should be advised if the urinary sodium excretion is high, as it appears to contribute to idiopathic hypercalciuria.

REFERENCES

1. R. A. L. Sutton, and J. H. Dirks, in:"The Kidney",
   B. M. Brenner and F. C. Rector, eds., W. B. Saunders,
   Philadelphia (1981).
2. C. R. Kleeman, J. Bohannan, D. Bernstein, S. Ling, and
   M. H. Maxwell, Proc. Soc. Ex. Biol. Med. 115:29 (1964).
3. M. Walser, Am. J. Physiol. 200:1099 (1961).
4. R. H. Flocks, J. Am. Mech. Assoc. 113:1466 (1939).
5. F. Albright, P. Henneman, P. H. Benedict, and A. P. Forbes,
   Proc. Roy. Soc. Med. 46:1077 (1953).
6. J. A. Thom, J. E. Morris, A. Bishop, and N. J. Blacklock,
   Br. J. Urol. 50:459 (1978).
7. W. G. Robertson, M. Peacock, P. J. Heyburn, F. A. Hanes,
   A. Rutherford, E. Clementson, R. Swaminathan, P. B. Clark,
   Br. J. Urol. 51:427 (1979).
8. P. N. Rao, C. Gordon, C. Davies, and N. J. Blacklock,
   Br. J.Urol. 54:575 (1982).
9. F. P. Muldowney, Kidney Int. 16:637 (1979).
10. R. A. L. Sutton and V. R. Walker, in:"Urolithiasis:Clinical and
    Basic Research", L. H. Smith, W. G. Robertson and
    B. Finlayson, eds., Plenum, New York (1980).

RESTRICTED CALCIUM DIET AND CALCIUM OXALATE UROLITHIASIS

Y. Berland, M. Olmer, M. Grandvuillemin, and
R. Calaf

Service de Néphrologie, Hôpital de la Conception, and
Laboratoire de Biochimie, Hôpital de la Timone
13005 Marseille, France

INTRODUCTION

Urinary excretion of oxalate plays an important role in the formation of calcium oxalate crystals[1] and stones[2]. Elevated oxaluria has been observed in stone-forming patients with hyper-calciuria[3,4]. This hyperoxaluria might be explained by an increase in the intestinal absorption of calcium leading to a decrease in the intestinal concentration of calcium thereby reducing the complexation of calcium with oxalate and favouring the intestinal absorption of oxalate[5].

We have studied a group of hypercalciuric patients with recurrent urinary lithiasis in order to assess the influence of dietary calcium restriction on oxaluria and on urinary supersaturation of calcium oxalate.

PATIENTS AND METHODS

Sixty stone-forming patients, 38 males and 22 females aged 38.8 $\pm$ 11 years (mean $\pm$ SD), with urinary calcium excretions > 0.1 mmol/kg/24 h were studied at the end of the two 4-day periods, period 1 (P1) and period 2 (P2). During P1, the patients were placed on a diet containing 1 g of calcium; during P2, 400 mg calcium were given daily. Oxalic acid intake was not modified between P1 and P2. All foodstuffs rich in oxalic acid were excluded. The daily sodium intake was 6 g.

Calciuria was measured by conventional methods and oxaluria by gas chromatography. The supersaturation of urine with respect to

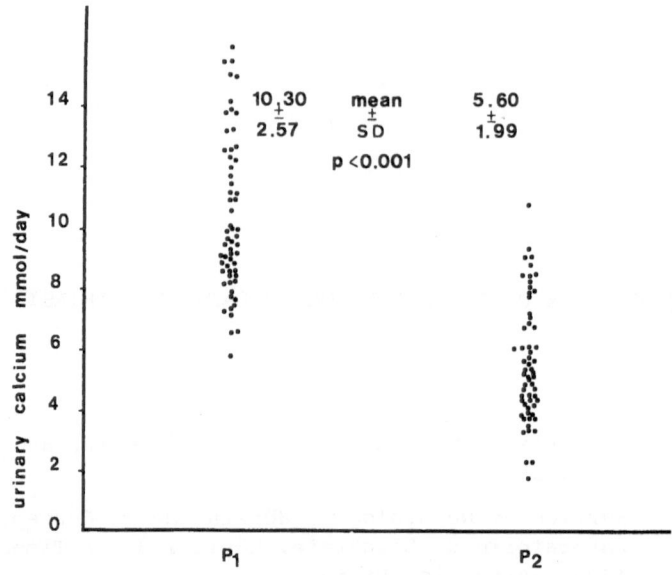

Fig. 1. Urinary calcium excretion during the 1 g (P1) and 400 mg (P2) calcium diets.

calcium oxalate was determined according to the procedure published by Marshall and Robertson[6].

RESULTS

The mean 24-h urinary calcium excretion during P2, following dietary calcium restriction, was significantly lower than that during P1 (5.6 $\pm$ 1.99 mmol/24-h vs 10.30 $\pm$ 2.57 mmol/24-h ($P < 0.001$)) (Fig. 1). The mean values of oxaluria were equivalent at the end of the two periods (during P1 : 0.40 $\pm$ 0.39 mmol/24-h; during P2 : 0.41 $\pm$ 0.28 mmol/24-h) (Fig. 2). The mean daily urinary volume measured during the 2 periods P1 and P2 was 1.670 $\pm$ 0.600 and 1.800 $\pm$ 0.810 litres respectively (n.s.). The urinary relative calcium oxalate supersaturation was on average 0.93 $\pm$ 0.21 during P1 and 0.84 $\pm$ 0.22 during P2 (n.s.) (Fig. 3). A value greater than 1, i.e. above the formation product, was noted in 21 patients during P1 and in only 12 patients during P2. Of the 12 patients, 9 presented a value greater than 1 at P1 while three had a value lower than 1. The increase of oxaluria between P1 and P2 explains the increase of the calcium oxalate relative supersaturation in these 3 patients. The mean urinary oxalate/calcium ratio increased significantly after dietary calcium restriction (during P1 : 0.041 $\pm$ 0.036; during P2 : 0.079 $\pm$ 0.66)($P < 0.05$).

434

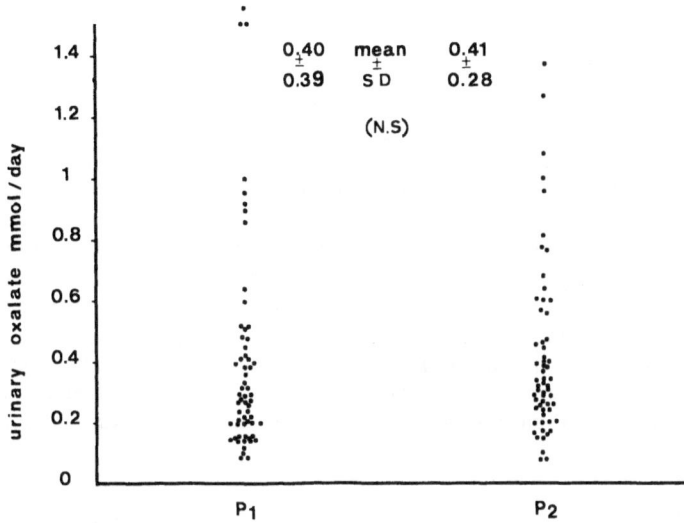

Fig. 2. Urinary oxalate during the 1 g calcium (P1) and 400 mg (P2) calcium diets.

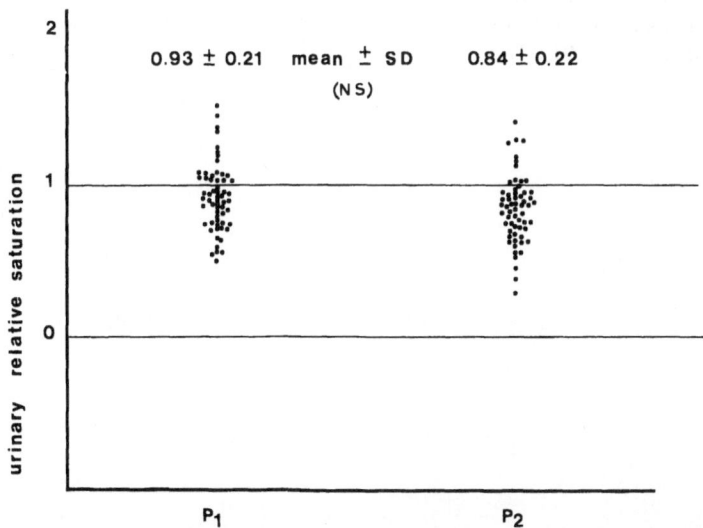

Fig. 3. Calcium oxalate urinary relative supersaturation during the 1 g (P1) and 400 mg (P2) calcium diets.

DISCUSSION

Oxaluria has an important effect on urinary calcium oxalate supersaturation[1]. Our results show that dietary calcium reduction from 1 g to 400 mg is not followed by an increase of oxaluria, whereas the calciuria decreases, such that the urine supersaturation with respect to calcium oxalate does not rise.

However, the increase of the oxalate/calcium ratio may promote the formation of crystals of greater dimensions[1] in patients whose urine is supersaturated with calcium oxalate. In our experience only 9 patients (i.e. 15%) might be exposed to this risk. This study confirms the results reported by Pak et al[7] that the imposition of a low calcium dietary regimen in stone-formers with hypercalciuria does not necessarily augment oxalate excretion.

REFERENCES

1. W. G. Robertson, D. S. Scurr, and C. M. Bridge, J. Cryst. Growth, 53:182 (1981).
2. B. Baggio, G. Gambaro, S. Favaro, and A. Borsatti, Nephron 35:11 (1983).
3. P. M. Zarembski and A. Hodgkinson, Clin. Chim. Acta 25:1 (1969).
4. W. G. Robertson and M Peacock, Nephron 26:105 (1980).
5. A. Hodgkinson, Clin. Sci. Mol. Med. 54:291 (1978).
6. R. W. Marshall and W. G. Robertson, Clin. Chim. Acta 72 (1976).
7. R. Galosy, L. Clarke, D. L. Ward, and C. Y. C. Pak, J. Urol. 123:320 (1980).

PYROPHOSPHATE EXCRETION IN VARIOUS GROUPS OF CALCIUM STONE-

FORMERS: EFFECT OF A CALCIUM-RESTRICTED DIET

P. Bataille, B. Lacour, J. B. Roullet, M. Finet, I. Grégoire,
P. Fiévet, and A. Fournier

Service de Néphrologie, Laboratoire de Biochimie, Hôpital
Necker, Paris, Laboratoire de Biochimie, C.H.U., Amiens
France

INTRODUCTION

The role of inhibitors of crystallization seems important since
urine is frequently supersaturated with respect to calcium oxalate
and calcium phosphate[1]. Inorganic pyrophosphate is one of several
ions in urine which can inhibit the precipitation of calcium salts
in vitro[2] but reports in the literature on the importance of this
inhibitor have been conflicting[3,4]. These discrepancies may be
explained by various factors which can affect pyrophosphate
excretion, such as the urinary excretion of calcium and the dietary
intake of phosphate[5].

The present study was undertaken to determine whether or not
pyrophosphate excretion is different in various groups of stone-
formers classified according to their calcium excretion and whether
or not calcium restriction, which induces a simultaneous phosphate
restriction because of the elimination of dairy products from the
diet, affects the urinary excretion of pyrophosphate.

METHODS

Twelve controls and 62 calcium stone-formers were studied on an
ambulatory protocol. They collected their 24-h urines on a free
diet and after 4 days on a low-calcium diet which provided
approximately 400 mg of calcium/day. In the 24-h urine
collections, performed on each diet, we measured creatinine,
calcium, phosphate, sodium and pyrophosphate. After calcium
restriction, blood samples were analyzed for calcium, phosphate, and
creatinine by AutoAnalyzer and alkaline phosphatase and parathormone

Table 1. Urinary Excretion of Phosphate and Pyrophosphate Before and After Calcium Restriction in Controls and in Various Groups of Ca Stone Formers (Mean ± SEM).

	n	Free Diet			Ca-Restricted Diet		
		Pi (mmol/day)	PPi (μmol/day)	PPi/Pi (10^{-3})	Pi (mmol/day)	Pi (μmol/day)	PPi/Pi (10^{-3})
Control	12	26 ± 1	43 ± 1.0	1.51 ± 0.2	22 ± 1	30 ± 5	1.17 ± 0.2
N Ca	27	30 ± 1	30 ± 0.3	1.08 ± 0.1*	29 ± 1	28 ± 1	1.05 ± 0.
DH	14	33 ± 2	29 ± 6.0	0.84 ± 0.2*	28 ± 1	25 ± 5	0.9 ± 0.2
IH	21	33 ± 2	27 ± 0.5$	0.84 ± 0.1**	°29 ± 1	22 ± 3 *o*	0.74 ± 0.1*

Difference between stone formers and controls: *P < 0.05, **P < 0.01.

Change induced by calcium restriction: P < 0.05.

NCa = normocalciuric; DH = diet-dependent hypercalciuria; IH = idiopathic hypercalciuria.

(C-terminal assay). Urinary pyrophosphate was determined by an enzymatic method with a centrifugal analyser (E.N.I. Gemsaec)[6].

From our previously published control values[7], we classified the 62 calcium stone-formers according to calcium excretion. Twenty-seven were normocalciuric (NCa) (calciuria $<$ 0.1 mmol/kg/day); 14 patients who were hypercalciuric on a free diet had a diet-dependent hypercalciuria (DH), a diagnosis based on the return to normal of urinary calcium excretion after calcium restriction, when compared to controls on the same restricted diet (calciuria $<$ 0.01 mmol/kg/day); and idiopathic hypercalciuria (IH) was found in 21 subjects who were hypercalciuric on a free diet and on a restricted diet (calciuria $>$ 0.1 mmol/kg/day on free diet; calciuria $>$ 0.07 mmol/kg/day on calcium restricted diet).

RESULTS

Table 1 shows the values of urinary pyrophosphate (PPi), phosphate (PO_4) and the pyrophosphate/phosphate ratio (PPi/PO_4) in controls and in the various groups of calcium stone-formers on a free diet and after calcium restriction. When compared to the control values, PPi was significantly lower only in IH group on both the free and calcium-restricted diets. Calcium-restriction induced a significant decrease (P $<$ 0.05) in PO_4 and PPi only in patients with IH. Because of the possible effect of the phosphate load on the excretion of PPi we determined the ratio PPi/PO_4 in each control and in each stone-former on both diets. On the free diet the PPi/PO_4 ratio was significantly lower in each group of patients when compared to the control values. After calcium restriction the PPi/PO_4 ratio remained significantly lower only in patients with IH. Calcium restriction induced no significant changes in this ratio. There were direct correlations between PO_4 and PPi in patients (r = 0.31, P $<$ 0.02) and in controls (r = 0.449, P $<$ 0.02) on their free diet. After calcium restriction, the correlation disappeared in controls (r = 0.27) but remained in stone formers (r = 0.36; P $<$ 0.02). The variations in PO_4 and PPi induced by calcium restriction were well correlated in the controls (P $<$ 0.01) and in the stone formers (P $<$ 0.01). There was a positive correlation between PO_4 and PPi only in the patients with IH, before and after calcium restriction (on a free diet: r = 0.400, P $<$ 0.02; after calcium restriction r = 0.60, P $<$ 0.01). The correlation between PO_4 and PPi induced by calcium restriction was found only in the group with IH (r = 0.53, P $<$ 0.02).

DISCUSSION

The correlations between PO_4 and PPi confirm that PO_4 and PPi excretions are closely linked in both normal subjects and stone formers. This link between PO_4 and PPi have been found previously especially after supplementation with orthophosphate[5]. The resulting increase in urinary pyrophosphate has been considered as the mechanism by which this treatment prevents recurrence of stone formation. The striking relationship between urinary PPi and PO_4 may depend upon a direct action of orthophosphate on the kidney. The infusion of orthophosphate directly into one kidney of the dog causes a greater increase in the excretion of PPi from the infused kidney as compared to the contralateral side[5]. This suggests that there is decreased tubular reabsorption of pyrophosphate owing to competition with orthophosphate for a common transport mechanism. The fact that the relationship between PO_4 and PPi excretion was strongest in the IH group further supports this hypothesis. This disorder is frequently associated with a decreased TRP[8] and thus the dependency of pyrophosphate excretion on the filtered load of PO_4 may be anticipated to be greater since the competition for tubular reabsorption is greater. A significantly lower excretion of PPi in urine was observed in this study only in patients with IH, but the urinary PPi/PO_4 ratio on a free diet was lower in all stone-forming groups when compared to controls. Russell and Fleisch[5] observed a decrease in PPi excretion in the urine only in male stone formers aged 30 to 40 years. This was not present in the other age groups of stone formers[5]. Although our study was not performed with a control population matched with respect to age and sex, our data are in agreement with those of Wikström et al[9] who noted a significantly lower PPi excretion in stone formers with impaired renal acidification capacity and possibly hypercalciuria since impaired renal acidification capacity is frequently associated with idiopathic hypercalciuria.

REFERENCES

1. B. E. C. Nordin and W. G. Robertson, Br. Med. J. 1:450 (1966).
2. H. Fleisch and S. Bisaz, Am. J. Physiol. 203:671 (1962).
3. R. G. G. Russell, N. A. Edwards, and A. Hodgkinson, Lancet, 1:466 (1964).
4. M. M. O'Brien, I. Uhlemann, and H. W. McIntosh, Canad. Med. Ass. J. 96:100 (1967).
5. R. G. G. Russell and H. Fleisch, in:"Proceedings of the Renal Stone Research Symposium", A. Hodgkinson and B. E. C. Nordin, eds., Churchill, London (1969).
6. J. B. Roullet, B. Lacour, A. Ullmann, and M. Bailly, Clin. Chem. 28:134 (1982).
7. P. Bataille, G. Charransol, A. Pruna, and A. Fournier, J. Urol. 130:218 (1983).
8. F. P. Muldowney, R. Freaney, and J. G. Ryan, Quart. J. Med. 49:193 (1980).
9. B. Wikström, B. G. Danielson, S. Ljunghall, M. McGuire, and R. G. G. Russell, Scand. J. Urol. Nephrol. Suppl. 61:1 (1981).

THE USE OF WHEAT BRAN TO DECREASE CALCIUM EXCRETION AND TO

TREAT CALCIUM OXALATE STONE DISEASE

K. Jarrar, V. Graef, and W. Guttmann

Dept. of Urology and Institute of Clinical Chemistry
and Pathobiochemistry, University of Giessen, F.R.G.

INTRODUCTION

There are conflicting reports on the effect of long-term administration of wheat bran on plasma calcium and the urinary excretion of calcium. Heaton and Pomare[1] gave their patients 38 g of bran daily for 4 to 9 weeks and found a significant decrease in plasma calcium. In contrast, Brodribb and Humphreys[2] administered 24 g of wheat bran daily for 6 months and described a significant decrease in calcium excretion without a change in plasma calcium. Other authors[3] have found that bulk material is able to bind calcium. In one-third of the patients with calcium oxalate stones idiopathic hypercalciuria is present and is usually treated by reduction of milk and milk products or by administration of thiazides. Based on these and other observations[4,5] we have used wheat bran to decrease the urinary excretion of calcium as a treatment for calcium oxalate stones.

METHODS

Twenty patients (9 male and 11 female) with idiopathic hypercalciuria and calcium oxalate stone formation were given 24 g of wheat bran daily. The patients took the wheat bran either in one portion in the morning or distributed in 2 or 3 portions over the day. One day before therapy, Na, K, Ca, P, creatinine and uric acid were determined in urine and plasma. In addition, Mg, citrate, oxalate, Fe, Zn and Ca were measured in 24-h urine collections. The same constituents were determined at intervals of 6 weeks for about 9 months. At the beginning of the study the patients had no stones and were symptom-free. Four patients stopped the treatment

Table 1. Effect of Wheat Bran on Urinary Composition in Calcium
Oxalate Stone Patients (mean $\pm$ SD).

Constituent	Before therapy (mmol/24 h)	During therapy (mmol/24 h)	P
Calcium	11.31 $\pm$ 5.30	6.06 $\pm$ 2.52	<0.02
Sodium	265.0 $\pm$ 95.3	280.9 $\pm$ 179.2	
Potassium	81.1 $\pm$ 39.6	76.3 $\pm$ 42.8	
Phosphorus	40.9 $\pm$ 14.9	33.1 $\pm$ 10.5	
Magnesium	3.78 $\pm$ 0.99	3.21 $\pm$ 1.85	
Citric acid	2.94 $\pm$ 1.82	2.38 $\pm$ 1.70	
Uric acid	6.15 $\pm$ 2.44	5.31 $\pm$ 2.16	
Oxalic acid	0.23 $\pm$ 0.17	0.25 $\pm$ 0.17	
Creatinine	20.1 $\pm$ 6.5	17.1 $\pm$ 6.8	
Fe (x 10^{-3})	19.6 $\pm$ 12.2	5.6 $\pm$ 2.9	<0.001
Zn (x 10^{-3})	12.0 $\pm$ 9.5	8.4 $\pm$ 5.6	
Cu (x 10^{-3})	1.7 $\pm$ 0.9	1.5 $\pm$ 0.5	

in the first weeks (diarrhoea and flatulence in two of them).
Therefore, only 16 patients could be treated and studied throughout.

RESULTS AND DISCUSSION

The mean values of the urinary constituents before and during
treatment are shown in Table 1. There was a marked fall in calcium
and iron excretion during treatment with wheat bran. In only one
patient did calcium excretion not change. He had colic followed by
passage of a calcium oxalate stone. Urinary oxalate in the 16
patients increased up to the 18th week of treatment and decreased

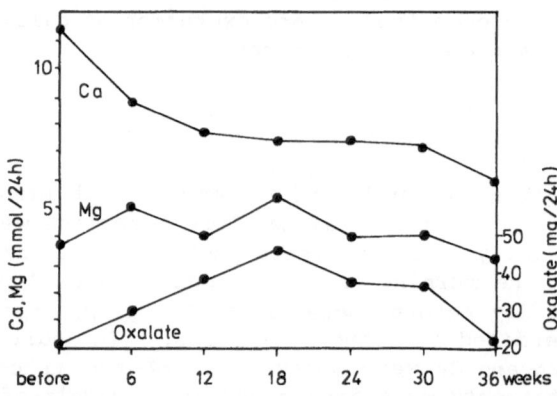

Fig. 1. Excretion of calcium, magnesium and oxalate during wheat
bran therapy.

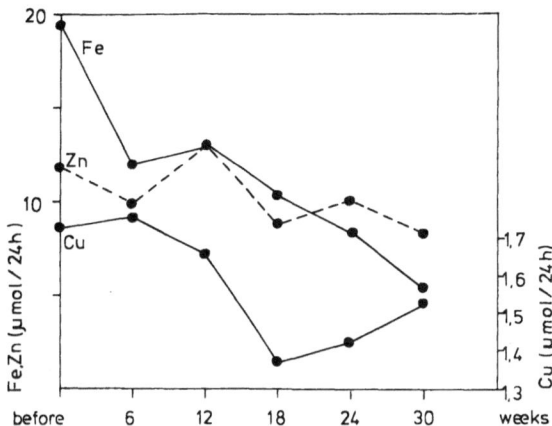

Fig. 2. Excretion of iron, zinc and copper during wheat bran
         therapy.

thereafter (Fig. 1).   No significant change was noted in the other
urinary constituents except iron (Fig. 2).   The decrease in iron
excretion is important, since it is known that iron stimulates the
growth of calcium oxalate and hydroxyapatite crystals.   There was
no change in the concentrations of the measured ions in serum.   All
patients except one were without stones and without complaints
following the wheat bran therapy and the obstipation disappeared in
part.

     This study shows that wheat bran therapy leads to a decrease of
the calcium and iron excretion.   Wheat bran is suitable for
reducing hypercalciuria in calcium oxalate stone formation and it is
a "natural" alternative to thiazide therapy.   We can recommend
it in the preventative therapy of calcium stones.

REFERENCES

1. K. W. Heaton and E. W. Pomare, Lancet 1:49 (1974).
2. A. I. M. Brodribb and D. M. Humphreys, Br. Med. J. 1:424 (1976).
3. W. P. T. James, W. J. Branch, and D. A. T. Southgate, Lancet
   1:638 (1978).
4. P. H. Henneman, P. H. Benedict, A. P. Forbes, and R. H. Dudley,
   New Engl. J. Med. 259:802 (1958).
5. P. J. R. Shaf, G. Williams, and N. A. Green, in:"Urolithiasis,
   Clinical and Basic Research", L. H. Smith, W. G. Robertson,
   and B. Finlayson, eds., Plenum, New York (1981).

Fig. 2. ... zinc and copper during wheat growth.

Since 1965, ... No significant change were noted in the other ... concentration during growth (Fig. 2). The decrease in zinc and copper in ... growth ... In knowledge from literatures, the ... calcium, potassium and hydroxyapatite crystallne, there was some visible concentration of ... the seedling form. In maize, all these ... ... and ... the grain loss ... and the distribution disappeared in part.

... ... some phase into wheat seed factory made to a decrease of ... calcium, ... potassium ... wheat from ... table. For ... observed ... a soluble oxidative urease formation and ... the result of a ... in wheat through ... the can ... ... in the cumulative therapy of cellular shoots ...

1. K. W. Henderson and D. Bronner, Cancer 3, 20 (1956).
2. E. L. A. McComb and O. W. Richardson, ... 3, ... 1965.
3. R. S. W. Jakes, W. I. Mayer, and O. W. ... R. L. ..., 122W (1973).
4. ... Newtonian, ... 2, ... and R. ..., Cancer Res., 3, 2 Cell, 750-174 1965.
5. P. L. Hart, J. Williams, R. L. ..., ..., ..., ...
   ... and R. ... ..., New York (1971).

CRITICAL ROLE OF OXALATE RESTRICTION IN ASSOCIATION WITH CALCIUM
RESTRICTION TO DECREASE THE PROBABILITY OF BEING A STONE FORMER:
INSUFFICIENT EFFECT IN IDIOPATHIC HYPERCALCIURIA

P. Bataille, A. Fournier, I. Grégoire, G. Charransol,
M. A. Hervé, and A. Pruna

Service de Néphrologie, Hôpital Nord, Amiens, Institute
d'Hydrologie, Hôpital Pitié-Salpêtrière, Paris, and
Unité de Mathématiques Appliquées de l'Université de
Picardie, Amiens, France

INTRODUCTION

Calcium and oxalate are the main urinary risk factors for
calcium stone formation. Many therapeutic measures have been tried
in an attempt to reduce the concentrations of these risk factors in
urine. A low calcium diet has been a popular form of therapy since
many authors have described the high incidence of hypercalciuria in
stone formers. Unfortunately, it is well-documented that calcium
restriction induces an increase in oxalate excretion[1-3].

Because of this inverse relationship between oxaluria and
calciuria after calcium restriction, we have studied the final
effect of a low calcium + low oxalate diet in stone formers by the
changes of the "probability of being a stone former", (the P_{SF} of
Robertson), a parameter which combines urinary oxalate and calcium
excretion[4].

MATERIALS AND METHODS

A total of 42 patients with calcium urolithiasis were studied
as out-patients. They collected 24-h urines on 4 regimens: (i) on a
free diet, (ii) after 4 days on a low calcium + low oxalate diet,
(iii) after an oxalate load (200 g of frozen spinach) while on
either a 1 g calcium diet or (iv) on a 400 mg calcium diet.
Calcium restriction was obtained by exclusion of all dairy products
and oxalate restriction by exclusion of foods with a high oxalate
content. Creatinine, calcium and oxalate were measured in the 24-h
urine collections. The probability of being a stone former (P_{SF})
was determined as published elsewhere[1,4].

Table 1. The Urinary Data on Various Diets.

Stone formers	Free diet			Low Ca + Low Ox diet			Oxalate load			
							lgCa		Low Ca	
	UCaV mg/day	UOxV mg/day	P_{SF}	UCaV mg/day	UOxV mg/day	P_{SF}	ΔUOx mg/day	P_{SF}	ΔUOx mg/day	P_{SF}
NCa	185	39	0.56	144***	44	0.44*	+6	+0.08	+25	+0.28
D.H.	403	42	0.80	166***	40	0.48**	+4	+0.06	+30	+0.36
I.H.	423	33	0.77	282***	39*	0.68	+6	+0.02	+25	+0.24

Significance of the difference between free diet and low Ca+ low Ox diet *P<0.05; **P<0.01; ***P<0.001. Significance of the variations of oxaluria and of P_{SF} with Ox load P<0.01.

RESULTS

Of the 42 patients 18 were normocalciuric (NCa) (calciuria < 4 mg/kg/day), 7 patients had a diet-dependent hypercalciuria (DH) in which the diagnosis was based on the normalization of calciuria after calcium restriction (calciuria < 3 mg/kg/day) and 17 patients had idiopathic hypercalciuria (IH) (i.e. calciuria > 4 mg/kg/day on a free diet, and calcium > 3 mg/kg/day on a calcium-restricted diet). The effects of the double dietary restriction on calcium and oxalate excretion, and on the P_{SF} are shown in Table 1 with the changes of oxalate and of the P_{SF} after an oxalate load while on 1 g calcium diet and on a calcium-restricted diet.

The P_{SF} decreased significantly only in NCa and DH with the combined Ca and Ox dietary restriction. In IH, the decrease in P_{SF} was not significant because oxalate excretion significantly increased when dietary calcium was restricted in spite of the concomitant oxalate restriction. The oxalate load significantly increased the P_{SF} in all subgroups only when dietary calcium was restricted.

DISCUSSION

Our data show that oxalate restriction does not prevent an increase in urinary oxalate excretion induced by calcium restriction in idiopathic hypercalciuric stone formers. Our results are different from those of Marshall et al[3] who found that in 7 hospitalized patients with a controlled low calcium + low oxalate diet reduced urinary calcium and prevented the increase in urinary oxalate. These opposite results may be explained by the difficulty in reducing dietary oxalate at home. Particularly in patients with hyperabsorption of calcium, as in idiopathic hypercalciuric patients, the smallest quantity of oxalate which is provided by the diet is no longer complexed by intraluminal calcium during a low calcium diet, and is then directly available for passive absorption in the colon.

This point of view is supported by the effects of the oxalate load performed on a high and low calcium diet. The increased oxaluria is four times greater during a low calcium diet than during a 1 g calcium diet, and would be able to induce peaks in concentration and crystalluria as observed by Finch et al[2].

In all calcium stone formers, concomitant oxalate restriction is critical to minimise the increase in oxalate excretion induced by calcium restriction. But in patients with idiopathic hypercalciuria, this measure is insufficient to decrease the P_{SF} significantly suggesting that additional measures are necessary.

REFERENCES

1. P. Bataille, G. Charransol, J. Gregoire, and A. Fournier, J. Urol. 130:218 (1983).
2. A. M. Finch, G. P. Kasidas, and G. A. Rose, Clin. Sci. 60:411 (1981).
3. R. W. Marshall, M. Cochran, and A. Hodgkinson, Clin. Sci. 43:91 (1972).
4. W. G. Robertson, M. Peacock, P. J. Heyburn, D. H. Marshall, and P. B. Clark, Br. J. Urol. 50: 449 (1978).

DIETARY TREATMENT OF HYPEROXALURIA FOLLOWING

JEJUNOILEAL BYPASS

B. Nordenvall, L. Backman, P. Burman, L. Larsson,
and H.-G. Tiselius

Dept. Surgery, Karolinska Institute at Danderyd
Hospital, Stockholm and Depts. of Clinical Chemistry
and Urology, University Hospital, Linköping, Sweden

INTRODUCTION

Hyperoxaluria is a common consequence of intestinal resection[1] and jejunoileal bypass operations[2]. It may result in renal failure due to oxalosis[3]. High intestinal absorption of oxalate is thought to be responsible for the hyperoxaluria[4,5]. Peroral supplementation with calcium reduces the degree of hyperoxaluria under "metabolic ward" conditions[6,7]. In patients living at home, however, the effect seems to be doubtful[8]. Diets low in oxalate[9] and fat[4] likewise decrease oxalate excretion under metabolic ward conditions. Little is known of the effect of such diets under out-patient conditions. The aim of the present investigation was to observe the effect of low-oxalate, low-fat diet on the urinary excretion of oxalate in patients with hyperoxaluria following jejunoileal bypass living at home.

MATERIALS AND METHODS

The observations were made on 10 patients who had undergone jejunoileostomy because of obesity. Three surgical techniques were used, viz. end-to-side jejunoileostomy[10], end-to-end jejuno-ileostomy[11] and bilio-intestinal bypass[12]. The operation reduced the length of the small intestine in continuity to about 10% of the original. Clinical data are presented in Table 1. Body weight was stable in all patients. Five patients had recurrent urolithiasis after the operation.

The studies were made under out-patient conditions. Each patient was given a diet low in oxalate and fat. Foods with high

Table 1. Data on 10 Patients with Jejuno-Ileal Bypass.

Case	Sex	Age (y)	Surgical method	Stones	Years after op.	Present weight	Weight loss (kg)
1	M	33	End-to-end	+	7	82	38
2	M	38	End-to-end	–	4	110	41
3	M	45	End-to-side	+	5	96	34
4	M	55	End-to-end	+	9	95	45
5	F	35	Bili-intestinal shunt	+	5	76	37
6	F	36	Bili-intestinal shunt	–	5	90	32
7	F	39	End-to-side	–	4	98	21
8	F	50	End-to-side	–	4	70	40
9	F	56	End-to-side	+	5	78	32
10	M	57	End-to-end	–	9	85	45

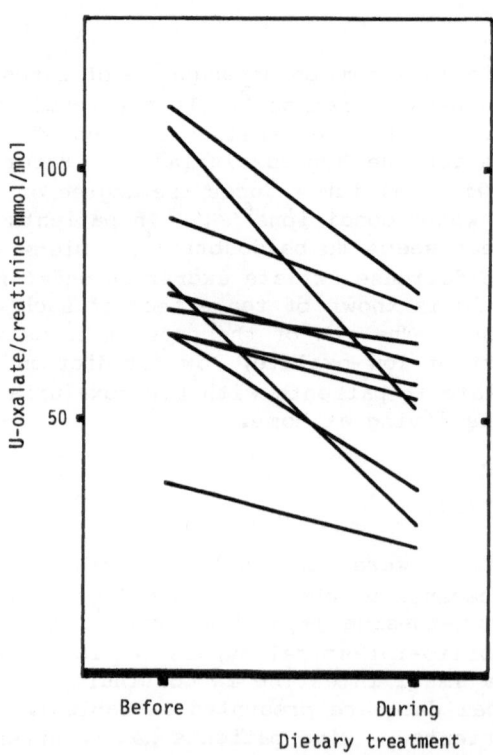

Fig. 1. Oxalate (mmol/mol creatinine) in 24-h urine specimens
before and during low-oxalate, low-fat dietary regimen
in 10 patients with jejuno-ileal bypass.

Table 2. Urinary Oxalate (mmol/24h) Before and During Dietary Regimen.

Case	Basal Diet		Low Oxalate+Low Fat	
	Day 1	Day 2	Day 8	Day 9
1	1.31	1.11	0.61	0.68
2	0.70	0.85	0.47	0.34
3	0.70	0.99	0.59	0.72
4	1.14	1.04	0.78	1.18
5	0.80	1.16	0.94	0.81
6	1.01	1.95	0.84	0.90
7	1.31	1.28	0.43	0.51
8	1.13	1.08	0.51	0.48
9	0.60	0.60	0.58	0.50
10	1.97	1.28	0.94	1.17
Mean	1.97	1.13	0.67	0.73
SEM	0.13	0.11	0.06	0.09

or moderate content of oxalate were excluded[13], and vegetarian dishes were declared to be undesirable. Only lean foods were allowed and a minimum of fat in cooking. Vitamin C supplements were not allowed. The composition of the diet before treatment was as previously reported[8]. The special diet reduced the oxalate and fat intakes by approximately 40 and 50% respectively.

Urine was collected as 24-h specimens on consecutive days before the dietary regimen was begun and also after one week on the diet. The plastic bottles used for the urine collection contained 90 mmol HCl to maintain oxalate in solution. From each sample, 250 ml was frozen at $-20^{\circ}C$ and analyzed at the end of the study, but within 3 weeks in all cases. Statistical analysis was carried out using Wilcoxon's test for paired observations[14]. Oxalate was determined using chromotropic acid[15]. The upper limit of normal was 0.45 mmol/24-h. The oxalate excretion was also expressed in relation to the creatinine clearance, to compensate for errors in urine collection. The upper limit of normal was 30 mmol/mol creatinine. Calcium and magnesium were analyzed by atomic absorption and creatinine by AutoAnalyzer with alkaline picrate.

RESULTS

All the patients had hyperoxaluria before the low oxalate-low fat dietary regimen (Table 2). During the treatment urinary oxalate excretion diminished in all patients ($P<0.01$) (Fig.1). The mean decrease was 30%. The mean urinary outputs of calcum and magnesium were unchanged during the study. The day-to-day variations in urinary volume and creatinine excretion were minimal.

DISCUSSION

The endogenous production of oxalate appears to be normal in patients with hyperoxaluria following jejuno-ileal bypass[5]. In order to reduce urinary oxalate, therefore, it is necessary to decrease the intestinal absorption of oxalate. One method is to bind oxalate in the intestinal lumen with calcium, magnesium, aluminium or cholestyramine. Our experience of these measures has been disappointing[8]. Reduction of dietary oxalate[9] or fat[4] can also reduce the urinary excretion of oxalate. To our knowledge, no studies have been made of this form of treatment in non-hospitalized persons with jejuno-ileal bypass. In the present study of low oxalate-low fat diet in 10 such persons, the urinary output of oxalate fell significantly, on average by 30%. If the rate of endogenous oxalate production is assumed to be constant at a level of 0.3 mmol/24 h[5], the results would imply a reduction of approximately 50% in oxalate absorption. Although the reduction in urinary oxalate was considerable in most of the 10 persons studied, it did not fall to normal. However, because of the importance of oxalate in altering the crystallization propensity of urine, even a minor decrease in oxalate may be beneficial in such cases[21]. It remains to be seen if the observed effect on oxalate excretion will be sufficient to prevent stone formation.

REFERENCES

1. J. W. Dobbins and H. J. Binder, in:"Progress in Gastroenterology", Vol. 3, G. B. J. Glass, ed., Grune & Stratton, New York (1977).
2. J. Gregory, K. Park, and H. Schoenberg, J. Urol. 117:631 (1977).
3. S. Das, B. Joseph, and A. Dick, J. Urol. 121:506 (1979).
4. H. Andersson and R. Jagenburg, Gut, 15:360 (1974).
5. B. Nordenvall, L. Backman, and L. Larsson, Scand. J. Gastroenterol. 16:395 (1981).
6. D. L. Earnest, H. E. Williams, and W. H. Admirand, Trans. Assoc. Am. Phys. 88:224 (1975).
7. J. Stauffer, Dig. Dis. 22:921 (1977).
8. B. Nordenvall, L. Backman, L. Larsson, and H-G. Tiselius, Acta. Chir. Scand. 149:93 (1983).
9. U. S. Chadwick, K. Modha, and R. M. Dowling, New Engl. J. Med. 289:172 (1973).
10. J. H. Payne and L. T. DeWind, Am. J. Surg. 118:141 (1969).
11. M. Buchwald and R. L. Varco, Surgery 70:62 (1971).
12. D. Hallberg and U. Holmgren, Acta. Chir. Scand. 145:405 (1979).
13. G. P. Kasidas and G. A. Rose, J. Human Nutr. 34:225 (1980).
14. G. W. Snedecor and W. G. Cochran, "Statistical Methods", 6thEdn, Iowa State University Press, Ames (1967).
15. H.-G.Tiselius, Invest. Urol. 15:5 (1977). 4:241 (1978).

THE STONE CLINIC EFFECT IN PATIENTS WITH

IDIOPATHIC CALCIUM UROLITHIASIS

D. H. Hosking, S. B. Erickson, C. J. Van den Berg,
D. M. Wilson, and L. H. Smith

University of Manitoba, Winnipeg, Canada and
Mayo Clinic, Rochester, Minnesota, U.S.A.

INTRODUCTION

Frequently, following initial assessment in a stone clinic, patients with idiopathic calcium urolithiasis do not demonstrate stone growth or new stone formation (metabolic activity)[1] during follow-up, although no specific drug therapy has been instituted. The only management which these patients have received consists of advice to increase their fluid intake and, when appropriate, to eliminate excessive intake of dairy products, protein, purines, oxalate, salt, and refined sugars[2-4]. The effect of these fluid and dietary recommendations alone may be referred to as the "stone clinic effect". The purpose of our study was to evaluate the extent of the "stone clinic effect" and to determine whether or not the metabolic activity of stone disease during follow-up was related to fluid intake.

MATERIALS AND METHODS

Patients with urolithiasis, referred to our stone clinic with inadequate radiological evidence of stone growth or new stone formation within the previous year and no documented passage of gravel within the previous year, are classified as having stone disease of indeterminate metabolic activity[1]. We reviewed the clinical courses of 108 patients with idiopathic calcium urolithiasis of indeterminate metabolic activity whose stone disease was initially treated with fluid and dietary recommendations alone. All patients were followed for over a year, had uninfected urine, and no identifiable disease which might be related to their stone disease. At the time of initial assessment, no patient was taking

453

thiazide diuretics, orthophosphates, acetazolamide, allopurinol or vitamin D compounds.

Patients were advised to drink approximately 8 oz (240 ml) of fluid hourly while awake to try and achieve a 24-h urine volume in excess of 2500 ml. It was recommended that half of the fluid should be water. Patients with hypercalciuria were advised to restrict their dairy product intake to one helping daily, and patients with hyperuricosuria were advised to limit their meat intake to one meal per day. When dietary questioning or urine biochemical evaluation suggested excessive intake of oxalate or salt, elimination of this excess was recommended.

The metabolic activity of the stone disease during the follow-up period was evaluated according to the criteria outlined by Smith[1]. The assessment of metabolic activity at follow-up was usually made with plain renal roentgenograms in conjunction with tomography of the kidneys without contrast.

For patients who did not demonstrate stone growth or new stone formation during the follow-up period (metabolically inactive), the follow-up period commenced with the first visit to the stone clinic. The follow-up period (for purposes of this study) ended either with the last visit at which renal roentgenograms were performed, or if for reasons unrelated to their stone disease, patients commenced thiazide or allopurinol therapy, at the time such therapy commenced.

Initial urine volumes were recorded on most patients at the time of initial assessment. In patients who were metabolically active at follow-up, the follow-up urine volume was determined as the mean of the urine volume at the time that metabolic activity was detected, and the preceding urine volume. In patients who were metabolically inactive during follow-up, the follow-up urine volume was calculated as the mean of the last two recorded urine volumes.

Hypercalciuria was defined as a 24-h urinary excretion of calcium > 300 mg in men and > 250 mg in women[5,6] or > 4 mg/kg in either sex[5]. Hyperuricosuria was defined as a 24-h urinary excretion of uric acid > 800 mg in men and > 750 mg in women[7,8].

RESULTS

There were 83 men and 25 women. Ninety-three of the patients had had or had passed > 1 urinary calculus. Fifty-four of the patients demonstrated no excessive excretion of calcium or uric acid, while the remainder were found to have hypercalciuria, hyperuricosuria or both.

During the follow-up period, 63 patients (58.3%) were metabolically inactive, with a mean follow-up duration of 62.6 $\pm$ 6.8 (mean $\pm$ SEM) months. Forty-five patients (41.7%) did demonstrate active stone growth or new stone formation during follow-up with a mean follow-up interval until metabolic activity was detected of 38.1 $\pm$ 4.2 months. Hypercalciuria was not associated with a higher incidence of metabolic activity at follow-up.

In 94 patients, data on initial and follow-up 24-h urine volumes were available. Although initial mean 24-h urine volumes were similar in patients who were metabolically active or metabolically inactive at follow-up, only the metabolically inactive group at follow-up showed a significant increase in mean 24-h urine volume ($P < 0.001$). In addition, the follow-up 24-h urine volume was significantly higher in the metabolically inactive group than in the metabolically active group.

One patient required surgery for a calculus formed during the follow-up period, while on conservative treatment. A small new calculus was identified in this patient 24 months after initial assessment and neutral orthophosphate prescribed. The medication was not taken by the patient and at follow-up one year later further stone growth had occurred and the calculus noted at the previous visit required surgical removal.

DISCUSSION

Our results show that 58% of our patients with idiopathic calcium urolithiasis of indeterminate metabolic activity showed no evidence of stone growth or new stone formation with a mean follow-up of over 5 years. Of those patients with hypercalciuria alone, over 70% were metabolically inactive during follow-up, and over 45% of patients with hyperuricosuria alone were metabolically inactive during follow-up.

Only one patient required surgery for a stone formed during the follow-up period suggesting that with careful follow-up, the risk of increased morbidity with an initial conservative approach is low.

Our observation that patients who were metabolically inactive at follow-up had a significantly higher mean 24-h urine volume at follow-up than metabolically active patients, is clinical support for the recommendation of increasing fluid intake in patients with stone disease.

In the majority of patients with idiopathic calcium urolithiasis of indeterminate metabolic activity, fluid and dietary recommendations alone constitute adequate therapy. Consequently, we feel that drug therapy in these patients is not indicated until

the effects of fluid and dietary recommendations alone on stone
growth or new stone formation have been evaluated.

REFERENCES

1. L. H. Smith, Urol. Clin. N. Am. 1:241 (1974).
2. L. H. Smith, C. Van den Berg, and D. M. Wilson, New Engl. J.
      Med. 298:87 (1978).
3. A. E. Broadus and S. O. Thier, New Engl. J. Med. 300:839 (1979).
4. J. Lien, Mod. Med. Can. 35:530 (1980).
5. A. Hodgkinson and L. N. Pyrah, Br. J. Surg. 46:10 (1958).
6. F. L. Coe and M. J. Favus, Adv. Intern. Med. 16:373 (1980).
7. A. B. Gutman and T.-F. Yü, Am. J. Med. 45:756 (1968).
8. F. L. Coe and A. G. Kavalich, New Engl. J. Med. 291:1344
      (1974).

456

DO STONE FORMERS ACCEPT DIETARY ADVICE?

P. N. Rao, A. Buxton, V. Prendiville, and
N. J. Blacklock

University Hospital of South Manchester
Manchester M20 8LR, U.K.

INTRODUCTION

Hypercalciuria, hyperoxaluria and hyperuricosuria are important risk factors for idiopathic urolithiasis[1]. It is essential to reduce these abnormalities in urine to minimise recurrence of stone formation. Phosphates and thiazides are commonly used to treat hypercalciuria. However, it is also important to correct the others as far as possible to prevent stone formation successfully. We have shown previously that reduction in the consumption of refined carbohydrates, animal protein, oxalate-rich foods and addition of fibre to the diet reduce urinary excretion of all the above risk factors[2]. Since the treatment for stone prophylaxis is a life-time measure, this form of dietary manipulation must be totally acceptable to the patient if it is to achieve its object. We report herein the results of a long-term compliance study of a group of stone-formers who were treated by dietary manipulation.

PATIENTS AND METHODS

A total of 62 idiopathic stone formers were studied (46 males and 16 females). Their dietary intakes were assessed by a questionnaire designed to determine the daily consumption of the main sources of cereal fibre, sugar and sugar products. Nine patients completed a pro-forma detailing animal protein intake over 4 days at home. The amount of the nutrients in the daily diet was calculated from food composition tables[3].

Following this initial dietary assessment, all patients received detailed advice from a dietitian to take fibre supplements, preferably in the form of soya bran, with each main meal of the day and were shown how to increase their fibre content of the diet in general.   They were advised to minimise their intake of sugar and sugar-containing foods and recommended to limit consumption of animal protein to approximately 40 g/day.   They were also asked to avoid excessive consumption of foods rich in calcium and oxalate, but the advice was not that of a "low calcium" diet[2].   Their dietary intakes were reassessed by the same method after a period ranging from 6 to 43 months (mean 16.6 months).

Statistical analysis was carried out using the Wilcoxon matched-pairs signed-ranks test.

RESULTS

There was a significant change in the dietary habits of the patients following advice (Table 1).   Three groups were identified: 43 (70%) of the patients were compliant since they incorporated all the recommended changes in their diet (Fig. 1);   16 (24%) were partially compliant since they changed their intake of sugar, fibre or meat but not all; only 4 (6%) were non-compliant.

DISCUSSION

The association between idiopathic urolithiasis and increased urinary excretion of calcium, oxalate and uric acid is well recognised.   Correction of these abnormalities can produce a reduction in the recurrence rate of stone formation and this is amply demonstrated in the case of hypercalciuria treated with either phosphates or thiazide diuretics[4,5].   Phosphates in any form are usually effective in absorptive hypercalciuria and thiazides are useful mainly in patients with a renal "leak" type of hypercalciuria[6]. Even if hypercalciuria is successfully controlled, stones continue to form unless other risk factors in the urine .   Although hypercalciuria is the most common disorder, investigation of a large

Table 1. Intake of Nutrients Before and After Dietary Advice.
         (Median (range) g/day).

Nutrients	Before Advice	After Advice	P
Sucrose and sucrose products	86 (12-408)	49.5 (4-158)	<0.001
Fibre	9 (1.3-27)	15 (5-34)	<0.001
Animal Protein (N=9)	56	57	ns

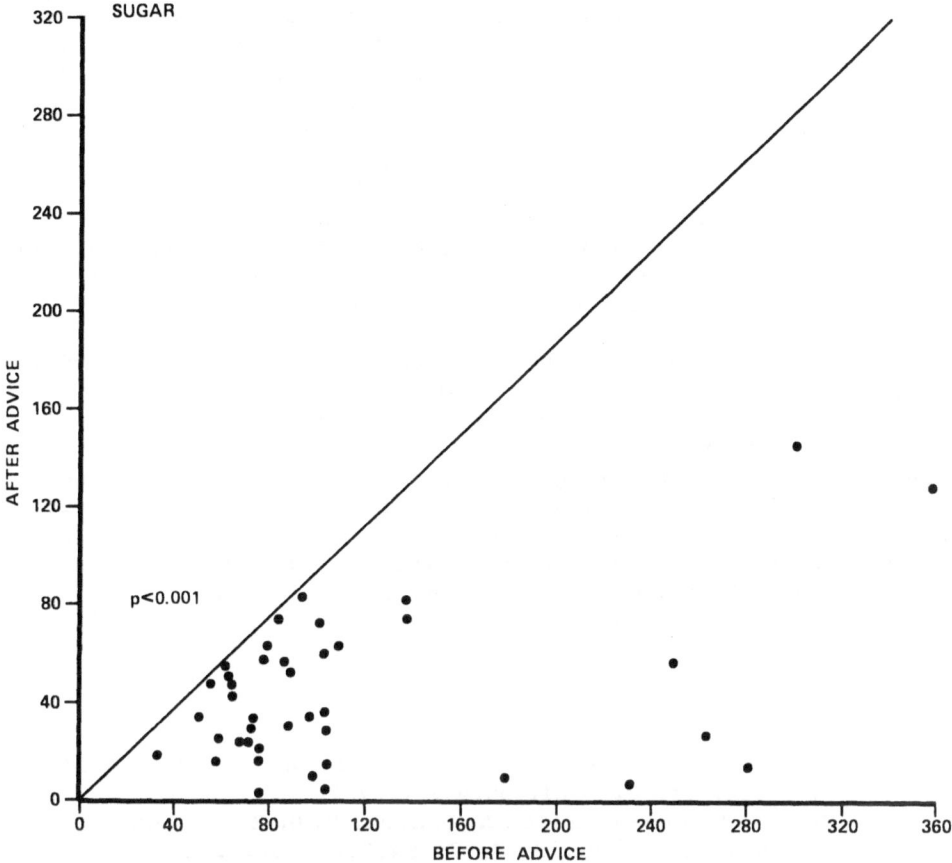

Fig. 1. Daily sugar consumption of the compliant group (g/day).

group of stone formers showed that more than one abnormality in the urine occurs in up to 16% of stone former[2]. Unfortunately, there is no medication which can simultaneously influence the excretion of all risk factors and it is difficult to use a separate drug for each abnormality in the urine. Furthermore, a long-term treatment with drugs is expensive and often associated with side-effects. It is also doubtful if patients take the medicines regularly.

The role of dietary factors in the pathogenesis of these disorders in the urine is well established[7,8]. There are several advantages in managing these urinary abnormalities by dietary manipulation. It is economical and without side-effects. It incorporates all the presently accepted principles of healthier eating[9] and is applicable not only to the patient but also the other members of the family. We have already shown that this form of treatment effectively reduces all the 3 main risk factors in the urine[2].

The use of dietary modification to influence urinary composition is not new as dietary calcium restriction has been in use for several years. The success of the treatment is of course dependent on compliance. Baker and Mallinson[10] found that urinary calcium could be controlled by calcium restriction in the long-term in only 14% of their patients, although up to 30% responded initially. They attributed this failure to non-compliance but they did not examine dietary habits objectively before and after advice. Furthermore, calcium restriction is effective only in patients who consume excess calcium[11] as dietary factors other than calcium are probably more important in inducing hypercalciuria[7,8].

For dietary advice to be effective, a simple "diet sheet" alone is inadequate. The advice given depends on each patient's normal dietary habits and may not be directly applicable to another patient. It is necessary to obtain a dietary assessment in the individual patient before giving detailed advice and it is useful to seek the help of a dietitian for this purpose. It is our practice to re-assess the patient on more than one occasion if there are no beneficial changes in urinary composition. Drug treatment is considered necessary only when we are satisfied that the patient is adhering to the advice.

REFERENCES

1. W. G. Robertson, M. Peacock, P. J. Heyburn, D. H. Marshall, and P. Clark, Br. J. Urol. 50:449 (1978).
2. P. N. Rao, V. Prendiville, A. Buxton, D. G. Moss, and N. J.Blacklock, Br. J. Urol. 54:578 (1982).
3. R. A. McCance and E. M. Widdowson, "The Composition of Foods", HMSO, London (1980).
4. P. J. Heyburn, W. G. Robertson, and M. Peacock, Nephron 32:314 (1982).
5. E. R. Yendt and M. Cohanim, Kidney Int. 13:397 (1978).
6. C. Y. C. Pak, J. Urol. 128:1157 (1982).
7. W. G. Robertson, M. Peacock, P. J. Heyburn, F. A. Hanes, A.Rutherford, E. Clementson, R. Swaminathan, and P. B. Clark, Br. J. Urol. 51:427 (1979).
8. J. A. Thom, J. E. Morris, A. Bishop, and N. J. Blacklock, Br. J.Urol. 50:459 (1978).
9. R. Passmore, D. F. Hollingsworth, J. Robertson, Br. Med. J. 1:527 (1979).
10. L. R. I. Baker and W. J. W. Mallinson, Br. J. Urol 51:181 (1979).
11. P. Bataille, G. Charransol, I. Grégoire, J. L. Daigré, B. Coevoet, R. Makdassi, A. Pruna, P. Locqquet, J. P. Suer, and A. Fournier, J. Urol. 130:218 (1983).

DRUG TREATMENT

THE PREVENTION OF CALCIUM STONES WITH THIAZIDES

E. R. Yendt and M. Cohanim

Dept. of Medicine, Queen's University
Kingston, Ontario, Canada

INTRODUCTION

Twenty-two years have now elapsed since we first started to use thiazides to prevent calcium stones[1,2]. However, despite the lengthy experience with the use of these agents, there is probably considerable disagreement concerning the exact role of thiazides in the management of the stone patient. Therefore, I have elected not to attempt a comprehensive review of this subject but rather to address some of the more controversial aspects of thiazide usage and to provide some updated information from our own clinic.

EFFICACY

First of all, I would like to deal briefly with the efficacy of thiazides. In 1973, we reported that our 10-year experience with thiazides indicated that the formation of new stones and growth of previously formed stones ceased completely in at least 90% of all patients who took hydrochlorothiazide (50 mg twice daily) on a regular basis[3]. Subsequent experience[4] has confirmed these earlier reports and we now have experience with these agents in over 500 patients. Confirmatory evidence has been published by others[5,6]. On reviewing the literature it is clear that such widespread success has not been uniformly possible with any other therapeutic agent[7]. Despite this impressive body of evidence, it is current fashion to accept only evidence from controlled clinical trials as proof of therapeutic efficacy. The results of two such trials have failed to demonstrate the efficacy of thiazides[8,9] although others, including some at this conference, have. However, a negative controlled clinical trial is not necessarily the final word concerning the efficacy of a therapeutic agent. There is a very high risk of missing a significant therapeutic effect simply because of inadequate sample size and follow-up period, the so called "Type II" or "beta" error[10]. Moreover, improper experimental design can also lead to erroneous conclusions. In many, if not most published studies dealing with the efficacy of therapeutic agents in stone prevention, adequate radiographic documentation of stone status by tomography at the time of initiation of treatment is lacking and there is usually no analysis of drop-outs or compliance. Our experience has repeatedly shown that a simple KUB X-ray or plain film of the abdomen may fail to detect small calcific calculi; moreover one cannot rely on reports from the X-ray Department to establish whether or not progression has occurred during therapy. Personal examination of all the films is necessary in every case.

MECHANISM OF ACTION

There is general agreement that thiazides reduce crystalluria and urinary supersaturation with calcium oxalate and calcium phosphate[11-13]. Undoubtedly these beneficial effects are largely due to the now well known hypocalciuric action of thiazides and of related diuretics such as chlorthalidone and metolazone. It was this action of thiazides which led to their initial employment in stone patients. However, in some patients the hypocalciuric action of the drug is not very impressive, yet stone formation ceases. This has prompted us to search for other actions of thiazides which might contribute to their therapeutic efficacy. In 1980, we reported that although urinary oxalate excretion does not fall during the first year of oxalate administration (and may actually rise slightly), a significant reduction does occur thereafter[14]. We have now expanded these observations to a much larger series of 77 patients followed for 1 to 8 years (total follow-up period 270 patient years) and have demonstrated a highly significant reduction of urine oxalate excretion (Table 1). This effect occurs in both normocalciuric and hypercalciuric patients and is also apparent in patients treated with 25 mg hydrochlorothiazide twice daily as well as in those given the full dose of 50 mg twice daily. We have suggested that the oxalate lowering effect of thiazides is due to diminished absorption of dietary oxalate secondary to the reduced absorption of dietary calcium which has been demonstrated in some patients during long-term thiazide therapy by both traditional balance[4] and isotopic techniques[15,16]. The oxalate lowering effect of thiazides is demonstrated dramatically in a patient who had overt hyperoxaluria, which was neither primary nor secondary to the generally recognized causes, but which, we believe, was due to hyperabsorption of dietary oxalate resulting from hyperabsorption of dietary calcium. Urinary oxalate excretion gradually fell to normal during long-term thiazide therapy but hyperoxaluria recurred when phosphates were substituted for thiazides.

Table 1. The 24-h Urinary Composition (mean $\pm$ SEM) of Patients with Calcium Stones before and after more than 12 months Treatment with Thiazides.

	n	Excretion (mg/day)			Concentration (mg/dl)		
		Control	Thiazides	P	Control	Thiazides	P
Volume (ml)	77a	1634	1801	n.s.			
Calcium	77a	309 $\pm$ 12.4	224 $\pm$ 11.4	<0.001	20.6 $\pm$ 0.9	13.2 $\pm$ 0.7	<0.001
Magnesium[b]	76	109 $\pm$ 3.7	122 $\pm$ 3.6	<0.02	7.3 $\pm$ 0.3	7.0 $\pm$ 0.3	n.s.
Citrate	53	561 $\pm$ 27	514 $\pm$ 32	n.s.	42.5 $\pm$ 3.4	29.3 $\pm$ 1.6	<0.001
Uric acid	53	763 $\pm$ 28	818 $\pm$ 38	n.s.	56.5 $\pm$ 3.8	48.5 $\pm$ 2.1	n.s.
Oxalate	77a	38.0 $\pm$ 1.5	28.8 $\pm$ 1.1	<0.001	2.7 $\pm$ 0.2	1.8 $\pm$ 0.1	<0.001

a Forty-seven of the patients were normocalciuric and 30 were hypercalciuric. Forty patients were treated with 25 mg hydrochlorothiazide twice daily and 37 with 50 mg hydrochlorothiazide twice daily.

b If values during the first three years of thiazide therapy are excluded, a significant change in urine magnesium can no longer be demonstrated.

The initial increase in urinary magnesium excretion with diuretic therapy[1] is a well recognized phenomenon[17]. Unlike the hypocalciuric effect, this action is not specific for thiazides. However, after the first 2 to 3 years of thiazide therapy, urinary magnesium excretion is not significantly higher than the pre-treatment values presumably due to the reduction in serum magnesium levels (and hence the filtered magnesium load) which occurs during long-term treatment[2,16]. It is of interest that the magnesiuric effect of thiazides is maximal during the initial phase of thiazide treatment at a time when the oxalate lowering effect has still not become established.

Although thiazides cause a sustained increase in urinary zinc excretion[18] by altering the renal tubular transport of this ion[19,20] the significance of this effect in relation to stone prevention is still uncertain. Zinc is a potent inhibitor of calcification of an organic matrix in vitro, especially in the presence of magnesium[21]. Zinc at concentrations approximating those found in normal urine has no effect on calcium oxalate crystal growth[22,23] but does inhibit calcium phosphate crystal growth to a relatively minor degree[23]. However, the effects of zinc on crystal growth in the concentrations resulting from thiazide administration and in the presence of magnesium have not been assessed.

In all the metabolic studies which we performed while patients were on constant diets, thiazides initially decreased urine citrate excretion by substantial amounts[22]. However, we[2] and others[9,16] have found that although urine citrate excretion is reduced by about 10% during long-term thiazide treatment, this effect is not statistically significant[9,16]. We have recently re-examined this question in a larger group of patients with essentially the same results. However, this slight reduction in urine citrate excretion when taken together with a slight (10%) but also statistically non-significant increase in urine volume which occurs during chronic thiazide therapy results in a highly significant reduction in urine citrate concentration (Table 1).

Our experience provides no basis for the fear that thiazide therapy might increase the risk of uric acid stone formation by promoting hyperuricosuria[24]. We found no acute changes in uric acid excretion during thiazide therapy during our early metabolic studies with patients on constant diets[22] and we[2] in agreement with most other workers[9,16] have found no increase in uric acid excretion during long-term thiazide therapy. We have seen only one patient who passed uric acid stones during thiazide therapy and he was passing both uric acid stones and calcium oxalate stones prior to treatment.

ARE THIAZIDES EFFECTIVE IN NORMOCALCIURIC PATIENTS?

This is another controversial issue. In our experience, thiazides have been just as effective in normocalciuric as in hypercalciuric patients[4] and Ljunghall et al[6] have reported a similar experience whereas others advocate restricting the use of thiazides to hypercalciuric patients[25]. There seems to be no a priori reason why thiazides should not be effective in normocalciuric patients since the thiazide induced changes in urinary composition are qualitatively similar in normocalciuric and hypercaliuric patients. Although Coe[5] suggested that thiazides were less effective in normocalciuric patients than in hypercalciuric patients, this has not been our experience. As a matter of fact, recent re-examination of this question in our clinic has provided impressive evidence of the efficacy of thiazides in normocalciuric patients. In 18 normocalciuric patients who had formed 89 stones and required 11 surgical operations during 165 pre-thiazide patient years, only 1 new stone was formed during 126 patient years of follow-up on thiazides. This occurred during a period of very poor compliance and no further progression has occurred in this patient since this problem was corrected.

IS IT NECESSARY TO SELECT PATIENTS WHO ARE SUITABLE FOR THIAZIDE THERAPY?

We have never attempted to do so and our high success rate suggests that this is unnecessary in the average nephrologic or urologic practice. We believe that thiazides are effective in any patient with calcium oxalate stones regardless of the presence or absence of hypercalciuria, the type of hypercalciuria or the presence or absence of hyperuricosuria. Thiazides are also effective in patients with medullary sponge kidney[4]. This philosophy of patient management has important economic implications by reducing the cost of unnecessary investigations.

PREPARATIONS AND DOSE

There has been considerable variability in the preparations and doses of thiazides used by various authors. In our initial trials, we used hydrochlorothiazide at the upper end of therapeutic dosage range whereas others have tended to use smaller equivalent doses of the various benzothiadiazides (Table 2). We now use smaller doses of hydrochlorothiazide (25 mg twice daily) in women and normocalciuric men but continue to use 50 mg twice daily for hypercalciuric men. A number of patients continue to form stones on the smaller doses but cease doing so on the larger doses. It is not known if one form of thiazide is more effective than another but this seems unlikely if equivalent doses are used. However, there

Table 2. Recommended Dosages of Various Thiazide Diuretics.

Thiazide	Range of Optimally Effective Oral Diuretic Dose in Man[29] (mg/day)	Daily Dose For Stone Prevention (mg/day)	Reference
Hydrochlorothiazide	25 - 100	100	Yendt & Cohanim
Bendroflumethiazide	2.5 - 15	5	Backman et al.
	-	5	Rose
Trichlormethiazide	2 - 8	4	Coe
	-	4	Pak et al.
Chlorthalidone	25 - 200	50	Pak et al.

may be some advantages (e.g. improved compliance, less nocturia) in using one of the longer acting benzothiadiazide preparations (e.g. trichlormethiazide) or related diuretics (e.g. metolazone) which need be administered only once daily.

SIDE-EFFECTS

The incidence of thiazide side-effects in our patients has been higher than that reported by others, perhaps because of the larger doses used in our early studies when side-effects occurred in 30 to 35% of patients; these were of sufficient severity to necessitate stopping treatment in 7% of our patients[4]. Fatigue is probably the commonest side effect and this does not always respond to potassium supplementation. Hypokalemia is almost a universal finding in patients who take 50 mg hydrochlorothiazide twice daily. If serum potassium levels remain normal with this dose poor compliance should be suspected. Normokalemia in patients with good compliance suggests an unusual resistance to thiazides and higher than usual doses of thiazides may be necessary to prevent stones in these patients who tend to be remarkably free from thiazide side-effects. Although potassium supplementaion has been considered unnecessary in thiazide-treated patients with serum potassium levels above 3.0 mEq/l in the absence of heart disease, digitalis therapy etc., there are both real and theoretical problems associated with this philosophy of management. Referring physicians tend to be concerned about any degree of hypokalemia and tend to implicate and treat this metabolic abnormality when subsequent unrelated illnesses occur. Potassium supplementation is also necessary before a general anaesthetic and hypokalemia often necessitates delaying surgery. There is also increasing concern that hypokalemia may be hazardous if the patient subsequently develops ischemic heart disease since hypokalemia has been shown to induce an increase in ventricular ectopic activity with the possibility of serious cardiac problems and sudden death[26]. Because of these considerations, there is an increasing tendency in our clinic to prescribe thiazides along with a potassium sparing agent. Of the various agents available, we prefer amiloride over triamterene (which may result in triamterene stones) or spironolactone (which may cause impotence). There is also the possibility that amiloride may potentiate the hypocalciuric action of thiazides but our experience to date in this regard has not been very impressive. Thiazides alone may cause decreased libido and impotence and this side-effect may not be recognized unless specific questions are directed to the patient. The significance of other thiazide induced metabolic changes such as hypomagnesemia is as yet uncertain. The observation by Ljunghall et al[16] that muscle magnesium content remains normal after three years' treatment is reassuring but the possibility of magnesium deficiency in some patients with a need for magnesium supplementation should still be kept in mind.

Although an increase in serum cholesterol and triglyceride levels during treatment of hypertensive patients with thiazides has been reported[27] subsequent studies showed that this was true only if there was an associated weight gain during treatment[28].

ACKNOWLEDGMENTS

This work was supported by grants from the Medical Research Council of Canada MT681.

REFERENCES

1. E. R. Yendt, R. J. Gagne, and M. Cohanim, Am. J. Med. Sci. 251:449 (1966).
2. E. R. Yendt, F. G. Guay, and D. A. Garcia, Can. Med. Assoc. J. 102:614 (1970).
3. E. R. Yendt, and M. Cohanim, Trans. Am. Clin. Climatol. Assoc. 85:65 (1973).
4. E. R. Yendt, and M. Cohanim, Kidney Int. 13:397 (1978).
5. F. L. Coe, Ann. Intern. Med. 87:404 (1977).
6. S. Ljunghall, U. Backman, B. G. Danielson, F. Fellström, G. Johansson, and B. Wikström, in:Urolithiasis:Clinical and Basic Research", L. H. Smith, W. G. Robertson, B. Finlayson, eds., Plenum, New York (1981).
7. E. R. Yendt, in:Stones, Clinical Management of Urolithiasis", R. A. Roth and B. Finlayson, eds., Williams & Wilkins, Baltimore (1983).
8. P. Brocks, C. Dahl, and H. Wolf, Lancet 2:124 (1981).
9. D. Scholz, P. O. Schwille, and A. Sigel, J. Urol. 128:903 (1982).

10. J. A. Freeman, T. C. Chalmes, H. Smith, and R. R. Kuebler,
    N. Engl. J. Med. 299:690 (1978).
11. D. V. Weber, F. L. Coe, J. H. Parks, M. S. L. Dunn, and
    V. Tembe, Ann. Int. Med. 90:180 (1979).
12. C. Y. C. Pak and R. A. Galosy, Am. J. Med. 69:681 (1980).
13. P. G. Werness, J. H. Bergert, and L. H. Smith, J. Crystal Growth
    53:166 (1981).
14. M. Cohanim and E. R. Yendt, Invest. Urol. 18:170 (1980).
15. U. Ehrig, J. E. Harrison, and D. R. Wilson, Metabolism 23:139
    (1974).
16. S. Ljunghall, U. Backman, B. G. Danielson, B. Fellström, G.
    Johansson and B. Wikström, in:"Urolithiasis:Clinical and
    Basic research", L. H. Smith, W. G. Robertson, and
    B. Finlayson, eds., Plenum, New York (1981).
17. R. A. L. Sutton and J. H. Dirks, in:"The Kidney", B. M. Brenner
    and F. C. Rector, eds., W. B. Saunders, Philadelphia (1982).
18. M. Cohanim and E. R. Yendt, Johns Hopk. Med. J. 136:137 (1975).
19. D. W. Watkins, L. D. Antoniou, and R. J. Shalhoub,
    Can. J. Physiol, Pharmacol. 59:562 (1981).
20. W. Victery, J. M. Smith, and A. J. Vander, Am. J. Physiol.
    241:F532 (1981).
21. E. D. Bird and W. C. Thomas, Proc. Soc. Exp. Biol. Med. 112:640
    (1963).
22. D. A. Garcia and E. R. Yendt, Can. Med. Assoc. J. 103:473
    (1970).
23. J. L. Meyer and E. E. Angino, Invest. Urol. 14:347 (1977).
24. C. Y. C. Pak, Tolentino, A. Stewart and R. A. Galosy,
    Invest.Urol. 16:191 (1978).
25. C. Y. C. Pak, P. Peters, G. Hurt, M. Kadesky, M. Fine,
    D. Reisman, F. Splann, C. Caramela, A. Freeman, F. Britton,
    K. Sakhaee, and N. A. Breslau, Am. J. Med. 71:615 (1981).
26. O. Holland, J. V. Nixon, and L. Kuhnert, Am. J. Med. 70:762
    (1981).
27. R. P. Ames and P. Hill, Am. J. Med. 61:748 (1976).
28. A. Helgeland, I. Hjerman, I. Holme, and P. Feren, Am. J. Med.
    64:34 (1978).
29. G. H. Mudge, in:"The Pharmacologic Basis of Therapeutics"
    6th edn., L. S. Goodman and A. Gilman, eds., Macmillan,
    New York, 1980.

EXPERIENCE WITH LONG-TERM THIAZIDE TREATMENT IN CALCIUM

OXALATE STONE DISEASE

C. Ahlstrand, H.-G. Tiselius, and L. Larsson

Depts. of Urology and Clinical Chemistry, University
Hospital, S-581 85 Linköping, Sweden

INTRODUCTION

The high recurrence rate of calcium oxalate (CaOx) stones makes
prophylactic treatment desirable. Available forms of medical treatment are directed toward the correction of one or several CaOx risk
factors. Although prophylactic treatment with thiazides has been
used for at least 20 years, reports on the clinical efficacy and the
biochemical effects are contradictory. For a rational choice of
therapy, it might be necessary to define biochemically those patients
in whom thiazide treatment will be most efficient.

PATIENTS AND METHODS

Eighty-five patients with either recurrent CaOx stone disease or
surgical removal of CaOx stones were treated with 2.5 or 5 mg of
bendroflumethiazide (BFT) daily. Twenty-six patients stopped treatment within 2 years because of side-effects. Fifty-nine patients
remained on treatment for a mean (+SD) period of 3.7 $\pm$ 1.0 years, 20
treated with 2.5 mg and 39 with 5 mg of BFT daily.

The patients were investigated biochemically before and during
treatment according to principles described previously[1]. The pre-
treatment evaluation showed that 38 patients had hypercalciuria, 10
hyperoxaluria, and 7 low urinary citrate. Rates of stone formation
were calculated for the pre-treatment and treatment periods. Stones
present in the urinary tract at the beginning of each period were
neglected. Formation of a new stone or growth of a stone by more
than 50% of its diameter were both classified as recurrent stone
formation. The pre-treatment recurrence rate after the first stone

471

episode and the recurrence rate during treatment were compared by means of life-table analysis.

RESULTS

Twenty-one of the 59 patients remained on treatment despite minor side-effects. Eight had recurrent stone formation, and another 2 had growth of stones. Recurrence was diagnosed after a mean (+SD) treatment period of 2.5 + 1.6 years. Patients who formed new stones had higher pre-treatment stone formation rates than those who did not. The mean stone formation rate decreased from 0.35 to 0.15 stones/year during daily administration of 5 mg of BFT (P < 0.001). With a daily dose of 2.5 mg of BFT it was not possible to demonstrate a positive effect with life-table analysis.

Urinary calcium was reduced by about 25% during treatment. A reduced calcium excretion (P<0.05) was observed also in patients with recurrent stone formation. Magnesium was transiently increased, whereas oxalate, citrate, urate and inhibition of CaOx crystal growth in diluted urine were all unaffected. Patients with recurrent stone formation had lower citrate excretion and higher calcium/citrate quotients both before and during treatment. Furthermore, the AP(CaOx)-index[2], an estimate of CaOx supersaturation in urine, was high both before and during treatment in patients with stone recurrences (Table 1).

DISCUSSION

The rate of stone formation in CaOx stone formers was apparently reduced during daily treatment with 5 mg of BFT. Side-effects were

Table 1. Urine Composition (Mean+ SEM) Before and After 1 Year of Treatment with BFT.

Urine Variable (mmol/mol Cr)	Patients with Recurrence		Patients without Recurrence	
	Before Treatment	During Treatment	Before Treatment	During Treatment
Calcium	555 + 45	455 + 37	616 + 26	525 + 33
Magnesium	326 + 57	382 + 94	329 + 17	383 + 17
Oxalate	24.8 + 2.2	22.9 + 2.2	26.6 + 1.2	27.1 + 1.1
Citrate	153 + 13	151 + 13	225 + 19	229 + 15
Ca/Mg	1.99 + 0.25	1.46 + 0.22	2.04 + 0.11	1.44 + 0.09
Ca/Citrate	3.71 + 0.41	3.10 + 0.42	3.49 + 0.32	2.69 + 0.21
AP(CaOx)-index	2.78 + 0.35	2.43 + 0.37	2.54 + 0.21	2.04 + 0.13

472

more frequent than expected. Patients with recurrences during treatment had higher pre-treatment stone formation rates and CaOx supersaturation levels. Furthermore, low urinary excretion of citrate and high calcium/citrate quotients appeared to be associated with a higher risk of recurrent stone formation. In contrast to previous reports[3] no effects were observed on urinary oxalate despite treatment for up to 5 years. Further long-term studies of biochemically well-defined patients are necessary before the exact role of BFT in stone prevention can be settled.

REFERENCES

1. H.-G. Tiselius, L. E. Almgård, and B. Sörbo, Eur. Urol. 4:241 (1978).
2. H.-G. Tiselius, Clin. Chim. Acta 122:409 (1982).
3. M. Cohanim and E. R. Yendt, Invest. Urol. 18:170 (1980).

THIAZIDE PROPHYLAXIS OF UROLITHIASIS:

A DOUBLE BLIND STUDY IN GENERAL PRACTICE

E. Laerum and S. Larsen

Institute of General Practice, University of Oslo
Oslo, and Nordic Statistical Center, Ciba-Geigy
Pharma A/S, Strømmen, Norway

INTRODUCTION

Since 1970 several clinical trials using thiazides have been performed - all showing a substantial reduction in the rate of stone recurrence[1-4]. The following objections, however, can be made against these studies. There were no adequate control groups and/or randomization, and the double blind technique and placebo comparison were not applied except in one case[5]. No prospective study has been reported on the treatment of the different types of urolithiasis in general practice. The present study was conducted to investigate, in recurrent calcium stone formers, the prophylactic long-term effect of hydrochlorothiazide versus placebo in a randomized double blind trial in general practice, and to see if the outcome of treatment is related to pre-treatment urinary calcium and uric acid excretion.

MATERIALS AND METHODS

The study was performed during 1977-81 in a group practice in a partly rural municipality in Norway. The patients comprised 50 (38 men and 12 women) from 93 recurrent stone formers encountered in general practice[6]. Cooperative patients of both sexes, over 15 years of age, with or without hypercalciuria (>6 mmol/24 h) and/or hyperuricosuria (>3.5 mmol/24 h) and with two or more stones were included if the most recent stone had occurred during the previous 2 years and was verified by X-ray examination, surgery or stone passage. The stones had to contain calcium oxalate alone or combined with calcium phosphate. Patients were excluded who had chronic and/or active urinary tract infection, pyelographically

475

verified urinary obstruction, uric acid or triple phosphate stones
or chronic diseases such as cancer or sarcoidosis. All patients were
advised to reduce a high salt intake as well as ingestion of food
rich in calcium, oxalate and purines. A high fluid intake was
recommended.   The patients were randomly grouped, 25 being
allocated to treatment with 25 mg hydrochlorothiazide (and 0.6 g
potassium chloride) twice daily and the other 25 given matching
placebo tablets.   Double-blind technique was used.   A plain
abdominal X-ray (additionally i.v. pyelography and tomography when
results were ambiguous) was taken yearly and at the end of the
trial.   On the basis of the X-ray descriptions a new stone was
lassified as verified or probable.   Passed stones, previously not
demonstrated by X-ray examination, were recorded as verified.

Table 1. Number of Patients with Verified or Probable New Stones
Formed during Treatment.

Stones Formed	Verified		Probable	
	Thiazide	Placebo	Thiazide	Placebo
0	19	15	21	21
1	2	3	1	4
2	0	4	0	0
3	0	3	0	0
4	0	0	1	0
5	0	0	0	0
6	1	0	0	0
7	1	0	0	0

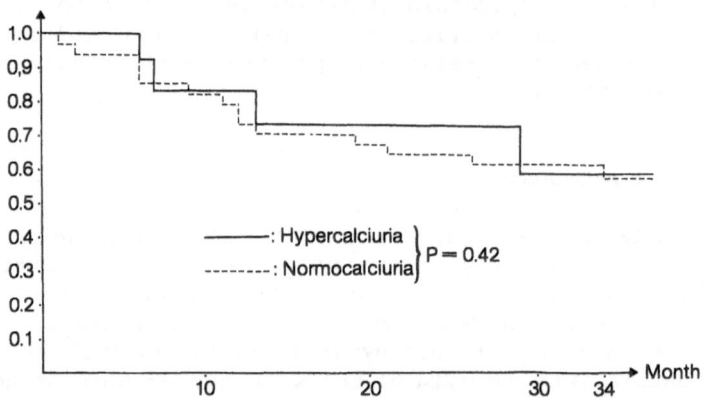

Fig. 1. The probability of not forming a new stone in 13 patients
with hypercalciuria and 25 with normocalciuria during a
median treatment period of 3 years with thiazide or
placebo, using a Kaplan and Meier plot.

476

Differences between groups were tested using the Wilcoxon
midrank sum test. Categorized data analysis was performed for
comparison of frequencies. The probability of forming new stones
was analyzed using Kaplan and Meier's method, and Gehan's test was
applied for comparison of groups.

RESULTS

The initial patient data were similar in the two treatment
groups (not shown). Two women in the thiazide group interrupted
the treatment for psychosocial reasons after 4 and 9 months
respectively, with no sign of recurrence. They were considered
drop-outs because the probability of forming a new stone while on
treatment was below 0.25. The expected median number of new stones
was reduced by 78% in the thiazide group and 59% in the placebo
group. In both groups the reduction was statistically significant
(P<0.01). The number of patients forming new stones in the
placebo-group (n=12, 48%) was more than twice the number in the
thiazide group (n=5, 22%) (P=0.05) (Table 1). The 95% confidence
interval of this difference was 28 to 60 in the placebo group and 8
to 44 in the thiazide group. If a new stone was formed, thiazide
had the effect of prolonging the stone-free interval by 52%. No
such prolongation of the stone-free period was observed in the
placebo group (P<0.01). The effect of thiazide was the same
whether the patient had hyper- or normocalciuria (Fig. 1). The
findings are similar with respect to time until a new stone is
formed and number of patients with new stones (0.25 < P < 0.42). The
probability of not forming a new stone was 64% in the hyperuricosuric group and 46% in the group with normouricosuria. (Not
significant, P=0.14). Two patients on thiazide showed a

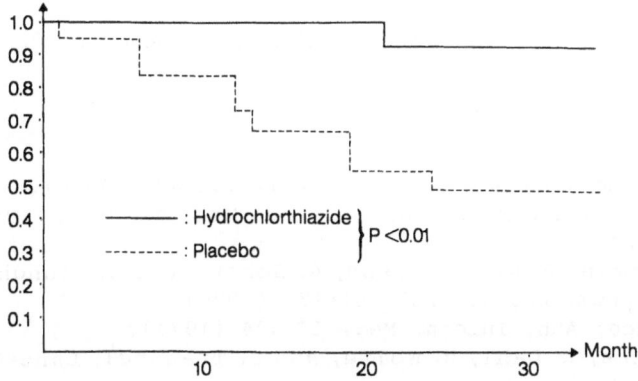

Fig. 2. Uric acid corrected probability of not forming a new stone
during a median treatment period of 3 years with thiazide
or placebo, using a Kaplan and Meier plot.

substantial increase in stone frequency and formed 6 (expected 1.3) and 7 (expected 2) stones respectively, during treatment. The probability of not forming a new stone, when corrected for uric acid, was 86% in the thiazide group and 45% in the placebo group (Fig. 2). One male patient experienced an attack of gout after 10 months of thiazide treatment, and one woman hypopotassaemia (K < 3 mmol/l). Otherwise there were few side-effects in either group.

DISCUSSION

There are several problems in assessing the prophylactic effect of a given treatment on stone formation. For example, calculation of the expected number of stones that will be formed during a treatment period may give too high a figure, since many patients will receive medical care when there is a peak of stone frequency. This may be misinterpreted as a reduction of stone recurrence as a result of the treatment. A better adherence to advice on how to prevent stone recurrence may also be of importance. This clearly demonstrates the necessity to include an adequate control group. It is considered essential to include the time until a new stone is formed and not only whether or not it actually did occur. Both factors are included by using Kaplan and Meier plot[7].

In contrast to the present findings, a recent Danish study with bendroflumethiazide showed no difference between a placebo and an actively treated group[5], but the average follow-up period was only 18 months. The present study suggests that thiazide has an equally beneficial effect in patients with or without hypercalciuria. It may be concluded that this is the first prospective, double-blind controlled clinical study showing that thiazide has a significantly more positive effect than placebo on stone prophylaxis.

ACKNOWLEDGEMENTS

This study was supported by Ciba-Geigy Pharma A/S, Norway.

REFERENCES

1. E. R. Yendt, Canad. Med. Assoc. J. 102:479 (1970).
2. E. R. Yendt and M. Cohanim, Canad. Med. Assoc. J. 198:755 (1978).
3. U. Backman, B. G. Danielson, G. Johansson, S. Ljunghall, and B. Wikström, Br. J. Urol. 51:175 (1979).
4. F. L. Coe, Ann. Intern. Med. 87:404 (1977).
5. P. Brocks, C. Dahl, H. Wolfe, and J. Transbøl, Lancet ii:124 (1981).
6. E. Laerum, Scand. J. Prim. Health Care 1:56 (1983).
7. E. L. Kaplan and P. Meier, J. Am. Stat. Assoc.. 53:457 (1958).

APPRAISAL OF METHODOLOGY IN STUDIES OF EITHER THIAZIDE OR

ORTHOPHOSPHATE THERAPY FOR RECURRENT CALCIUM UROLITHIASIS

D. N. Churchill

Faculty of Health Sciences, McMaster University
Hamilton, Ontario, Canada

INTRODUCTION

Thiazide diuretics and orthophosphates are generally considered effective in the prevention of recurrent calcium urolithiasis[1-12] but several randomized controlled clinical trials have failed to demonstrate this effectiveness[13-15]. These different conclusions may, in part, be explained by the various clinical research designs used. In order to evaluate this, clinical trials using these drugs to prevent recurrent calcium urolithiasis were examined from the viewpoint of clinical research methodology.

METHODS

The inclusion criteria were: (i) the study was an English language publication, (ii) the episodes of kidney stone recurrence were well-defined and (iii) drug treatment was clearly described. The research designs were classified as: (1) one group design with outcomes (stone episodes) measured before and after the intervention (drug), (2) one group design plus a non-equivalent comparison group with outcomes measured before and after the intervention, and (3) randomized controlled clinical trial. Within each of these designs the following methodologic and statistical problems were considered: (a) co-intervention, (b) statistical regression to the mean, (c) selection, (d) low statistical power and (e) heterogeneity of study subjects.

RESULTS

Sixteen studies (10 thiazide, 6 orthophosphate) met the inclusion criteria[1-15]. Eight[1-8] (4 thiazide, 4 orthophosphate) had a one group design, five[9-12] (4 thiazide, 1 orthophosphate) had a one group design with a non-equivalent comparison group and three[13-15] (2 thiazide, 1 orthophosphate) had a randomized controlled clinical trial design.

The 8 studies with a one group design[1-8] concluded that the intervention was effective. This result could have been due to changes in diet or an increase in fluid ingestion (i.e. co-intervention). Disease activity (e.g. stone frequency) will vary randomly around a mean activity level. If patients are referred for and receive drug treatment when disease activity is high, there will be a tendency to a spontaneous decrease in disease activity to the mean level regardless of treatment. This is known as statistical regression to the mean and is very likely operative in the one-group design.

Five studies with a one group design with a non-equivalent comparison group[9-13] are subject to a selection bias. The non-equivalent comparison group differs systematically from the treatment group when the former contains non-compliant patients and the latter does not[9-11]. If the treatment group is followed in a stone clinic and the comparison group is not, differential co-intervention will occur. Three of these studies using this design found the treatments effective but were subject to these biases[9-11]. Two of these studies found that both treatment and comparison groups had improved. There were compliant patients in both treatment and comparison groups and were both followed in a stone clinic[12].

The three studies with a randomized controlled clinical trial design[13-15] failed to reject the null hypothesis of no difference in stone episode rate between treatment and control group. The power, at the planning stage, was less than 30% for each study and the probability of a Type II error greater than 70%. The method described by Dunnett and Gent was used to assess power at the analysis stage[16]. In each case, the null hypothesis of a risk reduction of more than 50% in the stone recurrence rate was not rejected ($P > 0.05$). The possibility that a sub-group (e.g. hypercalciuric patients) within the total study group might be responsive to drug treatment (i.e. heterogeneity of study subjects) was not addressed.

DISCUSSION

Clinical trial designs which do not randomly allocate subjects to treatment and control groups are subject to the methodologic biases of co-intervention, statistical regression to the mean, and selection. The conclusion that drug treatment is effective is limited by these biases. On the other hand, the failure to demonstrate effectiveness in randomized controlled clinical trials does not necessarily mean that there is no effect. Larger studies, with appropriate stratification for risk, are required to provide sufficient statistical power to accept the null hypothesis of no significant clinical effect.

REFERENCES

1. D. S. Bernstein and R. Newton, Lancet 2:1105 (1966).
2. E. R. Yendt, Canad. Med. Assoc. J. 102:479 (1970).
3. L. H. Smith, W. C. Thomas, and C. D. Arnaud, in:"Urinary Calculi", L. Cifuentes Delatte, A. Rapado, and A. Hodgkinson, eds., Karger, Basel (1973).
4. B. Ettinger and F. O. Kolb, Am. J. Med. 55:32 (1973).
5. F. L. Coe and A. G. Kavalich, New Engl. J. Med. 291:1344 (1974).
6. E. R. Yendt and M. Cohanim, Kidney Int. 13:397 (1978).
7. M. Peacock, W. G. Robertson, P. J. Heyburn, A. E. J. Davies, and A. Rutherford, in:"Urolithiasis, Clinical and Basic Research", L. H. Smith, W. G. Robertson, and B. Finlayson, eds., Plenum, New York (1981).
8. G. Maschio, N. Tessitore, A. D'Angelo, A. Fabris, F. Pagano, A. Tasca, G. Graziani, A. Aroldi, M. Suriam, G. Colussi, A.Mandressi, A. Trinchieri, F. Rocco, C. Ponticelli, and L. Minetti, Am. J. Med. 71:623 (1981).
9. F. L. Coe, Ann. Intern. Med. 87:404 (1977).
10. U. Backman, B. G. Danielson, G. Johansson, S. Ljunghall, and B. Wikström, Br. J. Urol. 51:175 (1979).
11. S. Ljunghall, U. Backman, B. G. Danielson, B. Fellström, G. Johansson, and B. Wikström, in:"Urolithiasis, Clinical and Basic Research", L. H. Smith, W. G. Robertson, and B.Finlayson, eds., Plenum, New York (1981).
12. C. Y. C. Pak, P. Peters, G. Hurt, M. Kadesky, M. Fine, D.Reisman, F. Splann, C. Caramela, A. Freeman, F. Britton, K.Sakhaee, and N. A. Breslau, Am. J. Med. 71:615 (1981).
13. B. Ettinger, Am. J. Med. 61:200 (1976).
14. P. Brocks, C. Dahl, H. Wolf, and I. Transbøl, Lancet 2:124 (1981).
15. D. Scholz, P. O. Schwille, and A. Sigel, J. Urol. 128:903 (1982).
16. C. W. Dunnett and M. Gent, Biometrics 33:593 (1977).

THE EFFECTS OF ORTHOPHOSPHATE AND ION BINDERS

L. H. Smith

The Nephrology Research Unit, Mayo Clinic and
Mayo Foundation, Rochester, Minnesota, U.S.A.

The composition and amount of our daily diet along with intestinal absorption plays an important role in determining the composition of urine. The concentration of the major urinary ions is related, at least in part, to dietary intake[1-3]. With this in mind it is not surprising that compounds that complex normal dietary ions such as calcium, oxalate or phosphate within the intestinal tract and prevent their absorption have been used in the management of specific disorders complicated by the formation of urinary calculi. Shorr suggested the use of phosphate-binders in association with a low phosphate diet for the management of patients with phosphatic stones[4]. This program was suggested particularly for the control of struvite infection stones. Sodium phytate was used in conjunction with dietary calcium restriction for the management of idiopathic hypercalciuria by several groups[5,6]. Later, cellulose phosphate was suggested for the complexation of calcium although in the initial report it seemed to be most useful as adjunctive therapy to thiazide diuretics when suppressing hypercalciuria[7]. Since these early reports other compounds that can complex the important crystal ions within the intestinal tract have been suggested but characteristic of each has been their lack of specificity in terms of ion complexation resulting in multiple changes in the composition of the urine with both adverse and beneficial effects. As a result of these inter-related changes it is not sufficient to consider only the effect of these compounds on the specific ion of interest, i.e., calcium or oxalate. Instead, one must observe the effect on all of the major ions present in urine as well as the physical chemical factors including the state of supersaturation and inhibitors.

An example of this problem is illustrated by the treatment trials with cellulose phosphate in patients with idiopathic calcium urolithiasis. Backman et al reported the use of cellulose phosphate in 35 patients and compared these results with 29 untreated controls and 44 patients treated with thiazides[8]. After 2 years the recurrence rate with cellulose phosphate was 47% and the response was not different from the untreated controls. A subsequent study reported by Pak took into account adverse changes caused by the cellulose phosphate including reduced urinary magnesium and increased urinary oxalate[9]. Cellulose phosphate was used only in patients with documented absorptive hypercalciuria, the patients were given a low calcium-low oxalate diet and magnesium supplementation was used. With these changes the recurrence rate in 18 patients treated for an average of 2.4 years was 22% emphasizing the problem which may arise if one does not identify and correct the multiple alterations that may occur in the urine with these agents.

Orthophosphate, as a neutral sodium-potassium salt, was used initially as a potential complexor of dietary calcium[10]. In this role it had limited effect but when used in patients with idiopathic calcium urolithiasis, initial treatment trials were encouraging. Howard et al[11] reported its effective use in the control of stone formation and noted that urine from these patients that initially mineralized rachitic rat cartilage (evil urine) was converted to non-mineralizing urine (good urine) with the oral orthophosphate at a dosage to provide 2 g of elemental phosphorus per 24 h in divided doses. Since these initial observations there have been a number of reports that found this treatment program to be effective[12-16]. In one study, benefit could not be demonstrated but the acid potassium salt of orthophosphate was used at a maximum dose of 1.5 g of elemental phosphorus per 24 h[17]. This particular salt of phosphate reduces the urinary excretion of citrate and can increase hypercalciuria, changes that may explain the apparent lack of efficacy in that particular study[18].

Table 1. Types of Stone Formation Treatable with Orthophosphate.

Idiopathic calcium urolithiasis
    With hypercalciuria
    Without hypercalciuria
Primary hyperoxaluria
Type 1 renal tubular acidosis
Primary hyperparathyroidism
Sarcoidosis
Immobilization
Carbonic anhydrase inhibitor-induced stones

Orthophosphate has been used in a variety of clinical conditions complicated by the formation of calcium-containing stones within the urinary tract (Table 1). There would be limited indications with several of these conditions. In Type 1 renal tubular acidosis it has been used only in the limited group of patients who continue to form urinary calculi in spite of adequate replacement with alkali and electrolytes. In primary hyperparathyroidism it has been used in patients who were surgical failures and its only benefit has been in the prevention of further stone formation. It has no apparent beneficial effect on bone disease or other complications of hyperparathyroidism. In stone formation associated with the use of carbonic anhydrase inhibitors in patients with glaucoma it has been used only in those patients where the ophthalmologist felt there was a compelling need to continue the drug in the management of the eye problem. The greatest experience has been with patients who have idiopathic calcium urolithiasis and a small number of patients with the rare inherited disorder of primary hyperoxaluria. Reported below is our long-term experience with these two groups of patients.

A study was begun 21 years ago to evaluate the effectiveness of the neutral salt of orthophosphate in the prevention of urinary calculi in patients with idiopathic calcium urolithiasis. An earlier report on this study[12] was presented in Madrid in 1972. From this larger study was selected all of the patients who had formed at least one stone per year prior to initiation of treatment and had a minimum of 5 years of follow-up on treatment. In all of these patients the presence of metabolic activity in spite of increased fluid intake and elimination of dietary excesses (the stone clinic effect) was established prior to initiation of treatment[19]. This group included 37 patients with 31 males and 6 females. Hypercalciuria was present in 21 of the patients. Follow-up before treatment was 400 patient years and during treatment 445 patient years. The mean ($\pm$ SEM) follow-up before treatment was 10.8 $\pm$ 1.2 years and during treatment 12 $\pm$ 0.8. The median before treatment was 9.5 years and the median during treatment 11.8 years. The range before treatment was 1 to 30 years and the range during treatment 5 to 21 years. Before treatment the patients had formed 2,404 stones (6 stones per year per patient), during treatment they formed 60 (0.13 stones per year per patient). All of these new stones formed in three patients. In one, the new stone formation was stopped when the dosage of orthophosphate was increased to 2.0 g/24 h. In the other two, the new stone formation occurred after the patients had been under control on treatment for 3 and 5 years and they reduced the dosage of orthophosphate on their own volition. When the medication was increased to the original dose (2 g/24 h) stone formation stopped. Before treatment 1,041 stones (2.6 stones/year/patient) had been passed. During treatment 208 (0.5 stones/year/patient) stones were passed with the majority being old stones (Fig. 1).

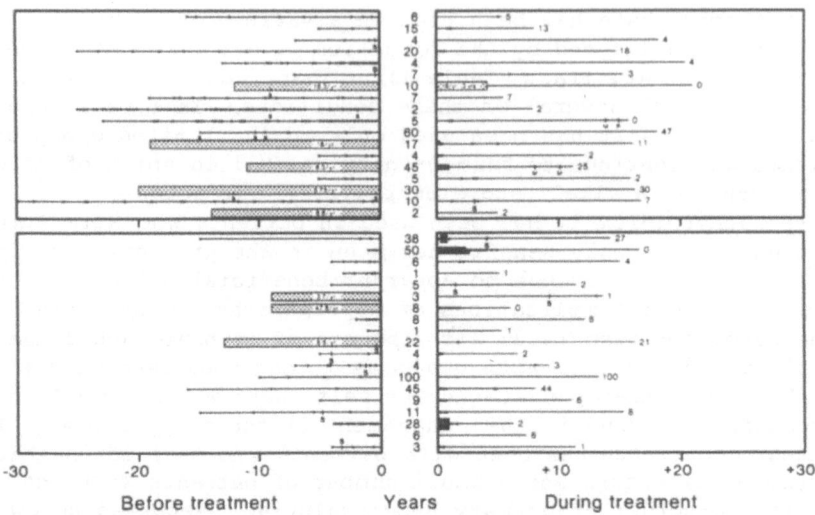

Before treatment   Years   During treatment

Fig. 1. Plot of stone formation before and during treatment. The
         numbers between the plots are the number of stones that
         each patient had when treatment was started. The number
         at the end of each of the treatment plots is the number of
         stones present at the time of the last follow-up.
         S = surgery; M = stone manipulation; P = percutaneous
         ultrasonic lithotripsy.

      The second group of patients had the rare inherited metabolic
disorder of primary hyperoxaluria. As historic control for this
group the review by Hockaday et al in 1964 established the natural
history of primary hyperoxaluria in untreated patients[20]. In that
report, 64 patients were described. The mean age of onset of
symptoms was 9.5 years. Of these patients only 30 were alive at the
time of the report; 34 patients who had died did so at a mean age
of 13.6 years with a range of less than 1 year to 34 years of age.
In 1966 a study was started in patients identified as having primary
hyperoxaluria. Treatment included the neutral salt of
orthophosphate to provide from 25 to 30 mg of elemental
phosphorus/kg/24 h in divided doses (2g/24h in adults) and
pyridoxine (150 to 200 mg/24 h). The study includes 14 patients,
10 females and 4 males. The mean age of onset of symptoms in this
group was 11.4 years with a range of 2 months to 22 years. The
mean age when the diagnosis was made was 18.1 years with a range of
2 to 39 years. One of the patients was initially detected at the
age of 39 during a family screen initiated because the diagnosis of
primary hyperoxaluria had been made in her sister. At that time
she had no history of urinary calculi and normal renal function.
During the 13 years of follow-up her status remains unchanged and
treatment has not been started in spite of persistent hyperoxaluria
and calcium oxalate crystalluria. In the 13 patients who were

486

placed on this treatment program the mean time of follow-up has been 9.7 ± 1.2 years, the range is 2.2 to 16.5 years. Prior to treatment, 14 surgical procedures had been carried out in 10 of these patients. This included nephrectomy in 4 and a successful cadaveric transplantation. It has now been 6 years since the cadaveric transplant was done and the patient has a serum creatinine of 0.9 mg/dl with an iothalamate clearance of 90 ml/min/1.73 m^2. Twelve of the 13 patients have had complete control of their stone formation. One patient has continued to accumulate stone mass slowly within his solitary kidney. In this patient the 24-h urine excretion rate of oxalate is consistently greater than 300 mg/day. One of the 12 patients who was under complete control developed a highly malignant breast cancer with recurrence after 3 months; at that time radiation and chemotherapy was instituted in another institution with cessation of pyridoxine and orthophosphate. At that time her serum creatinine was 0.9 mg/dl. Six weeks later she presented with a complete heart block and a serum creatinine of 15.8 mg/dl. Evidence of diffuse oxalosis rapidly developed and in spite of aggresive dialysis the patient died. In 6 of these patients there was evidence of loss of stone mass either as decrease in stone size or passage of old stones. In 4, control of their stone formation was temporarily lost during the period of increased growth during puberty. It was felt that this breakthrough in treatment was related to our failure to increase the dosage of orthophosphate to compensate for increased body weight. During the treatment period only 4 surgical procedures have been necessary in 3 patients. All of these were for old stones that had been present at the initiation of treatment.

As reported previously, the most common complication of orthophosphate treatment has been gastrointestinal intolerance[12]. This is usually in the form of diarrhea which is most common during the initial period of treatment. In most patients this subsides without further difficulty. In those patients where the problem is significant, dosage should be decreased 50% until the symptoms subside then gradually increased to treatment levels. Patients who have underlying gastrointestinal diseases including irritable bowel syndrome do not tolerate orthophosphate well and alternative approaches to treatment may be necessary. Hypertension can be aggravated with the sodium salt of orthophosphate. Patients who have stones present within the urinary tract at the time treatment is initiated may pass some or all of these stones. In an earlier report 40% of the patients treated lost stone mass and of those who did approximately one-half did so without symptoms[12]. This usually occurs within the first 6 months of treatment and is a phenomenon that will occur with any effective form of treatment.

The presence of secondary stone factors including obstruction or infection with struvite stone formation are absolute contraindications to orthophosphate treatment. In these situations the mechanism of stone formation is different and orthophosphate will not be effective. Also, adjustments are necessary in patients with reduced renal function. It should not be used in patients who have a GFR in the range of 30 to 50 ml/min, it can be used cautiously with frequent monitoring of serum creatinine, calcium and phosphorus. If the GFR is 50 ml/min, this treatment program can be used safely.

Orthophosphate therapy has beneficial effects on several physical chemical factors in the urine. The excretion rate of calcium (mmol/24 h) is reduced. This is associated with an increase in phosphate, citrate, and carbonate excretion as well as urine pH. This combination increases complexation of calcium resulting in an even greater decrease in the free calcium ion acivity and a significant decrease in the (free calcium ion/total calcium) ratio documenting the increase in complexation of calcium. These changes decrease supersaturation for the calcium oxalate crystal system without a change in the supersaturation of hydroxyapatite and brushite. Citrate and pyrophosphate increase and with the increase in urine pH, pyrophosphate becomes a more effective inhibitor in the calcium oxalate crystal system[21]. Crystalluria is decreased markedly and since the inhibitors are adsorbed to the crystal surface and effectively removed from solution, these inhibitors will remain in solution when crystalluria is decreased or eliminated. These two effects increase inhibition of crystal formation. It is thought that these two major effects acting together explain the apparent beneficial effect of orthophosphate. In the patients with primary hyperoxaluria pyridoxine did cause a significant decrease in the urinary excretion of oxalate providing an important added benefit. In 2 of the patients oxalate excretion was reduced to near normal. In 7 of the additional patients the decrease was in the range of 30%.

REFERENCES

1. W. G. Robertson, M. Peacock, P. J. Heyburn, F. A. Hanes, A. Rutherford, E. Clementson, R. Swaminathan, and P. B. Clark, Br. J. Urol. 51:427 (1979).
2. E. W. Vahlensieck, D. Bach, and A. Hesse, Urol. Res. 10:195 (1982).
3. L. H. Smith, C. J. Van Den Berg, D. M. Wilson, New Engl. J. Med. 298:87 (1978).
4. E. Shorr and A. C. Carter, J. Am. Med. Assoc. 144:1540 (1950).
5. P. H. Henneman, E. L. Carroll, and F. Albright, Ann. N. Y. Acad. Sci. 64:343 (1956).
6. W. H. Boyce, F. K. Garvey, and C. E. Goven, J. Am. Med. Assoc. 166:1577 (1958).
7. C. E. Dent, C. M. Harper, and A. M. Parfitt, Clin. Sci. 27:417 (1964).

8. U. Backman, B. G. Danielson, G. Johannson, S. Ljunghall, and B. Wikström, J. Urol 123:9 (1980).

9. C. Y. C. Pak, Invest. Urol. 19:187 (1981).

10. H. Spencer, L. Kramer, D. Osis, and C. Norris, J. Nutr. 108:447 (1978).

11. J. E. Howard, W. C. Thomas, T. Mukai, R. A. Johnson, and B. J. Pascoe, Trans. Assoc. Physcns. 915:301 (1962).

12. L. H. Smith, W. C. Thomas, and C. D. Arnaud, in:"Urinary Calculi", L. Cifuentes Delatte, A. Rapado, and A. Hodgkinson, eds., Karger, Basel (1973).

13. H. Fleisch, S. Bisaz, and A. D. Care, Lancet ii:1065 (1964).

14. N. A. Edwards, R. G. G. Russell, and A. Hodgkinson, Br. J. Urol. 37:390 (1965).

15. D. S. Bernstein and R. Newton, Lancet ii:1105 (1966)

16. W. C. Thomas, Kidney Int. 13:390 (1978).

17. B. Ettinger, Am. J. Med. 61:200 (1976).

18. K. Lau, C. Wolf, P. Nussbaum, B. Weiner, P. DeOreo, E. Slatopolsky, Z. Agus, and S. Goldfarb, Kidney Int. 16:736 (1979).

19. D. H. Hosking, S. B. Erickson, C. J. Van Den Berg, D. M. Wilson and L. H. Smith, J. Urol. 130:1115 (1983).

20. T. D. R. Hockaday, J. E. Clayton, E. W. Frederick, and L. HSmith, Medicine 43:315 (1964).

21. H.-G. Tiselius, Br. J. Urol. 53:470 (1981).

EFFECT OF ORTHOPHOSPHATE TREATMENT ON URINE COMPOSITION

IN IDIOPATHIC CALCIUM UROLITHIASIS

J. W. L. Wilson, P. G. Werness, and L. H. Smith

Nephrology Research Unit, Mayo Clinic and Foundation
Rochester, Minnesota, U.S.A, and Dept. of Urology
Queen's University, Kingston, Ontario, Canada K7L 2V7

INTRODUCTION

Oral neutral orthophosphate (OP) has been shown to be effective in the treatment of patients with idiopathic calcium urolithiasis (ICU)[1,2].

METHODS

In order to determine the effect of therapy on urine composition, we studied a group of 19 patients with ICU, on no treatment and while being treated with OP, in a dose providing the equivalent of 1.5 to 2.0 g of elemental phosphorus per day. Each study period was conducted in a clinical research unit, while the patients were consuming their normal diet and fluid intake, as determined by diet history.

Urine pH and major ions were determined (Table 1), and using the EQUIL program[3], supersaturation was calculated. To avoid large numbers, a form of the Gibbs free energy ΔG for transfer from supersaturated to saturated solutions was used to express supersaturation according to $\Delta G = -(RT/n)\ln SS$, where R is 8.314 joules/degree per mol, T is temperature in $^{\circ}K$, n is number of ions in the molecule and SS is relative supersaturation ratio. To eliminate the confusion of negative numbers, we arbitrarily defined a function DG to express supersaturation, where $DG = -\Delta G$. Inhibitors of crystal growth of calcium oxalate and hydroxyapatite were assayed using seeded crystal growth systems[4]. Crystalluria was assessed in each freshly voided urine sample, according to previously described techniques[5].

Table 1. Major Ions Analyzed and Assays Utilized in Orthophosphate Treatment Study.

Major Ions	Known Inhibitors	Inhibitor Assay	Crystalluria
Sodium	Pyrophosphate	Calcium Oxalate	2 ml freshly
Potassium	Citrate	Hydroxyapatite	voided urine
Calcium	Magnesium		
Oxalate			
Phosphorus			
Sulphate			
Uric Acid			
Ammonia			
CO_2 content			
Creatinine			
pH			

RESULTS

Urine volume, osmolality, and ionic strength did not change on therapy. Total urine calcium excretion decreased (mean change -0.25 mol/mol creatinine, $P < 0.001$), and ionized calcium concentration decreased (mean change -1.3 mmol/l, $P < 0.001$). The ratio, ionized calcium concentration to total calcium concentration, decreased (mean change -0.2, $P < 0.001$) indicating increased complexation of calcium with treatment. Total oxalate and urate excretion did not change, and total phosphate excretion increased (mean change +2.87 mol/mol creatinine, $P < 0.001$). Urine pH increased. Supersaturation decreased for calcium oxalate and uric acid, but did not change for hydroxyapatite, or brushite.

There was no change in inhibitor activity of calcium oxalate crystal growth; inhibitor activity of hydroxyapatite crystal growth increased (mean change +15 IU/l, $P < 0.005$). Excretion of the individual inhibitors pyrophosphate and citrate increased (mean change +3.0 mmol/mol creatinine and +0.05 mol/mol creatinine respectively, $P < 0.001$ for both). Magnesium excretion decreased (mean change -0.11 mol/mol creatinine, $P < 0.001$). Crystalluria score decreased (mean change -0.55, $P < 0.005$).

DISCUSSION

The beneficial changes of orthophosphate therapy included a decrease in urine calcium excretion with an increase in calcium complexation secondary to increased urinary phosphate, citrate and pH. This resulted in a decreased supersaturation of calcium oxalate, without an increase in supersaturation of the phosphate-containing phases, hydroxyapatite and brushite. The excretion of

492

the inhibitors pyrophosphate and citrate increased, as reflected by the increased inhibitor activity of hydroxyapatite crystal growth. Crystalluria decreased to normal.

Oral neutral orthophosphate salts have been shown to be effective in the treatment of idiopathic calcium urolithiasis, and we define the beneficial chemical changes that occur in the urine to decrease the tendency toward the formation and growth of urinary calculi.

REFERENCES

1. L. H. Smith, W. C. Thomas, and C. D. Arnaud, in:"Urinary Calculi", L. Cifuentes Delatte, A. Rapado, and A. Hodgkinson, eds., Karger, Basel (1973).
2. W. C. Thomas, Kidney Int. 13:390 (1978).
3. B. Finlayson, in:"Calcium Metabolism in Renal Failure and Urolithiasis", D. S. David, ed., Wiley, New York (1977).
4. J. L. Meyer and L. H. Smith, Invest. Urol. 13:36 (1975).
5. P. G. Werness, J. H. Bergert, and L. H. Smith, J. Cryst. Growth 53:166 (1981).

PHOSPHATE TREATMENT OF CALCIUM UROLITHIASIS

B. Wikström, U. Backman, B. G. Danielson, B. Fellström,
G. Johansson, S. Ljunghall, and L. Wide

Depts. of Internal Medicine and Clinical Chemistry
University Hospital, S-751 85 Uppsala, Sweden

INTRODUCTION

Dietary supplementation with orthophosphate was proposed as an alternative for prophylaxis of renal stone formation many years ago[1]. The rationale for this proposal is the documented effect of phosphates on reducing the urinary excretion of calcium, thus decreasing supersaturation of the urine. Phosphate intake has also been shown to increase the urinary excretion of inhibitors of stone formation, e.g. pyrophosphate[2]. A number of reports of prophylactic treatment with phosphate have been published. They have shown varying clinical results[3]. Since there is a great need for treatment alternatives in renal stone disease we undertook a study of the clinical and biochemical effects of long-term phosphate treatment. Since patients with renal acidification defects tend to have more severe stone disease[4], a special interest was placed on the clinical outcome in these patients.

MATERIALS AND METHODS

Sixty-four patients with idiopathic recurrent renal calcium stone disease were studied (51 males, 13 females, mean age 46 years (range 27 to 79)). Clinical and metabolic evaluation was performed in our out-patient stone clinic. Mean ($\pm$SD) urinary calcium was 8.6 $\pm$ 33 mmol/24 h. Therapy with phosphate was instituted irrespective of urinary calcium. Fifty-three calcium stone patients (43 males, 10 females) with no prophylactic treatment were used as controls. Their mean age was 46 years (range 32 to 76).

The short ammonium chloride loading test[5] was performed in 57 patients in the treatment group. The test disclosed 37 patients with normal acidification, 15 patients with proximal incomplete renal tubular acidosis (pRTA) and 5 patients with distal incomplete RTA (dRTA).

Neutral sodium-potassium orthophosphate salts were given as one tablet (Phosphate Sandoz) three times per day. This is equivalent to 1.5 g of phosphorus per day. Follow-up time was 1 to 5 years (mean 3.1). Patients were regularly followed in our stone clinic.

RESULTS

At the follow-up evaluation for this study, 51 (80%) of the patients remained free of relapse. The corresponding figure for controls was 31%. Stone episode rate during follow-up was significantly lower in treated patients than in controls (Table 1). There was no significant difference in the results of treatment between normocalciuric and hypercalciuric patients or between patients with different degrees of urinary acidification capacity (Table 2). In controls, the stone episode rate (stones per year) did not change significantly during follow-up.

During phosphate treatment TmP/GFR fell from 0.87 ± 0.11 mmol/l to 0.70 ± 0.20 (n=18, P<0.01). However, there were no significant changes in serum phosphate, calcium, alkaline phosphatase or parathyroid hormone in the treated patients. During phosphate treatment a significant increase was seen in urinary excretion of phosphate and pyrophosphate with a corresponding decrease in urinary calcium excretion.

In two patients an increase in serum parathyroid hormone concentrations was noted after treatment with phosphate 6 months and 2 years, respectively. A biochemical and metabolic evaluation of these patients suggested at least transient parathyroid stimulation in these patients and phosphate medication was stopped in one of the

Table 1. Clinical Results of Phosphate Treatment.

Group	Stone Episode Rate (stone episodes/year)	
	Before follow-up	During follow-up
Phosphate- treated (n=64)	0.56	0.07
Controls (n=53)	0.45	0.23

Table 2. Clinical Results of Phosphate Treatment on Stone Patients
and Patients with Acidification Defects.

	NC	HC	no RTA	pRTA	dRTA
Patients (n)	27	37	37	15	5
Follow-up (years)	77	115	106	42	12
Stones (n)	4	9	6	5	2
Stone episode rate (stones/year)	0.06	0.08	0.06	0.12	0.17
Patients with recurrence (n)	4	7	-	-	-

NC = normocalciuric; HC = hypercalciuric; no RTA = without RTA;
pRTA = proximal incomplete RTA; dRTA = distal incomplete RTA.

cases. In this case the development of hypertension also made
withdrawal of phosphate necessary.

Clinical side-effects were noted in 40% of the treated
patients. Gastrointestinal discomfort with gastric irritation,
loose stools and sometimes diarrhoea was seen in 35% of the patients
and aggravation of hypertension in 8%. Because of these side-
effects phosphate had to be withdrawn in 12% of the treated
patients.

DISCUSSION

In this study with long-term orthophosphate treatment
beneficial urinary biochemical effects were confirmed and a
satisfying clinical prophylactic effect was seen. These results
are similar to some recent reports on phosphate treatment[3,6], but
treatment failures have occurred[7]. Wider use of phosphate
treatment, however, may be limited because of the clinical side-
effects of orthophosphate intake. Development of secondary
hyperparathyroidism would be a serious side-effect of dietary
supplementation with phosphate. Mild parathyroid stimulation could
not be excluded in two cases in this study. Regular biochemical
evaluation to check for parathyroid stimulation should be performed
during phosphate treatment. However, other recent clinical studies
have not shown evidence of secondary hyperparathyroidism[3,6].

REFERENCES

1. F. Albright, W. Bauer, D. Claflin, and J. R. Cochriel, J. Clin.
   Invest. 11:411 (1932).

2. H. Fleisch, Kidney Int. 13:361 (1978).

3. L. H. Smith, P. G. Werness, C. J. Van den Berg, and D. M. Wilson, Scand. J. Urol. Nephrol. 53 (Suppl):253 (1980).

4. U. Backman, B. G. Danielson, G. Johansson, S. Ljunghall, and B. Wikström, Nephron 25:96 (1980).

5. U. Backman, B. G. Danielson, and M. Sohtell, Scand. J. Urol. Nephrol. 35 (Suppl):33 (1976).

6. P. J. Heyburn, W. G. Robertson, and M. Peacock, Nephron 32:314 (1982).

7. B. Ettinger, Am. J. Med. 61:200 (1976).

THE ROLE OF URATE AND ALLOPURINOL IN STONE DISEASE:

A REVIEW

B. Finlayson, R. C. Newman, and P. T. Hunter

Division of Urology, Dept. of Surgery, College of
Medicine, University of Florida, Gainesville
Florida 32610, U.S.A.

INTRODUCTION

In the past 20 years, many investigators have endeavored to
shed light on the role of urate and allopurinol in stone disease.
This discussion attempts to define what has been established.

URATE EXCRETION AND ALLOPURINOL IN URIC ACID AND URATE UROLITHIASIS

The uric acid content of urinary stones varies from 1 to 98%.
In predominantly uric acid stones, uric acid serves as the primary
precipitant and known crystallization inhibitors modulate it very
little[1]. Adult, uric acid stone-formers tend to have a urine more
acid than normal which increases the likelihood of uric acid
precipitation and stone formation. Infants physiologically excrete
high urinary uric acid levels. Children starved or fed a highly
acid ash diet excrete ammonia, and ammonium urate bladder calculi
may result.

The therapeutic effect of allopurinol on uric acid and urate
stones appears to result from a lowering of urinary urate excretion
which in turn allows stone dissolution. In short, the role of
urate excretion and allopurinol in uric acid stones seems
straightforward.

URIC ACID AND ALLOPURINOL IN CALCIUM OXALATE STONE DISEASE

This interaction is less clear. In fact, making sense of this
subject by reading the literature is a little like trying to pick up

499

a drop of mercury with one's fingers.   Past understanding has been based on the following:

1. There is an apparent increased incidence of calcium oxalate stones in gouty patients[2,3].

2. Close lattice matches between calcium oxalate and urates[4,5], suggest that some urates may catalyze the precipitation of calcium oxalate[4].

3. Based on the preceding observations, allopurinol has been used in calcium oxalate stone-formers and caused an apparent reduction in stone formation[6,7].   Other studies have demonstrated a similar effect, but they were not blind and therefore lacked statistical discriminating power[6,8-10].

4. The frequency of hyperuricosuria among calcium oxalate stone-formers varies from 10-30%[11,12] and is dependent on age[13] and geographic location[11,12].   Based on this fact, many infer that urinary urate promotes calcium oxalate stone formation. Unfortunately, data comparing the incidence of calcium oxalate stone disease in hyperuricosurics and the general population is not available.   The latter information seems essential to draw conclusions.

Taken together, these data are not conclusive and analysis of other factors seems warranted.

Data on the epitaxial factors of strain energy[14,15], nucleation[16-22] and seed crystal precipitation[23] are conflicting and cannot be compared owing to experimental variation.   In fact, the epitaxy hypothesis may be irrelevant, since the expected effects of an increase in crystallization by nucleation catalysis will be small when the ordinary washout time of the upper urinary tract is considered.

In vitro experiments have demonstrated that urate precipitates in urine can cause solution depletion of crystallization inhibitors like glycosaminoglycans (GAGs).   When the amount of urate precipitate required per day to deplete fractionally the urine of a given amount of inhibitor is calculated[24-28], it appears statistically that we are close to, but are not yet in, the region of plausibility for inhibitor depletion by urate precipitates.   In addition, there are some data which suggest that urates may interfere with inhibitor excretion.   The normal positive correlation between GAGs and urate excretion is negative in hyperuricosuric stone-formers[24].

Diet may play a role in the interaction of urate in calcium oxalate stone disease.   Both Simmonds and Hodgkinson observed that urinary oxalate excretion is positively correlated with purine intake[29,30].

500

The urate produced may serve as a mortar or cement by its presence in the "matrix" of seemingly pure calcium oxalate stones[31,32]. It is a common observation that hyperuricosuric calcium oxalate stone-formers have more frequent stone episodes and produce bigger stones than comparable groups of non-hyperuricosuric calcium oxalate stone-formers[12]. This phenomenon seems analogous to the effect of triamterene on calcium oxalate stones[33] in which triamterene does not necessarily initiate the process, but does aggravate the problem by becoming incorporated into the stone and accelerating growth rate. Since the advent of extracorporeal shock wave lithotripsy (ESWL) therapy, we have learned that 85% of the population can pass particles up to 3 mm asymptomatically[34]. A hyperuricosuric stone patient may be more likely to notice passage because of increased stone growth rate.

In the laboratory, calcium oxalate crystals stick to the tubular epithelium, possibly injuring the epithelium and acting as an encrustation platform. Dystrophic calcification in these epithelial tissues could lead to Randall's plaque formation[35-37]. Through the Vermeulen "trigger" process, we and others[38] postulate that urate precipitates will cause similar problems.

Other studies show that allopurinol has no specific effect on calcium oxalate precipitation[39,40] and does not reduce calcium excretion. The drug does reduce urinary oxalate and may directly increase inhibitor excretion[25]. Pak has shown that allopurinol does not reduce the calcium oxalate activity product ratio[41].

A new report by Ettinger is being presented at this conference. Although this study is double-blind, it is not yet rich enough in patients to be conclusive. It must be considered in minute detail, because considerable lines of inquiry could be justified or foreclosed depending on acceptance or rejection of the report's conclusion.

CONCLUSION

The role of urate and allopurinol in urate stone disease seems uncomplicated. Definitive substantiated information on the role of urate/allopurinol in calcium oxalate stone disease is not available at present, and therefore we cannot accept or reject the uric acid/allopurinol/calcium oxalate hypothesis. It is rarely possible to prove things in biology; however, progress is often made by disproving hypotheses and reducing the universe of discourse. Experimental efforts aimed at falsifying hypotheses should be helpful.

ACKNOWLEDGMENT

This work was supported by N.I.G. Grant AM 20586.

REFERENCES

1. O. Sperling, A. de Vries, and O. Kedem, J. Urol. 94:286 (1965).
2. E. L. Prien and E. L. Prien, Jr., Am. J. Med. 45:654 (1968).
3. A. B. Gutman, Am. J. Med. 45:756 (1968).
4. K. Lonsdale, Science 159:1199 (1968).
5. N. S. Mandel and G. S. Mandel, in:"Urolithiasis:Clinical and Basic Research", L. H. Smith, W. G. Robertson, and B. Finlayson, eds., Plenum Press, New York (1981).
6. M. J. V. Smith, J. Urol. 117:690 (1977).
7. F. L. Coe and L. Raisen, Lancet 1:129 (1973).
8. F. L. Coe, Ann. Int. Med. 87:404 (1977).
9. G. Brien and C. Bick, Eur. Urol. 3:35 (1977).
10. F. C. Berthoux, J. Jorge, C. Genin, J. C. Sabatrer, and H.Assenat, Min. Elect. Metab. 2:207 (1979).
11. B. Fellström, U. Backman, B. G. Danielson, G. Johnson, S. Ljunghall, and B. Wikström, J. Urol. 127:589 (1982).
12. F. L. Coe, "Nephrolithiasis Pathogenesis and Treatment", Yearbook Medical Publishers, Chicago (1978).
13. P. Schwille, N. Samberger, and B. Wach, Nephron 16:116 (1976).
14. B. Finlayson, Kidney Int. 13:344 (1978).
15. D. Turnbull and B. Vonnegut, Ind. Eng. Chem. 44:1291 (1952).
16. J. A. Venables and G. L. Price, in: "Epitaxial Growth, Part B", J. W. Matthews, ed., Academic Press, New York (1975).
17. M. J. Stowell, in:"Epitaxial Growth, Part B", J. W. Matthews, ed., Academic Press, New York (1975).
18. J. R. Burns and B. Finlayson, Invest. Urol. 18:2:133 (1980).
19. J. L. Meyer, J. Urol. 19:197 (1981).
20. F. L. Coe, R. L. Lawton, R. B. Goldstein, and V. Tembe, Proc. Soc. Exp. Biol. Med. 149:926 (1975).
21. C. Y. C. Pak and L. H. Arnold, Proc. Soc. Exp. Biol. Med. 149:930 (1975).
22. P. G. Koutsoukos, C. Y. Lam-Erwin, and G. H. Nancollas, Invest. Urol. 18:178 (1980).
23. L. Blomen, "Growth and Agglomeration of Calcium Oxalate Monohydrate Crystals", Ph.D. Thesis, Leiden (1982).
24. D. S. Scurr, C. M. Bridge, and W. G. Robertson, in:"Urolithiasis:Clinical and Basic Research", L. H. Smith, W. G. Robertson, and B. Finlayson, eds., Plenum Press, New York (1981).
25. R. Caudarella, F. Stefarri, E. Rizzoli, N. Malavolta, and G. D'Antuano, J. Urol. 129:665 (1983).
26. B. Finlayson and L. DuBois, Clin. Chim. Acta 84:203 (1978).
27. L. Leal and B. Finlayson, Invest. Urol. 14:278 (1977).

28. L. Cifuentes-Delatte, Crystalluria, in "Stones:Clinical Management of Urolithiasis", R. A. Roth and B. Finlayson, eds., Williams and Wilkins, Baltimore (1983).

29. H. A. Simmonds, K. J. VanAcker, C. F. Potter, D. R. Webster, G. P. Kasidas, and G. A. Rose, in:"Urolithiasis:Clinical and Basic Research", L. H. Smith, W. G. Robertson, and B. Finlayson, eds., Plenum Press, New York (1981).

30. A. Hodgkinson, "Oxalic Acid in Biology and Medicine", Academic Press, New York (1977).

31. P. J. Buscemi, E. P. Goldberg, S. R. Khan, R. L. Hackett, and B. Finlayson, in:"Urinary Calculus", J. G. Brockis and B. Finlayson, eds., PSG Publishing Co., Inc., Littleton (1981).

32. L. Cifuentes-Delatte, J. Bellamato, M. Santos, and J. L. Rodriguez-Minon, Eur. Urol. 4:441 (1978).

33. B. Ettinger, N. O. Oldroyd, and F. Sörgel, J. Am. Med. Assoc. 244:2443 (1980).

34. C. Chaussy, E. Schmiedt, D. Jocham, W. Brendel, B. Forssmann, and V. Walther, J. Urol. 127:417 (1982)

35. S. R. Khan, R. L. Hackett, B. Finlayson, and J. R. Konicek, Scan. Electron. Microsc. 3:155 (1981).

36. S. R. Khan, B. Finlayson, and R. L. Hackett, Am. J. Path. 107:59 (1982).

37. S. R. Khan, B. Finlayson, and R. L. Hackett, Urology 23:194 (1984).

38. F. L. Coe, Adv. Exp. Med. Biol. 128:439 (1980).

39. B. Finlayson and F. Reid, Invest. Urol. 15:489 (1978).

40. G. A. Rose, J. Roy Soc. Med. 75:897 (1982).

41. C. Y. C. Pak, "Calcium Urolithiasis:Pathogenesis, Diagnosis, Treatment", Plenum, New York (1978).

ALLOPURINOL TREATMENT IN UROLITHIASIS

B. Fellström

Dept. of Internal Medicine, University Hospital
S-751 85 Uppsala, Sweden

INTRODUCTION

A large number of prophylactic treatments have been used to
prevent stone formation in the urinary tract.   Treatment with
orthophosphate, thiazides and magnesium hydroxide have been shown to
be effective in preventing recurrence of calcium stone disease.
Allopurinol has been used in the treatment of both uric acid stones
and calcium oxalate stones.   A brief review of the theoretical
background and the results from various studies of allopurinol in
the treatment of urolithiasis will be given.

ALLOPURINOL

Allopurinol interferes with purine metabolism through
inhibition of xanthine oxidase, which stimulates both the
conversion of hypoxanthine to xanthine and xanthine to uric acid
(Fig. 1).   A large number of inhibitors of xanthine oxidase are
known, but allopurinol has proved to be the most important[1].   Both
allopurinol and its major metabolite oxipurinol are potent
inhibitors of the enzyme.   Allopurinol itself has a short
biological half-life of 2 to 3 h.   It rapidly becomes oxidized to
oxipurinol which has a half-life of 28 h. Only some 3 to 10% of the
administered dose of allopurinol can be recovered in the urine.
Serious side-effects of allopurinol therapy appear to be rare
during the 15 years that the drug has been in general use.
Potentially important drug-to-drug interactions involving
allopurinol, includes basically purine analogues such as 6-
mercaptopurine and azathioprine, which are inactivated by xanthine
oxidase.   Allopurinol treatment has been widely used in uric acid

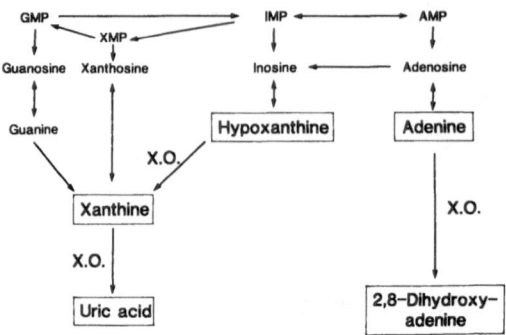

Fig. 1. Allopurinol is an analogue to hypoxanthine, and is both a
substrate for and an inhibitor of xanthine oxidase (xo).

over-production.   It has a well documented effect in the long-term
treatment of gout and uric acid nephropathy.   The use of
allopurinol in both uric acid and calcium oxalate stone disease
involves various aspects of uric acid metabolism, a brief summary of
which will be given.

PHYSIOLOGICAL ASPECTS OF URIC ACID

     Uric acid is the end-product of purine metabolism in man who
lacks uricase.   The precursors are basically endogenously
synthesized purines and the dietary content of nucleic acids in the
foodstuffs.   On a purine-free diet, uric acid excretion is about 2.5
mmol/24 h in man[2].   Two-thirds of the formed uric acid is excreted
in the urine and one-third through intestinal secretion to the gut[3].
The renal handling of urate is complex and involves almost complete
ultrafiltration in the glomeruli.   There is a 99% reabsorption of
the filtrate in the proximal tubuli of the nephron.   Tubular
secretion and the postsecretory reabsorption are the major transport
mechanisms deciding the final excretion of urate[4].   Urate clearance
is usually 6 to 12% of GFR.   There are also some rare hereditary
forms of deficiency in the tubular reabsorption of urate,
characterized by hypouricaemia, hyperuricosuria and renal stones[5].

PHYSICOCHEMICAL ASPECTS OF URIC ACID

     The importance of uric acid or urate salts in urolithiasis
depends upon the existence of a solid or colloidal phase in the
urine.   Uric acid is a weak acid (pK_1 = 5.7), and its solubility
increases when pH>5.7.   If pH is < 5.7, the solubility decreases and
the risk of uric acid crystals precipitating becomes important.   On
the other hand, when the free urate ion dominates, the
supersaturation levels of sodium acid urate, ammonium urate and

506

potassium urate increase. It has been shown that urine becomes supersaturated with sodium acid urate when the urate concentration 1.8 mmol/l (300 mg/l)[6]. The metastable range for sodium acid urate is, however, wide and the activity product is unlikely to exceed the formation product where crystals may form spontaneously. Whether or not the proposed intermediate colloidal phase exists in the urine has not been proven. As allopurinol causes a decreased production of uric acid and a decrease in its urinary excretion, urine will become less supersaturated with respect to both uric acid and the various urate salts.

URIC ACID LITHIASIS

In most countries pure uric acid lithiasis comprises about 5% of all renal stones[7], but there is some variation in the incidence between various countries. In Sweden, 2 to 3% of all stones are pure uric acid stones, whereas a higher incidence has been reported in Germany, France and, in particular, Israel. Successful treatment of uric acid lithiasis with allopurinol in combination with alkalinisation of the urine has been clearly proved[8].

URATE LEVELS IN CALCIUM STONE DISEASE

The incidence of renal stone formation in gout has been shown to be higher than in a non-gouty population[9]. This includes basically uric acid stones but also mixed uric acid and calcium oxalate stones. Hyperuricaemia does not seem to be a risk factor for calcium stone formation, however, as calcium stone formers do not have a higher serum urate than healthy controls[10,11].

Conflicting results have been reported on whether or not hyperuricosuria is a risk factor in calcium stone disease. There have been reports of calcium stone formers having a higher urinary urate than healthy controls[12,13], whereas in other studies no difference could be found[10,14]. Such a comparison also becomes difficult, as there are wide variations in the levels of urinary urate between various stone centres. A comparison of the frequency of hyperuricosuria suffers from the lack of unity in defining hyperuricosuria. The definition can be based either on statistical considerations (mean value + 2 SD) or on physicochemical grounds. Strauss and Coe reported that 36% of the patients were hyperuricosuric, using the limit 4.75 mmol/24 h in males and 4.45 mmol/24 h in females, a seemingly arbitrary level for hyperuricosuria[13]. In another study[15], 34% of the patients were considered hyperuricosuric (>3.6 mmol/24 h). In Italy[16], 48% of the patients had a urinary urate > 4.75 mmol/24 h. Apparently, there are large variations in urinary urate between various centres, and just as many definitions of hyperuricosuria as there are reports.

We used an arbitrary definition of hyperuricosuria in order to study the clinical characteristics of these patients. Ten percent of our patients had a urinary urate >4.5 mmol/24 h and had had more stone operations[14]. This is a finding that has also been reported previously[17] and points towards urinary urate being involved in the formation of larger aggregates in the urinary tract. There is also experimental evidence using an in vivo model supporting this clinical observation. The simultaneous induction of uricosuria and hyperoxaluria in the rat led to the formation of larger renal stones than hyperoxaluria alone[18].

POSSIBLE MECHANISMS FOR ALLOPURINOL IN CALCIUM STONE DISEASE

Several mechanisms have been proposed by which urate may play a role in the formation of calcium oxalate stones. However, these are all based on the existence of a solid or colloidal phase of uric acid or sodium acid urate which have not been proven to exist in the urine in calcium oxalate disease. The mechanisms include an anti-inhibition by urate through the binding of inhibitors of calcium oxalate crystal growth and aggregation[19]. Binding of both heparin and chondroitin sulphates to sodium urate crystals does take place and is potentiated in the presence of divalent cations[20]. Such binding apparently causes a reduction of the macromolecular inhibitors present in urine[19,21]. It was also demonstrated in vivo that a purine load decreased the formation product ratio (FPR) of calcium oxalate, whereas allopurinol treatment restored the original FPR[22]. The theory of growth of calcium oxalate on sodium urate microcrystals is based on structural similarities of the crystals and on in vitro studies of epitaxial growth[23]. Whether or not such a mechanism exists in vivo has not been proven. Sodium urate crystals are rarely observed in urine, although a mixture of urate and calcium oxalate has been found in 5% of stones.

Another mechanism by which allopurinol may have a beneficial effect in calcium oxalate stone disease is through a reduction in urinary oxalate excretion[24]. Whether this is linked to the suggested metabolic pathway of purine to oxalate or whether it involves a minor role of xanthine oxidase in the oxidation of glyoxylate to oxalate has not yet been settled.

ALLOPURINOL TREATMENT OF CALCIUM STONE DISEASE

In the assessment of the results of a clinical trial on prophylactic treatment in urolithiasis, one of the difficulties is the positive placebo effect. The positive effect of advice given to the patients regarding dietary restrictions and fluid intake also has to be considered in the evaluation of the effects by the active drug. Most studies that have been performed with allopurinol have been open studies with or without open control groups. This emphasizes the need of a randomized controlled study, before definite conclusions about the efficacy of allopurinol can be drawn. Nevertheless, a review of some of the reports on allopurinol treatment in calcium stone disease will be given. The study by Smith[25] was a randomized study where the only inclusion criterion was a serum urate >360 µmol/l. Both the allopurinol and the placebo groups were simultaneously given alkali. It was concluded that 60% of the patients in the allopurinol group were free of recurrence compared to 10% in the placebo group. In a recent update of the study, the conclusion has been revised and it was stated that no major difference could now be found between the groups[26]. Only a smnall group of patients with hyperuricosuria were considered to benefit from allopurinol treatment (Table 1).

Coe treated hyperuricosuric patients with 200 mg allopurinol daily and claimed a high frequency of remission. Patients who were both hyperuricosuric and hypercalciuric were treated with both allopurinol and thiazides. All patients were given advice regarding a reduction of dietary calcium and an increase of fluid ingestion. Independent of the pre-treatment metabolic classification, cases that relapsed had usually not been able to increase their urinary volume or had a persistent hypercalciuria[13,17]. No placebo group was used, however.

In a recent study by Pak[15], 47 patients were classified as hyperuricosuric and treated with 300 mg allopurinol. Patients with co-existing hypercalciuria were also given thiazides. All patients were given certain dietary restrictions and advice regarding fluid intake. Patients with hyperuricosuria alone had a remission rate of 85% during an average 1.7 year follow-up. A group of patients with absorptive hypercalciuria, treated only with dietary and fluid recommendations, served as a control group. Their remission rate was 91% in 1.8 years. No placebo control group was used. The conclusion was that allopurinol is generally beneficial.

Thirty calcium stone patients, of whom 50% were hyperuricosuric, were studied after 12 months' treatment with 300 mg allopurinol daily[27]. A generally beneficial effect was concluded, independent of whether or not the patients were hyperuricosuric prior to treatment. Apparently, a randomized study in 15 patients has been performed in the same centre, with half the patients on allopurinol and the other half on placebo for 3 years. They have reported, in this issue, an absence of beneficial effects of allopurinol treatment, independent of whether the patients were hyperuricosuric or not prior to treatment. In a multicentre study[16] all patients were given thiazides or amiloride. Forty-eight percent of the patients were hyperuricosuric and given 100 mg allopurinol in addition to the other treatment. No difference in the outcome, whether they were given allopurinol or not, could be

Table 1. Reports on Allopurinol Treatment in Calcium Stone Disease.

Investigator	Number of patients	Follow-up (years)	Free of recurrence	Simultaneous treatment or advice	Controls (number)	Investigators' conclusion
MJV Smith[25]	16 (92)	5	60%	alkali, fluid	alkali, fluid placebo (7)	positive
Coe[17]	90	3	91%	Tz in Hc diet, fluid	Tz in Hc diet, fluid (34)	positive
Miano[27]	30	1	60%	?	?	positive
Pak[15]	47	1.7	85%	Tz in Hc diet, fluid	Tz in Hc diet, fluid (21)	positive
Maschio[16]	277	1.6	90%	Tz or Amiloride	Tz or Amiloride (242)	negative
Strauss[13]	97	2	75%	Tz in Hc diet, fluid	Tz in Hc diet, fluid	positive
MJV Smith[26]	11	10	27%	alkali, fluid	alkali, fluid, placebo	doubtful
Miano[A]	8	3	-	-	placebo (7)	negative
Fellstrom[A]	31	2	51%	diet, fluid	diet, fluid (40)	negative
Robertson[A]	9	2-3	-	none	untreated (9)	doubtful
Wilson[A]	17	2.8	53%	diet, fluid	diet, fluid (21)	doubtful
Ettinger[A]	36	2	-	-	placebo (36)	positive

Tz = Thiazides; Hc = Hypercalciuria; A - Reported in this issue observed. In Uppsala 31 calcium stone patients were treated with 300 mg of allopurinol during a mean follow-up period of 2 years. Thirteen were hyperuricosuric prior to treatment (>4.5 mmol/24 h) and 12 patients were hypercalciuric (>7.5 mmol/24 h). Sixteen patients (51%) were free of recurrence after 2 years of treatment, irrespective of whether they were hyperuricosuric or not prior to treatment. A difference was found between patients that were hypercalciuric, where only 40% were free of recurrences after 2 years compared to 60% in patients with normocalciuria. In a control group of 40 patients without medical treatment, the degree of remission after 2 years' observation was 65%. Thus, we conclude that allopurinol treatment did not seem to be beneficial in this study.

Studies on allopurinol presented at this Conference have shown variable results. In one (Robertson et al), idiopathic stone patients were treated with 300 mg allopurinol. Their stone recurrence rate was only marginally reduced when compared with an untreated group of patients. No effect of allopurinol could be found in another series of idiopathic stone patients who were also given dietary advice (Wilson et al). In a controlled study, 72 calcium stone patients with hyperuricosuria were randomly assigned to allopurinol or placebo (Ettinger et al). A substantial decrease in the stone recurrence rate was seen in the placebo-treated patients, with an even more pronounced reduction in the allopurinol group. Finally, in a study of 126 calcium stone patients, treated with 300 mg allopurinol daily, it was concluded that relapses were common if extreme hypercalciuria was present (Ulshöfer et al). Thus, it seems as if allopurinol may be beneficial in calcium stone patients if they are hyperuricosuric, provided that no excess of urinary calcium co-exists, or that hypercalciuria has been treated simultaneously.

ACKNOWLEDGEMENTS

This work was supported by the Swedish Medical Research Council (nos. 2329, 6354), the Swedish Society of Medical Sciences and the Tore Nilsson Foundation.

REFERENCES

1. W. N. Kelley, Nephron 14:99 (1975).
2. B. Fellström, B. G. Danielson, B. Karlström, H. Lithell, S. Ljunghall, and B. Vessby, Clin. Sci. 64:399 (1983).
3. L. B. Sørensen and D. J. Levinson, Nephron 14:2 (1975).
4. H. S. Diamond and J. S. Paolino, J. Clin. Invest. 52:1491 (1973).
5. M. Frank, M. Many, and O. Sperling, Br. J. Urol. 51:88 (1979).

6. C. Y. C. Pak, O. Waters, L. Arnold, K. Holt, C. Cox, and D. Barilla, J. Clin. Invest. 59:426 (1977).

7. D. J. Levinson and L. B. Sørensen, in:"Nephrolithiasis, Pathogenesis and Treatment", F. L. Coe, ed., Year Book Medical Publishers, Chicago (1978).

8. A. de Vries, M. Frank, U. A. Liberman, and O. Sperling, Ann. Rheum. Dis. 25:691 (1966).

9. W. J. C. Currie and P. Turmer, Br. J. Urol. 51:337 (1979).

10. A. Hodgkinson, Br. J. Urol. 48:1 (1976).

11. B. Fellström, U. Backman, B. G. Danielson, G. Johansson, S. Ljunghall, and B. Wikström, J. Urol. 29:256 (1983).

12. W. G. Robertson, M. Peacock, P. J. Heyburn, D. H. Marshall and P. B. Clark, Br. J. Urol. 50:449 (1978).

13. A. L. Strauss, F. L. Coe, L. Deutsch and J. H. Parks, Am. J. Med. 72:17 (1982).

14. B. Fellström, U. Backman, B. G. Danielson, G. Johansson, S. Ljunghall, and B. Wikström, J. Urol. 27:589 (1982).

15. C. Y. C. Pak, P. Peters, G. Hurt, M. Kadesky, M. Fine, D. Reisman, F. Splann, C. Caramela, A. Freeman, F. Britton, K. Sakhaee, and N. A. Breslau, Am. J. Med. 71:615 (1981).

16. G. Maschio, N. Tessitore, A. D'Angelo, A. Fabris, F. Pagano, A. Tasca, G. Graziani, A. Aroldi, M. Surian, G. Colussi, A. Mandressi, A. Trinchieri, F. Rocco, C. Ponticelli, and L. Minetti, Am. J. Med. 71:623 (1981).

17. F. L. Coe, Ann. Intern. Med. 87:404 (1977).

18. F. Hering, K.-H. Bigalke, and W. Lutzeyer, in:"Purine Metabolism in Man", A. Rapado, R. W. E. Watts, and C. H. M. M. de Bruyn, eds., Plenum, New York (1979).

19. B. Fellström, U. Backman, B. G. Danielson, K. Holmgren, S. Ljunghall, and B. Wikström, Clin. Sci. 62:509 (1982).

20. B. Fellström, B. G. Danielson, F. A. Karlsson, and S. Ljunghall, in:"Urolithiasis and Related Clinical Research", P. O. Schwille, L. H. Smith, W. G. Robertson, and W. Vahlensieck, eds., Plenum, New York (1985).

21. J. E. Zerwekh, K. Holt, and C. Y. C. Pak, Kidney Int. 23:838 (1983).

22. C. Y. C. Pak, D. Barilla, K. Holt, L. Brinkley, R. Tolentino, and J. E. Zerwekh, Am. J. Med. 65:593 (1978).

23. C. Y. C. Pak and L. H. Arnold, Proc. Soc. Exp. Biol. Med. 149::930 (1975).

24. R. Scott, P. J. Paterson, A. Mathieson, and M. Smith, Br. J. Urol. 50:455 (1978).

25. M. J. V. Smith, J. Urol. 117:690 (1977).

26. M. J. V. Smith, in:"Proceedings of the European Dialysis and Transplant Association - European Renal Association", Vol. 20, A. M. Davison and P. J. Guillou, eds., Pitman, London(1983).

27. L. Miano, S. Petta, and M. Gallucci, Euro. Urol. 5:229 (1979).

FURTHER REDUCTION OF OXALATE EXCRETION BY ALLOPURINOL IN

STONE FORMERS ON LOW PURINE DIET

B. Tomlinson, S. L. Cohen, A. Al-Khader, G. P. Kasidas, and G. A. Rose

Dept. of Medicine, University College, Dept. of Chemical Pathology, St. Peter's Hospital, and Institute of Urology, London, U.K.

INTRODUCTION

Allopurinol may reduce calcium oxalate stone formation. Small elevations in urine oxalate are implicated in calculus production and increased dietary purine increases oxalate excretion[1]. Oxalate excretion has been reduced by allopurinol in some stone formers[2] but trials have been complicated by variations in oxalate excretion with changes in diet and doubts over oxalate methodology. Preliminary studies[3] have shown that allopurinol reduced urine oxalate in normal subjects and the effect was greater with a high purine intake.

PATIENTS AND METHODS

Eleven patients (10 males and 1 female) aged 28 to 55 entered the study. Each had formed at least two calculi which were radio-opaque or contained calcium oxalate. They had normal renal function and no obvious metabolic abnormality. Eight had a high urine calcium excretion at some stage and had been advised to reduce their calcium intake. The mean urinary calcium and urate excretion were 5.6 mmol/24 h and 4.64 mmol/24 h respectively while taking a low purine diet with moderate calcium restriction. Any drug treatment which might affect stone formation was stopped prior to the study. The patients were asked to restrict their purine, calcium and oxalate intake to approximately 450, 700 and 40 mg respectively for 8 weeks. Allopurinol (100 mg three times per day) was given during the third and fourth weeks and again during the seventh and eighth weeks after commencement of the diet. At the end of each 2-week period, 24-h urine collections were made. Oxalate and glycollate were measured enzymatically [4,5]. Creatinine, urate and calcium were

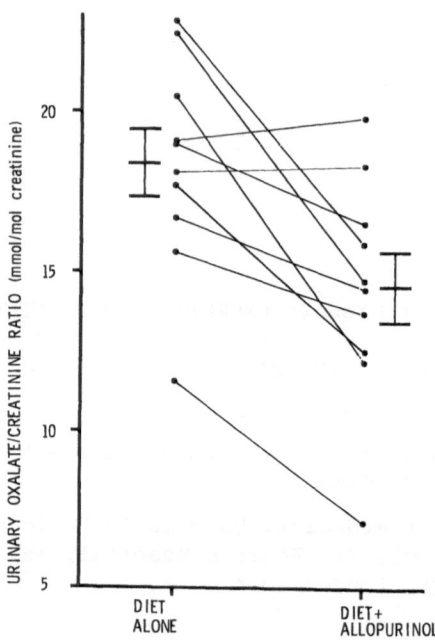

Fig. 1.   Urinary oxalate/creatinine ratio with and without
          allopurinol (means of 2 periods for each subject and
          group means + SEM).

measured by routine laboratory methods. Results from the two
control periods were compared by paired t-tests as were those from
treatment periods.   Where no significant change was found, results
from control periods were combined and means were compared to means
of treatment periods by paired t-tests.

RESULTS

    Ten patients completed the study.   There was no change in the
urinary excretion of the parameters studied between either of the
control periods or between the two periods of allopurinol treatment
Comparing control and treatment periods, urinary urate showed a
significant fall of 38% on allopurinol treatment (Table 1).   There
was a significant fall in mean urinary oxalate whether expressed as
mmol oxalate/24 h (P<0.002) or as an oxalate/creatinine ratio (P<
0.005) on giving allopurinol (Fig. 1).   There was no change in
urinary glycollate or calcium excretion. The mean 24-h oxalate and
urate excretions for each patient both on and off allopurinol showed
a significant correlation (r = 0.73; P<0.001) that persisted when
oxalate and urate excretion were expressed as ratios to creatinine
(r = 0.51;P<0.001; Fig. 2).

514

DISCUSSION

Our results show a significant fall in oxalate excretion during allopurinol treatment. Previous evidence, however, is conflicting. Pak et al[6] found no change in oxalate excretion in stone formers taking allopurinol on both high and low purine diets on an unspecified oxalate intake. Scott et al[2] showed a reduction in oxalate excretion in the half of their group of stone formers while taking an unspecified purine and oxalate intake. More recent studies with controlled purine and oxalate diets[3] have shown an increase in urinary oxalate following dietary purine loading confirming the work

Table 1. Urine Changes on Diet $\pm$ Allopurinol (Means $\pm$ SEM).

Excretion/	Diet			Diet + Allopurinol		
Week	1-2		5-6	3-4		7-8
Creatinine[a]	12.8 $\pm$ 1.0		14.0 $\pm$ 1.6	12.6 $\pm$ 1.2		13.7 $\pm$ 1.5 ***
Urate[b]	360 $\pm$ 27		320 $\pm$ 26	220 $\pm$ 28		200 $\pm$ 22
Calcium[b]	466 $\pm$ 74		344 $\pm$ 68	429 $\pm$ 74		451 $\pm$ 58 ***
Oxalate[b]	19.9 $\pm$ 1.8		16.9 $\pm$ 1.4	15.3 $\pm$ 1.6		14.1 $\pm$ 1.0
Glycollate[b]	18.7 $\pm$ 2.1		17.8 $\pm$ 1.7	22.0 $\pm$ 2.7		17.6 $\pm$ 1.2

[a] mmol/24-h; [b] μmol/mmol creatinine; Diet vs Diet + Allopurinol: *** $P < 0.0005$; ** $P < 0.005$.

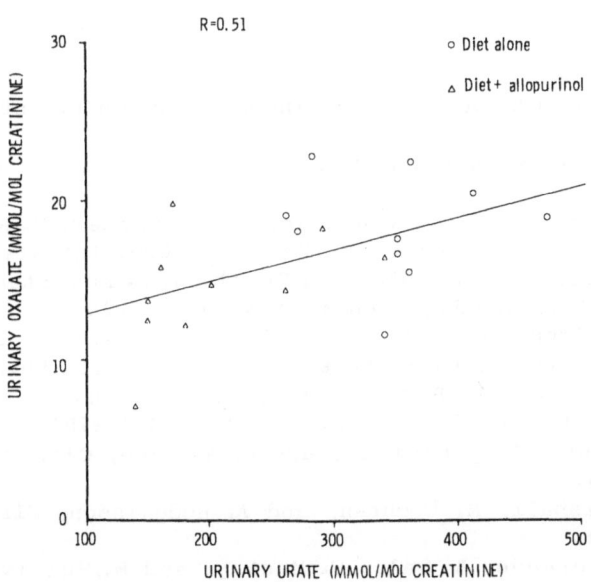

Fig. 2. Urinary oxalate/creatinine ratio plotted against urinary urate/creatinine ratio for each patient with and without allopurinol (each point represents mean of 2 results).

515

of Zarembski and Hodgkinson[1]. Oxalate excretion depends largely on oxalate intake[7] and shows an inverse relationshp with calcium intake[1,8], so it is important to control these factors in any study of changes in oxalate excretion. Oxalate balance appears to be controlled over relatively short periods and an oxalate load appears to be rapidly excreted[9], but changes in calcium intake may have a more prolonged effect and the calcium restriction in our study could have led to a progressive fall in calcium excretion but this was not demonstrated. If oxalate absorption had been reduced by allopurinol, more would remain in the gut to bind calcium which would then reduce urinary calcium so there is no evidence for this mechanism.

Zarembski and Hodgkinson[1] suggested a metabolic pathway from purine to oxalate and the demonstration of a relationship between urate and oxalate excretion supports this. The low purine intake of our patients should minimise any change in oxalate excretion resulting from effects upon purine metabolism or absorption, and the reduction in urinary oxalate may well have been greater if the patients had taken a high purine diet. If allopurinol does reduce calcium oxalate stone formation as suggested[2,10], it may do so by reducing urinary oxalate excretion.

ACKNOWLEDGEMENT

We would like to acknowledge the Wellcome Foundation Ltd. for financial assistance with this study.

REFERENCES

1. P. M. Zarembski and A. Hodgkinson, Clin. Chim. Acta. 25:1 (1969).
2. R. Scott, A. Mathieson, and A. McLelland, Br. J. Urol. 50:455 (1978).
3. H. A. Simmonds, K. J. Van Acker, C. F. Potter, D. R. Webster, G. P. Kasidas, and G. A. Rose, in:"Urolithiasis:Clinical and Basic Research", L. H. Smith, W. G. Robertson, and B. Finlayson, eds., Plenum, New York (1981).
4. P. C. Hallson and G. A. Rose, Clin. Chim. Acta 55:29 (1974).
5. G. P. Kasidas and G. A. Rose, Clin. Chim. Acta 96:25 (1979).
6. C. Y. C. Pak, D. E. Barilla, K. Holt, L. Brinkley, R. Tolentino, and J. E. Zerwekh, Am. J. Med. 65:593 (1978).
7. A. M. Finch, G. P. Kasidas, and G. A. Rose, Clin. Sci. 60(4):411 (1981).
8. R. W. Marshall, M. Cochran, and A. Hodgkinson, Clin. Sci. 43:91 (1972).
9. T. B. Hargreave, A. Sali, C. Mackay, and M. Sullivan, Br. J. Urol. 49:597 (1977).
10. F. L. Coe, Kidney Int. 13:418 (1978).

THE EFFECT OF LONG-TERM TREATMENT WITH ALLOPURINOL ON STONE RECURRENCE IN CALCIUM UROLITHIASIS

B. Ulshöfer, J. Zenke, W. Achilles, and G. Rodeck

Urologische Universitätsklinik und Poliklinik Marburg
Marburg a.d. Lahn, F.R.G.

INTRODUCTION

The role of uric acid (UA) in calcium lithiasis is not yet understood[1], but some clinical studies suggest that reducing UA excretion has a prophylactic effect on stone recurrence[2]. The results of allopurinol treatment are as varied as the indications for using it (hyperuricosuria[2], hyperuricemia[3], idiopathic calcium stone disease[4]). The decrease of UA in serum and urine, which seems to be the only effect of allopurinol, depends on the values prior to treatment, i.e. the higher the value before treatment, the greater the decrease during treatment[5]. The aim of the study was to evaluate whether or not potential treatment failures can be recognized from their biochemistry before treatment commences and how they differ from responders when stones recur.

METHODS

In an outpatient study, 60 recurrent calcium stone-formers were treated with 300 mg allopurinol/day (Zyloric). The patients were advised to take a fluid intake >1.5 litres/day and to avoid excessive calcium and/or oxalate intake. The minimal follow-up was 12 months. Stone recurrence was defined by X-ray or by proven passage of a stone.

RESULTS

Laboratory data before treatment are given in Table 1. Data from the last evaluation before treatment are contained in Table 2.

Table 1. Data from Calcium Stone-Formers Before Treatment with Allopurinol (mean ± SD).

	Urine Volume (ml/24h)	Ca/Cr (mol/mol)	Ua/Cr (mol/mol)	Age (years)	Stones (n)	Sex (m/f)
Without Stone Recurrence During Therapy (n=52)	1617 ±482	0.33 ±0.17	0.28 ±0.11	57.2 ±10.0	10.9 ±17.7	33/19
With Stone Recurrence During Therapy (n=8)	1457 ±452	0.39 ±0.30	0.34 ±0.06	51.6 ±12.1	16.8 ±13.3	7/1

Table 2. Data from Calcium Stone-Formers during Treatment with Allopurinol (mean ± SD).

	Urine Volume (ml/24h)	Ca/Cr (mol/mol)	UA/Cr (mol/mol)	Follow-up (months)
Without Stone Reurrence During Therapy (n=52)	1548 416	0.37 0.18	0.21 0.08	23.5 24.0
With Stone Recurrence During Therapy (n=8)	1681 362	0.49 0.12	0.21 0.04	30.9 19.3

Table 3. Frequencies of Hypercalciuria and Hyperuricosuria in Calcium Stone-Formers During Treatment with Allopurinol.

	24-h Urine Hyper-		2-h Fasting Urine Hyper-	
	calciuria	uricosuria	calciuria	uricosuria
Without Stone Recurrence During Therapy (n=52)	17/52 (32.7%)	5/52 (9.6%)	7/52 (13.5%)	17/52 (32.7%)
With Stone Recurrence During Therapy (n=8)	7/8 (88.0%)	0/8 (0.0%)	3/8 (37.5%)	4/8 (50.0%)
P	<0.005	n.s.	n.s.	n.s.

The frequencies of hypercalciuria (HCU) (Ca/creatinine (mol/mol)⩾ 0.4) and hyperuricosuria (HUU) (UA/creatinine (mol/mol) ⩾0.3 and UA/24 h ⩾4.0 mmol respectively) are shown in Table 3.

DISCUSSION

It would appear that the later failures on allopurinol treatment had higher Ca and UA excretions, more stones, a lower urine volume and were younger than those who responded to treatment, but the differences were not significant. UA excretion during treatment indicates that medication was taken regularly in both groups; the significant difference in the failures is explained entirely by their higher pre-treatment values. Although not significant, a marked increase in Ca excretion was evident in the non-responders. This was probably caused by relaxation of their diet after a long interval free from stones since their fasting 2-h urine calcium remained low. A distinct difference was evident in the frequency of marginal HCU, which occurred in 88% of failures but in only 32.7% of responders. As far as to the number of cases under consideration allows any conclusions to be drawn, it may be assumed that allopurinol has a beneficial effect on Ca-stone recurrence in cases of HUU; additional HCU requires additional treatment (e.g. thiazides or diet) to maintain the effect of allopurinol. As HCU may develop during therapy by neglecting dietary restrictions, it is important for the recognition of potential treatment failures to evaluate the patients carefully during treatment.

REFERENCES

1. B. Finlayson, in:"Urolithiasis and Related Clinical Research", P. O. Schwille, L. H. Smith, W. G. Robertson, and W.Vahlensieck, eds., Plenum, New York (1985).
2. F. L. Coe, Kidney Int. 13:418 (1978).
3. M. J. V. Smith, J. Urol. 117:690 (1977).
4. W. G. Robertson, M. Peacock, P. L. Selby, R. E. Williams, P. Clark, G. D. Chisholm, T. B. Hargreave, M. B. Rose, H. Wilkinson, D. C. Hammonds, and W. J. Gall, in: "Urolithiasis and Related Clinical Research, P. O. Schwille, L. H. Smith, W. G. Robertson, and W. Vahlensieck, eds., Plenum, New York (1985).
5. B. Ulshöfer, Akt. Urol. 15: (in press) (1984).

A PLACEBO CONTROLLED DOUBLE-BLIND STUDY OF ALLOPURINOL IN SEVERE RECURRENT IDIOPATHIC RENAL LITHIASIS. PRELIMINARY RESULTS

L. Miano, S. Petta, G. Paradiso Galatioto
S. Goldoni and A. Tubaro

Dept. of Urology, University of Rome, Italy

INTRODUCTION

Recently the possible role of mild disorders of purine, uric acid and/or urate metabolism in renal stone formation has been emphasised[1,2].   When urine pH increases above 5.7, uric acid dissociates to urate which can then form sodium urate in the presence of sodium ions.   When urinary pH approaches 6.0, the sodium urate/uric acid balance favours urate formation. Although the former is more soluble than the latter, sodium urate can precipitate if its urinary concentration increases sufficiently[3,4]. One hypothesis suggests that if the urine is metastable with respect to calcium oxalate and/or calcium phosphate, precipitation of these salts may be initiated through heterogeneous nucleation by sodium urate[5]. The second hypothesis is that a colloidal form of sodium urate binds certain crystal-inhibiting substances in urine, e.g. the glycosaminoglycans (GAGS), with a consequent decrease in the ability of urine to inhibit crystal growth and aggregation[6].   Previous clinical studies on calcium stone formers with disorders of uric acid metabolism have shown a marked reduction in stone formation with allopurinol. We therefore undertook a double-blind study in a group of patients with recurrent idiopathic calcium oxalate stones.

MATERIALS AND METHODS

Starting in 1978, 30 patients were entered into a double-blind study of allopurinol (300 mg/day) versus placebo. The criteria for entry included a minimum recurrence rate of 2 stone episodes per year for 3 years prior to entry.   Fifteen patients have so far completed 3 years observation, 8 receiving allopurinol and 7 with

521

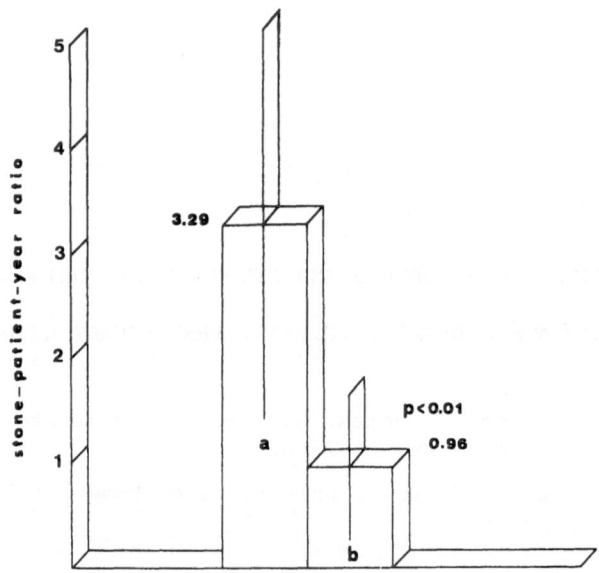

Fig. 1. Change in passage of stone/patient/year (a) before and
(b) during treatment with allopurinol.

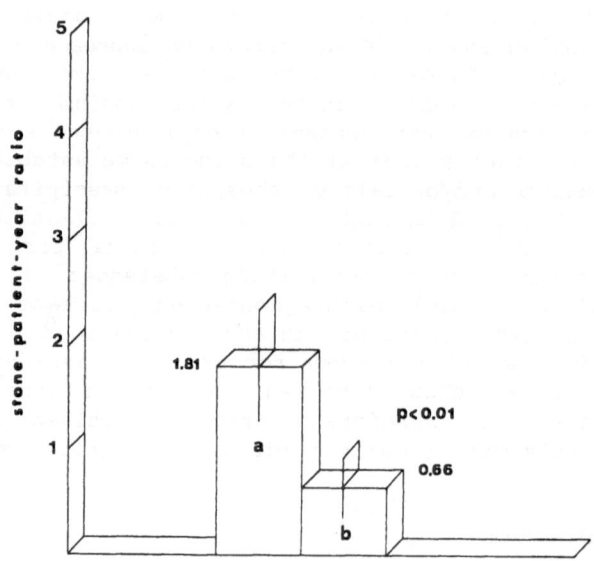

Fig. 2. Change in passage of stone/patient/year (a) before and
(b) during treatment with placebo.

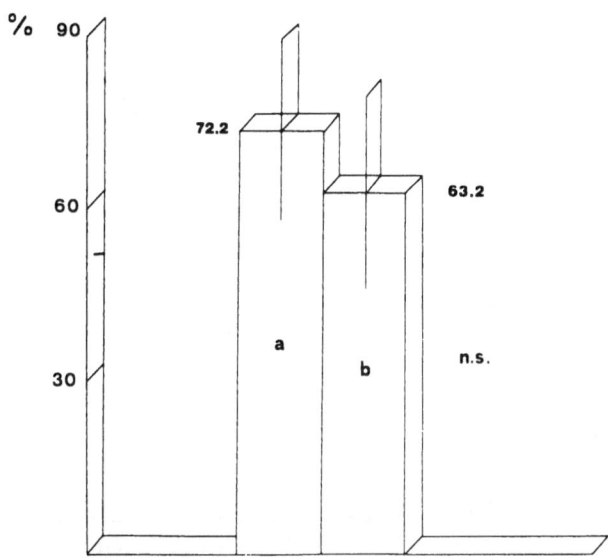

Fig. 3. Mean percent reduction in passed stones during treatment
with allopurinol (a) and placebo (b).

Table 1. Mean Laboratory Findings in the Treatment Groups.

Allopurinol Treatment	Basal	Treatment
Serum urate (mg/dl)	4.72 + 0.79	4.10 + 0.49
Urinary uric acid (mg/24 h)	513 + 136	444 + 103
Urinary calcium (mg/24 h)	203 + 34	210 + 44
Urinary volume (ml/24 h)	1314 + 497	1389 + 312
Placebo Treatment		
Serum urate (mg/dl)	4.10 + 0.70	4.34 + 0.55
Urinary uric acid (mg/24 h)	421 + 55	482 + 67
Urinary calcium (mg/24 h)	218 + 14	218 + 31
Urinary volume (ml/24 h)	1439 + 368	1653 + 413

placebo. Serum and urinary urate/uric acid and electrolyte levels
and various hepatic and renal function parameters were measured
every 3 months. Only one patient (in the placebo-treated group)
had a urinary infection at the beginning of the study and was given
antibiotic therapy. A low calcium and low purine diet was
recommended with a minimum water intake of 1500 ml/day.

RESULTS

    Figs. 1 to 3 show the frequency of stone passage over 3 years
prior to starting the trial and during the 3-year period of

treatment with allopurinol or placebo. Both allopurinol- and placebo-treated groups showed a significant reduction in the rate of stone formation during therapy (P<0.01). A greater reduction was found in the allopurinol-treated group compared with the controls but the difference is not yet significant. Neither intolerance to allopurinol therapy nor alterations in hepatic and/or renal function were observed. Comparison of the main laboratory findings showed no statistically significant differences in uric acid or calcium excretion or in serum urate before and during treatment between the two groups of patients (Table 1). A crystallographic study of urinary stones was performed before and during treatment in a sub-population of allopurinol-treated patients (4 patients). No changes in stone composition were found.

DISCUSSION

These preliminary results on idiopathic calcium oxalate stone formers are not as impressive as those described in our first report relating to patients with recurrent calcium oxalate stones with a high percentage of urate disorders[7]. The controls have also shown an improvement, probably attributable to recommendations on dietary and fluid intake, as shown in other studies. The results obtained are difficult to interpret because of the small number of patients who have so far completed the 3-year treatment period. The interpretation of the results is made more difficult because of the high number of stones passed per year in the allopurinol-treated group, compared with the controls. The study continues with the remaining patients still under double-blind conditions.

REFERENCES

1. G. Brien and C. Bick, Eur. Urol. 3:35 (1977).
2. F. L. Coe, Ann. Intern. Med. 87:404 (1977).
3. M. J. V. Smith, J. Urol. 117:690 (1977).
4. C. Y. C. Pak, O. Waters, L. Arnold, K. Holt, C. Cox, and
      D. Barilla, J. Clin. Invest. 59:426 (1977).
5. F. L. Coe, Kidney Int. 13:418 (1978).
6. W. G. Robertson, F. Knowles, and M. Peacock, in:"Urolithiasis
      Research", H. Fleisch, W. G. Robertson, L. H. Smith, and
      W. Vahlensieck, eds., Plenum, New York (1976).
7. L. Miano, S. Petta, and M. Gallucci, Eur. Urol. 5:229 (1979).

DRUGS AGAINST KIDNEY STONES: EFFECTS OF MAGNESIUM AND ALKALI

B. G. Danielson

Dept. of Medicine, University Hospital
S-751 85 Uppsala, Sweden

INTRODUCTION

During the 1920s it was reported that magnesium was able to increase the solubility of calcium oxalate in vitro and it was proposed that magnesium could be used in the prevention of kidney stones. Rats fed on a diet low in magnesium developed kidney stones within a short time. Precipitation, particularly of calcium phosphate (hydroxyapatite) crystals, occurred in the proximal tubules. This could also be achieved by feeding rats a diet deficient in vitamin B_6; but if at the same time the diet was supplemented with magnesium this prevented stone formation[1,2].

In order to determine whether or not magnesium depletion is a characteristic feature and cause of idiopathic calcium stone disease, a group of 70 patients was investigated with respect to different parameters of magnesium metabolism and compared with a group of healthy controls[3]. There was no difference in serum magnesium or magnesium excretion between stone formers and controls. Nor was there any difference in the body stores or in the retention of magnesium after an i.v. load. Finally, the fractional absorption of magnesium in the gut did not differ between stone formers and controls. From those studies it was concluded that magnesium depletion was not a common feature of calcium stone formers and probably not a common cause of idiopathic calcium stone disease. No signs of magnesium depletion were found in stone formers. The only abnormality was a low magnesium/calcium ratio in the urine and this was not due to a low excretion of magnesium. Rather, it was the result of a relatively high calcium excretion in relation to that of healthy controls (Fig. 1).

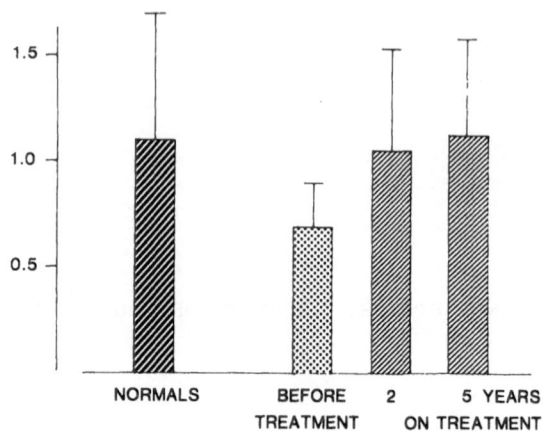

Fig. 1. The magnesium/calcium ratio in urine of stone formers and healthy controls before and on treatment with magnesium (mean + 1SD).

Magnesium reduces the formation of calcium-containing stones in experimental animals[1,2]. The stone prophylactic effect of magnesium has been explained as a result of several possible mechanisms. Magnesium binds oxalate in the gut, through which mechanism oxalate absorption is reduced. Magnesium also binds oxalate in the urine and acts as an inhibitor of calcium phosphate crystallisation in the urine. Prien and Gershoff[1] and Melnick et al[2] reported in 1974 that magnesium oxide combined with pyridoxine (vitamin B_6) had a prophylactic effect in kidney stone disease. However, magnesium has so far not found any common use as a prophylactic agent because of conflicting reports in the literature.

MAGNESIUM AS A STONE PROPHYLACTIC AGENT

It was considered relevant to study magnesium as a prophylactic agent against recurring formation of calcium-containing kidney stones. Seventy consecutive kidney stone patients, who on the average had had stone disease for 8 years with an average of 0.8 stones per year, were treated daily with 500 mg of magnesium in the form of magnesium hydroxide. These patients were followed for up to 7 years. The results showed that this form of treatment slightly increased serum magnesium for about one year, but after that the level returned to the pre-treatment value. Urinary magnesium increased by 1.5 to 2 mmol/24 h during treatment (Fig. 2). Serum calcium was slightly reduced during treatment, but no change in calcium excretion could be seen. As a consequence of the increased magnesium excretion and the unchanged calcium excretion the urinary magnesium/calcium ratio increased. Serum phosphate

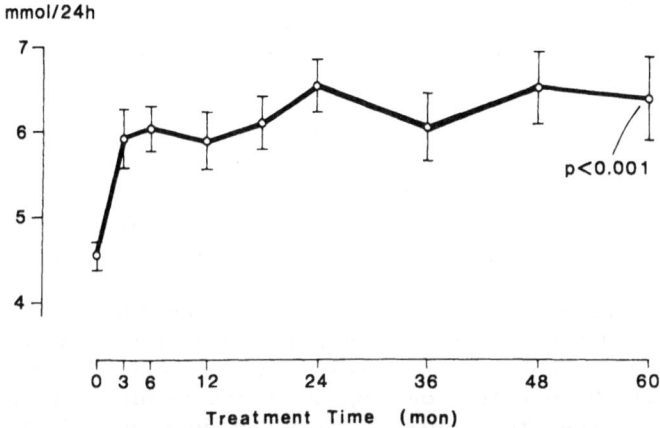

Fig. 2. Urinary magnesium in stone formers before and on treatment with magnesium.

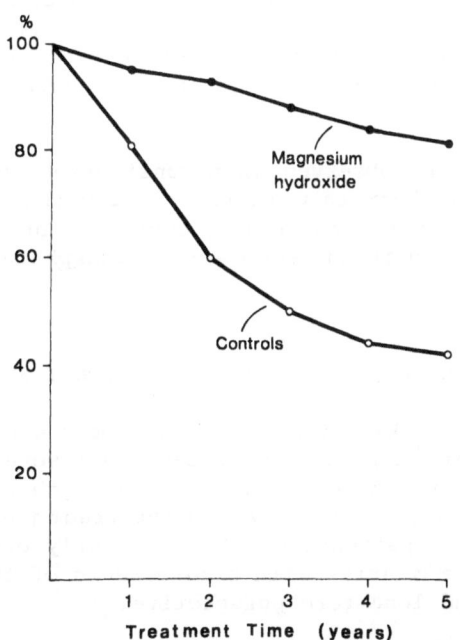

Fig. 3. Patients free of recurrences (%) on treatment with magnesium and in untreated group.

decreased slowly and following two years of treatment significantly lower values were found than at the start of treatment. The serum parathyroid hormone level was unchanged. The urinary excretion of citrate increased in the majority of patients to nearly normal levels, an effect for which no explanation has been found so far.

CLINICAL RESULTS

In order to evaluate better the clinical results of magnesium treatment, another group of patients was observed at the same time. This group consisted of 43 stone patients with a similar type and degree of stone disease, but they did not receive any form of treatment. They were only given the same general advice as the magnesium-treated patients. Following 5 years observation (Fig. 3) about 80% of the patients on magnesium treatment were free of recurrence. The stone episode rate had decreased from 0.8 to 0.08 stones per patient per year. In the control group without prophylactic treatment, only 40% were free of recurrence after 5 years of observation in spite of the fact that the stone episode rate was also reduced. Following 7 years of treatment, 75% of the treated patients in this group were still free of recurrence. Side-effects with the treatment were few and small. Only a few patients showed minor symptoms, such as diarrhoea, and dropped out of the treatment trial. As far as the rest of the patients were concerned, no side-effects were reported. Hypermagnesemia was not observed.

Caution must be observed when considering the possible use of magnesium in stone formers with recurrent urinary tract infection. It may be that an increased urinary excretion of magnesium would promote stone growth in the same way as phosphate treatment in this group of patients.

INDICATIONS FOR THE USE OF MAGNESIUM IN KIDNEY STONE DISEASE

Since recurring kidney stone disease may need long-term prophylactic treatment, it is important that several treatment alternatives are available. Thiazide and orthophosphate are the most frequently used alternatives in the treatment of calcium stones. For those patients who have an early onset of kidney stones, problems may arise with side-effects of the treatment in both the short and long-term perspective.

In patients with enteric hyperoxaluria and gastrointestinal disorders magnesium depletion may develop, with an increased risk of kidney stones. Magnesium depletion may perhaps also develop in some patients on long-term treatment with thiazides. It may become necessary to prescribe magnesium as a supplement in magnesium depletion due to gastrointestinal disorders or due to long-term thiazide treatment. Treatment with magnesium as a prophylactic agent as an alternative or a complement to thiazide or orthophosphate also seems to be possible.

The clinical effect of magnesium as a prophylactic agent appears to be good in our experience and its more wide-spread use as a prophylactic treatment in patients with recurring calcium-containing kidney stones seems justified. From our experience the dose should be in the range of at least about 250 mg of magnesium in the form of magnesium hydroxide once or twice daily. Whether or not other magnesium salts are better than the hydroxide is so far difficult to assess. The absorption of magnesium takes place along the small intestine with possible differences in absorption linked to different compounds.

Even if the clinical effect of magnesium as a prophylactic agent appears to be good according to our experience, others have not come to similar conclusions[4,6]. However, in none of these studies has it been stated how much magnesium actually was absorbed and excreted in the urine. It is essential in the evaluation of the treatment response of magnesium to assess the increase in magnesium excretion and relate the effect or the lack of effect to the magnesium excretion and to other risk factors such as urinary oxalate, citrate, calcium excretion, degree of inhibition, etc.

Although the clinical effect of magnesium as a prophylactic agent appears to be good in our experience, we have to remember that ours was an open study. Even if different clinical results concerning the efficiency of magnesium as a prophylactic agent have been obtained, one has to be cautious in the evaluation of such results since difference in the trial design, in the prescribed dose, in the form of magnesium given and in the mode of administration and absorption may influence the clinical results. A double-blind controlled study is therefore probably necessary in order to solve the question of the efficacy of magnesium as a prophylactic agent in kidney stone disease.

CITRATE EXCRETION IN STONE FORMERS

Urinary citrate forms soluble complexes with calcium, thus reducing the relative supersaturation of calcium-containing crystals and acts as an inhibitor of crystal growth of hydroxyapatite and calcium oxalate. Several investigations have shown that the urine excretion of citrate is reduced in stone formers, especially those with renal tubular acidosis (Fig. 4). The reduction is particularly pronounced in patients with distal RTA and even more so in patients with enteric hyperoxaluria[6]. In spite of the fact that a low citrate excretion is found in 20 to 30% of stone formers with

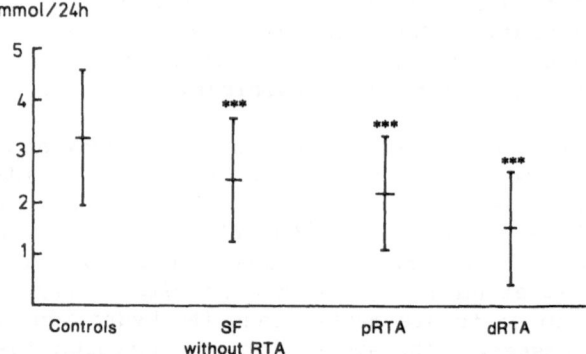

Fig. 4.   The average urinary citrate in healthy controls in
          idiopathic stone formers, stone formers with incomplete
          proximal RTA, incomplete distal RTA, and in patients with
          enteric hyperoxaluria.

calcium-containing stones, no relationship has so far been
demonstrated between the urinary excretion of citrate and the
severity of stone disease.   Several factors may influence the
urinary excretion of citrate including acid-base status, urine pH,
renal dysfunction, urinary tract infection and age.

     According to some investigators the urinary excretion of
citrate may be increased following an oral load of citric acid or
alkaline citrate, although other investigators have not found this[7].
From the literature, it is difficult to get a clear picture of what
dose has to be given and in which form citrate has to be
administered in order to obtain a substantial increase in urinary
citrate.   The effect of sodium-potassium citrate or potassium
citrate as prophylactic treatment has been reported[8].   An increased
citrate excretion and a reduction in calcium excretion and stone
incidence were found.   Pak has especially selected patients with
RTA and with chronic diarrhoeal syndromes and patients with low
urinary citrate in combination with e.g. hypercalciuria.   Treatment
with thiazide reduces urinary citrate but potassium citrate may be
used to complement thiazide treatment by increasing the previously
low urinary citrate levels to normal.

ALKALI TREATMENT

     Since the intake of alkali increases the renal excretion of
citrate, this treatment has been used as prophylaxis in patients
with calcium-containing kidney stone disease, particularly in
patients with a low citrate excretion.   We have used bicarbonate as
a prophylactic agent in a group of 19 stone formers with incomplete

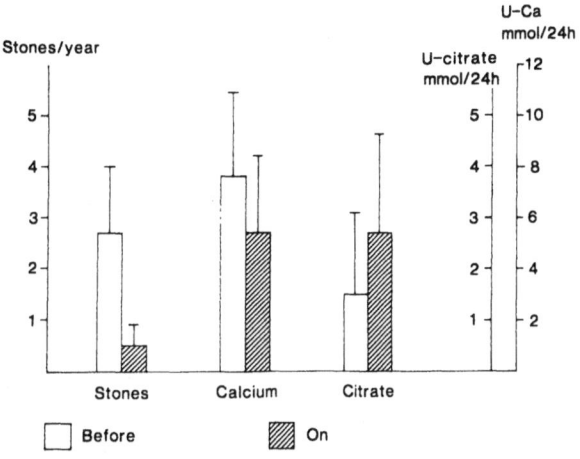

Fig. 5. The effect of treatment with bicarbonate on stone
recurrences, calcium excretion and citrate excretion in 19
patients with renal tubular acidosis.

or complete RTA (Fig. 5). They had had stone disease for an average
of 10 years and the mean pre-reatment stone episode rate was 2.5
stones/patient/year. The patients were observed for 4 years on
sodium bicarbonate (3 to 6 g/day). During treatment the stone
episode rate and urinary calcium excretion decreased; citrate
excretion increased significantly. Increasing the urinary citrate
seems to be one way of approaching the prevention of recurrent
kidney stone disease. This can be achieved by giving alkaline
salts like sodium bicarbonate or, alternatively, potassium citrate.
The long-term therapeutic effect as well as contra-indications,
side-effects and restrictions have to be further evaluated in
clinical trials.

REFERENCES

1. E. L. Prien and S. N. Gershoff, J. Urol. 112:509 (1974).
2. I. Melnick, R. R. Landes, A. A. Hoffman, and J. F. Burch,
   J. Urol. 105:119 (1971).
3. G. Johansson, Scand. J. Urol. Nephrol. Suppl.51:1 (1979).
4. D. R. Wilson, A. L. Strauss, and M. A. Manuel, Urol. Res. 12:39
   (1984).
5. B. Ettinger, J. Cotron, and A. Tang, Urol. Res. 12:49 (1984).
6. L. Backman, U. Backman, B. G. Danielson, and B. Nordenvall,
   Urol. Res. 12:36 (1984).

7. A. Faser, M. C. Gregory, G. A. Rose, and C. T. Samuell, Urol. Res. 12:64 (1984).
8. M. Butz, G. Karadzic, and H.-J. Dulce, Urol. Res. 12:40 (1984).

URINE COMPOSITION IN CALCIUM OXALATE STONE FORMERS

DURING TREATMENT WITH ALKALI

H.-G. Tiselius

Dept. of Urology, University Hospital
S-581 85 Linköping, Sweden

INTRODUCTION

There are several reasons for treating calcium oxalate (CaOx) stone-formers with alkali. The inhibition of CaOx crystal growth in diluted urine increases with increasing pH[1,2], and in urine with a high CaOx supersaturation the in vitro crystallization of CaOx is reduced when pH was above 6[3]. Consequently CaOx crystals are encountered only in urine with a low pH[4,5]. Furthermore urinary citrate, which is a determinant of the ion-activity product of CaOx[6] and an inhibitor of CaOx crystallization[7-9], is low in patients forming CaOx stones[10-12]. With this background it was of interest to study in more detail the effect of alkali on urine composition in a group of recurrent CaOx stone-formers.

MATERIALS AND METHODS

Fifteen patients with recurrent calcium oxalate stone disease (10 men, 5 women) were treated with 7.5 g of Renapur (Madaus & Co, West Germany) daily in 3 divided doses. This drug is a mixture of potassium citrate, sodium citrate, and citric acid, corresponding to a daily citrate supplement of about 28 mmol. Renapur was administered as a granulate dissolved in 100 to 150 ml of water. Twenty-four hour out-patient urine samples were collected before and after at least 4 weeks of treatment and analyzed for calcium (Ca), oxalate (Ox), magnesium (Mg), citrate (Cit), urate, creatinine (Cr), and inhibition of CaOx crystal growth in diluted urine (I_{GR}). All urine variables were related to urinary creatinine.

The AP(CaOx)-index was used as an estimate of CaOx supersaturation and calculated as previously described[6]. The CaOx-risk index had the following form:

$$\frac{(Ca/Cr)^{0.71} \times (Ox/Cr)}{(Mg/Cr)^{0.14} \times (Cit/Cr)^{0.10}}$$

The risk of CaOx crystallization was determined in fresh urine samples collected from 8 of the patients between 06.00 and 10.00, before and during treatment. After removal of crystals by acidification and re-establishment of the original pH, sodium oxalate was added to the urine until crystals occurred. The amount of oxalate required for formation of 100 crystals with a diameter of 3.5 to 5 μm as determined by a Coulter Counter, was used as a measure of the crystallization risk.

RESULTS

As shown in Fig. 1, urinary pH increased during treatment with Renapur. In all patients a higher Cit excretion (Fig. 2) was recorded during treatment (P<0.002), with an increment between 9 and 262%. Although urinary Ca was reduced in many patients a statistical difference was not recorded. However, the combined effects on urinary Ca and Cit resulted in a significantly reduced Ca/Cit-quotient (P<0.002). There were no effects observed on

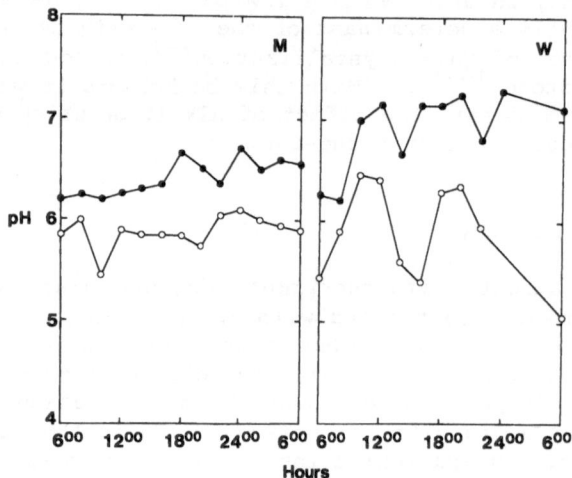

Fig. 1.   Diurnal variation of urine pH before (o) and during (●) daily administration of 7.5 g of Renapur to a male (M) and female (W) patient with CaOx stone disease.

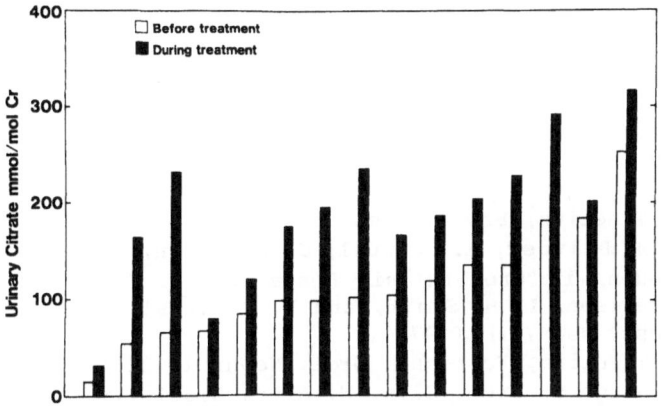

Fig. 2.   The 24-h urinary excretion of citrate in 15 CaOx stone
formers before and during treatment with Renapur.

urinary Mg, urate, or I_{GR}.   The CaOx-risk index was decreased in 11
of the 15 patients (P<0.05).   A slightly higher urine volume
(P<0.01) contributed to the significantly lower values of AP(CaOx)-
index (P<0.002).

Lower values of the risk of CaOx crystallization in 4-h urine
samples during treatment were observed in 6 of our 8 patients.

DISCUSSION

Administration of alkali as a mixture of potassium and sodium
citrate decreased CaOx supersaturation mainly by increasing urinary
citrate.   A similar effect of alkali on urinary citrate has also
been reported by other authors[13,14].   In addition, urine volume was
slightly higher, possibly as a result of the increased fluid intake
taken with Renapur.   It was not possible to find a clear effect on
I_{GR} which, however, was measured only at pH 6.0[7].   Recent
unpublished data have shown that citrate is a potent inhibitor of
CaOx crystallization in whole urine, and it is therefore possible
that the Ca/Cit quotient might be a good estimate of the effect of
alkali on urine composition in this respect.

Whereas an increased pH apparently reduces the risk of CaOx
crystallization, the risk of calcium phosphate (CaP) crystallization
will increase.   However, Cit is an inhibitor of both CaOx and CaP
crystallization, and it is possible that the increased Cit prevents
precipitated CaP from forming large crystals[3].   The patients
presented here have not been treated for periods of sufficient
length to draw any conclusions of effects on stone formation.
Although no new stone formation has been observed so far, remaining

concrements might grow.   It is therefore probably wise not to give
alkali to patients with residual concrements, and also to follow
carefully those patients treated in this way.

REFERENCES

1. H.-G. Tiselius, Br. J. Urol. 53:470 (1981).
2. O. L. M. Bijvoet, E. J. Will, J. van Aken, and H. van der
   Linden, in:"Urolithiasis Research", H. Fleisch, W. G.
   Robertson, L. H. Smith, and W. Vahlensieck, eds., Plenum
   Press, New York (1976).
3. H.-G. Tiselius, Fortschr. Urol. Nephrol. 22:184 (1984).
4. J. G. Gregory, Urol. Clin. N. Amer. 8:331 (1981).
5. C. Ahlstrand, H.-G. Tiselius, L. Larsson, Urol. Res. (1984)
   inpress.
6. H.-G. Tiselius, Clin. Chim. Acta 122:409 (1982).
7. H.-G. Tiselius and A.-M. Fornander, Clin. Chem. 27:565 (1981).
8. P. C. Hallson, G. A. Rose, and S. Sulaiman, Urol. Int. 38:179
   (1983).
9. W. G. Robertson, A. B. Latif, D. S. Scurr, A. M. Caswell, G. W.
   Drach, and A. D. Randolph, in:"Urinary Stone, R. Ryall, J. G.
   Brockis, V. Marshall, and B. Finlayson, eds., Churchill
   Livingstone, Melbourne (1984).
10. H.-G. Tiselius, in:"Urolithiasis:Clinical and Basic Research",
    L.H. Smith, W. G. Robertson, and B. Finlayson, eds., Plenum
    Press, New York (1981).
11. P. O. Schwille, D. Scholz, M. Paulus, W. Engelhardt, and A.
    Sigel, Invest. Urol. 16:457 (1979).
12. M. J. Nicar, C. Skurla, K. Sakhaee, and C. Y. C. Pak, Urology
    21:8 (1983).
13. M. Butz, Urologe A, 21:142 (1982).
14. K. Sakhaee, M. J. Nicar, H. Jacobson, and C. Y. C. Pak, Clin.
    Res. 30:403A (1982).

THE EFFECT OF ALKALINIZING AGENTS AND CHELATING AGENTS ON THE DISSOLUTION OF CALCIUM OXALATE KIDNEY STONES

J. G. Gregory, K. Y. Park, and T. C. Burns

St. Louis University School of Medicine, St. Louis
Missouri 63104, U.S.A.

INTRODUCTION

An attempt has been made to elucidate the role of alkalinization and chelation in the dissolution of both calcium oxalate
monohydrate crystals and stones. Dissolution by these agents has
been measured at various concentrations over the pH range from 4 to
8. The alkalinizing agents used were sodium orthophosphate and
sodium bicarbonate. The chelating agents were sodium
ethylenediaminetetraacetate (EDTA) and sodium citrate.

MATERIALS AND METHODS

Dissolution studies of calcium oxalate monohydrate (COM) were
performed by adding 100 mg of COM crystals (or 500 mg COM in the
studies involving Na_3PO_4 solutions) to 30 ml of various concentrations of chelating and alkalinizing agents in 20 x 150 mm culture
tubes. The suspension was stirred magnetically at room
temperature. A 1 ml sample was withdrawn from each tube after 1 h,
4 h, 24 h, 48 h, 72 h, and 96 h. After centrifugation at 1000 x g
for 5 min, the supernatants were analyzed for calcium by atomic
absorption spectroscopy and oxalate by gas chromatography[1].

Dissolution studies on calcium oxalate stones were conducted in
the same manner, except that renal stones ranging from 100 to 300 mg
were suspended at the mid-point of test tubes containing the
dissolution solutions.

RESULTS

Fig. 1 shows the linear correlations observed between both calcium and oxalic acid and the molar concentration of Na_2EDTA, corresponding to a 2.25 weight ratio between calcium and oxalic acid. Increasing the concentration of Na_2EDTA 10 times resulted in an approximately 3-fold enhancement of equilibrium solubility of COM crystals. The equilibium solubility of COM crystals was reached after 10 min at various concentrations of Na_2EDTA. Twenty-fold enhancement of the equilibrium solubility was obtained in 0.01M tetrasodium EDTA when compared to 0.01M disodium EDTA. Fig. 2 shows the dissolution of COM crystals in Na_2EDTA at various pH values. The crystals exhibited a low solubility at pH 4.27 which increased to a maximum above pH 6.31. Fig. 3 shows the dissolution profiles of calcium oxalate renal stones and COM crystals in 0.01 M Na_2EDTA solution at various pH values. The equilibrium solubility of calcium oxlate renal stones was reached after 48 h, and an approximately 20-fold enhancement of the equilibrium solubility was obtained at pH 6.31 compared to pH 4.27.

The dissolution of COM crystals was studied in 0.1 M citric acid at various pHs. The lowest solubility of COM crystals was shown to occur at pH 3.73 and the maximum at 6.72. The solubility of COM crystals was increased 5-fold in tetrasodium citrate solution when compared to monosodium citrate solution. Further increase in pH did not enhance the solubility of COM crystals. The solubility of COM crystals increased with increasing concentration of Na_3 citrate. Equilibrium solubility of COM crystals was obtained after 10 min at various concentrations of Na_3 citrate whereas that of calcium oxalate renal stones was only reached after 48 h. The solubility of calcium oxalate renal stones was somewhat higher than that of COM crystals.

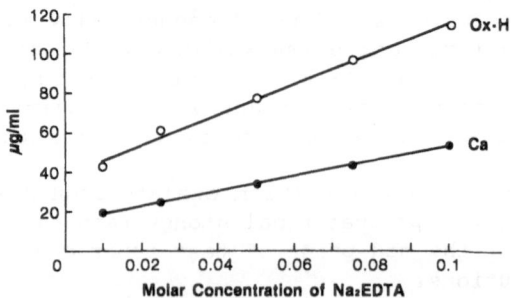

Fig. 1. Dissolution of calcium oxalate monohydrate crystals in Na_2EDTA.

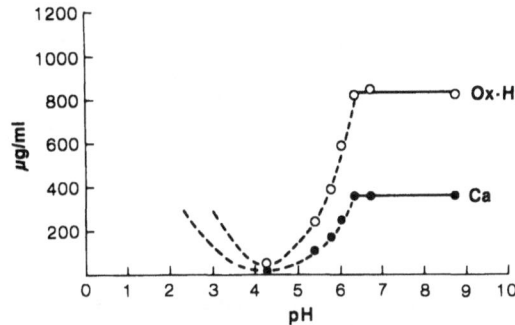

Fig. 2. Dissolution of calcium oxalate monohydrate crystals in 0.01 M Na_2EDTA in relation to pH.

The equilibrium solubility of COM crystals was reached after 48 h in sodium phosphate at various pHs. An approximately 50-fold enhancement of solubility was obtained in 0.1 M Na_3PO_4 when compared to 0.1 M Na_2HPO_4 solution. The dissolution of COM crystals in both Na_2HPO_4 and Na_3PO_4 solutions yielded low values of calcium (3.2-4.2 μg/ml) and high values of oxalate. The equilibrium solubility of CaOx stones was not obtained after 144 h either in Na_2HPO_4 or in Na_3PO_4. The solubility of CaOx renal stones in Na_2HPO_4 was decreased 5-fold in comparison with that of COM crystals, whereas, the solubility of CaOx renal stones in Na_3PO_4 was approximately 80-fold lower than that of COM crystals.

The dissolution of COM crystals in $NaHCO_3$ solutions produced low values of calcium (4.5-5.1 μg/ml) and high values of oxalate.

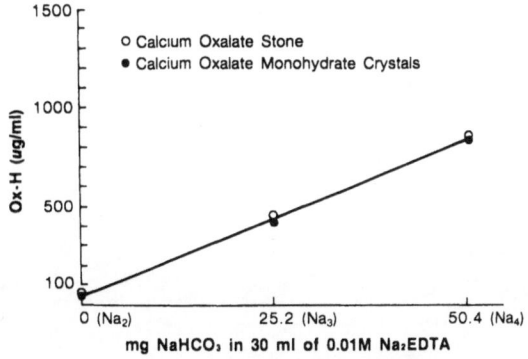

Fig. 3. Dissolution of calcium oxalate monohydrate crystals and calcium oxalate stones in 0.01 M Na_2EDTA and increasing calcium concentrations of $NaHCO_3$.

An equilibrium solubility was not obtained after 96 h. Increasing NaHCO$_3$ concentration did enhance the solubility of COM crystals. The equilibrium solubility of calcium oxalate renal stones was not obtained either in 0.2 M or 0.3 M NaHCO$_3$ solution after 96 h. The solubility of CaOx renal stones in NaHCO$_3$ was approximately 10-fold lower than that of COM crystals.

DISCUSSION

The results suggest that the rate of dissolution of calcium oxalate in chelating solutions depends upon the concentration of anions which affect the formation of a soluble calcium complex. Chelating agents, such as EDTA and sodium citrate, dissolve CaOx crystals preferentially when in the anion-enriched tetra- and trisodium form[2]. The marked difference between the solubility of COM crystals and renal stones in all solutions can be explained in terms of the difference in specific surface of crystals and stones. Further prevention of dissolution of renal stones is due to the crust formation of calcium carbonate or calcium phosphate that forms on the surface of stones placed in these solutions. The dissolution of formed calculi is greater by chelation than by alkalinization due to the absence of the dissolution/reprecipitation processes occurring on the stone surface in chelating solutions. It appears that alkaline solutions of citrate and EDTA are effective agents for calcium oxalate dissolution and should be considered for use in percutaneous chemolysis.

REFERENCES

1. K. Y. Park and J. G. Gregory, Clin. Chem. 26:1170 (1980).
2. B. S. Abeshouse and T. Weinberg, J. Urol. 65:316 (1951).

THE EFFECT OF ALKALINIZING AGENTS ON CALCIUM

OXALATE STONE FORMATION IN A RAT MODEL

J. G. Gregory, K. Y. Park, and T. C. Burns

St. Louis University School of Medicine
1325 South Grand Avenue, St. Louis
Missouri 63104, U.S.A.

INTRODUCTION

In an attempt to determine the relative efficacy of therapy to
reduce calcium oxalate stone formation in patients with enteric
hyperoxaluria, the effects of the alkalinizing agents sodium
bicarbonate, sodium orthophosphate and sodium citrate have been
studied with an experimental animal model capable of inducing rapid
enteric hyperoxaluric stone formation.

MATERIALS AND METHODS

Male Sprague-Dawley rats weighing approximately 100 g, were fed
powdered Purina laboratory chow supplemented with 4.65% ammonium
oxalate. Animals were allowed water ad lib. Animals fed the same
lithogenic diet were, in addition, given alkalinizing agents in
their drinking water for the entire 4-week treatment period
(Table 1). One animal from each treatment group was kept in a
metabolic chamber and urinary collections made daily. These were
analysed for urinary volume, pH, calcium, and oxalate[1]. At weekly
intervals, groups of 5 animals were sacrificed in a carbon dioxide
chamber. The kidneys were removed, frozen and cut longitudinally.
Postmortem examination of these sections of rat kidneys were made
both under the dissecting and light microscope.

RESULTS AND DISCUSSION

A group of 50 rats made hyperoxaluric by feeding a diet supplemented with ammonium oxalate produced calcium oxalate renal stones

541

Table 1. Alkalinizing Agents

Alkalinizing Agents*	Amounts (g/l)	Normality of Solution	pH of Solution
$NaHCO_3$	8.4	0.1	8.04
$NaHCO_3$	16.8	0.2	8.00
$Na_2HPO_4 \cdot 7H_2O$	13.4	0.1	8.89
$Na_2HPO_4 \cdot 7H_2O$	26.8	0.2	8.88
$Na_3citrate \cdot 2H_2O$	9.8	0.1	8.41
$Na_3citrate \cdot 2H_2O$	19.6	0.2	8.57

* Agents mixed in drinking water to which animals were given ad lib access.

Table 2. The Effect of Alkalinizing Agents on Incidence of CaOx Stone Formation.

Treatment	% Incidence of Kidney Stone		% Incidence of Bladder Stone
	1 Week	4 Weeks	4 Weeks
Control (stone-former)	90	100	30
0.1N Na_2HPO_4	30	30	1
0.2N Na_2HPO_4	20	30	0
0.1N $NaHCO_3$	20	30	0
0.1N $NaHCO_3$	0	20	0
0.1N $Na_3citrate$	10	15	0
0.1N $Na_3citrate$	0	0	0

* 5 rats sacrificed per week in each treatment group.

after 4 weeks in 100% of the animals and bladder stones in 30% (Table 2). The urine of stone forming animals contained 554 μg/ml of oxalate, 11.8 μg/ml of calcium oxalate crystals (Table 3). In addition to free stones, micro and macro deposits of crystals were seen at the papillary tip, the corticomedullary junction, and in the renal fornices.

A group of animals on this same lithogenic diet who were, in addition, orally supplemented with sodium bicarbonate or sodium orthophosphate for the 4-week treatment period showed a 30% incidence of renal stones and no bladder stones (Table 2). The urine of these animals contained 1070 μg/ml of oxalate, 34.5 μg/ml of calcium and a pH of 6.56, but rarely had calcium oxalate crystals (Table 3).

Table 3. Urinary Excretions (Mean $\pm$ SEM).

Treatment	No. Rats	Water Intake (ml/24h)	Volume (ml/24h)	pH	Oxalic acid (µg/24h)	Ca (µg/24h)
Normal	10	30 ± 3	18.0 ± 2	6.9 ± 0.3	1.67 ± 0.17	3.00 ± 0.29
Control (Stone-former)	50	55 ± 3	35.0 ± 3	5.7 ± 0.4	19.39 ± 1.44	0.41 ± 0.04
0.1N Na_2HPO_4	20	30 ± 2	17.0 ± 2	6.3 ± 1.2	17.92 ± 1.44	0.30 ± 0.03
0.2N Na_2HPO_4	20	31 ± 3	15.4 ± 2	6.7 ± 0.1	17.23 ± 2.06	0.29 ± 0.01
0.1N $NaHCO_3$	20	26 ± 4	12.9 ± 2	7.4 ± 0.2	14.32 ± 1.5	0.21 ± 0.03
0.2N $NaHCO_3$	20	28 ± 3	18.5 ± 3	7.8 ± 0.3	20.67 ± 4.14	0.57 ± 0.14
0.1N $Na_3citrate$	20	35 ± 2	14.5 ± 2	6.6 ± 0.1	15.52 ± 1.28	0.50 ± 0.05
0.2N $Na_3citrate$	20	29 ± 3	12.3 ± 2	7.4 ± 0.1	18.65 ± 2.52	0.39 ± 0.05

The mechanism by which alkalinizing agents may influence stone formation is triphasic: formation of stable soluble salts[2], crystal stabilization[3], and crystal dissolution[4]. We postulate that calcium oxalate crystal formation is inhibited at an alkaline pH by conversion of urinary acids to anionic forms and by the urinary clearance of a percentage of the administered salts as additional anions. These anions compete with oxalate for calcium and form stable soluble salts. Such does not occur at pH 5 because at this pH the predominant salt of calcium is calcium oxalate. In these experiments, sodium citrate has been shown to be a more effective drug for the prevention of calcium oxalate stone formation than either sodium bicarbonate or sodium orthophosphate.

Sodium citrate, sodium bicarbonate, and sodium phosphate affect stone formation by competitively reducing the chance of crystallization, stabilizing any formed crystals, and in time even bringing about slow crystal dissolution. They deserve to be considered as therapeutic agents of potential benefit in the treatment of calcium oxalate stone disease.

REFERENCES

1. K. Y. Park and J. G. Gregory, Clin. Chem. 26:1170 (1980).
2. J. G. Gregory, K. Y. Park, R. Wilt, and A. Feigl, in:"Urolithiasis Clinical and Basic Research", L. H. Smith, B. Finlayson, and W. G. Robertson, eds., Plenum Press, New York (1981).
3. J. G. Gregory, M. M. Hoy, K. Y. Park, and A. Fleigl, in:"Urolithiasis Clinical and Basic Research", L. H. Smith, B. Finlayson, and W. G. Robertson, eds., Plenum Press, New York (1981).
4. J. G. Gregory, K. Y. Park, and T. C. Burns, in:"Urolithisis and Related Clinical Research', P. O. Schwille, L. H. Smith, W. G. Robertson, and W. Vahlensieck, eds., Plenum Press, New York (1985).

A MULTICENTRE TRIAL TO EVALUATE THREE TREATMENTS FOR RECURRENT

IDIOPATHIC CALCIUM STONE DISEASE - A PRELIMINARY REPORT

W. G. Robertson, M. Peacock, P. L. Selby,
R. E. Williams, P. Clark, G. D. Chisholm,
T. B. Hargreaves, M. B. Rose, and H. Wilkinson

The General Infirmary, Leeds, Western General
Hospital, Edinburgh, Morriston Hospital, Swansea
and York District Hospital, York, U.K.

INTRODUCTION

Many attempts have been made in recent years to assess various forms of treatment for the prevention of recurrence of idiopathic calcium stones[1-5]. Because of the great variety of experimental designs employed, however, it is extremely difficult to decide which form of therapy is most likely to be successful in a given individual. Some trials have selected patients for specific therapy based on their pre-treatment urinary abnormalities, others have involved no such selective procedures. Some have prescribed their control patients a placebo, others have given no placebo, and others still have included no control patients in their studies. Some have given advice on dietary and fluid intake to their patients, others have not done so. In this study we have organised a multicentre trial to assess three forms of treatment currently being prescribed to recurrent idiopathic calcium stone-formers. These treated patients are compared with a group of similar patients who were receiving no treatment at all, not even advice on dietary and fluid intake.

METHODS

So far, 120 male recurrent idiopathic calcium stone-formers from 4 centres in the UK have been entered in the trial and followed up for between 3 and 5 years. The study included a period of observation before treatment during which the patients were assessed clinically and biochemically on their basal home diet to eliminate any with secondary calcium stones or with cystine, uric acid or infection stones. Two 24-h urines were collected from each patient prior to start of treatment and the urinary risk factors measured. The overall biochemical risk of stones (P_{SF}) was calculated[6]. Fasting blood and urine samples were also analyzed to assess each patient's state of calcium metabolism and renal function. The patients were then allocated at random to one of 4 treatment groups: (i) no treatment at all, not even dietary advice, (ii) allopurinol (300 mg Zyloric/day), (iii) thiazide diuretics (2.5 mg Centyl K t.d.s.), and (iv) orthophosphate supplementation (1 tablet Phosphate Sandoz, containing 0.5 g phosphorus, t.d.s.). The urinary risk factors were measured at regular intervals and all episodes of stone, defined as the passage or surgical removal of a stone, recorded. If any untreated patient formed more than two stones during "non-treatment", he was removed from the trial and given high fluids and dietary advice.

RESULTS

This preliminary report contains the data on the first 45 patients who were entered into the trial. The overall biochemical probability of forming stones (P_{SF}) was unchanged in the untreated group (basal 0.36 ± 0.09; untreated 0.30 ± 0.09) and in the allopurinol-treated group (basal 0.10 ± 0.07; allopurinol 0.34 ± 0.08), but was significantly reduced in both the thiazide-treated (basal 0.67 ± 0.08; thiazide 0.32 ± 0.09; P<0.01) and phosphate-treated groups (basal 0.71 ± 0.10; phosphate 0.30 ± 0.09; P<0.001). The corresponding recurrence rates in each of the 4 treatment groups before and during treatment are shown in Figs. 1 to 4. The data are presented in the form of cusum plots in which the ordinate represents the accumulated sum of stone episodes in the patients

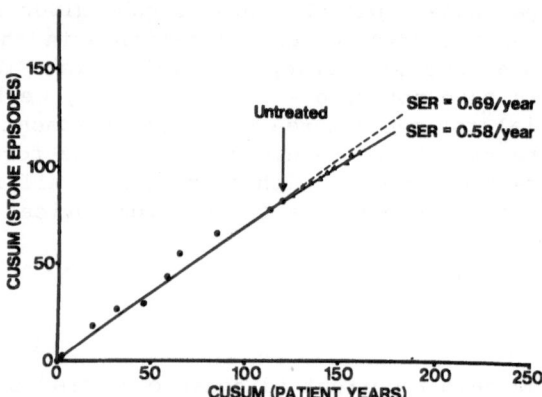

Fig. 1. A cusum plot of stone episodes against patient years before (●) and during (▲) "treatment" in a group of 9 untreated stone-formers.

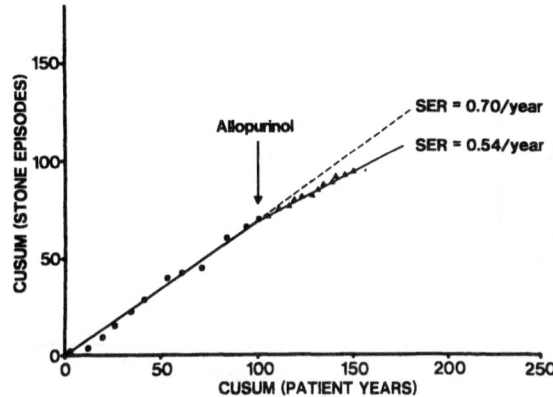

Fig. 2. A cusum plot of stone episodes against patient years in 12 stone-formers treated with allopurinol (Key as in Fig. 1).

under study, the abscissa represents the corresponding sum of patient years, and the slope represents the mean stone episode rate of the group. During treatment, the rate of stone recurrence was not reduced in the untreated group; it was marginally reduced in the group receiving allopurinol and was significantly reduced in each of the groups receiving thiazides or orthophosphate.

DISCUSSION

This preliminary report on the treatment of calcium stones is the first to include an untreated group of patients who received no

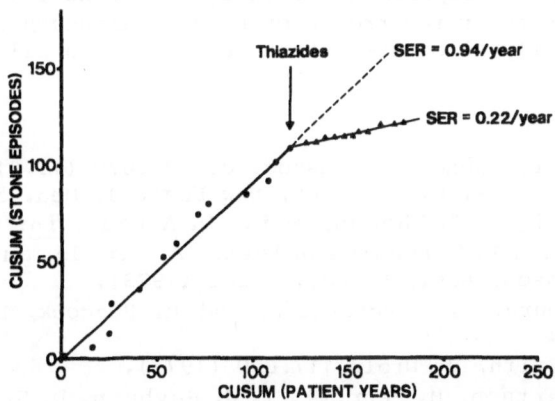

Fig. 3. A cusum plot of stone episodes against patient years in 13 stone-formers treated with thiazides (Key as in Fig. 1).

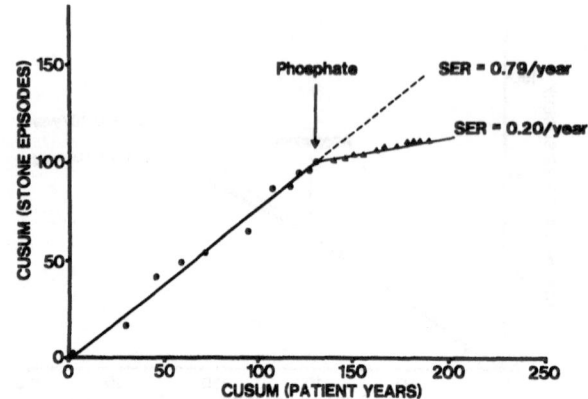

Fig. 4. A cusum plot of stone episodes against patient years in
11 stone-formers treated with orthophosphate (Key as in
Fig. 1).

advice on reducing their dietary intake of dairy foods, and oxalate-
rich foodstuffs or on increasing their fluid intake. The data
show that, in the following 2 to 3 years of "non-treatment", such
patients continue to form stones at approximately the same rate as
prior to "treatment".

Of the drug therapies, allopurinol appears at most to be of
marginal benefit to patients with calcium stones but, when the full
study is complete and we can analyze the response of each treatment
group in detail, it may be that we shall find that allopurinol is
effective in the sub-group of calcium stone-formers with
hyperuricosuria. The numbers are too small at the moment to draw
any conclusions on this possibility. On the other hand, thiazides
and orthophosphate supplements both appear to be effective in
reducing the rate of recurrence of stones, although neither
treatment totally eliminates stone recurrence in all patients.

REFERENCES

1. E. R. Yendt, Canad. Med. Assoc. J. 102:479 (1970).
2. F. L. Coe and A. G. Kavalich, New Engl. J. Med. 55:32 (1974).
3. L. H. Smith, W. C. Thomas, and C. D. Arnaud, in:"Urinary
   Calculi", L. Cifuentes Delatte, A. Rapado, and A.
   Hodgkinson, eds., Karger, Basel (1973).
4. P. J. Heyburn, W. G. Robertson, and M. Peacock, Nephron 32:314
   (1982).
5. M. J. V. Smith, J. Urol. 117:690 (1977).
6. W. G. Robertson, M. Peacock, P. J. Heyburn, D. H. Marshall, and
   P. B. Clark, Br. J. Urol. 50:449 (1978).

PROPHYLAXIS OF CALCIUM OXALATE STONES:CLINICAL TRIALS OF

ALLOPURINOL, MAGNESIUM HYDROXIDE AND CHLORTHALIDONE

B. Ettinger, J. T. Citron, A. Tang, and B. Livermore

Kaiser Permanente Medical Center, San Francisco, U.S.A.

INTRODUCTION

Despite numerous reports of kidney stone prophylaxis, there is still considerable controversy about the effectiveness of any regimen. Most published clinical trials suffer from one or more of the following faults: (i) lack of an adequate number of subjects, (ii) lack of an adequate follow-up time, (iii) lack of an objective end-point and (iv) lack of an adequate comparison group. We decided to carry out three double-blind controlled clinical trials to test adequately the effectiveness of magnesium hydroxide, chlorthalidone or allopurinol.

METHODS

Our study design incorporated the following elements: (i) adequate numbers of subjects, (ii) a 3-year duration of study, (iii) judgement of failure based on independent review by a referee and (iv) a 3-month "washout" period for magnesium hydroxide and chlorthalidone and 6-month "washout" period for allopurinol - sufficient time to allow treatment to bring about maximum chemical improvement.

We included subjects who had metabolically active calcium oxalate stone disease - forming at least two stones in the previous 5 years and at least one in the previous 2 years. Stone analyses were required to show 80% or more of calcium oxalate. We excluded subjects with chronic urinary infection, gastro-intestinal, renal, hepatic or cardiac disease.

The following dietary advice was given to all participants: reduce animal protein, increase fiber, reduce salt and refined sugar, increase water intake and avoid excessive dairy intake.

RESULTS

The first trial compared allopurinol, 100 mg 3 times per day, versus a placebo 3 times per day.   In addition to our usual entrance requirements, subjects entering this protocol were hyper-uricosuric (>800 mg/24 h for men, >750 mg/24 h for women) and normocalciuric (<300 mg/24 h for men, <250 mg/24 h for women or <4 mg/kg/24 h).

After an average duration of 29 months, the effectiveness of allopurinol was clearly documented.   Whereas 55% of placebo-treated subjects suffered recurrence, only 23% of allopurinol-treated subjects failed (P=0.01) (Fig.1).

Magnesium hydroxide in two doses, 325 mg bd and 650 mg bd was compared to a placebo.   Urinary magnesium was significantly increased by treatment, 53 mg and 86 mg respectively.   Despite the magnesiuria seen with therapy, survival analyses showed both doses were identical to the placebo (Fig. 2).

Chlorthalidone, in doses of 25 or 50 mg daily, was equally effective, reducing stone formation rates to 1/3 of those seen in the placebo-treated group.   Survival analysis showed P=0.05 and 0.04 for the 25 mg and 50 mg doses, respectively (Fig. 3).

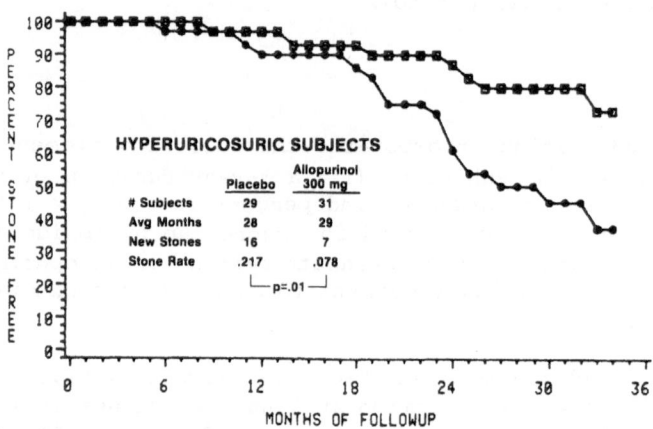

Fig. 1. Allopurinol study survival analysis double-blind protocol.
(● = placebo, □ = allopurinol).

550

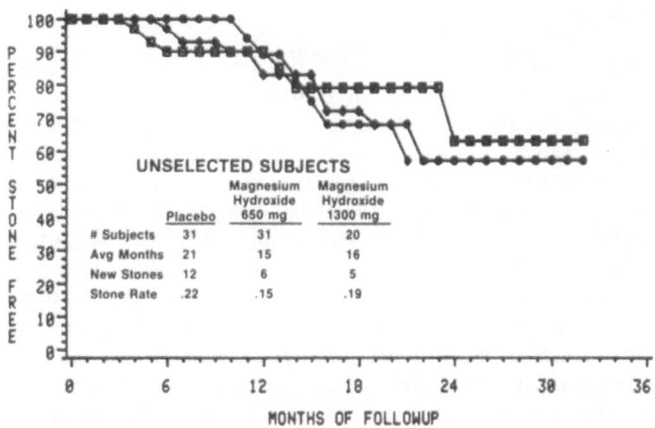

Fig. 2. Magnesium hydroxide study survival analysis double-blind
protocol. (o = placebo, □ = 650 mg, ◆ = 1300 mg).

Side-effects caused 25% of subjects on both doses to discontinue
therapy, usually in the first few weeks of treatment. Urinary
calcium was not changed in those subjects taking 25 mg but was
reduced by an average of 73 mg in those taking 50 mg daily.
Average urinary oxalate was reduced 13 mg in those taking 25 mg but
unchanged in those taking 50 mg of chlorthalidone daily. It is
possible that the beneficial effects of chlorthalidone were
moderated by different mechanisms at different dose levels.

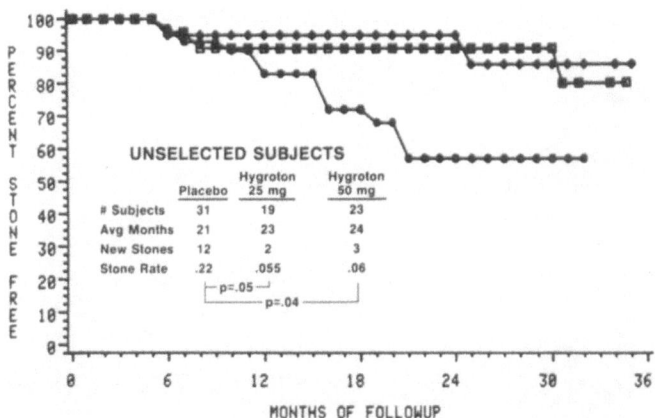

Fig. 3. Hygroton study survival analysis, double-blind protocol.
(● = placebo, □ = 25 mg, ◆ = 50 mg).

THE "CLINIC EFFECT"

Using an "historical control" design will strongly bias any stone prophylaxis trial towards a successful outcome . The pre-treatment stone rates of subjects assigned to various treatment groups in this study varied from 0.5 to 0.8 stones/patient/year. Those subjects observed on no treatment, on placebo or on ineffective treatment with magnesium hydroxide showed a reproducible and significant "reduction" in passage rate, to 0.2 stones per patient per year. Since no chemical changes were seen in placebo-treated subjects, we suspect that the stone rate observed during the study period is a true measure of the natural history of recurrent stones rather than a result of changes in diet or life style. Design and interpretation of stone prophylaxis studies should be modified in the future bearing in mind the "clinic effect".

THE EFFECTIVENESS OF LONG-TERM TREATMENT FOR

RECURRENT KIDNEY STONES USING THE DI METHOD

S. Perlberg, R. Azoury, Y. Wax,
N. Garti, and S. Sarig

Dept of Urology, Hebrew University, Hadassah Medical
Center, Jerusalem 91120, Israel

INTRODUCTION

The use of drugs to prevent recurrent kidney stone formation is largely empirical[1]. In this respect, thiazides[2] and phosphate[1] supplements have been found to be more successful than an increased fluid intake alone. Allopurinol is effective in patients suffering from hyperuricosuria and calcium oxalate (CaOx) stones[3]. However, more than 10% of patients continue to form stones, in spite of medication[1,2].

In this report we present a program of management of CaOx stone disease using the common drugs, phosphate, thiazides and allopurinol A newly introduced feature was to check the patient's response to medication about 10 days after starting treatment using our previously published Discriminating Index (DI) to control continuous treatment[4]. The treatment was continued if the response was positive, otherwise the patient was transferred to another treatment group. Patients whose DI failed to decrease on any of the 3 drugs, were excluded from the study.

MATERIALS AND METHODS

DI was measured as described by Sarig et al.[5]. Briefly, the method consists of the following: a solution containing 10% (v/v) urine is excessively supersaturated with calcium and oxalate ions. The crash precipitation profile of CaOx crystallization, as reflected by the decrease of calcium ion concentration, is measured by a calcium specific electrode. DI is defined as the ratio: $DI = \ln ([Ca^{+2}]_{0.5}/[Ca^{+2}]_{10})$ where the numerator and denominator

553

denote the concentrations of calcium after 0.5 and 10 minutes
respectively.   Values of DI < 0.66 are considered to be normal,
while DI values > 1.07 characterize stone formers.   Based on
statistical analysis, the change of DI in a patient from 1.0 or more
to below 0.66, resulting from treatment, was regarded in this study
as a criterion of success.   The rationale of using this criterion is
as follows, the drug increases the ability of urine to reduce CaOx
formation in vitro.   This we regarded as increasing the inhibitory
potential toward CaOx precipitation in urine[4,5].

This study included 55 patients with CaOx stones, 38 of whom
were recurrent stone formers.   Before commencing treatment, the DI
values of first morning urine specimens were determined, as well as
the collection of biochemical data from 24-h urine specimens in each
patient.   Phosphates, thiazide or allopurinol were prescribed
randomly.   Ten days after the start of treatment the DI was
checked.   If the response was positive the treatment was continued
and the dosage adjusted according to the DI.   If not, the patient
was prescribed another drug and the process repeated.   The duration
of the follow-up was 16 to 43 months.   We aimed at maintaining the
DI below 0.66, when this was achieved we considered the treatment
satisfactory, i.e. the urine response was kept within the normal
range.   The biochemical data were again checked while the DI
remained below 0.66.

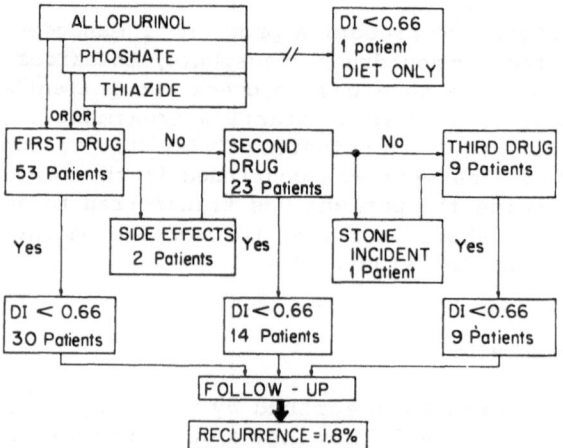

Fig. 1. The flow sheet of selected drug therapy according to the
         DI test.

RESULTS AND DISCUSSION

The scheme of treatment is presented in Fig. 1. One of the 3 drugs was prescribed at random for each of the 53 patients who had DI >1.07. In 32 cases the DI dropped below 0.66 indicating either corrected or compensated inhibitory characteristics to normal levels. Two patients with side-effects are mentioned below. The remaining 30 patients, 19 on phosphates, 8 on thiazides and 3 on allopurinol, continued treatment with the drug chosen initially. Twenty-three patients did not respond well and they, together with the 2 patients who had side-effects, were switched to another drug. The response was unsatisfactory in 9, who were successfully switched to the third drug, but one of these developed a stone during the adjustment of his medication.

Two patients, because of their continuing abnormal DI values, required a change of treatment. One, who had formed a stone while being treated with allopurinol for hyperuricemia, had a raised DI which fell when he stopped taking the drug. Other details are outside the scope of this report. The second did not respond to allopurinol according to the criteria of this study. He had an abnormally high uric acid excretion (1596 mg/24h) and was prescribed both allopurinol and thiazides. His final DI was 0.41 and his uric acid output fell to 682 mg/24h.

The present study includes recurrent and first time CaOx stone formers. In Fig. 2 the number of patient-years of 35 (out of 38) recurrent stone formers and their stone incidents are presented. The stone incidents prior to this study occurred despite all the

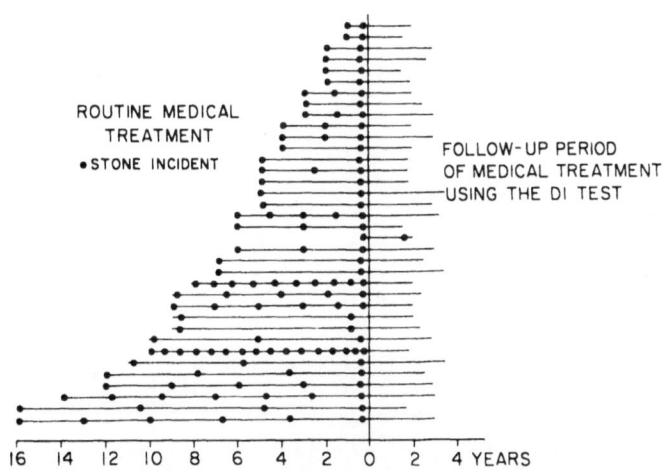

Fig. 2. Stone incidents of recurrent stone formers before and after proposed management of disease.

patients being on high fluid intake. For some of the patients the follow-up period exceeds the expected period of the next stone formation. The results to date are encouraging, since no recurrences of statistical significance have been encountered.

It is felt that further uninterrupted follow-up is necessary to confirm that the scheme of checking the DI value throughout drug treatment is to be recommended for the management of kidney stone disease.

REFERENCES

1. W. C. Thomas Jr., Kidney Int. 13:390 (1978).
2. E. R. Yendt and M. Cohanim, Kidney Int. 13: 397 (1978).
3. F. L. Coe and L. Raisen, Lancet 1:129 (1973).
4. S. Sarig, N. Garti, R. Azoury, S. Perlberg, and Y. Wax, J. Urol.129:1258 (1983).
5. S. Sarig, N. Garti, R. Azoury, Y. Wax, and S. Perlberg, J. Urol.128:645 (1982).

CALCIUM OXALATE STONE FORMERS FIVE YEARS LATER

J. Joost and A. Putz

Department of Urology, University of Innsbruck
Austria

INTRODUCTION

Only few prospective studies are available on calcium oxalate stone formers[1-4]. In 1976 a stone clinic was established in our department. Some of the questions arising at that time were: should single oxalate stone formers (SSF) undergo a complete metabolic check-up or not and which form of prophylaxis should they receive? How do recurrent stone formers (RSF) comply with the advice of a long-term treatment with a specific medication and how high is the recurrence rate? To answer these questions, a 5-year prospective study was started in 1977 (Table 1).

PATIENTS AND METHODS

Random assignment of patients provided 30 untreated SSF and 30 SSF who received non-specific treatment consisting of a high

Table 1. 5-year Prospective Study in Stone Formers.

	Recurrent	Single	Single
Patients (no)	30	30	30
Mean age (yr)	47	39	40
Stone analysis	oxalate	oxalate	oxalate
Metabolic disorders (no)	21 (70%)	4 (13.3%)	6 (20%)
Treatment	medication	diet, fluid	no
Controls after 5 years	26 (87%)	30 (100%)	26 (87%)
Patients with recurrence	8 (31%)	2 (6.7%)	1(3.8%)

Table 2. CaOx Stone Formers:Metabolic Disorders and Prophylaxis.

Metabolic disorders:	Single (n=26) no prophylaxis	Single (n=30) diet, fluid	Recurrent (n=26) medication
Hypercalciuria	3	4	11 Thiazide (50 mg/d)
Hyperuricosuria	0	0	2 Allopurinol (300 mg/d)
Hypocitraturia	1	1	4 Thiazide
Hypomagnesuria	0	1	1 Mg hydroxide (450 mg/day)
No disorder	22	24	8 Mg hydroxide

fluid intake (about 2 litres/day) coupled with a low calcium and oxalate diet. Both groups were sex- and age-matched. Thirty RSF who had passed at least 2 stones within the 5 years prior to treatment and at least one of which had been passed within the last year, received specific medication (Table 2). All patients underwent a complete metabolic check-up. Patients with primary hyperparathyroidism, urodynamic abnormalities or urinary infection were excluded. All stones, which were analysed by X-ray diffraction, consisted mainly of calcium oxalate mono- and dihydrate. Hypercalciuria was defined as more than 300 mg/day in men and 250 mg/day in women, hyperuricosuria as more than 800 mg/day, hypocitraturia as less than 1 mmol/day, and hypomagnesuria as less than 2.5 mmol/day. RSF and SSF receiving non-specific treatment were follwed at 6-month intervals. In 1982 all patients were called for a final assessment, comprising a medical history, urinalysis, blood analysis, 24-h urine and plain film.

RESULTS

In 1977 a metabolic abnormality was found in 21 (70%) of the 30 RSF and 10 (17%) of the 60 SSF (4 and 6 in each group). In 1982, 26 of the 30 RSF, all 30 of the SSF on therapy and 26 of the 30 SSF without treatment could be assessed. Of the 26 RSF only 5 (20%) still took their specific medication (2 allopurinol, 3 thiazide). All others had stopped medication after 2 to 3 years because of inconvenience and side-effects. Nevertheless, the stone passage rate, which was 0.5 within the 5 years before 1977, dropped to 0.09 during the follow-up period. Eight patients (30%), of whom 7 had a metabolic disorder (6 hyper-calciuria, 1 hypocitraturia), passed stones within the control period (Fig. 1). A metabolic abnormality (5 hypercalciuria, 4 hypocitraturia, 1 hypomagnesuria) was detected in 10 of the 18 patients without recurrence. One patient of the 26 SSF without

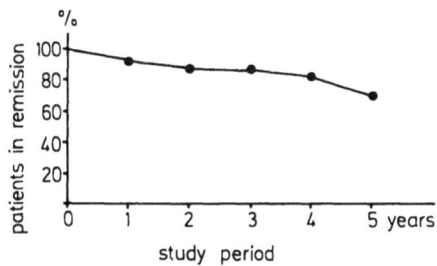

Fig. 1. Per cent of RSF without recurrence of urolithiasis during
5-year interval (n = 26 at entry).

treatment and 2 of the SSF with non-specific treatment had a
recurrence of stone formation. Hypercalciuria was found in the
first, whereas no abnormality could be found in the other two.

DISCUSSION

These clinical observations show that patients with a first
calcium oxalate stone episode do not need complete evaluation, as
metabolic disorders are rare and recurrence is low. It seems to
be sufficient to perform a urinalysis and to determine the serum
levels of calcium and creatinine. Over-consumption of meat,
dairy products and oxalate-rich food should be avoided and
increase in fluid intake recommended. An extremely restricted
diet is not advisable, as the treated and untreated group showed
no significant difference concerning the recurrence rate.

RSF, on the other hand, should undergo a strict metabolic
assessment, as disorders are high in this group (70%). Although
metabolic disorders seem to be lower in patients with remission
(10 of 18) than in those with recurrence (7 of 8), the difference
is not statistically significant. As might be expected,
compliance with drug therapy diminished rapidly after 2 to 3 years.
Nevertheless, the stone passage rate dropped significantly in the
5-year follow-up period and no increase in stone formation was
seen in those patients who had discontinued medication. This
reduction in the stone passage rate, however, may also be an
effect of advancing age[4]; in this respect an untreated control
group was lacking.

Another explanation might be the so-called "stone clinic
effect". It is commonly known that regular visits to a stone
clinic reduce the recurrence rate per se. According to some
investigators[5] this effect is explained by a stricter adherence to
diet and increase of fluid intake. In our RSF the average 24-h
volume of urine increased from 1200 to 1800 ml (P<0.01). At

present we treat recurrent stone formers suffering from metabolic abnormalities with specific drugs for a period of 2 years and discontinue therapy if no stone has formed again. Treatment is resumed in case of recurrent stone formation.

REFERENCES

1. R. E. Williams, Br. J. Urol. 35:416 (1963).
2. N. J. Blacklock, in:"Proceedings of the Renal Stone Research Symposium", A. Hodgkinson and B. E. C. Nordin, eds., Churchill, London (1968).
3. V. Marshall, R. H. White, M. C. de Saintonge, G. C. Tresidder, and J. P. Blandy, Br. J. Urol. 47:117 (1975).
4. B. Ettinger, Am. J. Med. 67:245 (1979).
5. D. H. Hosking, C. J. Van Den Berg, S. B. Erickson, D. M. Wilson, and L. H. Smith, Urol. Res. 12:26 (1984).

THE RELATIONSHIP BETWEEN CLINICAL OUTCOME AND URINE BIOCHEMISTRY DURING VARIOUS FORMS OF THERAPY FOR IDIOPATHIC CALCIUM STONE DISEASE

M. Marangella, A. Tricerri, M. Ronzani, C. Martini,
M. Petrarulo, P. G. Daniele, S. Torrengo, and F. Linari

Divisione di Nefrologia e Dialisi and Servizio di
Fisica Sanitari, Ospidale Mauriziano Umberto I, lst
Analisi Chimica Strumentale Università, Turin, Italy

INTRODUCTION

We have previously reported our experience with the long-term management of idiopathic calcium stone disease (ICaSD) and observed that the administration of drugs such as thiazides (HCT) and/or allopurinol (ALP) in addition to careful dietary management failed to give further benefit to the patient. The aim of this paper was to relate the clinical response to the biochemical and physico-chemical changes induced by three therapies in order to try to explain why different kinds of treatment provided similar results.

METHODS AND MATERIAL

A total of 138 patients were included in this study. All had experienced at least two stone episodes during the preceding two years. Only patients with ICaSD (as shown by IR stone analyses or by X-ray documentation of radio-opaque stones) and with normal renal function were admitted. All patients were instructed to eat a low calcium oxalate diet and to increase fluid intake. Then they were allocated at random into three treatment groups: group A of 49 patients treated by diet alone; group B of 34 patients treated by diet plus ALP (300 mg/day); and group C of 55 patients treated by diet plus HCT (50 mg/day) often in conjunction with amiloride and/or ALP. The stone history and main biochemical and physico-chemical parameters were recorded before and during treatment. Patients with less than 9 months follow-up were excluded. Samples from 24-h urine collections were analyzed for Ca, Mg, Na, K, ammonia, pH, Cl, citrate, sulfate, phosphate, urate and creatinine using routine methods. Oxalate was determined by a colorimetric procedure[2].

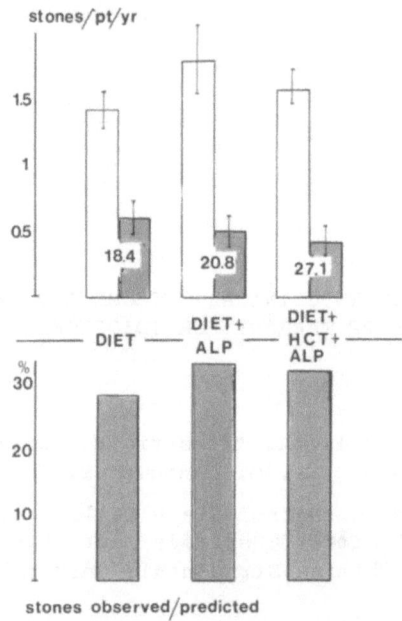

Fig. 1. Clinical follow-up before and during treatment.

Table 1. Clinical Outcome in the Three Treatment Groups (%).

Outcome	Group A	Group B	Group C	P (x^2)
No change	26	21	22	n.s.
Improvement	39	41	31	n.s.
Remission	35	38	47	n.s.

Urine supersaturation with calcium oxalate (β_{CaOx}) and brushite (β_{bsh}) were calculated by computer[3]. Statistical analyses were performed using the Chi-square or Student's t-test for matched pairs. Multivariate analysis was used to evaluate the correlation between the clinical and laboratory data.

RESULTS AND DISCUSSION

    The clinical outome is shown in Fig. 1. All three treatments significantly reduced the stone recurrence rate but the percent of patients in each group in whom improvement occurred did not differ (Table 1). Table 2 lists the biochemical and physico-chemical changes observed during treatment. Ca excretion significantly decreased in all groups; uric acid excretion decreased significantly only in groups B and C; urine volume increased

Table 2. Biochemical and Physical Chemical Changes during Therapy (Means ± SD).

	Group A		Group B		Group C	
	before	during	before	during	before	during
Ca (mmol/24h)	5.7 ± 2.3	4.7 ± 1.6**	5.5 ± 2.2	4.7 ± 1.6*	7.6 ± 2.6	5.7 ± 2.3***
Ox (mmol/24h)	0.46± 0.21	0.42± 0.17	0.53± 0.28	0.53± 0.16	0.52± 0.23	0.5 ± 0.18
Na (mmol/24h)	205 ± 82.5	178 ± 63.7	210.3± 67.1	188.6± 46.3	190.2± 65.6	195 ± 81.7
UA (mmol/24h)	3.2 ± 1.0	3.2 ± 0.8	3.9 ± 1.2	2.8 ± 0.9**	3.5 ± 0.9	2.8 ± 0.9***
Mg (mmol/24h)	2.9 ± 1.4	2.9 ± 1.2	3.3 ± 1.3	3.5 ± 1.6	3.6 ± 1.5	3.9 ± 1.6
Cit (mmol/24h)	3.9 ± 1.8	3.2 ± 1.2*	4.0 ± 2.0	3.9 ± 1.5	3.5 ± 1.7	3.4 ± 1.6
Vol (ml/24h)	1566 ± 572	1815 ± 643*	1588 ± 523	1710 ± 444	1693 ± 527	1837 ± 592*
pH	6.0 ± 0.53	6.2 ± 0.52	5.8 ± 0.59	5.7 ± 0.52	6.0 ± 0.49	6.2 ± 0.49
Ionic strength	0.19±0.09	0.16± 0.07*	0.23± 0.05	0.20± 0.06	0.19± 0.05	0.19± 0.07
β CaOx	8.65±6.6	6.55± 4.7	8.4 ± 3.1	7.4 ± 3.5	11.1 ± 5.7	8.7 ± 4.5*
β bsh	1.43±0.8	1.5 ± 1.1	1.1 ± 1	0.9 ± 0.6	2.2 ± 1.5	1.6 ± 1**

(*P<0.05; **P<0.01; ***P<0.001).

slightly in all groups; and β_{CaOx} and β_{bsh} decreased significantly only in group C. The variables which correlated best with clinical improvement were a high urine volume and a low calcium and oxalate excretion ($P < 0.05$).

The three different forms of therapy for ICaSD which have been used in this series have provided similar results in terms of reducing the rate of stone recurrence. Previous reports[4,5] have already noted the efficacy of these treatments, but in those trials patients were selected for a particular form of treatment. In this open study, the pre-treatment clinical and metabolic data were similar in the three groups and it is suggested that benefit can be obtained even when treatment is allocated on an unselected basis. In our hands, drugs such as HCT and/or ALP, do not seem to add significant benefit beyond that achieved by dietary management.

When the results were analyzed according to the biochemical and physico-chemical changes, few differences were observed in urinary composition during each of the three different forms of therapy. The decrease in stone activity during treatment correlated with both the increase in urine volume and the decrease in calcium and oxalate excretion. Since the effects of the three therapies on the above parameters were quite similar, it is suggested that this could be the reason why we failed to observe significant differences between these therapeutic approaches. Thus the decrease in uric acid excretion observed only in groups B and C did not seem to influence the results obtained in these patients as compared to patients in groups A in whom this change did not occur. Moreover, the comparable percentages of patients in which stone disease did not improve could be attributed to the inefficacy of our therapies on other urinary constituents such as magnesium, citrate or oxalate. Finally, a combined clinical biochemical follow-up suggests that the ability to maintain, rather than to achieve, a urine composition less conducive to stone formation, is important: the patient's compliance with a given therapy is critical in this regard.

REFERENCES

1. M. Marangella, A. Tricerri, S. Sonego, M. Ronzani, B. Fruttero, P. G. Daniele, M. Bruno, and F. Linari, in:"Proceedings of the European Dialysis and Transplant Association", A. M. Davison, ed ., Pitman, London (1983).
2. H. Baadenhuysen and A. P. Jensen, Clin. Chim. Acta 62:315 (1975).
3. P. G. Daniele and M. Marangella, Ann. Chim. 72:25 (1982).
4. C. Y. C. Pak, P. Peters, G. Hurt, M. Kadesky, M. Fine, D. Reisman, F. Splann, C. Caramela, A. Freeman, F. Britton, K. Sakhaee, and N. Breslau, Am. J. Med. 71:615 (1981).
5. F. L. Coe, Ann. Int. Med. 87:404 (1977).

BIOCHEMICAL ALTERATIONS IN URINARY STONE PATIENTS

ON CHEMOPROPHYLAXIS

Y. M. Fazil Marickar, H. Paul, S. Salahudeen,
and K. B. Nair

Depts. of Surgery and Biochemistry, Medical College
Hospital, Trivandrum, India

INTRODUCTION

Urinary stone formation is such a heterogeneous disorder that
no specific type of prophylaxis is uniformly effective in all
patients. Solubilization of potential components of calculi has
been the aim of prophylaxis[1]. The purpose of this study was to
identify the biochemical changes produced by various drugs used in
idiopathic calcium stone disease.

MATERIALS AND METHODS

Patients with calcium stones were investigated for urinary
calcium, uric acid and magnesium and serum uric acid. Thiazides,
as Hydrochlorothiazide 12.5 mg daily, were given to patients with
hypercalciuria. Allopurinol, in a dose of 100 mg thrice daily, was
given for hyperuricaemia and/or hyperuricosuria. A combination of
thiazides and magnesium was given for hypercalciuria along with
hypomagnesiuria. A combination of thiazides and allopurinol was
given to patients with hypercalciuria and hyperuricosuria and/or
hyperuricaemia. Magnesium, as magnesium trisilicate 100 mg three
times daily, was given for hypomagnesiuria. A few patients with
biochemical values in the normal ranges were also included in the
various drug regimes. Long-term studies were done at monthly
intervals for 2 to 6 months on urine calcium for the effect of
thiazides, thiazides + magnesium and thiazides + allopurinol, urine
uric acid for the effect of allopurinol and thiazides + allopurinol,
urine magnesium for the effect of thiazides + magnesium, and serum
uric acid for the effect of allopurinol and thiazides. Short-term
studies were performed at daily intervals for 4 to 10 days on urine

565

calcium for the effect of magnesium and urine magnesium for the effect of thiazides. For each observation, the results were expressed as a percentage of the pre-treatment results for that patient. The results were combined to give a mean ($\pm$ SEM) percentage excretion or serum concentration.

RESULTS

The long-term effect of thiazides on urinary calcium showed that the urinary excretion of calcium was reduced significantly in one month and the reduction persisted in the second and third months ($P < 0.05$). The values of the fourth and fifth months were not easily assessed because of the limited number of samples. The combination of thiazides + magnesium produced a significant decrease in urinary calcium in the second and third months ($P < 0.05$). The combination of thiazides + allopurinol showed a significant decrease in urinary calcium ($P < 0.01$) in the first, third, fourth and fifth months. According to Student's t-test, no statistical difference was observed between the biochemical changes produced by thiazides alone and thiazides + magnesium or thiazides + allopurinol.

Urinary uric acid was significantly reduced by allopurinol. Thiazides and allopurinol also produced a significant change. A statistically significant difference was noted between the effects produced by allopurinol and the combination of thiazides and allopurinol in the third ($P < 0.01$) and fourth ($P < 0.05$) months. Allopurinol alone produced a greater reduction than the combination. Serum uric acid was reduced significantly by allopurinol and this was maintained for 5 months. Thiazides produced no significant alteration in serum uric acid.

Urinary magnesium was significantly increased in the third and fifth months after the combination of thiazides + magnesium. Magnesium treatment increased urine calcium ($P < 0.05$) on the first and second days with no effect on days 3 through 10. Thiazides decreased urine magnesium on days 1 through 10.

DISCUSSION

Most of the studies of chemoprophylaxis reported for stone patients have been complicated and contradictory. Calcium stone formation is a complex problem and is influenced by the presence of other substances in urine[2]. The finding of a high uric acid excretion in the urine of calcium stone patients corroborates this view[3]. The role of magnesium in the inhibition of calcium oxalate crystallization has been stressed. The clinical state of the patient and the composition of the stone are important parameters on which the chemoprophylactic regime is to be based. The results of the present study indicate that thiazides, allopurinol and magnesium do produce significant alterations in urine biochemistry irrespective of the pre-treatment levels. Hence the problems remaining to be solved are, which drug is to be given, whether or not a combination of drugs is to be given, and how to counter the undesirable side-effects of the drugs.

It is surmised from the present observations, that magnesium should not be given alone to stone patients, as it produces hypercalciuria. Thiazides alone produce a significant early reduction of urinary mgnesium, and so it is ideal to supplement with magnesium. The absence of any significant effect of thiazides on uric acid is worth noting. The absence of any significant difference in the urine calcium excretion between patients on thiazides and those with thiazides + magnesium or thiazides + allopurinol indicates that drug combinations are not necessary for lowering urine calcium.

The action of allopurinol in dissolving uric acid stones is well-documented[4]. But its value for treating calcium stone formation is still being assessed. It is thus felt that, for a patient with a high urinary calcium, with or without hypo-magnesiuria, a combination of thiazides and magnesium should be given. If calcium stone formation is associated with a high uric acid level in the blood or urine, allopurinol should also be given. Idiopathic stone formers without any biochemical abnormality may be managed with dietetic advice alone, or treated with thiazides + magnesium or thiazides + allopurinol.

Intermittent chemoprophylaxis with drugs at the time of colic or stone episode has also been found to be of benefit. A long-term follow-up of patients on chemoprophylaxis has shown a significant reduction in the rate of stone incidents compared to pre-treatment levels.

ACKNOWLEDGEMENTS

The authors wish to thank the Principal, Medical College, Trivandrum, India for permission to use patient data, and Dr Gowenlock of the Biochemistry Department, Manchester Royal Infirmary, United Kingdom for help with the statistical analysis of the data.

REFERENCES

1. J. S. King, Clin. Chem. 17:971 (1971).
2. E. R. Yendt and M. Cohanim, Kidney Int. 13:397 (1978).
3. F. L. Coe, Kidney Int. 13:418 (1978).
4. B. Finlayson, Aust. N. Z. J. Surg. 50:8 (1980).

FIVE-YEAR TREATMENT IN HYPEROXALURIC STONE FORMERS

B. Pinto, F. J. Ruiz-Marcellán, and J. Bernshtam

Servicio de Urologia, Hospital Valle Hebrón and
Laboratorio de Exploraciones Metabólicas, Barcelona
Spain

INTRODUCTION

Gas chromatographic methods[1] show that hyperoxaluria is common in patients who have recurrent renal stones and that hyperoxaluria may be present alone or associated with hypercalciuria[2]. When hyperoxaluria was investigated using the absorption of ^{14}C-oxalate, hyperoxalemia and an increase in oxalate clearance were found[3]. However, a decrease in oxalate clearance was detected in patients with hyperoxaluria of which hyperabsorption seems to be the most frequent cause[2]. None of the patients with absorptive hyperoxaluria had intestinal disease[2,4]. In this paper we describe the results of treatment in these patients.

METHODS AND MATERIALS

From a group of 450 stone formers treated for 5 years, 69 hyperoxaluric patients were selected. A blind study was carried out in which calcium, magnesium, phosphate, urate and creatinine levels were determined in blood and 24-h urine samples[5]. Urate, phosphate and creatinine clearance levels were calculated. Oxalate was also determined in the 24-h samples[1]. Urinary pH, ammonia and titratable acidity were measured in a 2-h sample. The presence of hyperoxaluria alone or associated with hypercalciuria was confirmed in 3 additional 24-h determinations.

The different types of hyperoxaluria were investigated by intravenous administration of 4 µCi ^{14}C-oxalate and calculation of blood oxalate, oxalate clearance and excretion rate of the radio-activity[3,4]. Oxalate absorption and excretion were measured 1 week later in a 48-h urine sample after oral administration of 2 μCi ^{14}C-oxalate together with 250 mg sodium oxalate[3].

In patients with calcium oxalate stones the type of hypercalciuria was investigated by oral administration of 25 μCi [45]calcium while the patients were maintained on a 400 mg calcium intake for 12 days[6]. Patients with synthesis hyperoxalemia were given 6 g oral succinimide daily, while those with increased or decreased oxalate clearance received 1 g orthophosphate and 10 g magnesium chloride orally. The same treatment was given to a borderline group. Patients with hyperoxaluria and hyperabsorption of oxalate were managed with 15 g oral diethylaminoethanol cellulose daily[4]. Cellulose phosphate (15 g/day) was also administered to patients with hyperabsorption of calcium. Every 3 months, 24-h urinary oxalate and calcium levels were determined. Radiologic controls were performed every 6 months. If present, urinary infection was treated according to the antibiogram results.

RESULTS

A daily excretion of >40 mg oxalate was considered to be hyperoxaluric. Of the 450 patients treated for 5 years, hyperoxaluria was present in 69 (15.3%), while 41 (9.1%) had hyperoxaluria alone and 28 (6.2%) had hyperoxaluria and hypercalciuria.

Among the patients with hyperoxaluria alone, the main findings were oxalate hyperabsorption, hyperoxalemia and alterations in oxalate clearance (Table 1). In the borderline hyperoxaluric subgroup oxalemia, oxalate clearance and absorption were normal. The patients with both hyperoxaluria and hypercalciuria had the double defect of oxalate and calcium hyperabsorption (Table 2).

Table 1. Oxalate Metabolism Data in Patients with Hyperoxaluric Renal Stones (mean ± SD).

	Patients	Oxalemia (μg/100ml)	^{14}C-Oxalate Excretion From Oral Dose (%)	Oxalate Clearance (ml/min/ 1.73m^2)	Oxalate Creatinine Clearance
Absorptive hyperoxaluria	21	12.7± 8.9	31.0+24	166+56	1.2+0.4
Hyperoxalemia	9	72.7+36.0	2.5+1.5	84+56	0.5+0.3
Clearance increase	4	7.6± 3.7	3.6+2.1	308+55	2.7+1.0
Clearance decrease	3	18.5± 6.8	4.1+1.8	71+13	0.6+0.1
Borderline	4	20.0± 8.0	5.3+1.9	218+73	2.0+0.8

570

Table 2. Oxalate and Calcium Metabolism in 28 patients with Hyperoxalocalciuria.

	Oxalate	Calcium	Ratio
Oxalemia (µg/100 ml)	18.6 $\pm$ 4.1	–	–
% ^{14}C-oxalate excretion	43.0 $\pm$ 12	–	–
Clearance (ml/min/1.73m^2)	187.0 $\pm$ 43	0.82 $\pm$ 0.06	–
Ox/creatinine clearance	–	–	1.30 $\pm$ 0.3
% ^{45}Ca urinary excretion	–	14.20 $\pm$ 1.6	–
Urinary Ca (mg/24 h)	–	346.00 $\pm$ 68	–
Urinary Ca/creatinine	–	–	0.09 $\pm$ 0.04

Table 3. Effect of Treatment on Metabolic Findings (mean $\pm$ SD).

	Oxaluria (mg/24h)		Calciuria (mg/24h)	
	Before	During	Before	During
	Treatment		Treatment	
Absorptive hyperoxaluria	65 $\pm$ 18	24 $\pm$ 5	182 $\pm$ 22	173 $\pm$ 14
Hyperoxalemia	187 $\pm$ 175	69 $\pm$ 60	166 $\pm$ 41	180 $\pm$ 24
Clearance	61 $\pm$ 15	18 $\pm$ 6	181 $\pm$ 14	175 $\pm$ 19
decrease	82 $\pm$ 32	31 $\pm$ 14	172 $\pm$ 21	188 $\pm$ 15
Borderline	44 $\pm$ 9	33 $\pm$ 10	190 $\pm$ 16	169 $\pm$ 31
Hyperoxaluria and hypercalciuria	61 $\pm$ 14	23 $\pm$ 8	346 $\pm$ 68	167 $\pm$ 39

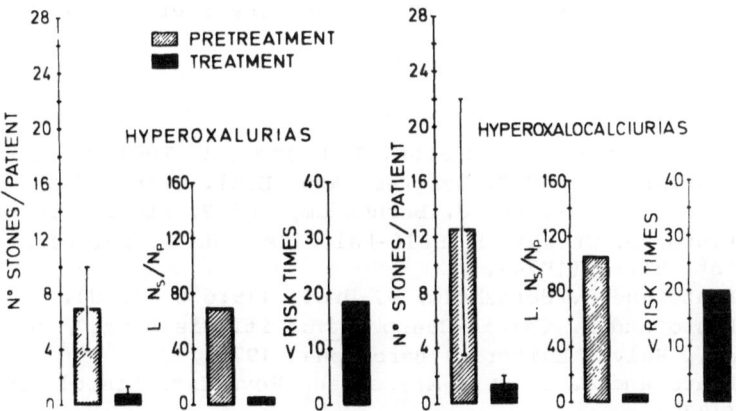

Fig. 1. Results of treatment in patients with hyperoxaluria (for key see text).

The risk of stone formation in each group was calculated from the equation: risk=(L x Ns) / Np, where L is the length of time (years) of disease or treatment, Ns is the number of stones and Np the number of patients. The pre-treatment-to-treatment risk ratio indicated that the risk of stone formation decreased through the treatment period in both groups of patients (Fig 1). Oxaluria decreased appreciably throughout the treatment period. Treatment was most effective in the group with hyperabsorption and increased clearance of oxalate (Table 3). However, oxaluria in the hyperoxalemic group was affected only slightly by treatment. In fact, most of these patients remained hyperoxaluric throughout treatment.

The age of the patients when the disease occurred, the duration of the disease and the duration of treatment were similar in both groups.

DISCUSSION

A urinary oxalate excretion of >40 mg/day was present in 69 of the 450 patients with stones (15.3%). The mechanism by which these patients hyperexcreted oxalate is complex. However, hyperabsorption, either alone or associated with hypercalciuria, seems to be the main cause. None of the patients with absorptive hyperoxaluria had bowel disease. Hyperoxalemia was the second most common cause of hyperoxaluria, perhaps through a higher rate of oxalate synthesis. A third group of patients had abnormalities in oxalate clearance.

Patients with absorptive hyperoxaluria were treated with diethylaminoethanol cellulose, whereas the synthesis and excretive groups were treated with succinimide or with a combination of phosphate and magnesium, respectively. The patients with absorptive hyperoxaluria responded best to treatment. Succinimide given to the hyperoxalemic (synthesis) group was the least effective treatment.

REFERENCES

1. M. T. Duburque, J. M. Melon, J. Thomas, E. Thomas, R. Pierre, C. Charransol, and P. Desgrez, Ann. Biol. Clin. 28:95 (1970).
2. F. J. Ruiz-Marcellán, J. Bernshtam, and B. Pinto, (In press).
3. B. Pinto, G. Crespi, F. Solé-Balcells, and P. Barcelo, Kidney Int. 5:295 (1974).
4. B. Pinto and J. Bernshtam, J. Urol. 119:630 (1978).
5. B. Pinto and E. Garcia-Cuerpo, in:"Litiásis Renal", B. Pinto, ed., Salvat Editores, Barcelona (1976).
6. B. Pinto and F. J. Ruiz-Marcellan, Rev. Esp. Fisiol. 35:311 (1979).

THE INFLUENCE OF FLURBIPROFEN ON CALCIUM EXCRETION AND

VITAMIN D3 IN RECURRENT CALCIUM LITHIASIS - A DOUBLE BLIND STUDY

A. C. Buck, C. J. Davies, R. Brown, R. Y. Sabur, and
K. Murray

Dept. of Urology, Welsh National School of Medicine
Cardiff, U.K.

INTRODUCTION

Idiopathic calcium stone formation occurs against a background
of subtle abnormalities in the crystalloid composition of urine and
poorly defined disorders of calcium metabolism. It is now
recognised that hypercalciuria is a major predisposing "risk" factor
in urolithiasis and in most cases it is secondary to calcium
hyperabsorption. The vitamin D metabolite, $1,25-(OH)_2D_3$, stimulates
intestinal calcium absorption and bone resorption and $1,25(OH)_2D_3$
levels are indeed raised in stone formers, although the factors
responsible for this abnormality remain obscure. Recent in vitro
experiments[1] suggest that prostaglandins may regulate renal 1α-
hydroxylase activity synthesising $1,25-(OH)_2D_3$. The aim of this
study was to evaluate the effect of prostaglandin inhibition with
Flurbiprofen on urinary calcium excretion and vitamin D_3 metabolism
in a selected group of recurrent idiopathic stone formers.

PATIENTS AND METHODS

Forty recurrent idiopathic stone formers were entered into a
double blind, cross-over trial of Flurbiprofen versus placebo.
These were 38 males and 2 females with a mean ($\pm$ SD) age of 44 ± 11
years (range 23 to 62 years).

The measurement of renal threshold phosphate concentration[2]
(T_mPO_4/GFR) , and tubular reabsorption of calcium[3] (T_mCa/GFR) was
begun with a timed 2-h urine collection. Blood was drawn at the
mid-point of the collection for a haematological and biochemical
screen which included blood urea, creatinine, electrolytes, calcium,

phosphate, uric acid, magnesium, parathyroid hormone (PTH) and 1,25-$(OH)_2D_3$. This was followed by three consecutive 24-h urine collections which were analysed for calcium, oxalate, phosphate, urate, sodium and magnesium excretion together with a measurement of creatinine clearance (GFR).

The patients were then randomly allocated to two groups: one of which received Flurbiprofen 50 mg tablets t.d.s. for 4 weeks and the other group received an indistinguishable placebo tablet under the same regime. During the fourth week, whilst on the first phase of treatment the patient again attended the clinic for all the investigations to be repeated as before. At the conclusion of the first assigned treatment the patient was switched to the alternative therapy for a period of 4 weeks and the investigations again repeated at the end of this second treatment phase.

Statistical analysis of the effects of placebo and Flurbiprofen on the various parameters measured was by the non-parametric Wilcoxon Rank Sum test for paired samples.

RESULTS

Six patients were withdrawn from this study for protocol violations and drug intolerance. The data from 34 patients were available for analysis.

The mean ($\pm$ SEM) baseline urine calcium excretion was 7.06 $\pm$ 0.437 mmol/24 h. Of the group, 14/34 patients were hypercalciuric (24-h urine calcium excretion $>$7.5 mmol/24 h), with a mean urine calcium excretion of 9.66 $\pm$ 0.38 mmol/24 h. There was a statistically significant reduction in urine calcium excretion with Flurbiprofen to 5.09 $\pm$ 0.4 mmol/24 h ($P < 0.01$). A slight fall in

Table 1. Biochemical Data (mean $\pm$ SEM)

	Initial	Placebo	Flurbiprofen
Serum			
PTH (ng/ml)	0.45 $\pm$ 0.12	0.46 $\pm$ 0.14	0.39 $\pm$ 0.09
Calcium (mmol/l)	2.34 $\pm$ 0.02	2.33 $\pm$ 0.02	2.27 $\pm$ 0.05
Phosphate (mmol/l)	0.98 $\pm$ 0.03	0.97 $\pm$ 0.03	0.96 $\pm$ 0.02
Creatinine (umol/l)	98.82 $\pm$ 3.24	96.34 $\pm$ 3.61	98.53 $\pm$ 3.03
Urine			
T_mPO_4 (mmol/l GF)	0.98 $\pm$ 0.04	1.01 $\pm$ 0.04	0.98 $\pm$ 0.03
T_mCa/GFR (mmol/l GF)	1.94 $\pm$ 0.04	1.89 $\pm$ 0.03	1.89 $\pm$ 0.03
Magnesium (mmol/24 h)	4.63 $\pm$ 0.23	4.47 $\pm$ 0.21	4.31 $\pm$ 0.25
Oxalate (mmol/24 h)	0.16 $\pm$ 0.02	0.14 $\pm$ 0.02	0.14 $\pm$ 0.02
Volume (l/24 h)	1.55 $\pm$ 0.07	1.48 $\pm$ 0.07	1.48 $\pm$ 0.07

urine calcium excretion occurred with placebo but this was not statistically significant. Phosphate and urate excretion were both reduced with placebo and Flurbiprofen. Urine sodium excretion and creatinine clearance (GFR) did not fall significantly with Flurbiprofen. There was no correlation between urinary sodium and calcium excretion in this study.

The $1,25-(OH)_2D_3$ values before treatment were 45.32 ± 5.03 ng/l. Following treatment with Flurbiprofen the mean value was 36.9 ± 4.16 ng/l (P<0.01). With placebo the mean $1,25(OH)_2D_3$ fell to 43.11 ± 4.43 ng/l but this was not significantly different from the initial values. Serum calcium, phosphate, PTH, T_mPO_4/GFR and T_mCa/GFR values, together with other urine parameters, were within the normal range and did not change significantly with either Flurbiprofen or placebo (Table 1).

DISCUSSION

$1,25(OH)_2D_3$, synthesised exclusively in the kidney, is the principal regulatory hormone that determines the capacity of the gut for active calcium transport. Circulating $1,25(OH)_2D_3$ levels have been found to be raised in stone formers with absorptive hypercalciuria[4,5], and a positive correlation has also been observed between $1,25-(OH)_2D_3$ levels and urine calcium excretion[6]. A number of variable factors are regarded as regulating the synthesis of $1,25(OH)_2D_3$ in the kidney; parathyroid hormone (PTH) both directly and by causing hypophosphataemia, promotes the synthesis of $1,25-(OH)_2D_3$, $1,25-(OH)_2D_3$ is strongly product inhibited and low serum calcium levels can stimulate renal 1α-hydroxylase [9]. Whilst there is experimental evidence in support of these mechanisms, it has not been possible to demonstrate abnormalities in serum calcium, phosphate, parathormone, cAMP or T_mPO_4/GFR in idiopathic stone formers. This would suggest that additional regulatory mechanisms may be involved in the synthesis of this hormone[10]. Recently, Wark et al[1] using in vitro preparations of chick renal tubules have shown that renal prostaglandins may act as local regulators of the 1α-hydroxylation reaction synthesising $1,25(OH)_2D_3$ in the kidney. Renal prostaglandins are now well recognised as important autocoids participating in the complex regulation of water and electrolyte excretion by the kidney[11]. Our previous studies have indicated that renal prostaglandins can influence calcium excretion and that PG synthetase inhibition with NSAIDs reduces urinary calcium excretion in both experimental animals and hypercalciuric stone formers[12].

In the assessment of any beneficial effect of drug treatment in idiopathic hypercalciuria it is important to eliminate the bias of both a placebo and a "clinic" effect which are well documented in this condition[13-16]. Flurbiprofen is a potent cyclo-oxygenase inhibitor and was used in this double blind, placebo controlled study to evaluate its effect on circulating $1,25(OH)_2D_3$, urinary calcium excretion and other parameters of renal function. This study has shown that Flurbiprofen significantly reduced both urinary calcium excretion and circulating $1,25(OH)_2D_3$ levels. Notable, however, was the reduction in urate and phosphate excretion with placebo and active compound which probably reflects self-imposed dietary modifications by the patient under these investigative conditions. In this study serum calcium, phosphate, PTH and T_mPO_4/GFR were within the normal range and no change was seen in any of these analytes coincidental with a fall in $1,25(OH)_2D_3$ with Flurbiprofen. This suggests that the response to Flurbiprofen is mediated by a mechanism independent of parathyroid hormone activity. However, it is not possible from the present study to deduce the mechanism of these effects, and clearly further investigations are needed to define the precise role of prostaglandins and their inhibitors in regulating calcium homeostasis.

REFERENCES

1. J. D. Wark, R. G. Larkins, J. A. Eisman, and K. R. Wilson, Clin. Sci. 61:53 (1981).
2. R. J. Walton and O. L. M. Bijvoet, Lancet 2:309 (1975).
3. M. Peacock and B. E. C. Nordin, J. Clin. Path. 21:353 (1968).
4. R. A. Kaplan, M. R. Haussler, L. J. Deftos, H. Bone, and C. Y. C. Pak, J. Clin. Invest. 59:756 (1977).
5. F. H. Shen, D. J. Baylink, R. L. Mielsen, D. J. Sherrard, J. L. Ivey, and M. R. Haussler, J. Lab. Clin. Med. 90:955 (1977).
6. A. E. Broadus, R. L. Horst, R. Lang, E. T. Littledike, and H. Rasmussen, New Engl. J. Med. 302:421 (1980).
7. M. Garabedian, M. F. Holick, H. F. DeLuca, and I. T. Boyle, Proc. Nat. Acad. Sci. 69:1673 (1972).
8. Y. Tanaka and H. F. DeLuca, Proc. Nat. Acad. Sci. 71:1040 (1974).
9. H. F. DeLuca ;and H. K. Schnoes, Ann. Rev. Biochem. 45: 631 (1976).
10. J. Lemann, in:"Contemporary Issues in Nephrology", F. L. Coe, B. M. Brenner, and J. H. Stein, eds., Churchill Livingstone, New York (1980).
11. M. J. Dunn and V. L. Hood, Am. J. Physiol. 233:F169 (1977).
12. A. C. Buck, C. J. Lote, and W. F. Sampson, J. Urol. 129:421 (1983).
13. B. Ettinger, Am. J. Med. 61:200 (1976).
14. M. J. V. Smith, J. Urol. 117:690 (1977).
15. P. Brocks, C. Dahl, H. Woolf, and I. Transbøl, Lancet 2:124 (1981).
16. D. H. Hosking, S. B. Ericson, C. J. Van den Berg, D. M. Wilson, and L. H. Smith, J. Urol. 130:1115 (1983).

THE INHIBITION OF EXPERIMENTAL NEPHROCALCINOSIS WITH

A PROSTAGLANDIN SYNTHETASE INHIBITOR

A. C. Buck

Dept. of Urology, The Welsh National School of
Medicine, Cardiff, U.K.

INTRODUCTION

Investigation into the pathognesis of idiopathic renal calculi
has focused mainly on the physiochemical aspects of urinary
crystallisation[1-3]. However, the presence of microscopic foci of
intranephronic calcification suggests that the pathogenesis of stone
formation begins within the interstitial tissues and the renal
tubular cells, and it is this lesion which is regarded as the
precursor of the calcium oxalate stone[4-7]. An explanation for the
mechanism of stone formation should endeavour to relate the physico-
chemical and anatomical concepts of calculogenesis.

Prostaglandin activity is an important factor in the mechanism
of hypercalciuria in recurrent stone formers[8]. Prostaglandins may
also be concerned with the membrane transport of calcium and non-
steroidal anti-inflammatory drugs have been shown to inhibit
calcium-binding by cell membranes and to block calcium deposition in
bone[9-12]. The aim of this study was to establish an animal model
of experimental nephrocalcinosis and to see whether or not this
lesion could be prevented by pretreating the animals with a
prostaglandin synthetase inhibitor.

MATERIALS AND METHODS

Experiments were performed in 50 female rats of an inbred PVG
strain. The animals were divided into 4 groups. Group 1 (15
rats) were given Ca gluconate (1.5 ml of a 10% solution) by intraperitoneal injection daily for 10 days to induce nephrocalcinosis[13].
Group 2 (15 rats) received indomethacin (10 mg/kg body weight) in

buffered saline by gastric intubation in a divided dose at 09.00 and 16.00 daily for 4 days before commencement of the i.p. Ca gluconate injections and indomethacin continued during the 10-day course of Ca gluconate. Group 3 (10 rats) were given flurbiprofen (2 mg/kg body weight) in buffered saline prior to the course of the i.p. Ca gluconate under the same regime as in the animals in Group 2. A sham control group of 10 rats (group 4) received 1.5 ml of 0.9% NaCl by i.p. injection. At the end of 10 days (Group 1 and 4) and 14 days (Group 2 and 3) the rats were killed by exsanguination under ether anaesthesia and serum separated for the estimation of calcium.

Both kidneys were removed. One kidney was fixed in buffered saline and examined for differential localisation of calcium by contact microradiography of freeze-dried sections and histology by means of von Kossa staining for calcium phosphate. The other kidney was used for quantitative analysis of elemental calcium by means of energy dispersive analysis of X-rays (EDAX) and by chemical analysis using atomic absorption spectroscopy.

RESULTS

Extensive cortical calcification was seen as radio-opaque flecks in microradiographs of the kidneys in all the animals given i.p. calcium gluconate (Group 1). In both the indomethacin- and flurbiprofen-treated rats minimal calcification was seen at the junction of the inner medulla and base of the renal papilla. Calcification was absent from the kidneys of rats receiving i.p. saline alone.

Cortical deposition of calcium phosphate was demonstrated by the von Kossa technique to be present in the kidney sections of all the rats treated with i.p. Ca gluconate. In rats pre-treated with flurbiprofen, cortical calcification was absent and only minimal calcification seen in the tubular basement membrane at the medullo-papillary junction. Calcification was not seen in the kidney sections of rats treated with indomethacin or normal saline.

X-ray fluorescence results were expressed as counts/sec/g of tissue. In the rats given i.p. Ca gluconate alone, the mean ($+$SEM) count was 306.57 ± 27.27 counts/sec/g. The indomethacin-treated rats had a significantly lower count 153.16 ± 9.5 ($P < 0.005$), as did the flurbiprofen-treated animals, 152.37 ± 10.7 ($P < 0.005$). The concentration of calcium in the kidneys of rats given i.p. saline was 48.13 ± 6.57 counts/sec/g ($P < 0.001$).

Quantitative calcium analysis by atomic absorption spectroscopy was performed in animals given Ca gluconate alone, indomethacin-treated animals and in the rats receiving i.p. normal saline. The mean calcium content of rats given Ca gluconate alone was

578

0.2 ± 0.033 mmol/g dry weight. The animals treated with indomethacin had a mean calcium of 0.144 ± 0.012 mmmol/g. The sham control animals receiving i.p. normal saline had a mean calcium of 0.0074 ± 0.0007 mmol/g.

The serum levels of calcium at the time of death showed that animals given i.p. gluconate were hypercalcaemic with a mean serum calcium of 2.72 ± 0.44 mmol/l. Indomethacin- and flurbiprofen- treated animals had low serum calcium levels (2.18 ± 0.20 mmol/l and 2.14 ± 0.17 mmol/l respectively). The mean serum calcium in animals given i.p. saline was 2.61 ± 0.14 mmol/l.

DISCUSSION

There are essentially two theories of calculogenesis: the physico-chemical and the anatomical. However, the relationship between these two processes remains obscure. Our previous studies suggest that renal prostaglandins influence urinary calcium excretion indicating the importance of these hormones in the hyper-calciuria associated with idiopathic urolithiasis[8]. The present study shows that experimental nephrocalcinosis is effectively prevented by treating the animals with a prostaglandin synthetase inhibitor. From this study it is not possible to determine the exact mechanism of this inhibitory action, which could be due to indomethacin and flurbiprofen preventing the development of hyper-calcaemia, as the rats receiving these drugs were found to have low serum calcium levels in comparison with those given Ca gluconate alone. Alternatively, inhibition of intra-renal prostaglandin synthesis could be the process preventing the deposition of calcium within the kidney.

The interdependence between Ca^{2+} ions and prostaglandin metabolism is well recognised. The influence of Ca^{2+} on prosta-glandin synthesis may be mediated through an action of this cation to stimulate the release of free arachidonic acid from tissue lipids stores by activation of the enzyme phospholipase A2[14-16]. It has also been suggested that increase in cytosolic Ca^{2+} derived from extracellular and intracellular pools may represent a common pathway through which the action of various stimuli initiate arachidonate release to subsequent prostaglandin conversion[17,18]. Acute changes in cellular calcium homeostasis, such as a rise in cytosolic Ca^{2+} which would occur in hypercalcaemia, may not only provide a primary trigger for initiation of arachidonate release, but also alter the structural arrangement of phospholipids rendering them more susceptible to cleavage by Ca^{2+} dependent acyl hydrolases[18].

To relate these events to stone formation in man it would be necessary to identify the predisposing factors of nephrolithiasis which could interact to produce the pathophysiological changes resulting in increased renal prostaglandin synthesis. Elevated calcium concentration within the renal tubular cell and interstitial tissues resulting from an increased delivery of Ca^{2+} to the excretory system, which would occur in absorptive hypercalciuria, could interface with key enzymes of intermediatry metabolism, such as Na-K-ATPase of cell membranes causing cellular death[19]. Precipitation of Ca salts within the damaged interstitial tissues and tubular epithelial cells is a common finding in the kidneys of patients with renal stones. Whilst this lesion is almost invariably present in stone formers, it is not uncommon in the non-stone former as well. Cellular injury associated with this lesion together with a secondary inflammatory response could be the challenging event stimulating the synthesis and release of prosta-glandins, as indeed, they are known to be important mediators of inflammation in other tissues. Therefore, this microscopic "anatomical" lesion could, by its ability to trigger prostaglandin synthesis, be acting as a mechanism for the abnormal urinary profile as well as providing the stimulus to 1α-hydroxylase activity in the kidney as has recently been suggested[20].

REFERENCES

1. C. Y. C. Pak, J. Clin. Invest. 48:1914 (1969).
2. S. Bisaz, R. Felix, W. F. Neumann, and H. Fleisch, Min. Electrol. Metab. 1:74 (1978).
3. B. Finlayson, Kidney Int. 13:344 (1978).
4. R. J. Carr, Br. J. Urol. 26:105 (1954).
5. R. S. Malek and W. H. Boyce, J. Urol. 109:551 (1973).
6. E. L. Prien, J. Urol. 114:500 (1975).
7. C. K. Anderson, in:"Urinary Calculous Disease", J. E. A. Wickham, ed., Churchill Livingstone, London (1979).
8. A. C. Buck, C. J. Lote, and W. F. Sampson, J. Urol. 129:429 (1983).
9. P. W. Reed, Fed. Proc. 36:673 (1977).
10. B. J. Northover, Br. J. Pharmacol. 48:496 (1973).
11. E. R. J. Sudmann and P. F. Marton, Acta Orthop. Scand. 46:588 (1976).
12. S. Dekel and M. J. O. Francis, J. Bone Jt. Surg. 63B:173 (1981).
13. J. Fourman, Br. J. Exp. Pathol. 40:464 (1959).
14. A. Kalisker and D. C. Dyer, Europ. J. Pharmacol. 19:305 (1972).
15. P. A. Craven, R. Briggs, and F. R. DeRubertis, J. Clin. Invest. 65:529 (1980).
16. D. Gosh and J. Dutta, J. Biosci. 4:7 (1982).
17. T. V. Zenser and B. B. Davis, Am. J. Physiol. 235:F213 (1978).
18. P. A. Craven, R. K. Studer, and F. R. DeRubertis, J. Lab. Clin. Med. 99:806 (1982).
19. F. J. Epstein and R. Whittam, Biochem. J. 99:232 (1966).
20. J. D. Wark, R. G. Larkins, J. A. Eisman, and K. R. Wilson, Clin. Sci. 61:53 (1981).

CLINICAL MANIPULATION OF URINARY GAGS -

A NEW METHOD OF STONE PREVENTION (?)

R. W. Norman, D. S. Scurr, W. G. Robertson, and
M. Peacock

MRC Mineral Metabolism Unit, The General Infirmary
Leeds LS1 3EX, U.K.

INTRODUCTION

Urinary polyanions are known to be potent inhibitors of calcium oxalate (CaOx) crystal growth and agglomeration[1-3]. These include glycosaminoglycans, ribonucleic acid and non-polymerised Tamm-Horsfall mucoprotein [2-4]. The excretion of these macromolecules tends to be lower in the urine of recurrent CaOx stone-formers than in the urine of normal subjects[4]. Unfortunately, it has not so far been possible to increase this fraction in urine with a view to preventing the recurrence of CaOx stones.

Sodium pentosan polysulphate (SPP) (mol.wt. 5000 daltons) is a semi-synthetic polyanionic analogue of heparin and is partially excreted in urine following oral administration. If the excreted products are sufficiently large and active, significant inhibition of CaOx crystallization should occur. This could constitute a potential new form of therapy for the prevention of recurrent CaOx stone disease.

The purpose of this study was to quantitate the inhibitory activity of SPP in vitro, to study the mechanism of this inhibition and to measure changes in the urinary zeta potential and risk factors following oral administration.

METHODS

The inhibitory activity of increasing concentrations of SPP on the crystal growth rate, the degree of agglomeration of

581

crystals and the amount of CaOx precipitated were measured in a continuous crystallizer at urinary levels of CaOx superaturation[5]. The zeta potential produced by the SPP on the surface of CaOx crystals was measured in 10% urine using a Zeta Meter[4].

In a separate study, SPP (10 mg/kg) was fed by oral gavage daily for 13 days to 4 pigmented rats of the PVG strain. The animals were housed in individual all-glass metabolism cages suitable for the separate collection of urine and faeces. The collection vessels were surrounded with carbon dioxide. Twenty-four-hour urine collections were made on days 1 and 13 and were analysed for changes in the zeta potential.

Finally, 24-h urine samples were collected in sterile containers without preservative from 6 normal male volunteers aged

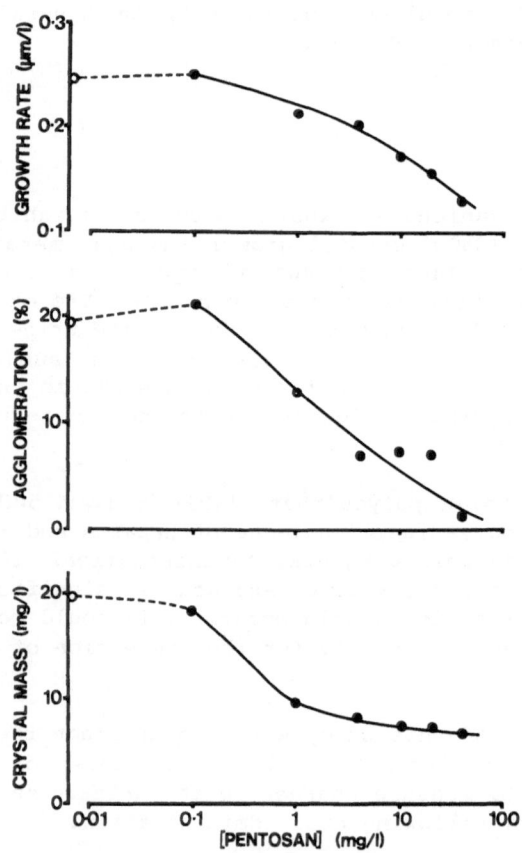

Fig. 1   Effects of SPP on the rate of crystal growth, the degree of agglomeration and the mass of CaOx crystals precipitated using a continuous crystallizer.

24-46 (mean 34 years) before SPP, after a single oral bolus of SPP
(500 mg) and after 10 days of oral SPP (250 mg twice daily). Each
specimen was analysed for volume, pH, calcium, sodium, uric acid,
alcian blue precipitable polyanions and creatinine by methods
previously described[5]. Oxalate and sulphate were measured by
ion-chromatography[6]. The zeta potential was measured as above.

RESULTS

     At lower molar concentrations, SPP clearly decreased the
crystal growth rate, the degree of agglomeration of crystals and
the amount of CaOx precipitated in vitro (Fig. 1). These
inhibitory effects can be largely explained by adsorption of SPP
on the CaOx crystal surface as indicated by the increase in the
negative zeta potential produced on the crystal surface (Fig. 2).

     The animal study showed an increase in the inhibitory
activity of urine as reflected by an increase in the negative zeta
potential from -15.5 + 0.9 mV (mean + SEM) to -20.5 + 0.9 mV.

     The human study confirmed a significant increase in the
negative zeta potential from -18.4 + 0.8 mV to 20.0 + 0.5 mV
(P<0.02) after the oral bolus and from -18.1 + 0.7 mV to -20.4 +
0.5 mV (P<0.05) after the 10-day course. There was also a
significant decrease in the 24-h urinary oxalate from 0.396 + 0.029
mmol to 0.339 + 0.030 mmol (P<0.05) after the chronic load. None of
the other measured urinary constituents was changed.

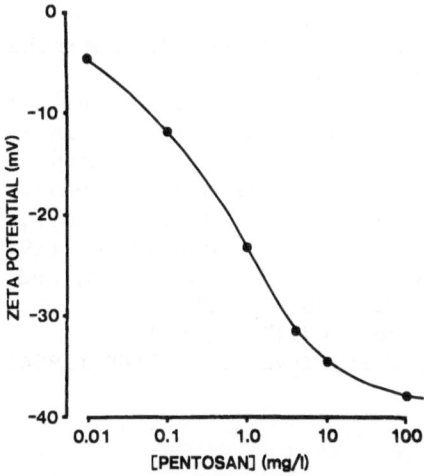

Fig. 2   Effect of SPP on the zeta potential on the surface of
          CaOx crystals.

DISCUSSION

While it is accepted that the two main chemical factors which determine the risk of forming calcium oxalate stones are the degree of supersaturation and the level of protective inhibitory activity against crystallization, most clinicians emphasize the reduction of supersaturation in their treatment protocols. Few attempts have been made to increase the macromolecular inhibitory activity[7,8].

SPP is a highly charged glycosaminoglycan-like substance which actively inhibits CaOx crystallization in vitro. Furthermore the inhibitory activity of urine as measured by the zeta potential increases following oral administration in vivo. An unexpected finding was a decrease in the 24-h urinary excretion of oxalate. This combination of effects may offer a novel approach to the prevention of CaOx stones.

ACKNOWLEDGEMENTS

The authors wish to thank Hazelton Laboratories, Harrogate, UK, who assisted with the animal studies. R. W. Norman was funded by the Medical Research Council of Canada.

REFERENCES

1. W. G. Robertson, M. Peacock, and B. E. C. Nordin, Clin. Chim. Acta 43:31 (1973).
2. W. G. Robertson, D. S. Scurr, and C. M. Bridge, J. Crystal Growth 53:182 (1981).
3. R. L. Ryall, R. M. Harnett, and V. R. Marshall, Clin. Chim. Acta 112:349 (1981).
4. W. G. Robertson, A. B. Latif, D. S. Scurr, A. M. Caswell, G. W. Drach, and A. D. Randolph, in:"Urinary Stone", R. Ryall, J. G. Brockis, V. Marshall, and B. Finlayson, eds., Churchill Livingstone, Melbourne (1984).
5. W. G. Robertson, M. Peacock, P. J. Heyburn, D. H. Marshall, and P. B. Clark, Br. J. Urol. 50:449 (1978).
6. W. G. Robertson, D. S. Scurr, A. Smith, and R. L. Orwell, Clin. Chim. Acta 126:91 (1982).
7. A. J. Butt, J. Urol. 67:450 (1952).
8. G. P. Kerby, J. Clin. Invest. 33:1168 (1954).

TREATMENT OF HYPEROXALURIA IN PATIENTS WITH JEJUNOILEAL BYPASS:

EFFECTS OF CALCIUM, ALUMINUM, MAGNESIUM AND CHOLESTYRAMINE

B. Nordenvall, L. Backman, L. Larsson, and
H.-G. Tiselius

Dept. of Surgery, Karolinska Institute at Danderyd
Hospital, Stockholm and Dept. of Clinical
Chemistry and Dept. of Urology, University Hospital
Linköping, Sweden

INTRODUCTION

Hyperoxaluria and calcium oxalate stones are common following intestinal resection[1] and jejunoileal bypass operations[2,3]. A high intestinal absorption of oxalate appears to be responsible for the hyperoxaluria[4,5]. Diets low in oxalate[5] and fat[4] have been recommended to reduce oxalate excretion, but may be difficult to adhere to because of unpalatability[6]. Oral administration of calcium[7], aluminium[6], magnesium[8] and cholestyramine[9] have been reported to decrease oxalate excretion in patients with enteric hyperoxaluria, but none of these studies was performed under ambulatory conditions. This study describes the effects of these treatments on the urinary composition of patients with hyperoxaluria after jejunoileal bypass operation under out-patient conditions.

MATERIALS AND METHODS

Seven patients with hyperoxaluria (3 women and 4 men, age 25 to 54 years) were investigated. They had been operated on with an end-to-end jejunoileostomy with ileocaecostomy because of obesity[10] 3 to 6 years prior to the study. The present body weights were stable at 58 to 120 kg; the post-operative weight loss was 40 to 63 kg. All were studied as out-patients. They were instructed to take the substances with meals and to follow their usual diet.

Study 1 was performed during two 7-day periods. During the first period the patients were given 38 mmol Ca/day (1.5 g) as Ca gluconate and Ca lactate in 3 divided doses, and during the second period 113 mmol of Ca/day (4.5 g) in 3 divided doses.

The regimen in Study 2 was as follows: (a) Al dihydroxide, $Al(OH)_2NaCO_3$ was given in doses of 0.8 g five times daily (28 mmol Al/day); (b) Mg oxide was given in doses of 0.4 g twice daily (20 mmol Mg per day); (c) Cholestyramine was given in doses of 4 g four times daily. Each 7-day regimen was followed by a free interval of 7 days. Serum and urine samples were collected before the study and at the end of each test period.

Urine samples were collected during two consecutive 24-h periods in plastic bottles, one containing 90 mmol HCl and the other without any additive. The acidified sample was analysed for oxalate[11], Ca[12] and Mg[13] and the other for citrate[14]. Creatinine was analyzed in both samples by the alkaline picrate method. All variables were related to creatinine excretion[15]. The reference limit in mmol/mol creatinine was for oxalate < 30, Ca < 600, Mg < 200 and for citrate < 150 mmol/mol creatinine.

Table 1. Urinary Excretion (Median) in 7 Patients with Jejunoileal Bypass during Administration of Calcium.

Excretion (mmol/mol Cr)	Control	Calcium Supplement	
		38 mmol	113 mmol
Oxalate	68	80**	65
Calcium	178	182	290**
Magnesium	120	232*	150
Citrate	68	52	183*
Ca/Mg ratio	1.5	1.0*	2.0*
Inhibition index	0.58	0.55	0.55

*$p < 0.05$; **$p < 0.01$.

Table 2. Urinary Excretion (Median) in 7 Patients with Jejunoileal Bypass during Treatment.

Excretion (mmol/mol Cr)	Control	Aluminium	Magnesium	Chole-styramine
Oxalate	68	70	72	80*
Calcium	178	263**	306	126
Magnesium	120	224**	292*	206
Citrate	68	64	44	28*
Ca/Mg ratio	1.5	1.5	1.2*	1.6
Inhibition index	0.58	0.58	0.58	0.59

*$p < 0.05$; **$p < 0.01$.

RESULTS

Administration of 113 mmol Ca resulted in a significant rise in serum Ca from 2.25 + 0.03 mmol/l (mean + SEM) to 2.34 + 0.02,P ‹0.001) and a concomitant drop in serum P from 1.02 + 0.10 mmol/l to 0.81 + 0.05 (P‹0.05). Serum Mg and creatinine were not altered by either of the two Ca doses. Urinary oxalate was significantly increased during administration of 38 mmol Ca daily, but not with the higher dose of 113 mmol (Table 1). The Ca/Mg ratio was decreased with the lower dose of Ca mainly attributable to the higher excretion of Mg (Table 1). The higher Ca dose increased urinary excretion of Ca and the Ca/Mg ratio (Table 1). Citrate excretion was significantly increased during administration of 113 mmol Ca. Urinary creatinine did not change during the study.

Al had no significant effects on serum Ca, P, Mg or creatinine. The urinary excretion of oxalate was not decreased, but both Ca and Mg excretion increased significantly (Table 2) and the Ca/Mg ratio remained at the pre-treatment level. Urinary citrate was unaffected. Mg had no significant effects on serum Ca, P, Mg, or creatinine. No effect was observed on the urinary excretion of oxalate or citrate but urinary Mg was significantly increased and the Ca/Mg ratio decreased (Table 2). Cholestyramine had no significant effects on serum Ca, P, Mg or creatinine, but significantly increased urinary oxalate excretion. Urinary Ca, Mg and the Ca/Mg ratio were unaffected but citrate excretion was significantly increased (Table 2).

DISCUSSION

The endogenous production of oxalate appears to be normal in patients with hyperoxaluria following jejunoileal bypass[16]. In order to decrease the urinary excretion of oxalate it is necessary to influence the intestinal absorption of oxalate, either by reducing the amount of free oxalate in the intestinal lumen[17], or with a high intake of Ca[7]. Our results do not support these observations, for reasons not fully understood. In the present study we have not administered Ca in doses higher than 113 mmol. As it was, administration of 113 mmol of Ca increased urinary Ca and this might add to the overall risk of stone formation, an effect reported previously by other authors[7].

Administration of Al antacids, by forming complexes with oxalate, has been suggested as an alternative treatment for enteric hyperoxaluria[6]. In the present study we found no effect on urinary oxalate after administration of 28 mmol of Al. Possibly the Al was bound to phosphate. An increased urinary excretion of Ca as a result of phosphate depletion following Al administration[18] might explain the observed increased urinary Ca in these patients.

Using 25 mmol Mg supplements, Barilla et al[8] reported decreased oxalate excretion in a metabolic ward study. We obtained no effect with a daily dose of 20 mmol Mg oxide, in agreement with the findings of Gregory et al[3].

Cholestyramine might influence oxalate absorption in two ways. Firstly, it can bind oxalate; secondly, the increased absorption of oxalate brought about by bile salts may be counteracted by the formation of bile salt-cholestyramine complexes. In contrast, we found an increased urinary oxalate excretion during administration of 16 g of cholestyramine/day. The reason for this is not clear.

There is an increased risk for recurrent stone formation, oxalate deposits and renal failure attributable to hyperoxaluria in patients with jejunoileal bypass[19]. In our hands, neither Ca, Al, Mg nor cholestyramine reduced oxalate excretion.

REFERENCES

1. J. W. Dobbins and H. J. Binder, in:"Progress in Gastroenterology", Vol. 3. G. B. J. Glass, ed., Grune and Stratton, New York (1977).
2. L. Backman, B. Nordenvall, and D. Hallberg, Urol. Res. 7:189 (1979).
3. J. Gregory, K. Park, and H. Schoenberg, J. Urol. 117:631 (1977).
4. H. Andersson and R. Jagenburg, Gut 15:360 (1974).
5. D. L. Earnest, G. Johnson, H. E. Williams, and W. Admirand, Gastroenterology 66:1114 (1974).
6. D. L. Earnest, H. E. Williams, and W. H. Admirand, Trans. Assoc. Am. Physcns. 88:224 (1975).
7. J. Q. Stauffer, Dig. Dis. 22:921 (1977).
8. D. E. Barilla, C. Notz, D. Kennedy, and C. Y. C. Pak, Am. J. Med. 64:579 (1978).
9. J. Q. Stauffer, M. H. Humphreys, and G. J. Wie, Ann. Int. Med. 79:383 (1973).
10. M. Buchwald and R. L. Varco, Surgery 70:62 (1971).
11. H.-G. Tiselius, Invest. Urol. 15:5 (1977).
12. D. L. Trudeau and E. F. Freier, Clin. Chim. 13:101 (1967).
13. J. L. Hansen and E. F. Freier, Am. J. Med. Tech. 33:158 (1967).
14. B. W. Greenbaum and N. Pace, Microchem. J. 15:673 (1970).
15. H.-G. Tiselius, L. E. Almgard, L. Larsson, and B. Sorbo, Eur. Urol. 4:241 (1978).
16. B. Nordenvall, L. Backman, and L. Larsson, Scand. J. Gastroenterol. 16:395 (1981).
17. M. J. Binder, Gastroenterology 67:441 (1974).
18. M. Lotz, E. Zisman, and F. C. Bartter, New Engl. J. Med. 278:409 (1968).
19. S. Das, B. Joseph, and A. Dick, J. Urol. 121:506 (1979).

RELATIVE MERIT OF VARIOUS NONSURGICAL TREATMENTS OF

INFECTION STONES IN DOGS

D. F. Senior, W. C. Thomas Jr., J. M. Gaskin,
and B. Finlayson

Dept. of Medical Sciences, College of Veterinary
Medicine, University of Florida, Gainesville
Florida 32611, U.S.A.

INTRODUCTION

Dietary management, urease inhibition and antibiotic treatment can control growth and recurrence of infection stones. Although urease inhibition and antibiotic treatment have also induced stone dissolution in a few patients, complete dissolution by these means is not common. Recently a stone dissolution (S/D) diet (Table 1) combined with antibiotic treatment has been shown to induce rapid dissolution of experimental and spontaneous infection stones in the dog[1]. Flurofamide is a novel potent urease inhibitor, excreted in the active form in the urine[2]. We compared the relative super-saturation of struvite (RSS) in urine when the S/D diet, flurofamide, and antibiotic treatment, alone or in combination, were given to dogs with experimental infection stone disease.

MATERIALS AND METHODS

Large fragments of a struvite stone were implanted into the bladder of 6 female mongrel dogs (20 kg body wt) by cystotomy. Before implantation the stone fragments were autoclaved and soaked for 2 h in a broth culture of urease-positive Staphylococcus aureus.

The dogs were treated with each of the following dissolution strategies for 14 days: (i) normal control diet; (ii) S/D diet; (iii) control diet plus flurofamide (5 mg/kg p.o. t.i.d.); (iv) S/D diet plus flurofamide; (v) control diet plus antibiotic (amoxicillin with clavulanic acid (4:1) at 10 mg/kg p.o. b.i.d. based on amoxicillin content); (vi) S/D diet plus antibiotic; (vii) S/D diet plus antibiotic plus flurofamide. Water intake was ad libitum.

589

Table 1. Composition of S/D Diet

Nutrient	Analysis (% as fed)	Daily Intake (g/kg/day)
Protein	1.5	0.67
Fat	6.4	2.87
Carbohydrate (NFE)	19.7	8.8
Fiber	0.7	0.3
Ash	1.3	0.58
Calcium	0.06	0.027
Phosphorus	0.04	0.018
Magnesium	0.04	0.002
Sodium	0.35	0.15
Energy	1.54 (Kcal/g)	69 (Kcal/kg/day)

During each treatment period, radiographic and bacteriological persistence of the infection stone model was verified.

Urine was collected into dry ice-chilled containers for 48 h, then rapidly thawed in a microwave oven. After pH measurement, the urine was acidified to pH = 1 with concentrated HCl, allowed to stand for 30 min, mixed, and frozen until analysed for ammonium, magnesium, phosphate, sulfate, calcium, oxalate, citrate, sodium, and potassium. The computer program EQUIL was used to estimate the relative supersaturation (RSS) in urine[3]. Statistical analysis was performed using Student's t-test.

RESULTS

The S/D diet alone reduced urinary RSS to below saturation and was more effective than both control diet plus flurofamide ($P < 0.005$) and control diet plus antibiotic ($P < 0.02$) (Table 2). Of the combination treatments, the S/D diet plus flurofamide reduced urinary RSS more than the S/D diet plus antibiotic ($P < 0.02$). The

Table 2. Relative Supersaturation of Urine for Struvite and Urinary pH (n=5). F = flurofamide; AB = antibiotic.

	RSS mean	SD	pH mean	SD
Control diet	16.3	± 11.4	7.67	± 0.25
S/D diet	0.519	± 0.57	6.67	± 0.31
Control diet + F	4.12	± 2.02	6.77	± 0.36
S/D + F	0.032	± 0.022	5.80	± 0.16
Control diet + AB	3.64	± 2.22	6.88	± 0.16
S/D diet + AB	0.215	± 0.144	6.40	± 0.24
S/D diet + AB + F	0.039	± 0.049	5.94	± 0.29

590

Table 3. Urinary Composition (n=5). F = flurofamide; AB = antibiotic.

	Mg^{2+} (μg/ml)		NH_4^+ (mg/ml)		PO_4^{3-} (μg/ml)	
	mean	SD	Mean	SD	Mean	SD
Control diet	47.6 $\pm$ 13.5		1.06 $\pm$ 0.43		1140 $\pm$ 495	
S/D diet	29.3 $\pm$ 7.9		0.55 $\pm$ 0.22		414 $\pm$ 163	
Control diet + F	152.2 $\pm$ 44.7		0.77 $\pm$ 0.31		1558 $\pm$ 472	
S/D diet + F	68.9 $\pm$ 21.8		0.51 $\pm$ 0.14		539 $\pm$ 238	
Control diet + AB	144 $\pm$ 19.7		0.62 $\pm$ 0.08		1526 $\pm$ 180	
S/D diet + AB	45 $\pm$ 20.1		0.54 $\pm$ 0.15		547 $\pm$ 106	
S/D diet + AB + F	30.7 $\pm$ 10.1		0.50 $\pm$ 0.14		410 $\pm$ 121	

Table 4. Urea: Serum Levels, Daily Output, Urinary Concentration
(mean $\pm$ SD). F = Flurofamide; AB = antibiotic.

	Serum Urea (mg/dl)	Daily Output (mmol)	Urinary (mmol)
Control diet	20.4 $\pm$ 2.1	52.2 $\pm$ 4.2	205 $\pm$ 57
S/D diet	6.2 $\pm$ 1.3	24.2 $\pm$ 7.6	27 $\pm$ 5
Control diet + F	18.2 $\pm$ 2.6	93.2 $\pm$ 20.4	250 $\pm$ 42
S/D diet + F	8.2 $\pm$ 1.5	42.8 $\pm$ 10.1	52 $\pm$ 6
Control diet + AB	21.2 $\pm$ 4.3	105.6 $\pm$ 24.2	279 $\pm$ 55
S/D diet + AB	6.6 $\pm$ 0.9	30.9 $\pm$ 5.7	47 $\pm$ 6
S/D diet + AB + F	5.8 $\pm$ 0.8	14.6 $\pm$ 5.3	22 $\pm$ 11

addition of antibiotic to the S/D diet plus flurofamide did not
further reduce urinary RSS. Each of the strategies had a similar
effect in decreasing urinary pH. Of the combination strategies, the
S/D diet plus flurofamide produced a lower urinary pH than did the
S/D diet plus antibiotic ($P < 0.01$), and the S/D diet plus flurofamide
plus antibiotic was not more effective than was the S/D diet plus
flurofamide (Table 2). Urinary NH_4^+ was reduced by all strategies
to a similar extent. When the S/D diet was fed, urinary Mg^{2+}
tended to be lower. While the dogs received the S/D diet, urinary
PO_4^3 was reduced by 60% (Table 3). During S/D diet feeding, sodium
output was increased, citrate output was reduced, and calcium,
oxalate, potassium, and sulphate outputs were unchanged. However,
the urinary concentrations of all constituents were lower on the S/D
diet because urine volume was doubled. Serum and urine urea were
reduced on the S/D diet (Table 4).

DISCUSSION

Theoretically, the RSS of urine determines the rate of growth
or dissolution of struvite stones. Strategies that reduce the RSS

would be expected to cause the fastest rate of stone dissolution. The S/D diet was the only single strategy to reduce RSS to less than 1. By reducing phosphate intake, the Shorr regimen has proved effective in the control of infection stones in man. The S/D diet reduces phosphate and magnesium excretion and, in addition, reduces RSS by increasing urine volume. When the S/D diet was supplemented with flurofamide or antibiotic, RSS was further reduced; flurofamide appeared to have the greatest additive effect. The addition of antibiotic to the S/D diet plus flurofamide did not further reduce urinary RSS. This suggests that direct urease inhibition may be more effective than antibiotic treatment in stone dissolution and that, if effective urease inhibition is achieved, antibiotic treatment may not further enhance the rate of stone dissolution.

Urinary ammonium concentration and excretion were reduced to a similar extent by all strategies, but the reduction was not great. The S. aureus used in this study was not a potent producer of urease, because the urinary pH on the control diet was 7.67. Some ammonium may have been lost from urine during the freeze-thaw process before acidification. The reason for the reduced ammonium excretion in dogs fed the S/D diet is not clear. Urinary urea was markedly reduced, but not low enough to inhibit urease activity based on the known Michaelis constant for bacterial ureases[4]. However, the K_M value for the urease produced by the S. aureus in this study is not known. Both phosphate and urea excretion were lower in the second of two consecutive S/D diet feeding strategies. The 14-day duration of each strategy may have been too short for proper equilibration because the diets were so dissimilar.

REFERENCES

1. C. A. Osborne, S. U. Abdullahi, J. R. Leissinger, D. J. Polzin, N. E. Hauer, J. S. Klausner, R. M. Hardy, A. B. Kuzma, and C. J. Gidlund, Minn. Vet. 22:14(1982).
2. D. E. Millner, J. A. Anderson, M. E. Appler, C. E. Benjamin, J. G. Edwards, D. T. Humphrey, and E. M. Shearer, J. Urol. 127:346 (1982).
3. B. Finlayson, in:"Calcium Metabolism in Renal Failure and Nephrolithiasis", D. S. David, ed., Wiley, New York(1977).
4. I. J. Rosenstein, J. M. Hamilton-Miller, and W. Brumfitt, Infect. Immun. 32:32 (1981).

EFFICACY AND SAFETY OF NON-STEROIDAL ANTI-INFLAMMATORY DRUGS IN URETERAL COLIC: A DOUBLE-BLIND CONTROLLED TRIAL

G. Comeri, G. P. Radice, R. Duvia, V. Manganini,
and G. Monza

Dept. of Urology, St. Anna Hospital
Como, and Medical Dept., Ciba-Geigy, Origgio, Italy

INTRODUCTION

The management of pain from ureteric colic (UC) has depended until now upon antispasmodic agents (AA) and, if ineffective, opiates. However, the high failure rate with AA and the risk attached to opiates makes this approach inadvisable. It has recently been proposed that UC be treated with indomethacin[1], a non-steroidal anti-inflammatory drug (NSAID), which inhibits PG biosynthesis thereby counteracting the effects of PGE_2 on ureteric wall tone and glomerular filtration rate, both of which increase the pressure above the stone and evoke pain[2,3].

METHODS

In this randomized, double-blind (DB), between-patient trial, the efficacy and toleration of intramuscular injection of 2 potent NSAIDs, diclofenac (D) 75 mg/3 ml and indomethacin (I) 50 mg, were compared with the most used preparation in Italy, a combination (C) of noramidopyrine (1 g) + pitofenon (0.4 mg) + fenpiverine (0.04 mg). For pain assessment, a 100 mm analogue chromatic continuous scale (ACCS) was used, because of its higher sensitivity in comparison with VAS[4]. Patients were followed for at least 2 days. The diagnosis was confirmed by urine analysis, i.v. pyelogram or voiding of a calculus. Patients allergic to salicylate or pregnant were excluded. Pain intensity was measured with ACCS at the start of the study and 30, 60, 120, 180, 240 and 300 min after treatment. Patients received i.m. injection of D, I or C, according to a randomization list. If the pain intensity did not decrease by 50% within 60 min, the patient received a second injection of the same

593

drug, always in DB manner.   If a patient, after the second
administration, did not experience a decrease of pain intensity, he
was considered to be a treatment failure.   Statistical analysis was
performed either with parametric or non-parametric tests, according
to the distribution and the quality of data.

RESULTS

Forty-six patients were given D, 49 I and 49 C, the 3 treatment
groups being homogeneous for age, sex, weight, height, severity and
duration of initial pain (Table 1).   Thirty-six patients on D, 33
on I and 28 on C needed a single injection to obtain complete relief
of pain, while 7, 10 and 15 patients respectively required a second
administration.   Three patients on D, 6 on I and 6 on C were
treatment failures.   The comparison between the number of
administrations within the 3 treatment groups showed a significant
smaller consumption on D compared with C (P<0.05), while no

Table 1. Basal Data on Patients in Various Treatment Groups
          (mean $\pm$ SD).

Parameter	Diclofenac	Indomethacin	Combination	P
Age (yr)	46.3 $\pm$ 15.73	43.6 $\pm$ 15.14	45.7 $\pm$ 15.43	n.s.
Weight (kg)	72.3 $\pm$ 12.87	68.5 $\pm$ 12.23	67.6 $\pm$ 13.20	n.s.
Height (cm)	166.9 $\pm$ 8.15	166.8 $\pm$ 7.11	167.8 $\pm$ 7.50	n.s.
Duration of pain (h)	5.8 $\pm$ 5.03	4.9 $\pm$ 4.5	5.2 $\pm$ 47	n.s.
Initial pain (ACCS, mm)	81.1 $\pm$ 11.37	83.7 $\pm$ 15.72	84.2 $\pm$ 12.64	n.s.

Table 2. Mean Pain Decrease (ACCS) within 30 min (Basal Values
          minus Values at 30 min).

Treatment	Pain Decrease (Basal-30 min)		n	P
	Mean	95% confidence limits		(Tukey test)
Diclofenac	67.7	76.20 59.19	46	
Indomethacin	63.8	71.67 55.98	49	<0.01 <0.01
Combination form	52.7	59.79 45.60	49	<0.01

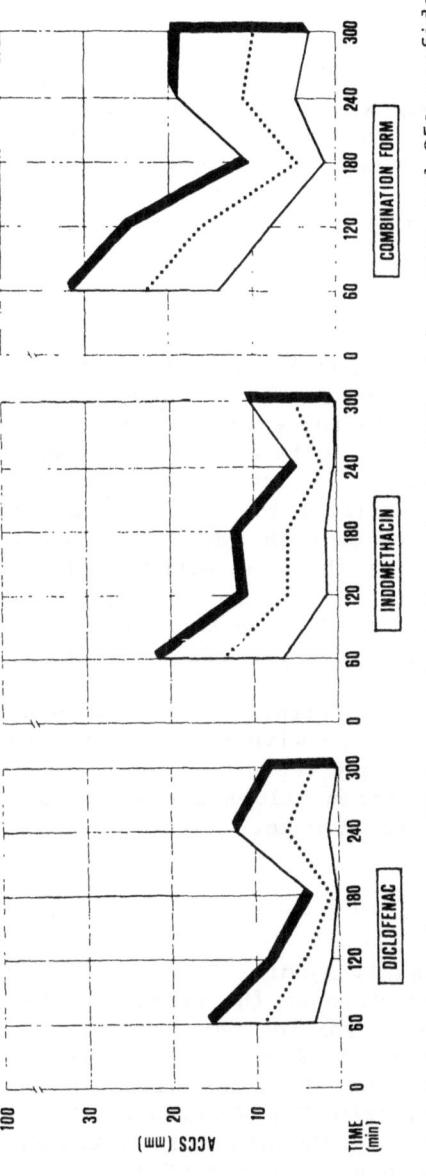

Fig. 1. Pain intensity at different times (60 min to 300 min) : mean and 95% confidence
limits are shown for each treatment group.

difference was detected between I and C. Complete relief of pain at 30 min (ACCS = 0) was obtained in 67% (31/46) of patients on D, 53% (26/49) of pts on I and 35% (17/49) of pts on C (P<0.01). The analysis of variance of pain decrease within 30 min showed a significant difference between-treatments (P<0.05). In addition, by the Tukey test both D and I proved to be clearly superior to C (P<0.01) (Table 2).

Within 1 h, 81%, 67% and 49% of patients, respectively, were free of pain (P<0.01, χ^2 test). The analysis of variance (F-test) of pain intensity at the different times, showed a significant difference (P<0.01) between-treatment and between-time (Fig. 1).

No side-effects from any of the treatments were reported.

DISCUSSION

Both indomethacin and diclofenac confirmed a quick onset of action with a high potency, clearly superior to both placebo and narcotic-spasmolitic in releaving UC[1,5,6]. In this trial D and I showed practically equal efficacy, with a trend in favour of D, in respect to both rapidity of action and number of administrations required. On the contrary, the antispasmodic component of C did not have any advantage over the NSAID component, which is probably the one responsible for the weak activity of this association. Despite the tradition of combining an analgesic with an antispasmodic agent, and despite the evidence that this drug relaxes smooth muscle, it does not seem clinically beneficial.

Intramuscular administration slightly reduces the percentage of patients on I free of pain within 30 min (53% in this study compared with about 70% previously reported when administered i.v.[1]). On the other hand, i.m. injection allows nurses to use these drugs for a first management of UC at home.

REFERENCES

1. D. Holmund and S. G. Sjödin, J. Urol. 120:676 (1978).
2. F. Kiil, "The Function of the Ureter and Renal Pelvis", W. B. Saunders, Philadelphia (1957).
3. E. W. Horton, Physiol. Rev. 49:122 (1969).
4. E. Grossi, C. Borghi, E. L. Cerchiari, T. della Puppa, and B. Francucci, Clin. Exp. Rheumatol. 1:337 (1983).
5. S. O. A. Lundstam, K. H. Leissner, L. A. Wahlander, and J. G. Kral, Lancet 1:1096 (1982).
6. A. Vignoni, A. Fierro, G. Moreschini, M. Cau, A. Agostino, E. Daniele, G. Toti, and E. Grossi, J. Int. Med. Res. 11:303 (1983).

METHODS AND RESULTS OF CONSERVATIVE EXPULSION OF URINARY CALCULI

D. Bach, A. Hesse, W. Vahlensieck, J. Joost,
H. D. Lehmann, G. Wegner

Depts. of Urology, Ulm Federal Army Hospital, Ulm
Bonn University Medical School, Bonn, Holweide
Municipal Hospital, Cologne, F.R.G. and Innsbruck
University Medical School, Innsbruck, Austria

INTRODUCTION

Consideration of the pathophysiology of the transit of a urinary calculus is a prerequisite to achieve successful expulsion of the urinary calculus by medication. Stone incarceration leads to local stretching and ischemia of the ureteral wall. This elicits acute pain and colic. If urinary stasis occurs, then there is additional pain from renal congestion. In the context of the viscero-visceral reflex or of the axonal reflex and the central counter-regulation via the sympathetic nervous system, the frequency of peristaltic contractions rises with simultaneous reduction of their amplitude[1]. If the urinary stasis is maintained because of incarceration of the calculus, especially from the stone-fixing mucosal edema that occurs immediately, then only frequent wave movements can be discerned with low, ineffective amplitude. The effective filtration pressure for urinary calculus expulsion is also lacking. Only a relief of pressure will restart ureteral peristalsis. The intestinal paresis often observed as a result of ureteral colic also results from this sympathicotonic reaction.

Initially, an effective spasmoanalgesic (e.g. pentazocine or novamine sulfone) is administered intravenously to interrupt the colic. If the acute phase of colic has subsided and spontaneous passage of the calculus appears possible, further therapeutic measures are designed to expel the concrement. To facilitate the transit of the stone, regular administration of spasmoanalgesics at intervals is to be recommended, i.e. a "continuous spasmoanalgesia"[2]. The spontaneous passage of the calculus can be accelerated by adjuvant measures including application of heat, edema treatment, enhancement of diuresis and movement therapy. The use of the various possible drugs in "continuous spasmoanalgesia" must be oriented to the constitution and tolerance of the patient. For the same effectiveness, the preparation with the least side-effects and costs is to be preferred. Taking these aspects into account, we carried out a multicenter, prospective, randomized therapeutic study to compare effectiveness of classical continuous spasmoanalgesia with pyrazolone-containing drugs with that achieved by administration of the phytotherapeutic, Urol[R] (Table 1).

Table 1. Composition and Effects of Urol[R] (Hoyer, D-4040 Neuss, F.R.G.)

Substance	Amount/capsule	Effect
Extr.Rad.Rubiae tinct spir (Root of Rubia tinctorum)	67.500 mg	Litholytic
Extr.Sem.Ammeos visnagae spir. (Bishop's weed)	37.875 mg	Myotropic-spasmolytic
Extr.Herb.Virgaurea spir. (Goldenrod)	71.000 mg	Myotropic-spasmolytic, diuretic
Extr.Rad.Taraxaci or herb.spir. (Dandelion)	73.625 mg	Diuretic
Aescin (Isolated from horsechestnut)	15.000 mg	Antiedematous
Total	265.000 mg	

Table 2. Average Ureteral Calculus Transit Times in Relation to the Form of Therapy. (A distinction was made between a transit time (beginning of therapy up to freedom from stone in controls) which can be precisely determined is to be distinguished from the calculated transit time.)

Form of Therapy	n	Average Transit (days)	Transit Time (determined precisely)		Unnoticed Stone Passage (calculated transit time)	
			n	average transit time (days)	n	average transit time (days)
Spasmoanalgesia (Group I)	47	18.3	25	16.3	22	20.3
Urol[R] (Group II)	50	17.1	20	13.3	30	20.9

MATERIALS AND METHODS

Over a period of 18 months, 111 patients with calcium-containing ureteral calculi capable of spontaneous passage were included in the study. In accordance with a randomization plan, 55 patients were treated with the amidopyrine derivative Novalgin[R] (30 drops t.i.d.) and Baralgin[R] (1 suppository t.i.d.) (Group I) and 56 patients were treated with the phytotherapeutic Urol[R] (2 capsules t.i.d.) alone (Group II) after acute colic had been eliminated by suitable spasmoanalgesics. The treatment was continued until the ureteral concrement was passed spontaneously. If intercurrent colic had to be treated by parenteral application of a spasmoanalgesic, the patient was removed from the study.

RESULTS

In the final evaluation, there were 47 patients in Group I and 50 patients in Group II. Fourteen patients (8 from Group I and 6 from Group II) had to be taken out of the study because the calculus had to be removed instrumentally (n = 5) or surgically (n = 7). Two patients had previously discontinued the therapy for unknown reasons.

In the patients treated with classical spasmoanalgesics (Group I), the ureteral concrement passed spontaneously in 85.5% (47 of 55) of the cases; in the Group II treated with Urol[R] alone, this was possible in 89.3% (50 of 56) of the cases.

If the cases with a calculus transit time which could be determined precisely and those with a calculated transit time (beginning of therapy up to freedom from calculus at check-up) are added, then there were no appreciable differences between the average transit times of Groups I and II (Table 2). If only the cases with a transit time which could be determined precisely are evaluated,

Table 3. Duration of Ureteral Calculus Expulsion in Relation to the Form of Therapy.

Form of Therapy	n	Average Treatment Time (days)				
		1 - 5	6 - 10	11 - 20	21 - 30	31 +
Spasmo-analgesia (Group I)	47	13(27.7%)	11(23.4%)	6(12.8%)	9(19.1%)	8(17%)
Urol[R] (Group II)	50	15(30%)	13(26%)	7(14%)	8(16%)	7(14%)

then the calculus is passed an average of three days earlier in the group treated with Urol[R]. About half of all ureteral concrements passed within the first ten days in the two therapy groups (Table 3). The level of localization of the calculus in the urinary tract in the two groups did not have any influence on the rate of spontaneous passage.

DISCUSSION

Classical continuous spasmoanalgesia has been a constituent of medicative therapy for the expulsion of urinary calculi for decades. In terms of the criterion "nihil nocere", drugs are to be preferred that are effective but at the same time have few side-effects and are cheap. In these terms, we tested Urol[R], a combination preparation consisting of various phytotherapeutically active agents. Spasmolytic effectiveness[3-5], enhancement of diuresis[6] and litholytic efficacy[7] were demonstrated for this preparation. Due to the aescin contained in the preparation, there was a simultaneous flushing out of edema.

The rate of urinary calculus expulsion of 89.3% achieved with application of Urol[R] alone is somewhat superior to that achieved by classical continuous spasmoanalgesia (85.5%). According to the lterature, expulsion rates averaging 81% with a mean transit time of 13.1 days are achieved with Urol[R] [8,9]. Under classical spasmoanalgesia, the expulsion rates were between 36%[10] and 80%[11]. The average transit time with Urol[R] medication alone is more favorable (13.3 days) than under classical continuous spasmoanalgesia (16.3 days). Further advantages of Urol[R] monotherapy are the simple form of application (capsules), the absence of side-effects and lower cost.

REFERENCES

1. G. Rutishauser, "Druck und Dynamik in den oberen Harnwegen", Steinkopff, Darmstadt (1970).
2. W. Vahlensieck, Dtsch. Med. Wschr. 95:529 (1970).
3. J. Westendorf, Fortschr. Urol. Nephrol. 14:13 (1979).
4. J. Westendorf and W. Vahlensieck, Arzneim.-Forsch. 31:40 (1981).
5. J. Westendorf, Therapiewoche 33:936 (1983).
6. K. Bandhauer, Akt. Urol. 1:42 (1970).
7. M. Gebhardt, Forschr. Urol. Nephrol. 14:34 (1979).
8. H. J. Schneider, Fortschr. Urol. Nephrol. 20:406 (1982).
9. H. Ziemer, Dtsch. Med. Wschr. 101:1908 (1976).
10. K. Bandhauer, Akt. Urol. 1:42 (1970).
11. H. Madersbacher, J. Frick, and G. Bartsch, Fortschr. Urol. Nephrol. 5:199 (1975).

SURGICAL TREATMENT

MODERN STRATEGIES IN STONE SURGERY, WITH SPECIAL EMPHASIS

ON PREVENTION OF STONE RECURRENCE

G. Rutishauser and A. N. Egilmez

Division of Urology, Dept. of Surgery, University of
Basle/Kantonsspital, CH-4021 Basle, Switzerland

INTRODUCTION

Some 100 years after the first successful surgical intervention
for kidney stones (by Morris 1880 and Czerny 1880), we can begin to
consider whether the age of open surgery in urinary stone disease is
slowly coming to an end[1]. New promising non-surgical therapeutic
methods, such as the shockwave-stone-disintegration, already provide
an alternative to surgery in some 75% of kidney stone cases. They
significantly reduce the period of hospitalisation and the time lost
from work, with the advantage of complete avoidance of surgically-
induced chronic renal failure[2]. Progress in transurethral stone
manipulation, combined with ureteroscopy and ureteroscopic stone
management[3] and the rapid development and spread of percutaneous
stone treatment since 1977[4], are other serious challenges to open
stone surgery.

There is no doubt that the so-called "non-surgical", non-
invasive or semi-invasive endoscopic techniques are "in" and the
simple pyelo- or ureterolithotomies will probably be "out" some day
in the near future. However, open surgery will retain an important
place in the treatment of complicated kidney stones and we should
not overlook the fact that the past years have also brought rapid
change and much progress in open surgical stone treatment. The
goals have remained the same: complete removal of the stone and all
stone particles at the time of operation; preservation of as much
functional kidney parenchyma as possible; restoration of abnormal
pre-operative renal anatomy (secondary to obstruction); and
correction of all possible abnormalities in the collecting system
which could contribute to recurrent stone formation. These aims
remain the guidelines for the general strategy of stone surgery and

603

we will now discuss some of the latest encouraging improvements
concerning tactical and technical aspects.

WHAT IS THE BEST APPROACH TO THE STONE-BEARING KIDNEY?

The selection of an appropriate approach to the kidney in a
given stone patient requires consideration not only of the general
goals of stone surgery, but also of numerous other factors
concerning the patient's history, general condition and anatomy.
There are 3 main ways to approach the stone-bearing kidney: (i) the
anterior (generally transperitoneal) incision with the patient in a
supine position; (ii) the lateral or flank incision with the patient
in a flexed lateral 70° decubitus; and (iii) the dorso-lateral
incision with the patient in a strictly lateral or slightly prone
90 to 110° position.

The flank approach with its numerous subcostal, costal or
intercostal variations[5] is by far the commonest used for stone
surgery though there are situations which make this position
impossible or undesirable. The posterior dorso-lateral approach
has been favoured in recent years on both sides of the Atlantic[6].
This incision has some important advantages, such as minimal
muscular transsection and consequently minimal post-operative pain.
But even if some authors propose it for almost all stone situations,
others - including ourselves - find that access to the kidney can be
limited. The abdominal transperitoneal approach may be the second
choice in infected cases. It has the disadvantage that because of
the vascular anatomy, the kidney has often to be mobilized
completely to gain access for pyelotomy. Nevertheless, for rare
cases of simultaneous treatment of bilateral nephrolithiasis[7] or
anomalies such as horse-shoe kidneys[8], the anterior approach is -
without question - the best one. The incision can be a midline
longitudinal or a transverse subcostal chevron-type one. As local
and general problems differ from patient to patient, the so-called
"best approach" has to be selected for every case after carefully
analysing and ranking both the patient's and his kidneys' problems
in view of the goal to be attained.

WHAT IS THE BEST WAY TO REMOVE STONES?

Extended pyelolithotomy, popularised by Gil-Vernet[9], allows the
removal of large calculi extending into the major calices. This
operation has become the procedure of choice for all branched
calculi with their main part in the renal pelvis and is generally
the first step in staghorn calculus surgery. In branched stones
that extend into the secondary ramifications of the lower calix
system, the arched Gil-Vernet-type pyelotomy can be continued
posteriorly downwards into the lower pole as a Resnick-type

pyelonephrotomy[10]. As the artery to the inferior renal segment parallels - but does not cross - the infundibulum of the lower calix, it is possible to continue the nephrotomy into the secondary calyces with only minimal risk of arterial damage and bleeding. In most cases, there is no need for arterial clamping and hemostasis is not a problem. Since these procedures give us the possibility of removing even caliceal stones with relative ease, and without sacrificing renal tissue especially in the lower part of the kidney, the question is whether there is still a place for partial nephrectomy in modern stone surgery?

Partial nephrectomy has been used frequently in localised polar stone disease. The procedure was promoted by Semb[11] and it was reasoned that it would also significantly reduce the recurrence rate. Indeed, in a series of papers prior to 1980, the results of partial nephrectomy compared favourably with those of other techniques. If the recurrence rates appeared relatively low, the follow-up time was often very short, sometimes only a few months whereas the average interval for stone recurrence lies somewhere between 5 and 10 years. In recent years, however, Wald et al[12] found a true ipsilateral recurrence rate of 24% after 6 years following partial resection, which approached the recurrence rate of simple pyelolithotomy. In the light of these and other criticisms[13] and with the development of new nephron-saving nephrotomy techniques, the indications have become much more rigorous. Partial nephrectomy still remains relatively important in stone surgery, not for simple caliceal stone disease but for calculi associated with scarred, hydronephrotic or poorly draining caliceal systems. If reserved for these types of disease, the results compare favourably with pyelo-nephrolithotomy as the ipsilateral recurrence rate is less than 10 to 15% within 5 to 6 years, depending on the selection of cases[14-15].

IS THERE A PLACE FOR COAGULUM-PYELOLITHOTOMY IN STONE SURGERY?

The technique of injecting coagulable material into the renal pelvis to entrap and remove renal calculi surgically was developed by Dees[16]. Enthusiasm for this method was limited initially owing to its relative complexity and to the price and scarcity of the necessary material. In recent years there has been a "renaissance" of coagulum pyelolithotomy[18]. This probably reflects the scientific interest in the development of better coagula[17] rather than the real need for the method in every day stone surgery.

The preferred source of fibrinogen is now cryoprecipitate, a human blood fraction prepared inexpensively from single-donor fresh frozen plasma. The other ingredients which form the stone-embedding coagulum are bovin thrombin, calcium chloride and methylene blue to colour the clot. These materials are prepared in two syringes, one with the fibrinogen and the other with thrombin and calcium and are injected simultaneously in adequate proportions until the renal pelvis is filled to capacity. After a few minutes, the coagulum is carefully extracted through a pyelotomy. The main indication for coagulum pyelolithotomy is multiple small stones especially in an enlarged intrarenal system and its main advantage is that all free stones, regardless of size and position, can be removed together with a success rate of 80 to 95% depending on the case selection[19].

However, there are limitations to the method; for example, the relation in size between stone and infundibulum or the adherence of stones to the calyceal wall. It is our experience that good indications are rather infrequent and that coagulum pyelolithotomy needs expertise and practice and is likely to be not very successful if used only on rare occasion. We do not think, therefore, that the method is a "conditio sine qua non" in modern stone surgery.

HOW ARE STAGHORN CALCULI TREATED TODAY?

In Central Europe, about 15 to 20% of kidney stones are composed of struvite and carbonate-apatite and form in the presence of urea-splitting bacteria. These stones usually occur as staghorn calculi and cause renal damage from infection and obstruction that finally leads to renal destruction[20]. A "wait-and-see-policy" that is advocated from time to time is not realistic, even with unilateral staghorn stones. Regrowth after surgery is not inevitable and renal function is usually improved even in cases with incomplete preoperative clearance. Extended pyelo-nephrolithotomy and partial nephrectomy may permit complete extraction of these dendritic calculi, provided that in partial nephrectomy, the resection plane is high enough to include the renal pelvis. However, for the majority of patients, some sort of "anatrophic" nephrotomy is necessary. The term "anatrophic" means that the incisions do not transect intrarenal arteries and therefore do not cause parenchymal atrophy. The prototype of an "anatrophic" nephrolithotomy is the one proposed by Boyce et al[21-22]. They identify the relatively avascular plane - known as Brodel's line - between the posterior and the anterior renal segment by clamping the posterior segmental artery and injecting methylene blue intravenously. After occlusion of the main renal artery, the capsule of the ischemic kidney is incised longitudinally and the parenchyma is dissected in the direction of the hilum. The nephrotomy should ideally enter the collecting system at the base of the posterior infundibula.

As this type of surgery needs considerable time, measures have to be taken to preserve the function of the ischemic kidney. It has been shown that in normothermic arterial occlusion, 20 to 30 min is the maximum tolerable period before permanent renal damage occurs, even if the patient is in excellent hydration and protective measures such as the administration of mannitol have been utilised. If intrarenal surgery requires a longer period of ischemia, some form of hypothermia is necessary. The most popular method is surface cooling with sterile ice slush. Applied correctly it permits a core temperature of 20 to 25°C to be reached in about 20 min. The level of hypothermia can be maintained without much difficulty and protects renal function for about 3 hours. Surface hypothermia has some problems: the possibility of tissue damage by direct contact with the ice, the possibility of body-cooling and last but not least, impediment of the surgeon. However, other forms of hypothermia, for example, transfemoral renal artery perfusion cooling, are far from being free of danger and pitfalls and are only possible in hospitals where arteriorgraphic facilities are available near the operating theatre[23].

The problems connected with hypothermia are the reason why various pharmacologic agents such as diuretics like mannitol or furosemide, alpha-blockers like proprandolol-derivatives to prevent vasoconstriction, renin-antagonists like saralasin, membrane stabilising substances like trasylol and ATP-presvering drugs like inosine, have been tried. Until now, there is no pharmacological regime that has proved to be as effective and as harmless for extended ischemic renal surgery as some type of cooling[24].

Significant progress in surgical stone treatment comes from technical developments for easier and better intraoperative visualisation of stones and for the localisation of intrarenal vessels. Intraoperative radiography is mandatory in stone surgery. The conditions for X-ray examination during the intervention may not always be good, but the use of newer equipment and film material has significantly improved the efficiency of this indispensable imaging method[25]. We are very satisfied with the Renodor equipment (Renal radiography unit, Siemens AG, Erlangen) (developed from a dental X-ray unit) where the emitting electrode can be positioned in the wound. The use of mammography-films makes it possible to identify calculi with a diameter less than 3mm. If bigger stones have to be checked, the use of Polaroid-Land high speed films saves time. If radiography shows a small stone fragment left behind, peroperative nephroscopy with one of the modern instruments can be useful for localisation and removal by irrigation or by forceps[26]. We use a rigid type nephroscopy (Wolf GmbH, Knittlingen) which gives us a better orientation than the flexible choledochoscope-type-nephroscopes which are on trial.

Intraoperative ultrasound imaging[27,28] has made stone finding in the kidney much easier. The necessary experience is acquired quickly by those who use ultrasonography in daily clinical work. Combined with a searching needle, which adds a "third" dimension to the two dimensional B-scan, even radiotranslucent stones can be localized rapidly. We use a short focus 5 Mhz probe (Aloka Co. Ltd., Tokyo). This type retains some of the accuracy of the 7 to 10 Mhz probes proposed and has the advantage that the scans are much easier to interpret.

The combined use of Doppler sonography[29] and B-mode ultrasound scanning[30] means that clamping of the renal artery and consecutive hypothermia can be avoided in many cases. This combination has opened a new era of planned, selective avascular nephrolithotomy. Once the calculus is localised, the Doppler stethoscope is applied on the kidney surface and the intraparenchymal vessels in the nephrotomy area are localised and mapped on the surface. The stone-bearing calyx can now be opened with a radial nephrotomy in a relatively avascular plane and with a low risk of vessel injury. This newer technology has moved the strategy of staghorn stone surgery away from large longitudinal nephrotomies to the more physiologic intrasinual pyelotomy, combined with small avascular radial nephrotomies in the normothermic organ. As the change has essentially taken place during the last 5 years, it is certainly not yet possible to evaluate long-term results, but the low stone recurrence rates published up to now are promising[30-31]. Unfortunately, the goal of complete surgical removal of stones and subsequent eradiation of infection is not always achieved. The residual stone rate lies somewhere between 5 to 25% and the recurrent stone rate after 5 years amounts to some 30%. Infection will persist in spite of correct antibiotic treatment in about 20 to 40% of patients. These figures emphasise that surgery itself is not the complete answer for the local treatment of infected kidney stones.

A promising comprehensive approach to this complex problem has been published recently by Silverman and Stamey[32]. These workers leave a small polythene nephrostomy tube routinely in all kidneys operated on for infected staghorn calculi and irrigate for 1 to 4 weeks with a 10% hemiacridin solution (Renacidin). Before the tube is removed, the kidney is screened by plain film tomograms. Using this procedure, any residual struvite particles, together with entrapped bacteria, are dissolved and washed out. Combined with a vigorous and appropriate antibiotic medication and careful follow-up, this comprehensive treatment in a group of 46 patients resulted in an excellent 2 to 30% recurrence rate (one recurrence) after a mean period of 7 years.

WHAT IS THE PLACE FOR EXTRACORPOREAL SURGERY IN THE TREATMENT OF KIDNEY STONE DISEASE TODAY?

Bench surgery in the treatment of stones is very seldom necessary and is perhaps the least well defined of all indications

608

for extracorporeal kidney surgery. This type of treatment has only rare indications such as kidneys with staghorn calculi and a history of multiple previous surgery, with stenosis of the pyeloureteral junction or with an associated reno-vascular problem[33,34]. However in really difficult cases, bench surgery has some compelling advantages: complete mobility of the kidney with excellent possibilities of transpyelic stone removal (and consequently avoidance of nephrotomies); perfect X-ray conditions; easy and atraumatic nephroscopy and irrigation; easy access to secondary branches of the renal arteries for dye-injection to mark nephrotomy incision-lines. Apart from these arguments autotransplantation allows the efficient handling of pyelo-ureteral strictures. For patients, where every possible treatment fails to prevent stone recurrences, Petterson[35] has recently proposed autotransplantation with direct pyelo-cystostomy for promotion of spontaneous stone-evacuation. It is probable that this type of neo-communication between pelvis and bladder avoids some problems inherent to the ileal ureter, indicated by Goodwin[36] for this condition, but nothing can be said yet about long-term results.

Today, as there is excellent transplantation surgery in many medical centers of the western world, explantation, preservation and implantation are standardised, relatively low risk procedures. If this could be a temptation to use bench surgery more often in kidney stone disease, the final decision should be based on the knowledge that there are very few renal stone situations that cannot be dealt with by an "in situ" procedure and the crucial questions should always be if - and if so why - extracorporal surgery in this particular patient is likely to result in better prognosis.

The indications, problems and pitfalls of the new methods are far from being known. Today, we are only in the enthusiastic phase of shock-wave stone destruction and of transcutaneous endoscopic stone manipulation. It is therefore difficult to foresee the place of stone surgery in the future, but as I said initially, there are many reasons to believe that it will retain a distinct place in stone treatment. Apart from stone bearing kidneys with pre-existing or consecutive pathology which cannot be dealt with by either extracoporeal shockwave therapy or by percutaneous endoscopic manipulaion, it seems to me that the infected staghorn calculus will remain one of the indications for open operation in the future because our new techniques give us an excellent chance of removing all stone debris, with an acceptable risk of septic complications and with a relatively short period of hospitalisation.

But as Albert Einstein said: "never think too much on the future; it will come early enough and tell you what you wished to know".

REFERENCES

1. W. F. Braasch, in:"Treatment of Urinary Lithiasis", A. J. Butt, eds., C. C. Thomas, Springfield (1960).
2. C. Chaussy and E. Schmiedt, Urol. Clin. N. Amer. 10:743 (1983).
3. J. L. Huffmann, D. H. Bagley, H. W. Schoenberg, and E. S. Lyon, J. Urol. 130:31 (1983).
4. E. A. Wickham and R. A. Miller, "Percutaneous Renal Surgery", Churchill Livingstone, Edinburgh (1983).
5. K. A. Kropp, Urol. Clin. N. Amer. 10:617 (1983).
6. R. F. Gittes and A. Belldegrun, Urol. Clin. N. Amer. 10:625 (1983).
7. J. W. Demler, M. A. Dennis, and B. Finlayson, J. Urol. 129:263 (1983).
8. E. Proca, Br. J. Urol. 53:201 (1981).
9. J. M. Gil-Vernet, Urol. Int. 20:255 (1965).
10. M. J. Resnick, Urol. Clin. N. Amer. 8:585 (1981).
11. C. Semb, Acta Chir. Scand. 109:360 (1955).
12. U. Wald, M. Caine, and H. Solomon, Urology 11:338 (1978).
13. C. K. Anderson, Proc. Roy. Soc. Med. 67:459 (1974).
14. J. F. Redmann, Urol. Clin. N. Amer. 10:677 (1983).
15. R. J. Bates, J. A. Heaney, and W. Kerr, Urology 17:409(1981).
16. J. E. Dees, J. Urol. 56:271 (1946).
17. H. Klosterhalfen, L. V. Wagenknecht, and R. Busch, Eur. Urol. 7:206 (1981).
18. S. Marshall, Urol. Clin. N. Amer. 10:659 (1983).
19. C. P. Fischer, L. P. Sonda, and A. C. Diokno, J. Urol. 126:432 (1981).
20. J. P. Blandy and M. Singh, J. Urol. 115:505 (1976).
21. M. J. V. Smith and W. H. Boyce, J. Urol. 99:521 (1968).
22. J. P. Spirnak and M. J. Resnick, Urol. Clin. N. Amer. 10:665 (1983).
23. M. Marberger and W. Stackl, in:"Current Trends in Urology", Vol. 1, M. J. Resnick, ed., Williams & Wilkins, London (1981).
24. A. G. Novick, Urol. Clin. N. Amer. 10:637 (1983).
25. F. F. Marshall, Urol. Clin. N. Amer. 10:629 (1983).
26. E. J. Zingg and A. Futterlieb, Br. J. Urol 52:333 (1980).
27. J. H. Cook and B. Lytton, J. Urol. 117:543 (1977).
28. B. Lytton, J. Urol. 130:213 (1983).
29. S. R. Bryniak and A. E. Chesley, J. Urol. 126:295 (1981).
30. H. Riedmiller, J. Thüroff, P. Alken, and R. Hohenfellner, J. Urol. 130:224 (1983).
31. C. R. J. Woodhouse, C. R. Farrell, A. M. I. Paris, and J. P. Blandy, Br. J. Urol. 53:520 (1983).
32. D. E. Silverman and T. A. Stamey, Medicine 62:44 (1983).
33. R. K. Lawson, J. Urol. 123:301 (1980).
34. A. C. Novick, Urol. Clin. N. Amer. 8:299 (1981).
35. S. Petterson, H. Brynger, C. Henrikson, A. E. Nilson and T. Ranch, Br. J. Urol. 55:154 (1983).
36. W. E. Goodwin and A. T. K. Cockett, J. Urol. 85:214 (1961).

OPERATIVE URETERORENOSCOPY FOR ENDOSCOPIC REMOVAL OF

URETERIC CALCULI

K.-H. Bichler, D. Erdmann, P. Schmitz-Moormann,
and S. Halim

Dept. of Urology, University of Tübingen, D-7400
Tübingen, and Dept. of Pathology, University of Marburg
D-3500 Marburg, F.R.G.

INTRODUCTION

Progress in the miniaturization of optical systems has made ureteroscopy possible. As well as the flexible instruments used in gastroenterology, we also employ inelastic metal instruments which allow optical control of the ureter as described by Perez-Castro and Pineiro[1]. We first reported our experience with this technique in 1981[2] and others have followed[3,4]. Two aspects have to be taken into consideration in the application of ureterorenoscopy: (i) the technique of inserting the instrument; and (ii) the manipulation in the ureter and application of ultrasound to fragment concrements. The use of ultrasound in the ureter seems particularly problematic because of possible damage to the urothelium. In order to test the direct effect of ultrasound on the urothelium we carried out some animal experiments. For anatomical reasons, we could not test the direct effect of ultrasound on the ureteric wall in dogs and so used the bladder wall instead, assessing both the immediate and long-term effects (after 40 days).

RESULTS

The animal experiments showed the following immediate alterations in the bladder wall after ultrasonic application for 30 to 180 sec. Defects occurred in the epithelium with blood extravasation and there was some haemorrhaging in the adjacent submucosa, dependent on the degree of the duration of application. In the long-term we found no pathological changes after 30 sec of ultrasonic radiation. Submucosal fibrosis was found in some cases after ultrasonic stimulation for 60 sec or more and, occasionally,

611

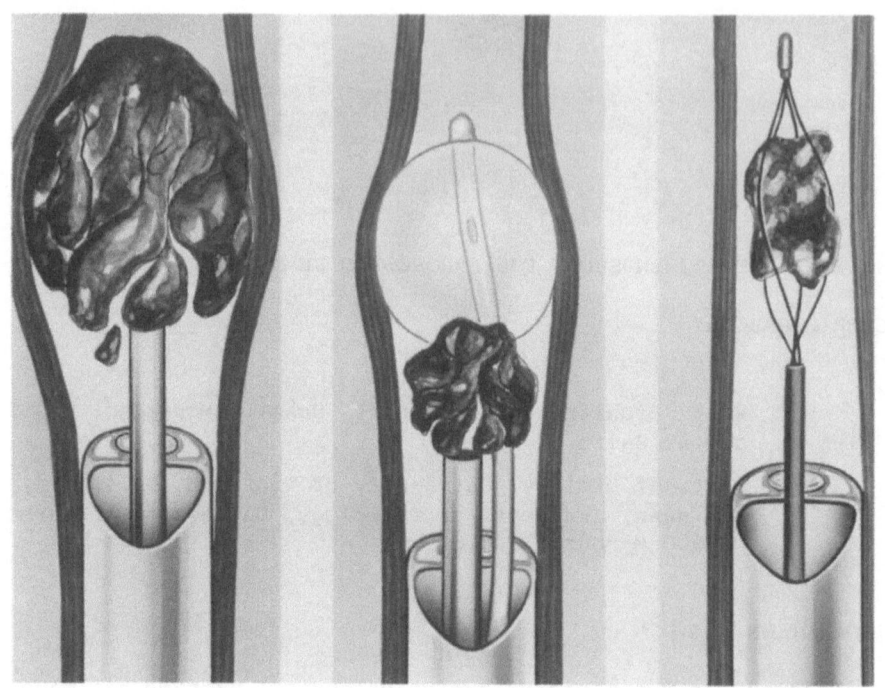

Fig. 1. Ultrasonic application for the fragmentation of ureteral
stones and extraction with a Dormia basket.

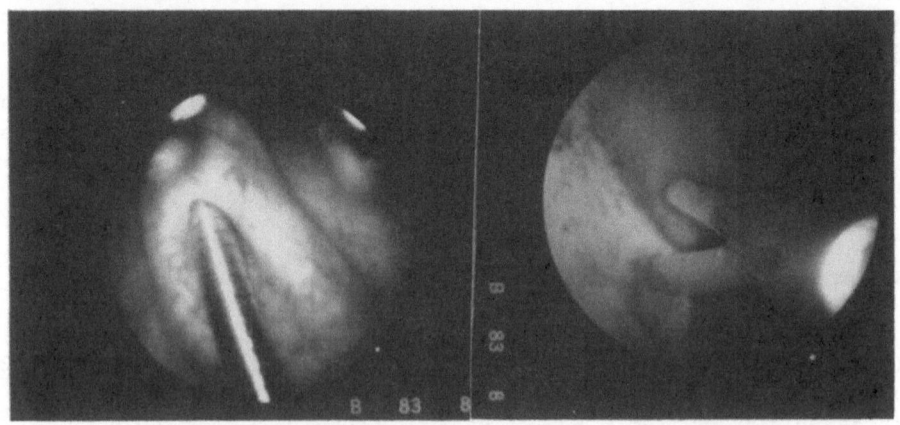

Fig. 2. Dilatation of slitting of the ostium of the ureter,
endoscopic view.

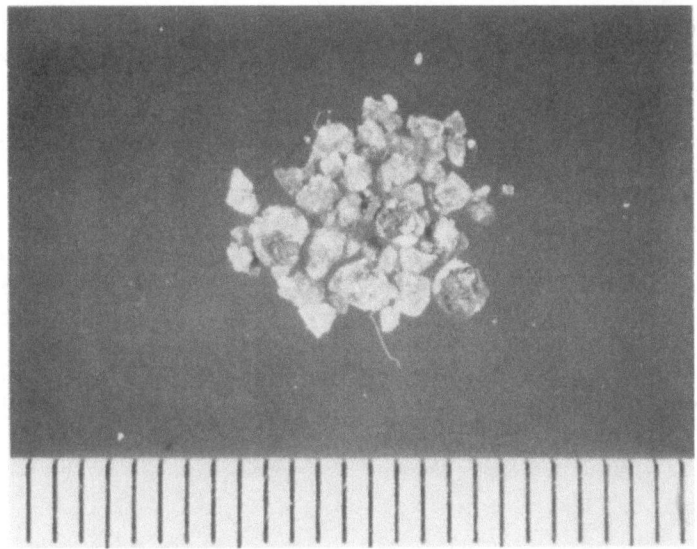

Fig. 3.   Remains after ultrasonic destruction of distal ureteral
          stone.

after even longer duration, the adjacent musculature was affected.
Furthermore, epithelial atrophy was observed in the area exposed to
ultrasonic radiation.   There was no indication of changes in the
muscle fibres, in the adventitia or in the vessels.

Based on these results and in association with Wolf
(Knittlingen, FRG), we developed a ureteroscope that allows
optically controlled application or ultrasound, as well as other

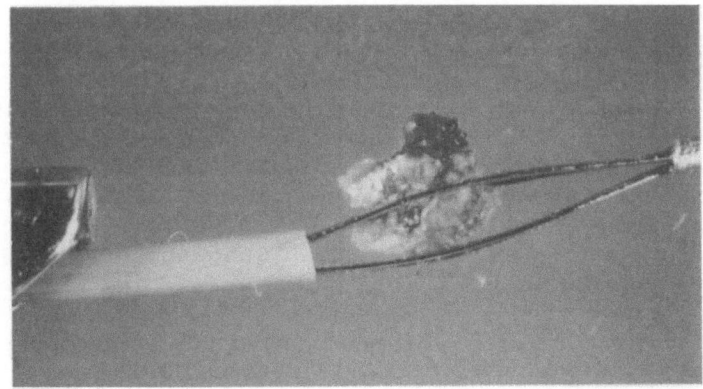

Fig. 4.   Stone extraction by means of a Dormia basket.

techniques for stone extraction.   It is a ureteroscope of
11.5 Charriere with a large oval wash and tube canal allowing
simultaneous application of two additional instruments e.g. an
ultrasonic probe and a balloon-catheter to focus the ureteral stone,
or a Dormia stone extractor (4 Charriere) and a Zeiss loop (Fig. 1).
Often the ureteral ostium reacted to the insertion of a
ureteroscope. To insert the instrument, dilatation of the ostium of
the ureter (10-12 Charriere) was necessary, and sometimes we had to
slit the ostium up to 2 - 3 mm using endoscopic scissors (Wolf,
Knittlingen) (Fig. 2).   When cutting with this instrument, we found
no resulting vesico-ureteral reflux.   Previous studies have already
demonstrated that slitting the top of the ostium up to 4 mm in
length does not cause reflux[5].   The clean cut obtained with a pair
of scissors seems to be more controllable and better for the healing
of the wound than the use of diathermy[6].

DISCUSSION

So far we have successfully extracted concrements from the
distal ureter using the ureteroscope coupled with various methods
for removing stones in 18 patients.   Fig. 3 shows the ultrasonic
fragmentation of a distal ureteric stone in a 29-year-old man.   In
Fig. 4 stone extraction by means of a Dormia basket in a 32-year-old
patient is demonstrated.   Our experience indicates that this is an
improvement in the treatment of distal ureteric stones.   Depending
on the size of the ureteric concrement, different strategies are
necessary to extract the concrement in toto (e.g. with a Dormia
basket) or to break up the concrement by means of ultrasound so that
the fragments can pass spontaneously through the ureter.
Ureteroscopy is indicated for concrements lodged in the distal
ureter where efforts to extract it with a Zeiss-loop have been
unsuccessful. It seems worthwhile to attempt optically controlled
disintegration or extraction of the stone by means of a ureteroscope
in one session.   This may be important in patients who are poor
surgical risks and where open ureterolithotomy can be avoided.

REFERENCES

1. E. Perez-Castro and J. A. Pineiro, Eur. Urol. 8:117 (1982).
2. M. A. Reuter, R. Harzmann, K.-H. Bichler, and St. H. Fluchter,
     Veeerhdl. Dtsch. Ges. Urol., Berlin (1981).
3. M. Bush, P. Guinan, and J. Lanners, Urol. Clin. N. Am. 9:131
     (1982).
4. J. L. Huffmann, D. H. Bagley, H. W. Schoenberg, and
     E. S. Lyson, J. Urol. 7:31 (1983).
5. H. H. Baur, Personal communication (1972).
6. W. Bischoff, "Ostotom ein neues Gerat zur Ostiumschlitzung",
     Verhdl. Dtsch. Ges. Urol., Wiesbaden (1983).

RENAL AUTOTRANSPLANTATION WITH DIRECT PYELOCYSTOSTOMY IN

PATIENTS WITH RECURRENT RENAL CALCULI

C. Henriksson, T. Ranch, A. E. Nilson, and
S. Pettersson

Dept. of Urology and Diagnostic Radiology
Sahlgrenska sjukhuset, University of Göteborg
S-413 45 Göteborg, Sweden

INTRODUCTION

Despite adequate prophylactic treatment, many stone patients continue to form stones and require repeated lithotomies. The recurrence rate may even increase with time because of post-operative scarring and obstruction. Bilateral stones are common and parenchyma-saving surgery should therefore be performed whenever feasible. Extended pyelolithotomy[1], nephrolithotomy under hypothermia[2] and anatrophic nephrotomy[3] have improved the completeness of stone removal. These methods, however, do not promote spontaneous stone passage. The use of autotransplantation of the kidney and a direct pyelocystostomy, described in the present report, aims at radical stone removal and constitutes a reprequisite for future spontaneous stone passage. The procedure has also been recommended for the treatment of urothelial tumors of the upper urinary tract[4] and after unsuccessful pyeloplasty[5]. A preliminary report on this procedure in treating patients with recurrent stones was given in 1981[6].

PATIENTS AND METHODS

Eight male patients, aged 34-61 years (mean 47 years), have been operated on since 1979 (details on request from authors). They had a 12- to 41-year history of stone disease before auto-transplantation. They had undergone between 2 and 9 conventional ipsilateral lithotomies. Two patients had a single kidney, one of them because of congenital aplasia, the other because of nephrectomy for a staghorn calculus. In another patient only half of the kidney remained at the time of the autotransplantation because of

previous partial nephrectomies for recurrent stones.   Four patients
had had urinary infections.   Two patients had been treated with
bendroflumethiazide (Salures-K^R) without apparent effect on the
recurrence rate.   In a patient with cystinuria (No. 8) α-mercapto-
propionylglycine (Thiola^R) seemed to have had no effect.

The pre- and post-operative examinations included ^{51}Cr-EDTA-
clearance, ^{132}I-hippuran renography including split kidney function
determination, maximum urinary osmolality, intravenous pyelography,
renal angiography, urethrocystoscopy, cystometry and urinary flow
rate determination.

Three patients had a staghorn calculus, the others multiple
calculi in the kidney to be autotransplanted.   The GFR of this
kidney was above 24 ml/min/1.73 m^2 in all patients.   Three patients
had medullary sponge lesions and 3 had an ipsilateral ureteric
stricture.   Two patients had multiple renal arteries.   Pre-
operatively all patients had a normal cystometry and flow rate.

The operation was carried out with the patient in the supine
position and employing two separate incisions.   Low molecular
weight dextran and mannitol were given per-operatively.   A careful
nephrectomy was performed.   Perfusion and preservation of the
kidney until implantation was carried out according to our routine[7].
On the work bench the ureter and renal pelvis were resected leaving
a brim allowing an anastomosis to the urinary bladder.   Contact
radiographs were taken and the stones were removed via the pelvis or
multiple nephrotomies.   The kidney was implanted in the ipsilateral
iliac fossa with its long axis almost tranverse.   In order to get a
position of the kidney allowing direct anastomosis between the renal
pelvis and bladder, the renal vessels were anastomosed to the
external iliac vessels except in one patient with multiple renal
arteries, where the internal iliac artery was also used.   The
urinary bladder was extensively mobilized.   An anastomosis with a
diameter of 1 to 2 cm was created between the bladder and renal
pelvis using running absorbable sutures.

Post-operatively the urinary bladder was drained by an indwelling urethral catheter and prophylaxis against thrombosis with
low molecular weight dextran and antibiotics were given.

RESULTS

The early postoperative course was complicated in one patient
(No. 3) by kinking of the artery requiring a new anastomosis with an
additional period of warm ischemia, and in another patient by
vascular thrombosis indicating transplantectomy.   This kidney had a
considerably reduced parenchyma after previous partial
nephrectomies.

Table 1. Glomerular and Tubular Renal Function Before and After
Autotransplantation and Pyelocystostomy.

Patient No	Preop		Postop		Last follow-up		Observation time, months
	GFR	Osm	GFR	Osm	GFR	Osm	
1	53	421	48	684	56	465	59
2	36	787	27	627	30	733	57
3	78	639	54	423	48	621	45
4	29	760	--	---	--	---	--
5	24	643	34	731	28	617	35
6	28	599	25	684	25	613	31
7	47	ND	37	584	34	460	26
8	49	655	52	756	52	842	9

GFR:calculated glomerular filtration rate of transplant,
ml/min/1.73 m^2BSA.
Osm:maximum urinary osmolality (μmol/kg); ND:not determined.

After a few weeks the general condition of each patient was
good and none of them complained about the unusual site of the
kidney. Two patients spontaneously passed stones. In another
patient two minor recurrent stones were recently diagnosed. None
developed hyper-tension. Renal function was mainly unchanged in
all patients except the one in whom a re-anastomosis had to be
undertaken (Table 1). In this patient the GFR was reduced from 78,
pre-operatively, to 54 ml/min post-operatively and remained at about
this level. Occasional asymptomatic bacteriuria occurred in 3
patients with the same kind of bacteria as pre-operatively. IVPs,
performed regularly, showed a normal collecting system. Cystometry
was normal in all cases. The follow-up time after autotransplantation was 9 to 59 months (mean 37 months).

DISCUSSION

When medical prevention of stone recurrence fails the patient
has to undergo repeated operations and often, finally, nephrectomy.
Goodwin et al[8] recommended the 'ileum ureter' in patients with
recurrent stones and obstruction to allow spontaneous passage of
stones. However, this procedure is complicated by electrolyte
disturbance, hydronephrosis, infection and renal insufficiency[9,10].
Renal autotransplantation and direct pyelocystostomy does not seem
to have any of these disadvantages. The free reflux of urine from
the bladder to the pelvis has so far not been found to deteriorate
the ranal function. At cystopyelography only a transient dilation
of the intrarenal collecting system has been observed. It is,
however, advisable to diagnose and eliminate promptly even a slight

intravesical outflow obstruction. Also in patients treated by auto-transplantation and pyelocystostomy for other disease, i.e. urothelial tumor and hydronephrosis, the renal function has remained unchanged at follow-up[4,5].

Renal autotransplantation with direct pyelocystostomy should be considered in patients with multiple recurrent stones in the upper urinary tract, especially when obstruction has developed.

REFERENCES

1. J. P. Blandy and G. C. Tresidder, Br. J. Urol. 39:121 (1967).
2. J. E. A. Wickham and V. K. Mathur, Br. J. Urol. 43.648 (1971).
3. M. J. V. Smith and W. H. Boyce, Trans. Am. Ass. Genito. Surg. 59:18 (1967).
4. S. Pettersson, H. Brynger, C. Henriksson, S. L. Johansson, A. E. Nilson, and T. Ranch. Cancer (in press).
5. S. Pettersson, H. Brynger, C. Henriksson, S. L. Johansson, A. E. Nilson, and T. Ranch, J. Urol. 130:234 (1983).
6. S. Pettersson, H. Brynger, L. E. Gelin, A. E. Nilson, and T. Ranch, Scand. J. Urol. Nephrol. Suppl. 60:39 (1981).
7. S. Pettersson, in:"International Perspectives in Urology: Renal Preservation", M. Marberger and K. Dreikorn, eds., Williams & Wilkins., Baltimore (1983).
8. W. E. Goodwin, C. C. Winter, and R. D. Turner, J. Urol. 81:406 (1959).
9. D. D. Creevy, Surgery 58:497 (1965).
10. E. A. Tanagho, J. Urol. 113:796 (1975).

THREE-DIMENSIONAL INTER-OPERATIVE RENAL RADIOGRAPHY BY MEANS OF

A COMBINATION OF POLAROID FILMS AND INTENSIFIER SCREENS

J. Braun and R. Hofmann

Dept. of Urology, Technical University of Munich
8000 Munich 80, F.R.G.

INTRODUCTION

In kidney stone surgery, it is desirable to achieve complete
removal of all stones from the kidney with minimal damage to the
parenchyma. The exact position of the concrements in the kidney,
however, often cannot be determined by pre-operative X-ray
investigation. The techniques available for intra-operative stone
localization include pyeloscopy, intra-operative ultrasound with
high-frequency scanprobes and intra-operative X-ray examination,
normally using a mammography X-ray film. For development, the film
must be brought to the processing machine in the radiological
department and back to the operation theatre resulting in loss of
time for the surgeon. In 1980, Koshiba et al[1] reported the use of
polaroid X-ray equipment for intra-operative examination, but,
in our experience, this was unsatisfactory. We therefore developed
a time-saving procedure for intra-operative X-ray examination using
a combination of polaroid films and intensifier screens.

MATERIALS AND METHODS

A small single film plate from the plastic frame of a commercially available polaroid film pack, normally containing 8 films,
was constructed for the use of a polaroid single film that can be
developed in a polaroid daylight processing box (Fig. 1(a)). The
intensifying screen is permanently fixed to the film box opposite
the light-sensitive part of the polaroid film. The other part of
the polaroid film is placed against the back of the plate, protected
by the rear-wall. This film plate is loaded in a darkroom, packed
in a foil and sterilized by gas. We also constructed a new

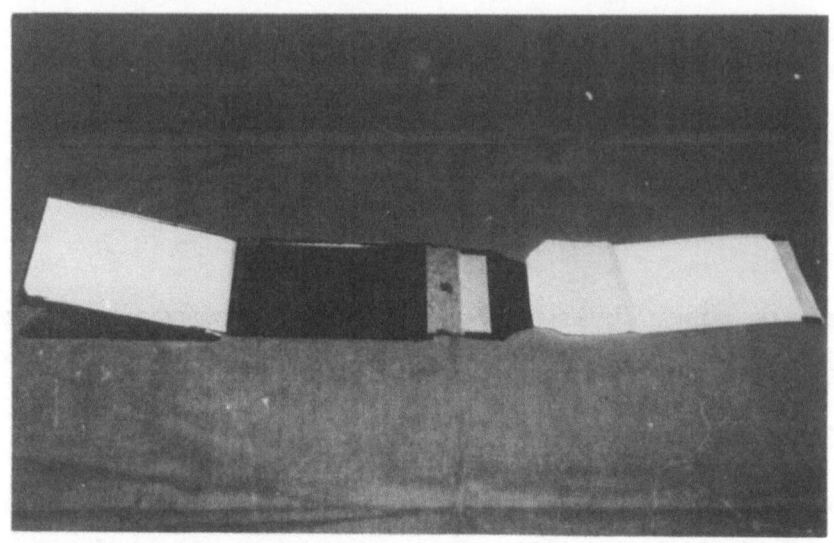

Fig. 1 (a). Polaroid single film box with film (right) and
intensifier screen left.

plateholder to position and change these film plates intraoperatively, consisting of a reticle positioned in front of the
exposed kidney and a filmholder parallel to the reticle behind the
kidney (Fig. 1(b)).

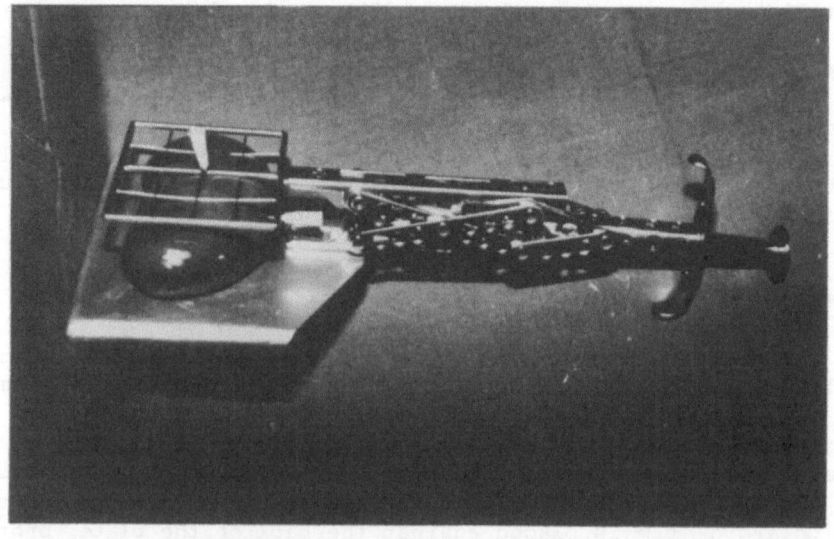

Fig. 1 (b). Plateholder with kidney - the reticle before and film
box behind the kidney.

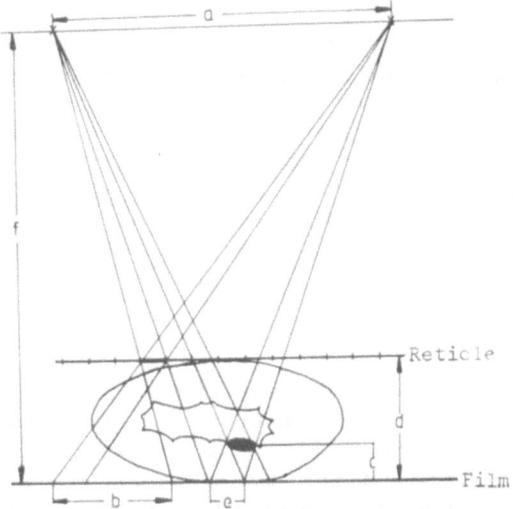

Fig. 2.   Sketch of the X-ray arrangement of twin-imaging, a = shift of the X-ray tube; b = shift of the reticle image; c = distance of stone to film surface; d = distance of reticle to film surface; e = shift of the stone image; f = distance of X-ray tube to film-surface.

Table 1. Calculation of the Distance between Stone and Film Surface.

$$c/e = (f - c)/a$$
$$\text{and}\quad d/b = (f - d)/a$$
$$\therefore\quad e(f - c)/c = b(f - d)/d$$
$$\therefore\quad c = de(f - c)/bd(f - d)$$
$$\text{but}\quad (f - c)/(f - d) \sim 1 \text{ if } f \text{ is large}$$
$$\therefore\quad c = de/b$$

Table 2. Comparison Between Various Films and Intensifier Screens.

Intensifier screen	Film Type		
	611	657	655
Kodak Universal	(+)	+	(+)
Kodak Lanex	++	++	+
Dupont Cronex	++	++	+
Agfa 8-46 U 1 Back	+	++	+
Agfa 8-41 E 1 Tube	+	++	+
Agfa 5-40 L 1	+	+	+
Agfa 4-46 A 1	+	++	+
Agfa 2-45 G 2	+	++	+

621

Double irradiation of the kidney at different angles, first published by Melchior and Lang[2], shows a twin-image of the reticle and the stone. Movement of the calculus and of the reticle in the picture after double X-ray exposure leads to an exact localization of the stone (Fig. 2). The position of the stone can be estimated easily or calculated exactly using a simple mathematical formula (Table 1) and then marked with pins. Different intensifier screens and various types of polaroid films have been tested (Table 2).

RESULTS

Rare earth intensifier screens in combination with the polaroid film type 667 proved to be the best. The quality of the pictures is as good as conventional radiographs on mamography films and can even visualize tiny stone fragments or poorly opaque calculi with a vastly reduced X-ray dose. Only 0.8 roentgen on the film surface is necessary, obtainable with an exposure of 3 mAsec at 35 kV. To obtain normal exposure times and dosages applicable to any X-ray apparatus, a copper filter of 0.3 mm or 1.0 mm thickness has to be used. To obtain optimal results under these conditions the X-ray apparatus was adjusted to 45 kV/15 mAsec or 65 kV/10 mAsec.

DISCUSSION

The polaroid X-ray film technique combined with rare earth intensifier screens offers a simple method for visualizing kidney stones in the exposed kidney during surgery. After about one minute a distinctive X-ray polaroid photograph can be obtained under daylight conditions in the operating theatre. The necessary equipment is cheap and the construction is simple for any precision toolmaker. The double X-ray exposure technique is an easy method for the exact intra-operative localization of calculi in the kidney.

ACKNOWLEDGEMENT

This paper is dedicated to Prof. Dr. W Mauermayer.

REFERENCES

1. K. Koshiba, A. Ishibashi, and S. Mashimo, J. Urol. 124:586 (1980).
2. H. Melchior and G. Lang, Urol. Int. 36:390 (1981).

DISSOLUTION OF PHOSPHATE STONES BY PERCUTANEOUS

NEPHROSTOMY AND LOCAL IRRIGATION

P. Froeling, C. Boetes, and S. Strijk

Dept. of Internal Medicine (Division of General
Internal Medicine), and Diagnostic Radiology
St. Radboud University Hospital, Nijmegen
The Netherlands

INTRODUCTION

A high urine pH plays a critical role in the origin and growth
of phosphate-containing calculi. Conversely, phosphate stones may be
dissolved in more acid solutions. In 1943, Suby and Albright[1]
reported the dissolution of phosphatic calculi in situ by the
retrograde introduction of a citrate solution containing magnesium
(Suby's solution or Solution G). Chemolysis of renal calculi by
local irrigation has been used as postoperative adjuvant treatment
but may also be considered as an alternative to the surgical removal
of the stones, especially in patients who are poor surgical risks or
when surgical removal is no longer possible[2].

The application of the solvents may be performed through
endoscopically introduced ureteral catheters or by percutaneous
nephrostomy. The second procedure has the advantage that the
patients are not confined to bed and that there is no outflow
obstruction in the ureter caused by a catheter.

The present report summarizes our results on local irrigation
(without operation) in 17 kidneys through a percutaneous nephrostomy
catheter, using solution G or R as the stone solvent.

PATIENTS AND METHODS

Table 1 summarizes the patient data and the results of treatment. Most patients previously had had one or more operations on
the relevant kidney, at least 6 months before treatment. No patient
had signs of urinary tract obstruction or urosepsis. In most

623

Table 1. Clinical Data and Results

Case	Kidney	Stone	Previous Operations	Irrigation (days)	Culture	Fever (>38.5°C)	Serum Creatinine (µmol/l) Before	After	Stone Dissolution
1	R	C	0	35	+	–	91	95	o
2	R	S	0	22	–	+	78	76	**
3 a	L	CP	2	22	–	+	75	68	*
b	R	CP	2	24	–	–	80	79	**
4 a	L	SP	1	67	–	–	170	162	**
b	R	SP	1	101	–	–	167	153	**
5	R	SP	0	19	–	–	113	90	***
6	R	SP	4	79	–	+	72	74	**
7	L	S	2	10	–	–	75	62	***
8	L	C	1	19	+	+	59	64	o
9	L	S	1	39	+	–	84	75	***
10	L	S	1	25	+	+	65	69	**
11	R	SM	0	55	+	+	139	135	**
12	R	SP	2	34	–	–	60	50	***
13	R	SP	0	15	+	–	132	95	***
14	R	SP	2	12	+	+	75	61	***
15	R	SP	1	32	+	–	92	93	***
Mean				36.5			96	88	

R = right; L = left; C = calyceal; S = staghorn; P = phosphate; M = mixed; o = no dissolution;
* = little dissolution; ** = >2/3 dissolution; *** = total dissolution.

patients operative removal of the stones had been judged to be impossible or very difficult, or was rejected because of the general condition of the patient. The mean age was 45 years (24 to 72). After the exclusion of coagulation disorders, percutaneous nephrostomy was performed using local anesthesia and the technique described by Hellsten et al[3] and Stables et al[4].

All patients received antibiotic treatment for the first 14 days. The second day after the introduction of the nephrostomy catheter, irrigation treatment was started if, after a fluoroscopic check (nephrostomogram and plain radiograph), the position of the catheter proved to be correct. During the treatment period all the patients were ambulatory. Nine patients were treated partially on an out-patient basis (mean 34 days). A radiological check was performed at least once weekly or in the event of fever, hemorrhage or pain, presumed to be caused by obstruction or by leakage along the catheter. Irrigation was performed with either solution G or R indiscriminately (without obvious differences of effects, complaints or other complications). The irrigation fluid was administered as an undiluted solution or diluted one to two times with saline. The flow was gradually increased from 50 to 200 ml/h, depending on the complaints of the patients and possible signs of outflow obstruction. The administration of the irrigation fluid was performed by continuous drip infusion. Treatment was terminated after total stone dissolution, or when, in spite of good position of the catheter, no further stone dissolution could be observed for a period of one week.

Table 2.   Stone Dissolution in Relation to Stone Type.

Type of Stone	Stone Dissolution				
	o	*	**	***	n
Shape					
Staghorn			6	7	13
Calyx stones	2	1	1		4
Composition					
Phosphate stone		1	5	7	13
Mixed stones			2		2
Unknown	2				2

RESULTS AND CONCLUSIONS

In 2 patients no reduction of stone size could be obtained. These 2 patients had stones localised in the calices. Complete stone dissolution was achieved in 7 patients (Table 2). All these patients had large staghorn calculi. Eight patients had positive urine cultures at the start of the treatment. Only 4 developed a temporary fever reaction during irrigation. Four other patients with negative urine cultures at the start of the irrigation period also developed a temporary fever. In no patient was GFR decreased at the end of the treatment.

In 9 patients exchange of the catheter was performed one or more times for different reasons during the irrigation period, in most cases to improve the position of the catheter in relation to the stone(s). The most common noticed side-effect was dysuric pain, which could be alleviated by diluting the irrigation fluid with saline. Hypermagnesemia was not encountered.

In conclusion this treatment proved to be a safe and good alternative to surgical removal of staghorn calculi especially when operation is judged to be impossible or contraindicated. This approach also can be used in the presence of a positive urine culture. Although it may take a long time to dissolve the stones, in most patients it proved to be possible to perform the treatment partially on an out-patient basis. Deterioration of the kidney function did not occur in any of our patients.

REFERENCES

1. H. I. Suby and F. Albright, New Engl. J. Med. 288:81 (1943).
2. S. P. Dretler, R. C. Pfister, and J. H. Newhouse, New Engl. J. Med. 300:341 (1979).
3. S. Hellsten, J. Hildel, P. Link, and U. Ulmsten, Eur. Urol. 4:282 (1978).
4. D. P. Stables, N. J. Ginsberg, and M. L. Johnson, Am. J. Roentgenol. 130:75 (1978).

A DIRECT COMPARISON OF THE LITHOLYTIC CAPACITY OF RENACIDIN AND
SOME NEW CALCIUM OXALATE AND/OR PHOSPHATE DISSOLVING IRRIGATION
SYSTEMS

P. Leskovar, E. Vogel, and A. Rozehnal

Urologische Klinik und Poliklinik der Technischen
Universität München, München, F.R.G.

INTRODUCTION

There are two possible systems for chemolitholysis, oral
(systemic) and local (instrumental). Oral dissolution of urinary
stones is successful only for uric acid calculi. Local
chemolitholysis may be used for urate, cystine and phosphate,
especially struvite, calculi. But, oxalate concrements cannot be
dissolved by this means. Our approach to oral chemolitholysis,
especially of "young" phosphate calculi, is based on increasing the
Ca^{2+}-binding capacity of urine by the stimulation of the tubular
secretion of citrate. This is achieved by the reversible,
competitive inhibition of tubular intramitochondrial citrate-
oxidizing enzymes or by the renal elimination of compounds which
complex urinary Ca^{2+}. In instrumental chemolitholysis our
experiments have focused on new irrigation solutions that may be
capable of dissolving, not only struvite, but also calcium oxalate
and apatite calculi. From direct comparisons of litholytic rates,
the practicability of calcium oxalate dissolution by irrigation in
stone-patients as well as the average expected treatment-time may be
predicted. Struvite calculi are known to be dissolved by
hemiacidrin on an average within 10 days[1-4]. By alternation of
calcium- and oxalate-binding irrigation systems, calcium oxalate
calculi could be dissolved at the same dissolution rate as struvite
concrements treated with hemiacidrin.

MATERIALS AND METHODS

Our study consisted of the gravimetric analysis of more than
1000 single calculi, subdivided according to their composition as

determined by X-ray diffraction and according to their size (2,4,6 and 10 mm diameter). In total we have tested 44 single and combined irrigation systems. As reference solutions, we used hemiacidrin (Renacidin) and citrate. The concentrations were 0.001, 0.005, 0.010, and 0.250 mol/l; the pHs of the solutions were 4.0 and 8.0, respectively. The flow rate was 1.0 ml/min. The preselection of test substances (44 out of 80) depended on their ability to inhibit crystal growth and aggregation in metastable and unstable Ca-oxalate and Ca-phosphate solutions[5,6].

Table 1. Dissolution of Calcium Oxalate Calculi by Test Solutions (0.1 mol/l) on (a) Struvite and (b) Oxalate Concrements, Measured under Identical Experimental Conditions.

Stone	Test Solution	Dissolution (%)	Stone	Test Solution	Dissolution (%)
MAP	Hemiacidrin	53.9	CaOx	MgEDTA/NaPP	46.4
CaOx	Hemiacidrin	10.0	CaOx	TI/TIV/TV/	
CaOx	TI	48.5		MgEDTA/ZnEDTA	67.0
CaOx	TIV	70.1	CaOx	Fe citrate	50.5
CaOx	TV	57.2	CaOx	Fe gluconate	50.4
CaOx	TVI	73.3	CaOx	Mg gluconate	56.7
CaOx	MgEDTA	55.2	CaOx	Methylsuccinate	56.9
CaOx	FeEDTA	50.1	CaOx	Sabacinate	50.8
CaOx	NaPP	57.7	CaOx	Trimellithate	58.6
			CaOx	Tricarballyalate	42.6

Flow rate = 1 ml/min; t= 32 h + 32 h (0.1 mol/l Fe/Al sol).
TI = nitrilotriacetate
TIV = 1,2-cyclohexylene-dinitrilo-tetraacetate
TV = diethylene-triamine-pentaacetate
TVI = bis(aminoethyl)-glycolether-N,N,N',N'-tetraacetate
PP = polyphosphate

Table 2. Dissolution of Struvite Calculi.

Stone	Test Solution	Dissolution (%)	Stone	Test Solution	Dissolution (%)
MAP	Hemiacidrin	52.5	MAP	TVI	85.2
			MAP	FeEDTA	77.5
MAP	TI	66.1	MAP	MgEDTA	67.0
MAP	TIV	74.6	MAP	TI/TIV/TV/	
MAP	TV	64.6		MgEDTA/ZnEDTA	68.7

Flow rate = 1 ml/min; t = 64 h; pH = 8.0.

RESULTS

The new irrigation systems were compared with hemiacidrin under the same experimental conditions. In some experiments, the dissolution rate of struvite in the presence of hemiacidrin was compared with the effect of test solutions on calcium oxalate concrements in relation to concentration, pH and alternation of irrigation system as well as to the size of calculi. An example of these experiments is shown in Table 1.

In other experiments, the efficiency of struvite dissolution in the presence of the test substances was directly compared with that of hemiacidrin to find out if chemolysis of struvite concrements could be increased by alternative irrigation solutions (Table 2). In addition, the possibility that litholytic effects, comparable with those of hemiacidrin, could be attained with other irrigation systems at lower concentrations of active ingredients, was tested under standardized conditions (Table 3). The advantages of irrigation in comparison with the stationary treatment of calculi, as well as the importance of the alternating irrigation by cation- and anion-binding solutions were shown on some model substances (Tables 4 and 5).

Table 3. Combined Irrigation Systems Chelating Calcium and Oxalate.

Stone	Test Solution	Dissolution (%)	Stone	Test Solution	Dissolution (%)
MAP	Hemidacidrin (0.1M)	44.2	MAP	TIV (0.01M)	85.7
CaOx	TIV (0.01M)	53.5	CaP	TIV (0.01M)	35.5
CaOx	TIV (0.01M)	48.0	CaP/MAP	TIV (0.01M)	63.7

Flow rate = 1 ml/min; t = 32 h + 32 h with 0.01M Fe/Al sol.

Table 4. Advantages of the Alternating Irrigation (AI) on Dissolution of Calcium Oxalate Calculi, in Comparison with the Stationary Stone Treatment (SST).

Type	Test Solution	Time Days	Dissolution (%)	Type	Test Solution	Time Days	Dissolution (%)
SST	TI	7	12.7	SST	Oxalacetate	7	7.7
SST	TI	14	17.1	SST	Oxalacetate	14	8.2
SST	TI	28	22.7	SST	Oxalacetate	28	11.0
SST	TI	56	28.7	SST	Oxalacetate	56	15.4
AI	TI	1.4+1.4	46.2	AI	Oxalacetate	1.4+1.4	28.0

Flow rate = 1 ml/min; concentration 0.01 M.

Table 5. Advantages of a Combined Stone Irrigation by Calcium- and Oxalate-Binding Compounds on Calcium Oxalate Stone Dissolution.

Test	Test Solution	Dissolution (%)	Test	Test Solution	Dissolution (%)
1	Hemiacidrin (0.01M)	7.0	5	Citrate (0.01M)	9.1
2	As in 1, but with alt	28.0	6	As in 5, but with alt.	24.3
3	Hemiacidrin (0.10M)	10.0	7	Citrate (0.10M)	18.6
4	As in 3, but with alt	54.8	8	As in 7, but with alt	43.3

Flow rate = 1 ml/min; t = 64 h (Tests, 1,3,5,7) or t = 32 h + 32 h alternation (Tests 2,4,6,8); pH 8.0.

DISCUSSION

In the past there have been several attempts to dissolve calcium-containing calculi. Stahler used citric acid (7%, pH 3.8); Otto replaced it by Solution G; Suby reported on the partial dissolution of phosphate stones by a Mg + citrate solution; Elliot et al used EDTA; Gaca used citric acid, NH_4 citrate and lactic acid. Timmermann and Kallistratos[7] treated 260 stone patients with EDTA-based irrigation solutions. In our own experiments we were interested in a wide range of new irrigation systems for calcium oxalate and phosphate calculi. Some of the tested compounds have Ca stability constants far greater than that of Ca-EDTA. The others are characterized by extremely high stability constants with oxalate. By alternating both classes of compounds in the irrigation system, a high dissolution rate of Ca oxalate calculi could be achieved, comparable with the rate of struvite dissolution in the presence of hemiacidrin.

REFERENCES

1. G. Royle and J. C. Smith, Br. J. Urol. 48:531 (1976).
2. N. J. Nemoy and T. S. Stamey, J. Urol. 116:693 (1976).
3. S. Jacobs and R. F. Gittes, J. Urol. 115:2 (1976).
4. B. Fam, A. B. Rossier, S. Yalla, and S. Berg, J. Urol. 116:696 (1976).
5. P. Leskovar, P. Allgayer, and A. Siebert, Aktuelle Nephrol. Wiss. Inf. 2:329 (1979).
6. P. Leskovar, Aktuelle Nephrol. Wiss. Inf. 1:149 (1979).
7. A. Timmermann and G. Kallistratos, J. Urol. 95:469 (1966).

POSTOPERATIVE RECURRENCE OF IDIOPATHIC CALCIUM UROLITHIASIS

K. Matsushita, K. Tanikawa, M. Ohkoshi, K. Okada,
Y. Katsuoka, H. Kinoshita, and N. Kawamura

Dept. of Urology, Tokai University School of Medicine
Iseharashi, Kanagawa, Japan

INTRODUCTION

High recurrence rates have been reported in idiopathic calcium stone disease[1]. Repeat surgery is often very difficult in previously operated patients, particularly in those who have undergone nephrolithotomy. We continue to make every effort to detect causes of the stone disease for prevention of recurrence in surgically treated patients.

METHODS

We followed up 307 patients with calcium urolithiasis of unknown etiology from February 1975 to December 1982. We sent questionnaires to 271 patients who had been hospitalized for treatment of stone disease during that period. Relevant data were extracted from the hospital records of 307 patients and from the completed questionnaires from 115 of the 271 patients contacted.

RESULTS

The mean recurrence rate of calcium stones in 307 subjects was 16.6% (51/307) at 29.0 months of follow-up. Of the total, 165 underwent 181 stone surgeries. In this operated group the true recurrence rate was 24.3% (44/181). With regard to type of operation, a high incidence of true recurrence was observed after nephrolithotomy (Table 1). In 132 of 142 unoperated patients, stones passed spontaneously. After their passage, recurrent calculus formation was noted in 7 cases (7/132, 5.3%) (Table 2).

In 53 operated patients we measured the rate of urinary calcium excretion of a single voided urine and of total daily output. Seventeen of them had postoperative recurrence, while 36 were free of recurrent stones. We classified hypercalciuria as a calcium/creatinine ratio (Ca/Cr) in a single voided urine >0.2 and a 24-h urinary calcium excretion >4 mg/kg body weight[2,3]. Hypercalciuria demonstrable on the basis of both criteria was more frequently observed in the operated group with postoperative recurrence than in that without postoperative recurrence (Tables 3 and 4).

Table 1. Relationship of Recurrence to Type of Operation.

Operation	Recurrence	
Nephrolithotomy	9/19	(31%)
Pyelolithotomy	13/51	(25%)
Ureterolithotomy	19/85	(22%)
Partial Nephrectomy	1/6	(16%)
Nephrectomy	2/10	(20%)
All operations	44/181	(24.3%)

Table 2. Recurrence Rate of Calcium Stone in the Operated and Unoperated Groups.

Recurrence	Operated Group	Unoperated Group
Recurrence	44	7
No Recurrence	137	125
Recurrence Rate[*]	24.3%	5.3%

$^{*}\chi^2$ = 22.637; P<0.005.

Table 3. Incidence of Hypercalciuria in Surgically Treated Patients with Respect to Postoperative Recurrence.

Ca/Cr (mg/dl) of Single Voided Urine	No. of Cases with Postop. Recurrence	No. of Cases without Postop. Recurrence
Ca/Cr >0.2	13	13
Ca/Cr <0.2	4	23

χ^2 = 7.52;P<0.01.

632

Table 4. Biochemical Data in Surgically Treated Patients with Respect to Postoperative Recurrence (mean ± SEM).

	Patients with Postop. Recurrence (n=46)	Patients without Postop. Recurrence (n=119)
Serum calcium (mEq/l)	4.92 ± 0.21	4.93 ± 0.25
No. with Hypercalcemia	0	2
No. with Hyperuricemia	5/46 (10.9%)	9/119 (7.5%)
No. with Hypercalciuria*	11/29 (37.9%)	12/84 (14.2%)

*χ^2= 7.43; P<0.01.

DISCUSSION

In Japan the incidence of recurrent urolithiasis is reported to be 35% at two years and 68.4% at 5 years of follow-up[4]. In our study we estimated an incidence of recurrent calcium stone disease to be 16.6% at 29.0 months of follow-up. It may be that in Japan urolithiasis other than calcium stone also recurs at a considerably high incidence rate.

The reasons why the incidence of recurrence was higher in the operated patients than in the unoperated may be multifactorial. We excluded false recurrences by examining an IVP obtained in the early post-operative period. It is possible that stones of low density are missed when they are obscured by overlying intestinal contents. Trauma to urothelium caused by surgical intervention cannot be neglected. Necrotic debris, reactive inflammatory exudates and bacterial infection may contribute to early post-operative recurrent stone formation. However, in the long-term follow-up those factors are of little importance. In this setting various metabolic abnormalities usually more or less involved in the pathogenesis of nephrolithiasis must be taken into account. We demonstrated that a higher incidence of hypercalciuria in the surgically treated patients may be one of the factors contributing to the increased incidence of postoperative recurrent stone formation. Whether or not hypercalciuria is induced by surgery of the kidneys remains to be investigated.

REFERENCES

1. F. L. Coe, "Nephrolithiasis, Pathogenesis and Treatment", Year Book Medical Publishers, Chicago (1978).
2. K. Matsushita, M. Hayakawa, T. Fujioka, and K. Odajima, J. Japan. Urol. Assoc. 72:590 (1981).

3. A. Hodgkinson and L. N. Pyrah, Br. J. Surg. 46:10 (1958).
4. O. Yoshida, J. Jap. Urol. Assoc. 70:975 (1979).

VII. ANALYTICAL METHODS
URINE AND PLASMA ANALYSIS

ADVANCES IN ANALYSIS OF URINARY OXALATE:

THE ASCORBATE PROBLEM SOLVED

G. A. Rose

St Peter's Hospitals and the Institute of Urology
London, U.K.

INTRODUCTION

Urinary oxalate is more critical than urinary calcium for calcium urolithiasis[1], but still not measured in most laboratories. Despite many new recent methods (Table 1), none has found general acceptance[2-5]. One particular difficulty concerns ascorbate. In 1933, it was reported that ascorbic acid could be oxidised to oxalate[6]. Stage 1, thought to be oxidation of ascorbate to dehydroascorbate, is catalysed by nitrite and by Fe^{3+}. In steps 2 and 3 (alkaline pH only) the latter converts to 2,3-diketogulonate and then to oxalate plus threonate. This important fact, forgotten for 50 years, was rediscovered simultaneously elsewhere[7] and here. Since several promising methods have used alkaline conditions, serious errors could be introduced by ascorbate in urine, particularly in the summer time when several mmols per day may be present. We have therefore investigated this conversion in a number of methods and found ways of preventing it. Fortunately, the oxalate decarboxylase method[2], operates at pH 3.5, where physiological ascorbate in urine does not yield detectable oxalate and it can be used as a reference method for studying the conversion. Figs. 1 and 2 show the conversion of ascorbate to oxalate under various conditions of time and pH. Fortunately, methods of preventing these conversions have recently been found. In the presence of oxygen, nitrite catalyses the oxidation of ascorbate to dehydroascorbate[8], which is stable in acid, but not in alkaline conditions. Fe^{3+} forms an unstable complex with ascorbate which quickly converts to Fe^{2+} and dehydroascorbate[9]. Rather surprisingly, and for reasons unknown, ferric chloride prevents conversion of ascorbate to oxalate. Perhaps the iron forms a stable complex with the intermediate diketogulonate.

637

Table 1. Some Recent Methods for Measurement of Urinary Oxalate.

Method	Problems
1. Instrumental	Equipment expensive
Gas Chromatography[18-21]	Needs sample preparation and/or derivative manufacture. Interference by ascorbate never checked.
Isotachophoresis[22,23]	Rather non-specific and could be interference. Ascorbate never checked.
Ion Chromatography[10]	Alkali elution causes ascorbate interference (see text).
HPLC[16]	Proven interference from ascorbate (see text).
HPLC[18]	Ascorbate depresses response.
2. Oxalate Decarboxylase	Enzyme expensive commercially but easy and cheap to make oneself.
Measuring CO_2 generation	
Warburg[24]	Cumbersome
diffusion[2,24-26]	Simple and specific but needs high level of skill and cannot be automated.
radioenzymatic[27]	Very cumbersome.
electrode[28]	Slow response, needs further development.
Measuring formate generation[15,27,35]	Needs two enzymes. May need preliminary precipitation. Commercial kit available (see text)
3. Oxalate Oxidase	Commercially available enzyme but expensive
Measuring peroxide generation[9,11,14]	Interference from many substances (see text).
Measuring CO_2 generation[29]	Very difficult to automate
4. Isotope	
Radio-isotope[30-33]	Tedious.
Stable isotopes[34]	Tedious and requires gas chromatography mass spectrometry.

ION CHROMATOGRAPHIC METHOD

Measurement of urinary oxalate by ion-chromatography (Dionex, USA) was thought to be satisfactory[10], but because of elution at pH 10.5 from the anion-exchange column any ascorbate present might be converted to oxalate. Fig . 3 shows that this is so leading to

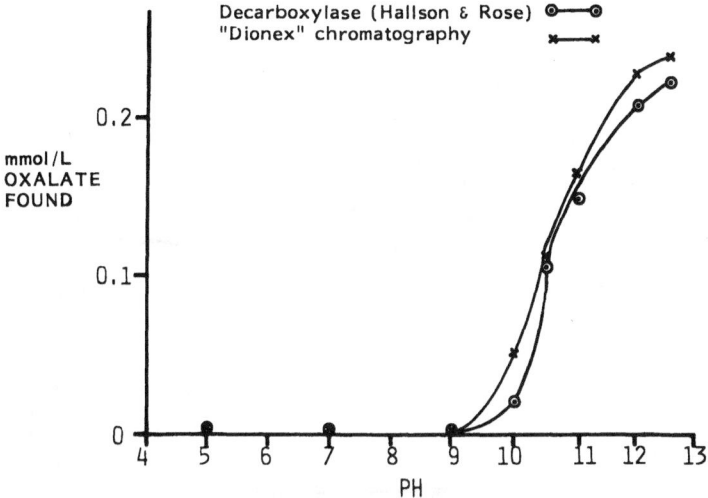

Fig. 1. Effect of pH on conversion of ascorbate to oxalate in simple aqueous solutions at room temperature.

a blurred peak coinciding with that of oxalate. This conversion is suppressed by addition of Fe^{3+} to the urine without disturbing the oxalate peak. The correlation between urinary oxalate by Dionex and oxalate decarboxylase methods is good when the Fe^{3+} step is included.

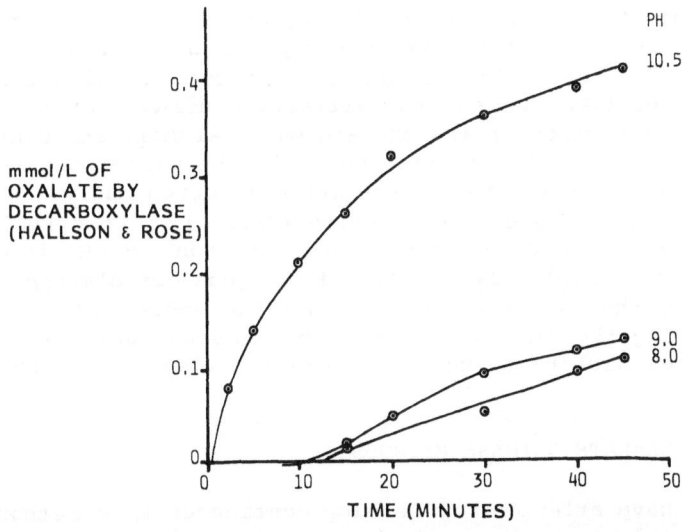

Fig. 2. Time course of in vitro conversion of ascorbate to oxalate in aqueous solution at 3 pH values and room temperature.

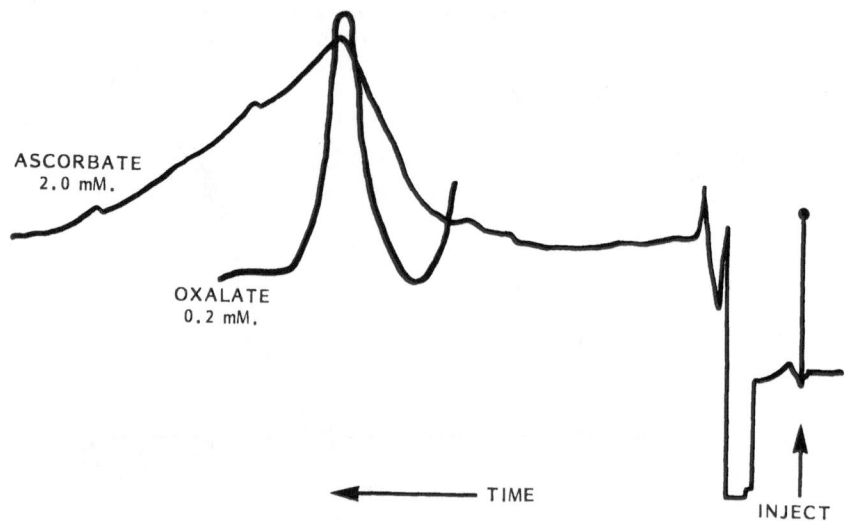

ASCORBATE
2.0 mM.

OXALATE
0.2 mM.

← TIME

INJECT

Fig. 3. "Dionex" ion-exchange chromatograms for oxalate and
ascorbate superimposed to show coincidence of the peaks
but increased width of the latter.

OXALATE OXIDASE METHOD (SIGMA KIT)

Various oxalate oxidase preparations have been described[11-13],
and methods devised for oxalate assays based upon their use[7,12,14].
Most have utilised the hydrogen peroxide generated as the basis for
colorimetric methods.   Problems have arisen in urine because of
various interfering substances which include common cations[11],
ascorbic acid, (competing oxygen receptor) and unknown
inhibitors[14,15] of oxalate oxidase.   The commercial kit marketed by
Sigma (Poole, U.K.) seemed most attractive using a simple separation
step with adsorption of the oxalate on to alumina and elution with
sodium hydroxide.   Our first results in the winter seemed good but
in summer the Sigma method gave obviously erroneously high results
apparently due to ascorbate in urine (Fig. 4).   When $FeCl_3$ was
first added to the urine (final concentration 7.6 mM) inteference by
ascorbate was completely suppressed and good correlation with the
reference method was restored.   Hence the modified Sigma kit
incorporating the $FeCl_3$ addition step seems an ideal method for
laboratories wishing to undertake small numbers of assays.

AUTOMATED OXALATE OXIDASE METHODS

Many have attempted to develop continuous flow methods for
oxalate based upon nylon coils bearing immobilized oxalate oxidase
in conjunction with peroxidase and formation of coloured dyes in

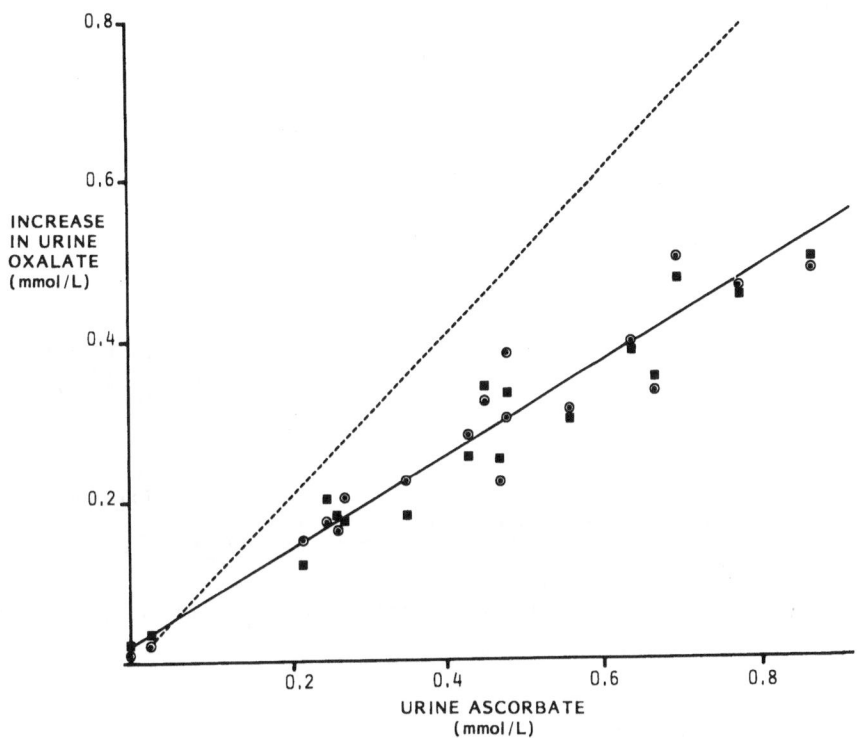

Fig. 4. Six urine samples were assayed for ascorbate with and
         without additional ascorbate. Urinary oxalate was assayed
         by oxalate decarboxylase[2] to find the true value and by
         oxalate oxidase using alumina extraction.

response to the hydrogen peroxide generated. None has previously
been satisfactory without preliminary separation steps to remove
interfering substances. Precipitation of oxalate as its calcium
salt[14] is cumbersome, and ascorbate might convert to oxalate during
the period overnight at pH 8.0. Removal of inhibitors of oxalate
oxidase from alkaline urine by charcoal[7], will very efficiently
convert ascorbate to oxalate and an "ascorbic acid.....
concentration of 1.5 mmol/l gave an apparent oxalate concentration
of 1.3 mmol/l when treated by our method". Their method is
unsuitable for patients taking citrus fruits.

     We have developed a new continuous flow automated method for
oxalate that is suitable for urine with very little preliminary
treatment. A 5-m nylon coil bears 10 IU immobilized oxalate
oxidase (Boehringer Corp). One volume of 50 mM sodium nitrite
added to 10 vols of neat urine at pH 3.5 prevents ascorbate
interference. A 50-fold dilution with pH 3.5 (0.05 M) citrate
buffer prevents inhibition by cations or other unknown inhibitors.

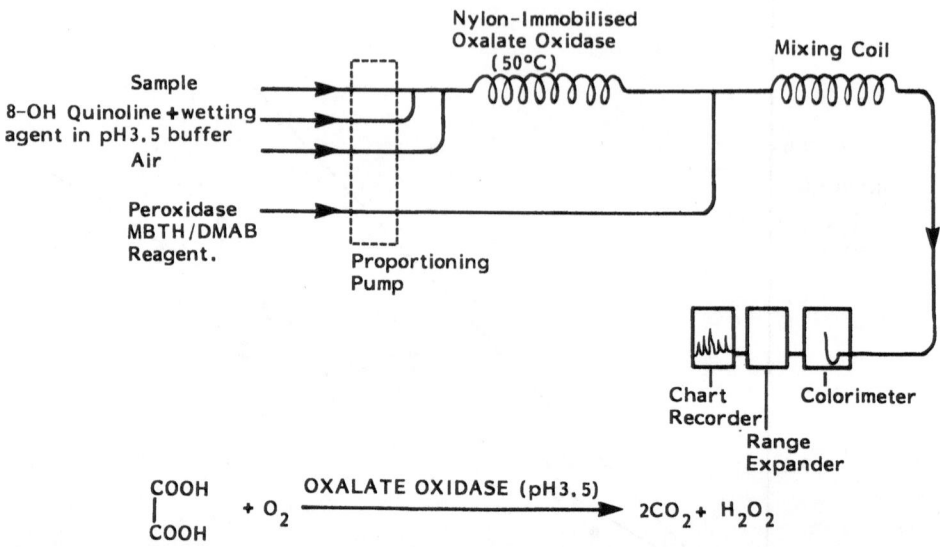

Fig. 5.   Flow chart for AutoAnalyzer method for urinary oxalate.

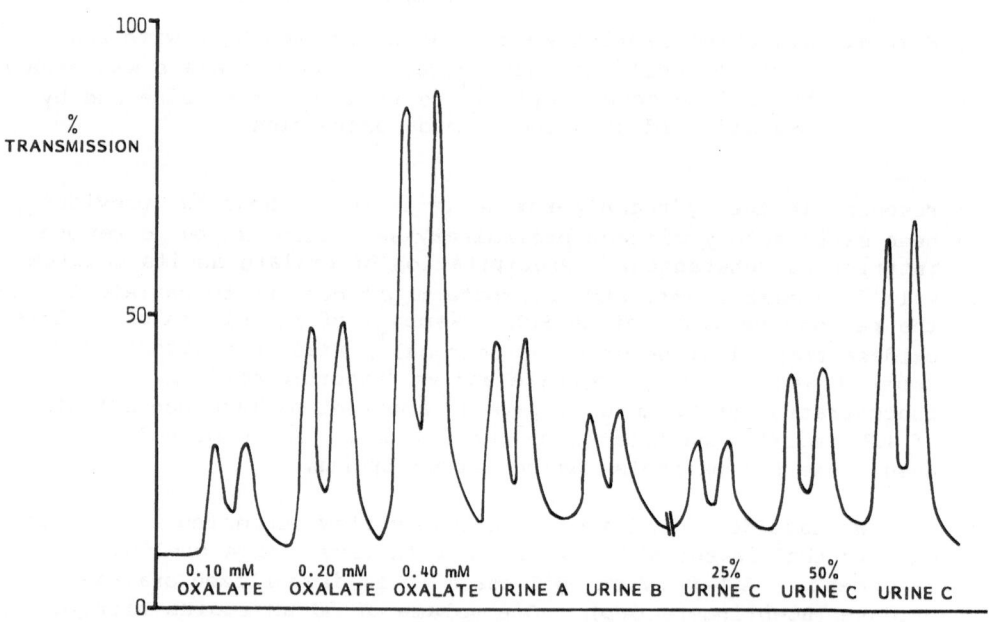

Fig. 6.   Peaks obtained from AutoAnalyzer method for urinary oxalate
at 30 samples/h.   The coil was 6-months-old.

Sufficient sensitivity is obtained by the long coil bearing the immobilized enzyme, and a 10 x scale expander between the colorimeter and the chart recorder of the AAI Auto Analyzer used at a sample speed of 30/h. The flow chart is shown in Fig. 5 and tracings of the peaks in Fig. 6. The correlation coefficient between the new and the reference method in 60 samples with oxalate concentrations of 0.02 to 0.8 mmol/l was 0.986 (y = 0.98x + 0.007). In our opinion this is now the method of choice for a laboratory wishing to undertake large numbers of urinary oxalate assays. Although the coil needs specialist preparation, it will last for many months and the procedure can be performed easily by relatively junior staff.

OTHER METHODS

Oxalate decarboxylase generates both carbon dioxide and formate from oxalate. Formate can be measured with formate dehydrogenase as a second enzyme[2,3,5] (Boehringer Co, Mannheim). However, the use of two enzymes is expensive. Moreover, ascorbic acid does partly suppress the final absorbance change. High performance liquid chromatography has been used as a method of measuring oxalate. One method[16], used a colour reagent with heating to 130°C for 15 min, which could lead to conversion of ascorbate to oxalate[17]. Another method, avoiding alkaline pH values, showed interference with ascorbate and "ascorbic acid concentrations exceeding 1.4 mmol/l gave a negative interference of 10%".

ACKNOWLEDGMENTS

The author expresses his gratitude to Dionex (U.K.) Ltd. for the loan of their instrument, to the Sigma Chemical Co. for their oxalate kits, and to Technicon Instruments Co. Ltd. for the gift of a range expander.

REFERENCES

1. W. G. Robertson and M. Peacock, Nephron 26:105 (1980).
2. P. C. Hallson and G. A. Rose, Clin. Chim. Acta 55:29 (1974).
3. G. A. Rose "Urinary Stones:Clinical and Laboratory Aspects", MTP Press, Lancaster (1982).
4. A. Hodgkinson. "Oxalic Acid in Biology and Medicine", Academic Press, London (1977).
5. G. A. Rose, W. G. Robertson, and R. W. E. Watts, eds., "Oxalate in Human Biochemistry and Clinical Pathology". Wellcome Foundation, London (1979).
6. R. W. Herbert, E. L. Hirst, E. G. U. Percival, R. J. W. Reynolds, and F. Smith, J. Chem. Soc. 1270 (1933).

7. J. E. Buttery, N. Ludvigsen, E. Braiotta, and R. R. Pannall, Clin. Chem. 29:700 (1983).

8. C. L. Walters, in:"Ascorbic Acid:Chemistry, Metabolism and Uses", R. A. Seib and B. M. Tolbert, eds., Amer. Chem. Soc. Adv. in Chem. 200 (1982).

9. G. S. Lawrence and K. J. Ellis, J. Chem. Soc. 1667 (1972).

10. M. Menon and C. J. Mahle, Clin. Chem. 29:369 (1983).

11. J. Chiriboga, Arch. Biochem. Biophys. 116:516 (1966).

12. M. F. Laker, A. F. Hofmann, and B. J. D. Meeuse, Clin. Chem. 26:827 (1980).

13. D. M. Obzansky and K. E. Richardson, Clin. Chem. 29:1815 (1983).

14. N. Potezny, R. Bais, P. D. O'Loughlin, J. B. Edwards, A. M.Rofe, and R. J. Conyers, Clin. Chem. 29:16 (1983).

15. M. Hatch, Bourke, E., and J. Costello, Clin. Chem. 23:76 (1977).

16. H. Hughes, L. Hagen, and R. A. L. Sutton, Analyt. Biochem. 119: 1 (1982).

17. N. Fituri, N. Allawi, M. Bentley, and J. Costello, Eur. Urol. 9:312 (1983).

18. A. DiCorcia, R. Samperi, G. Vinci, and G. O'Ascenzo, Clin. Chem. 28:1457 (1982).

19. B. G. Wolthers, and M. Hayer, Clin. Chim. Acta 120:87 (1982).

20. C. J. Farrington and A. H. Chalmers, Clin. Chem. 25:1993 (1979).

21. D. J. Tocco, A. E. W. Duncan, R. M. Noll, and D. E. Duggan, Analyt. Biochem. 94:470 (1979).

22. W. Tschope, R. Brenner, and E. Ritz, J. Chromatog. 222:41 (1981).

23. N. Schwendtner, W. Achilles, W. Engelhardt, P. O. Schwille and A. Sigel, J. Clin. Chem. Clin. Biochem. 20:833 (1982).

24. G. G. Mayer, D. Markow, and F. Karp, Clin. Chem. 9:334 (1963).

25. J. D. Sallis, M. F. Lumley, and J. E. Jordan, Biochem. Med. 18:371 (1977).

26. M. Bishop, H. Freudiger, U. Largiader, J. D. Sallis, R. Felix, and H. Fleisch, Urol. Res. 10:191 (1982)

27. D. J. Bennett, F. E. Cole, E. D. Frohlich, and D. T. Erwin, J. Lab. Clin. Med. 91:822 (1978).

28. R. K. Kobos and T. A. Ramsey, Anal. Chim. Acta. 121:111 (1980).

29. G. Kohlbecker, L. Richter, and M. Butz, J. Clin. Chem. Clin. Biochem. 17:309 (1979).

30. T. D. R. Hockaday, E. W. Frederick, J. E. Clayton, and L. H. Smith, L. Lab. Clin. Med. 65:677 (1965).

31. D. A. Gibbs and R. W. E. Watts, J. Lab. Clin. Med. 732:901 (1969).

32. S. Johansson and R. Tabova, Biochem. Med. 11:1 (1974)

33. O. P. Foss, "In Vitro Procedures with Radioisotopes in Medicine", IAEA, Vienna (1969).

34. D. E. Duggan, R. W. Walker, R. M. Noll, and W. J. A. Vandenheuval, Analyt. Biochem. 94:477 (1979).

35. J. Yriberri and S. Posen, Clin. Chem. 26:881 (1980).

A COMPARISON OF THREE METHODS FOR MEASURING URINARY OXALATE -

WITH A NOTE ON ASCORBIC ACID INTERFERENCE

D. S. Scurr, N. Januzovich, A. Smith, V. J. Sergeant and W. G. Robertson

Mineral Metabolism, The General Infirmary, Leeds LS1 3EX

INTRODUCTION

The measurement of urinary oxalate has become recognized as important in the investigation of patients with urinary stones[1-3]. With the advent of a new kit for the rapid enzymatic quantitation of oxalate, it is appropriate to compare the results obtained using the kit with those from other published techniques[4,5].

METHODS

Twenty-four-hour urines were collected from 25 male stone-formers (including 2 with primary hyperoxaluria). The urines were collected with 1 ml 20% (v/v) hibitane as preservative, shaken well, aliquoted and stored at $-20^{\circ}C$ prior to analysis. As far as possible, the oxalate content of each sample was measured by each of 3 methods, the colorimetric method of Hodgkinson and Williams[4], the ion-chromatographic (IC) method of Robertson et al[5] (as modified to prevent interference by ascorbic acid[6]), and the method outlined by Sigma for the determination of oxalate using oxalate oxidase[7]. A further 20 urines were collected and analysed using a modification of the Sigma technique in which 1 ml aliquots of urine were first acidified to pH 1 (instead of 3) with 1 ml of 1 M HCl. This permits more complete dissolution of any calcium oxalate crystals present in the urine than under the conditions recommended by Sigma[7].

Since ascorbic acid interferes with any oxalate method in which urine is alkalinised[6,8,9], we added increasing concentrations of ascorbic acid up to 17 mmol/l to a urine (pH 5.75) and measured oxalate by the original[5] and modified[6] IC procedures.

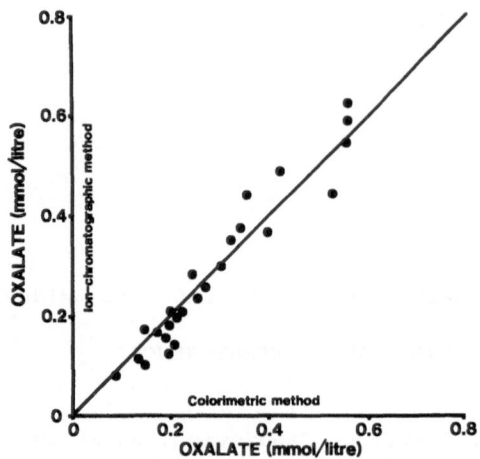

Fig. 1. A comparison of urinary oxalate concentration as measured
by ion-chromatography and by colorimetry.

RESULTS AND DISCUSSION

The comparison of oxalate concentrations in 25 urines measured
by the modified[6] IC method and the colorimetric method[4] is shown in
Fig. 1.   The good relationship between the two techniques confirms
our earlier published data[5]. The comparison of the oxalate
concentrations in 20 urines measured by the original Sigma method[7]
and the modified IC method[6] is shown in Fig. 2.

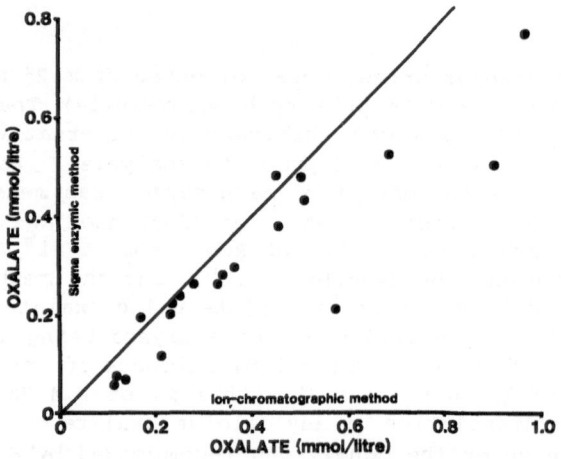

Fig. 2. A comparison of urinary oxalate concentration as measured
by the original Sigma method and by ion-chromatography.

646

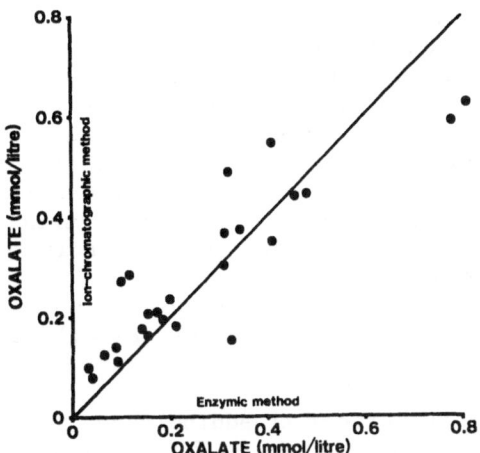

Fig. 3.   A comparison of urinary oxalate concentration as measured
by ion-chromatography and by our modified Sigma method.

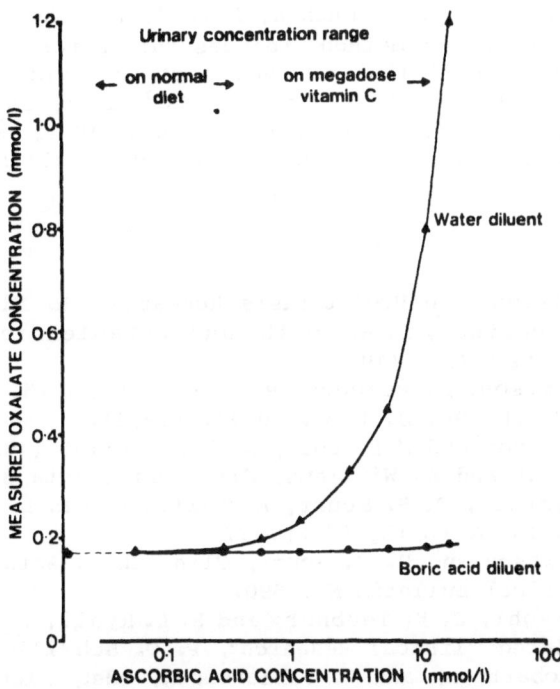

Fig. 4.   The measured oxalate concentration in urine in relation to
added ascorbic acid concentration by the original (water
diluent) and modified (boric acid diluent) ion-
chromatography techniques.

This demonstrates that the original enzymatic method underestimates oxalate on average by about 2 to 15%, but at higher oxalate concentrations the error may be as much as 50%. Amendment of the Sigma procedure to ensure dissolution of any calcium oxalate crystals present, improved the comparison between the methods considerably (Fig. 3). In the light of other studies, however, this relatively good agreement may be fortuitous. Firstly, an overestimate of oxalate may arise from the oxidation of ascorbate during the alkaline wash stage of the extraction of oxalate (and ascorbate) from urine on to alumina. Secondly, an underestimate of oxalate may occur because of incomplete extraction (85 to 90%) of oxalate from urine on to alumina during the 5 min recommended by Sigma (unpublished results). These errors will tend to cancel each other out.

Fig. 4 shows the effect of adding ascorbic acid to urine on the original[5] and modified[6] procedures for measuring urinary oxalate. Within the normal physiological range of urinary ascorbate, the error on urinary oxalate by the original method[5] is very small (<2%). Even at the upper limit of urinary ascorbate on a high vitamin C diet the error is only about 6%. However, in individuals taking megadose supplements of vitamin D (1 to 5 g/day) the error on urinary oxalate could be as much as 1 mmol/l. The boric acid diluent of the modified method[6] reduces this error to 0.014 mmol/l. It is important to note that prevention of the oxidation of ascorbate to oxalate by the addition of Fe^{3+} ions, as recommended for some methods[9], must be avoided when using IC since Fe^{3+} ions will rapidly poison the ion-exchange separator column.

REFERENCES

1. H. E. Williams, in:"Urolithiasis Research", H. Fleisch, W. G. Robertson, L. H. Smith, and W. Vahlensieck, eds., Plenum, New York (1976).
2. W. G. Robertson, M. Peacock, P. J. Heyburn, D. H. Marshall, and P. B. Clark, Br. J. Urol. 50:449 (1978).
3. W. G. Robertson and M Peacock, Nephron 26:105 (1980).
4. A. Hodgkinson and A. Williams, Clin. Chim. Acta 36:127 (1972).
5. W. G. Robertson, D. S. Scurr, A. Smith, and R. L. Orwell, Clin. Chim. Acta 126:91 (1982).
6. W. G. Robertson and D. S. Scurr, Clin. Chim. Acta 140:97 (1984).
7. Sigma Technical Bulletin No. 590.
8. B. C. Mazzachi, J. K. Teubner, and R. L. Ryall, in:"Urolithiasis and Related Clinical Research", P. O. Schwille, L. H. Smith, W. G. Robertson, and W. Vahlensieck, eds., Plenum, New York (1985).
9. G. A. Rose, in:"Urolithiasis and Related Clinical Research", P. O. Schwille, L. H. Smith, W. G. Robertson, and W. Vahlensieck, eds., Plenum, New York (1985).

THE EFFECT OF ASCORBIC ACID ON URINE OXALATE MEASUREMENT

B. C. Mazzachi, J. K. Teubner, and R. L. Ryall

Depts. of Clinical Biochemistry and Surgery
Flinders Medical Centre, Bedford Park, Australia

INTRODUCTION

We report that conditions employed in the pre-treatment of the urine are crucial to the correct estimation of oxalate. Interference of ascorbic acid, a common urinary constituent, has been noted in a number of different methods. After systematic investigation of the steps in our assay, we have found that this interference is associated with the pre-treatment conditions, particularly any pH adjustment with alkali, pH of precipitation, and collection and storage of urine. We describe conditions for assay which give minimal interference by ascorbic acid and which are applicable to all urinary oxalate methods.

MATERIALS AND METHODS

Urinary oxalate was measured by gas-chromatography of dimethyl oxalate, after overnight precipitation of oxalate from urine using calcium chloride and ethanol[1].

Twenty-four-hour urine collections were put into bottles either without stabliser (plain collection) or containing 50 ml of 3 mol/l HCl (acid collection). Prior to oxalate measurement all urine specimens were adjusted to pH < 1.6 and mixed well.

The effect of altering the pH of precipitation was studied as follows. (L+)ascorbic acid (Merck, Darmstadt, FRG) was added to acid collections to a final concentration of 0, 1, 5 or 15 mmol/l. Samples were assayed for oxalate after precipitation at pH values of 5, 6, 7 and 8.

649

The rate of increase in measured oxalate at alkaline pH was measured as follows. Samples of urines with added ascorbic acid as above were alkalinised to pH 9, using 1 mol/l NaOH, for periods of 0, 1, 5 and 30 min, then immediately readjusted to pH 5 for overnight precipitation.

The effects of collection and storage of urine were studied by taking aliquots of an acid collection with added ascorbic acid as above and storing them for one month at $-70^\circ C$, $-20^\circ C$, $4^\circ C$ and room temperature. These were assayed for oxalate after precipitation at pH 5. In a further study, urine collections were obtained from two women (A and B) who had been taking daily doses of 4 g ascorbic acid. Each voided sample collected over a 24-h period was halved: one half was put into a plain bottle and the other into an acid bottle. Each half was then aliquoted and stored at $-70^\circ C$, $-20^\circ C$, $4^\circ C$ and room temperature. Aliquots were assayed for oxalate after storage for 0, 2, 9, 15 and 29 days at the above temperatures. Plain aliquots were acidified immediately prior to assay.

RESULTS AND DISCUSSION

The pH of precipitation used in various urinary oxalate methods ranges from pH 5 to 8. As ascorbic acid can form oxalate on standing in solution, especially under alkaline conditions[2], we determined the effect of pH of precipitation on urinary oxalate measurement in the presence of ascorbic acid. Consistent results were obtained for all urines studied. For example at pH 7, 15 mmol/l added ascorbic acid caused more than a 200% increase in measured oxalate above the basal level of 0.2 mmol/l, and this rose to more than 300% at pH 8. A 20% increase was obtained with only 1 mmol/l added ascorbic acid at pH 8. However, with precipitation at pH 5 and 6, there was minimal increase in measured oxalate (pH 5 <10%, pH 6 <15%) with up to 15 mmol/l added ascorbic acid. As normal levels of ascorbic acid in urine range from 0 to 3.4 mmol/day and may reach 16 mmol/day in subjects taking oral ascorbic acid[3], pH 7 or 8 should not be used for precipitation of oxalate due to possible in vitro formation of oxalate from ascorbic acid. We chose pH 5 for all further precipitation of oxalate from urine, which gave good analytical recoveries of 95.8% (SD 3.8%, n = 50), and between-run coefficients of variation for two urine controls of 5.4% (oxalate = 0.23 mmol/l) and 4.4% (oxalate = 0.58 mmol/l), where n = 19 in each case.

Investigation of the rate of increase in measured oxalate in the presence of ascorbic acid at alkaline pH showed this to be very rapid (Fig. 1). When urine samples containing 1 mmol/l added ascorbic acid were exposed to pH 9 for only 1 min, an increase of 50% above the basal oxalate value resulted. This increased to more than 200% after exposure for 30 min. With higher levels of added

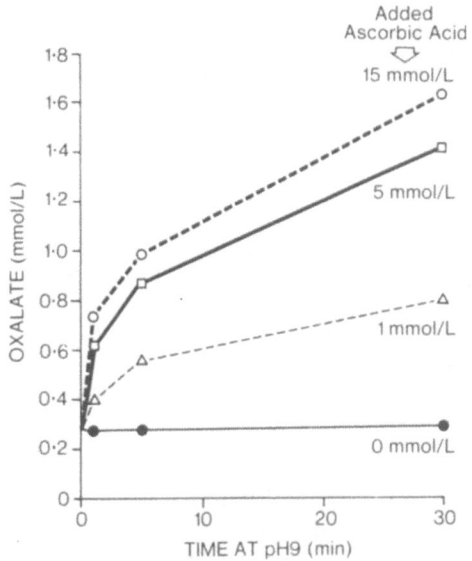

Fig. 1. The rate of increase in measured oxalate on alkalinisation
to pH 9 of urine with added ascorbic acid levels of 0 (●),
1 (△), 5 (□), or 15 (o) mmol/l.

ascorbic acid the rate of increase was even more rapid.   These
results confirm and extend previous comments on spontaneous
decomposition of ascorbic acid to oxalate in vitro.   Thus, if urine
is made alkaline for even a short time prior to oxalate measurement,
ascorbic acid present will cause a falsely elevated result.   Hence
use of dilute alkali and constant mixing are required when adjusting
pH, to prevent localised regions of high pH.

        Stability of stored urine for measured oxalate is also
affected by the prsence of ascorbic acid.   Acidified urine was
stable for oxalate when stored for one month at -70^oC or -20^oC with
up to 15 mmol/l added ascorbic acid.   However, this level of
ascorbic acid resulted in a 30% increase in measured oxalate with
storage at 4^oC, and a 55% increase at room temperature.   The type
of collection is also important with storage as shown in Fig. 2 for
plain and acid collections from subject A taking oral ascorbic acid.
The acid collection was stable for oxalate at -70^oC, -20^oC and 4^oC,
but increased by over 30% after storage for 9 days at room
temperature.   The plain collection, however, was markedly unstable
at both 4^oC and room temperature, but was stable for up to one month
at -70^oC.   Similar stabilities of urine for measured oxalate were
found with subject B.   Consequently, to ensure minimal increase in
measured oxalate from ascorbic acid plain urine collections should
be stored at -70^oC and acid collections at -20^oC or -70^oC (stable
for one month.   Currently there is a large range of methods for

651

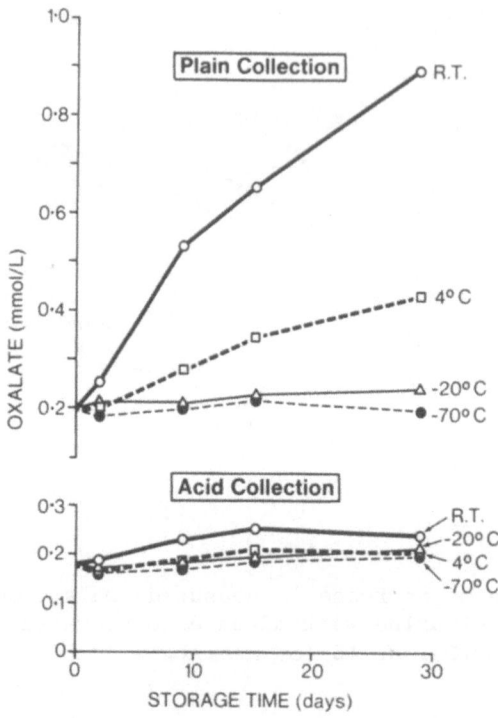

Fig. 2. The stability with respect to measured oxalate of a 24-h
urine collection equally divided between plain and acid
bottles from subject A taking oral ascorbic acid, with
storage over a one month period at $-70^\circ C$ (●), $-20^\circ C$ (▲),
$4^\circ C$ (□), and room temperature R.T. (o).

urinary oxalate measurement[4]. Many of these methods subject the
urine to pH values of 7 or above prior to assay, giving inaccurate
oxalate measurement in the presence of any ascorbic acid.

REFERENCES

1. B. C. Mazzachi, J. K. Teubner, and R. L. Ryall, Clin. Chem.
   30:(1984) (in press).
2. B. M. Tolbert, M. Downing, R. W. Carlson, M. K. Knight, and
   E. M. Baker, Ann. N. Y. Acad. Sci. 258:48 (1975).
3. C. Hughes, S. Dutton, and A. S. Truswell, J. Human Nutr. 35:274
   (1981).
4. M. F. Laker, in:"Advances in Clinical Chemistry" Vol. 23,
   A. L. Latner and M. K. Schwartz, eds, Academic Press, New
   York (1983).

SPONTANEOUS IN VITRO GENERATION OF OXALATE FROM L-ASCORBATE IN

SOME ASSAYS FOR URINARY OXALATE AND ITS PREVENTION

G. P. Kasidas and G. A. Rose

Institute of Urology and St Paul's Hospital
24 Endell Street, London WC2, U.K.

INTRODUCTION

Erroneously high levels of urinary oxalate were noticed in the summertime with the Sigma enzymatic oxalate assay[1]. It was thought that L-ascorbate might be responsible for this artifactual increase since L-ascorbate may be oxidised to oxalate via dehydroascorbate and diketogulonate[2]. We therefore studied this conversion in conditions used in some of the assays for urinary oxalate.

METHODS

Aqueous solutions of L-ascorbate and urine samples with and without added L-ascorbate were processed by the alumina extraction step as used in Sigma oxalate kit[1] for separating urinary oxalate. Oxalate levels in the alkali extracts were measured by four different assays:- (i) A routine enzymatic oxalate decarboxylase assay[3]; (ii) the Sigma oxalate kit assay[1]; (iii) a newly developed automated oxalate assay[4] using immobilised oxalate oxidase. Oxalate is oxidised during transit through a nylon tube with covalently attached oxalate oxidase. The H_2O_2 formed from the oxidation of oxalate is quantitated colorimetrically at 580 nm using peroxidase, 3-methylbenzothiazolinonehydrazone and 3-dimethyl-aminobenzoic acid. This assay is accurate (mean recovery of added oxalate in spiked urine samples is 93 $\pm$ 11 %), reproducible (within batch CV 3.5%; between batch CV 5%) and relatively rapid (15 samples/h). The detection limit for this assay ($<$1.0 μmol/l oxalate) permitted the dilution of the samples by 1/50 with normal levels of urinary oxalate. This assay correlated well (r = 0.99 and y = 0.99x - 0.003) with the oxalate decarboxylase[3] assay when

653

110 urine samples were separately assayed by the two methods. (iv) Dionex ion-chromatography[5].

L-ascorbate in aqueous and urine samples was measured by titration with 2,6-dichlorophenolindophenol (DCPIP)[6].

The following two procedures were used for the removal of interference by L-ascorbate: (i) One volume of 74 mM $FeCl_3$ in 3 M HCl was mixed with 10 volumes of sample, diluted 1/25 and assayed for oxalate by ion-chromatography and by the Sigma kit after alumina extraction. (ii) One volume of 50 mM $NaNO_2$ in pH 3.5, 0.05M citrate buffer was added to 10 volumes of sample and vortex mixed. Nitrite treated samples were diluted 1/50 with pH 3.5, 0.05 M citrate buffer and assayed directly with the automated oxalate assay.

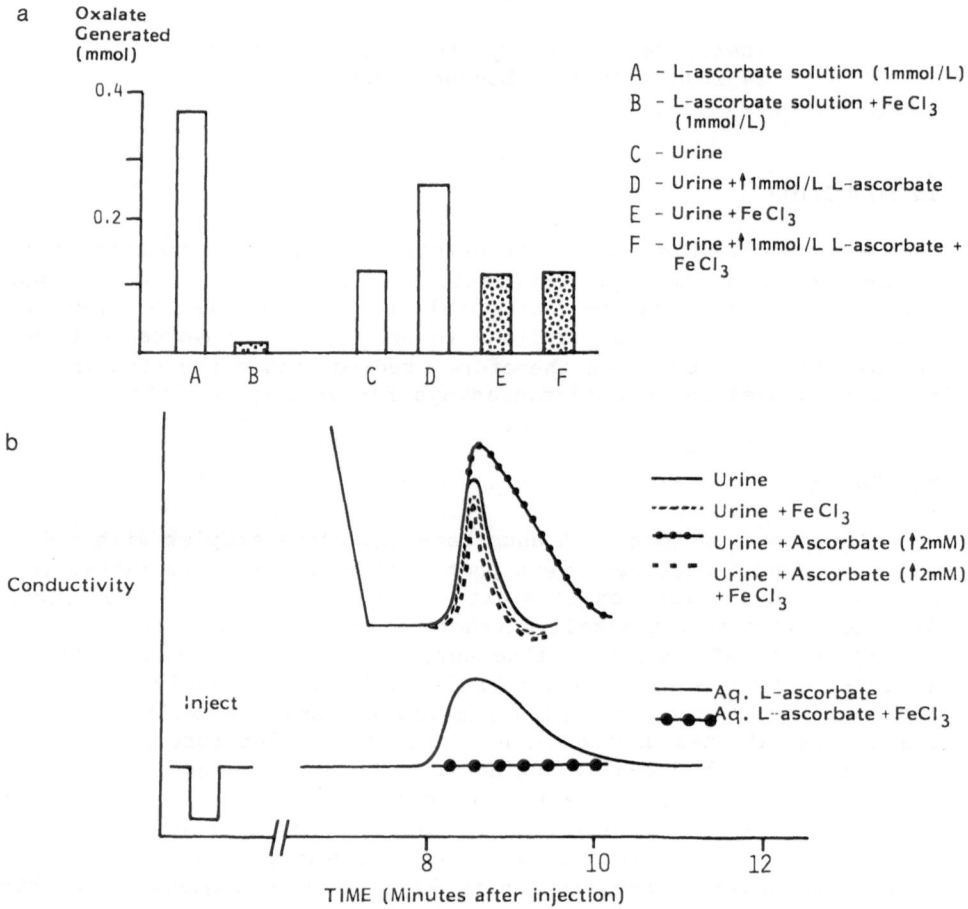

Fig. 1. (a) Removal of L-ascorbate interference with acidic $FeCl_3$ in (a) Sigma assay and (b) the Dionex assay.

RESULTS AND DISCUSSION

With the oxalate decarboxylase assay[3], conversion of
L-ascorbate to oxalate did not occur and it was used as a reference
method to study the conversion in other assays. The conversion of
L-ascorbate to oxalate increases with increasing pH[4] and is enhanced
by activated charcoal. The conversion of L-ascorbate to oxalate
following alkaline elution of acidic components adsorbed onto
alumina was 83% and 63% complete in aqueous solutions and urine
respectively[4]. In the Dionex assay, 2 mM (352 mg/l) L-ascorbate
increased the oxalate peaks by 30% and 44% in aqueous solutions and
urine respectively.

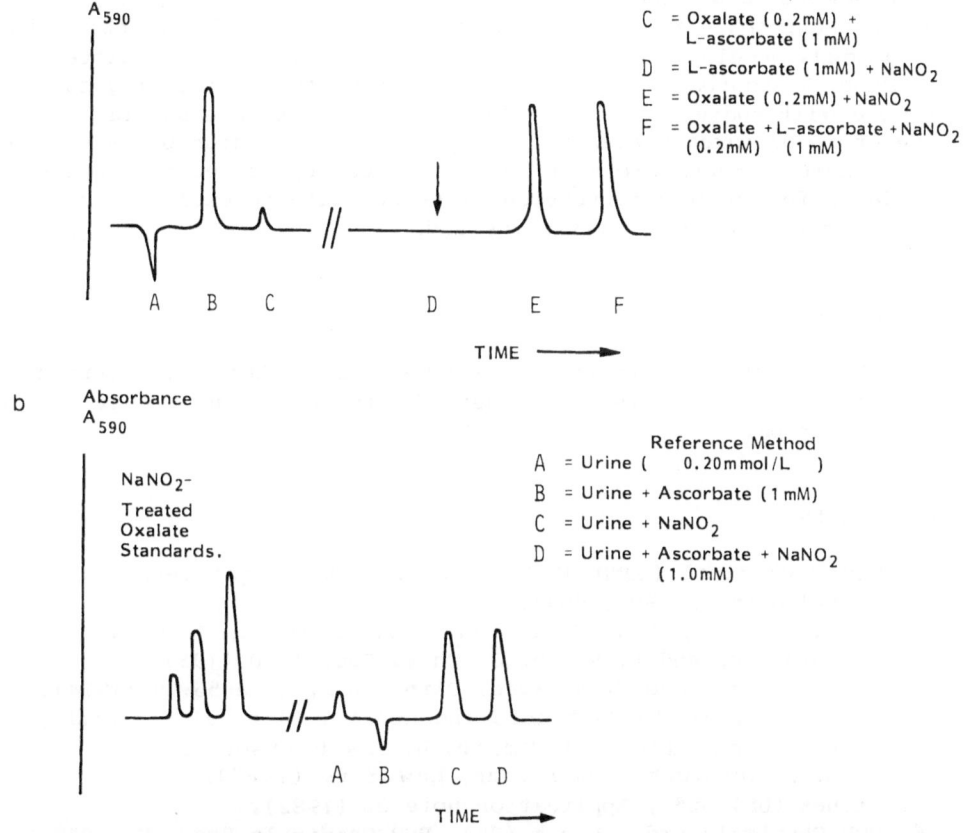

Fig. 2. (a) The elimination of L-ascorbate interference with $NaNO_2$
in the automated assay; (b) as in (a) but with urine. $NaNO_2$
treated oxalate standards (0.1, 0.2, 0.4 mmol/l) and urine
L-ascorbate with and without $NaNO_2$ are shown.

Preliminary studies demonstrated that acidic ferric chloride removed L-ascorbate (DCPIP tritation[6]) in aqueous solution and in urine. As seen in Fig. 1, the prior removal of L-ascorbate by acidic ferric chloride does not interfere with the assay of oxalate in samples by either the Sigma Kit[1] or Dionex ion-chromatography[5].

Preliminary studies demonstrated that $NaNO_2$ removed L-ascorbate (DCPIP titration). Fig. 2 shows that when oxalate was assayed by the newly developed automated assay, treatment by $NaNO_2$ eliminates interference from ascorbate, without affecting the oxalate level in either aqueous solutions or urine.

Because of the ease with which L-ascorbate is converted to oxalate, especially under alkaline conditions, normal urinary levels of L-ascorbate will give serious interference in oxalate assays which use alkaline pH[1,5,7,8] thus making them unsuitable. Here we have demonstrated that Sigma[1] and Dionex[5] methods could be used after L-ascorbate in urine is removed with acidic ferric chloride. In a newly developed automated assay using immobilised oxalate oxidase, L-ascorbate interference is eliminated by treating the sample with sodium nitrite. All assays for oxalate should therefore be investigated for the possible conversion of L-ascorbate to oxalate. Furthermore, it may be necessary to reconsider the evidence for in vivo conversion of L-ascorbate to oxalate since this might have occurred in vitro instead.

ACKNOWLEDGMENTS

We are grateful to the Sigma Chemical Co. Ltd. for providing us with their oxalate kits and Dionex (UK) for the loan of their IC 16 chromatograph.

REFERENCES

1. Sigma Chemical (LOND) Co.Ltd. (Poole, UK). Sigma Technical Bulletin No 590 (1983).
2. R. W. Herbert, E. L. Hirst, E. G. V. Percival, R. J. W. Reynolds, and F. Smith. J. Chem. Soc. 1270 (1933).
3. P. C. Hallson and G. A. Rose, Clin. Chim. Acta 55:29 (1974).
4. G. A. Rose, in:"Urolithiasis and Related Clinical Research", P. O. Schwille, L. H. Smith, W. G. Robertson, and W. Vahlensieck, eds. Plenum, New York (1985).
5. Dionex (UK) Ltd., Application note 36 (1982).
6. BDH Chemicals Ltd., Poole (UK), BDH Chemicals Prod. No. 23021.
7. J. E. Buttery, N. Ludvigsen, E. A. Braiotta, and P. R. Pannall, Clin. Chem. 29:700 (1983).
8. M. F. Laker, A. F. Hofmann, and B. J. D. Meeuse. Clin. Chem. 26:877 (1980).

ENZYMATIC ASSAY OF OXALATE USING OXALATE OXIDASE FROM

SORGHUM LEAVES

C. S. Pundir, R. Nath, and S. K. Thind

Dept. of Biochemistry, Postgraduate Institute of
Medical Education and Research, Chandigarh-160012, India

INTRODUCTION

Estimation of oxalate in biological fluids using plant and moss
enzyme has met with limited success owing to the inhibition of the
enzyme activity by sodium ions normally present in these fluids[1-4].
In this communication, we report on the separation and partial
purification of a highly active oxalate oxidase from sorghum leaves
which is not inhibited by sodium ions in physiological
concentrations and is suitable for direct estimation of oxalate in
urine and other biological fluids.

MATERIALS AND METHODS

The enzyme was isolated from the leaves of 10- to 12-day-old
seedlings of Sorghum vulgare L. which were frozen at $-20^{\circ}C$ using the
method of Chiriboga[2]. The supernatant after centrifugation at
15000 x g was further purified with 30 to 65% ammonium sulphate and
the pellet collected at 10000 x g used as the source of the enzyme.
This preparation was stored at $0-4^{\circ}C$. Assay of the enzyme was
based on the formation of H_2O_2 which was estimated colorimetrically
by the reaction with 4-aminophenazone and the peroxidase system[5].
Preliminary assay of the enzyme showed a pH optimum of 5.0 and a
temperature optimum of $45^{\circ}C$. Activation (150%) of the enzyme was
noted with Fe^{2+} ($5 \times 10^{-4}M$) and FAD ($1 \times 10^{-5}M$). A K_m of 2.4×10^5
mol/l was obtained under optimal conditions[6]. Sodium ions (up to
0.2M) had no effect on the activity of this enzyme compared with the
same enzyme from other sources (Table 1). A simple specific and
sensitive method of oxalate assay has been devised using this
enzyme.

657

Table 1. Comparative Effect (in %) of Na^+ on Oxalate Oxidase Activity.

Added NaCl (mmol)	Bougainvillea enzyme[7]	Barley enzyme	Sorghum enzyme[5]
20	–	–59	0
40	–	–75	0
60	–	–81	+4
80	–	–84	–4
100	–50	–	+4
200	–	–	0

– = Inhibition; + = Stimulation. The enzyme was incubated with 1 μmol of oxalate, 80 μmol of sodium succinate, 1 μmol of $FeSO_4$ and NaCl at pH 5 and $40^{\circ}C$ for 10 min.

The colour reagent was prepared as described by Bais et al[6] and consisted of 0.05 g of 4-aminophenazone, 0.1 g of phenol and 1 mg of horseradish peroxidase per 100 ml of 0.4M sodium phosphate buffer at pH 7.0. It was stored in the amber-coloured bottle at $4^{\circ}C$. Fresh reagent was prepared each week.

Either fresh or stored urine was diluted in a proportion of 1:10 with 0.05M sodium succinate buffer, pH 5.0. The reaction mixture consisted of 0.05M sodium succinate buffer at pH 5.0, containing 1.8 ml of Fe^{2+} ($10^{-4}M$), diluted urine (0.1 ml) and enzyme in a total volume of 2.0 ml. Appropriate controls were run with each assay. After incubation at $45^{\circ}C$, for 10 min, 1.0 ml of colour reagent was added to each tube and the tubes shaken and allowed to stand at room temperature ($\sim 32^{\circ}C$) for 30 min. The colour intensity was read at 520 nm and the values of oxalate in urine samples read from the standard curve of oxalate concentration versus units of enzyme activity, where one enzyme unit is defined as the amount of enzyme required to generate 1 nmol of H_2O_2/min under the standard conditions of assay. Protein was estimated according to the standard Lowry method.

RESULTS AND DISCUSSION

In the range of 0 to 1 μmol oxalate, linearity was observed for enzyme activity. Pre-incubation of enzyme with NaCl up to 0.2 M concentration had no effect on its activity (Table 2). So far oxalate oxidase reported from other plant sources has been shown to be NaCl-sensitive and more than 50% inhibition was observed in the presence of 0.1 M NaCl. The lack of sensitivity to NaCl of the sorghum oxalate oxidase suggests that it is better suited than the

Table 2. Effect of Na^+ on Assay of Oxalate in Urine.

Added NaCl mmol/l	Activity of oxalate oxidase (μmol H_2O_2/10 min)
0.05	0.115
0.10	0.110
0.15	0.110
0.20	0.120
No addition (control)	0.110

The diluted urine (0.1 ml) was incubated in presence of 80 μmol sodium succinate (pH 5.0), 1 μmol of $FeSO_4$, enzyme protein (0.3 mg) and NaCl, at a final volume of 2.0 ml at 40°C for 10 min.

Table 3. Values of Urinary Oxalate in 7 Healthy Men as Determined by Sorghum Oxalate Oxidase.

Sample	Urine oxalate concentration (μmol/l)	% Recovery of added 10 nmol oxalate
1	210	103
2	310	99
3	290	98
4	300	100
5	320	95
6	280	102
7	290	96
Mean $\pm$ SD	280 $\pm$ 34	99 $\pm$ 2

The diluted urine (0.1 ml) was incubated with 80 μmol of sodium succinate (pH 5), 1 μmol $FeSO_4$ and 0.3 to 0.4 mg enzyme protein (30 to 65% $(NH_4)_2SO_4$ ppt) at 40°C for 10 min.

same enzyme from other sources to the direct estimation of oxalate in urine and other biological fluids.

The assay is sensitive to concentrations of urinary oxalate as low as 0.01 μmol/sample and is highly reproducible. The measured recovery of 10 nmol of oxalate added to urine was 99% (Table 3). The addition of NaCl to urine up to 0.1 M concentration had no influence on the measured oxalate concentration.

REFERENCES

1. J. Chiriboga, Biochem. Biophys. Res. Commun. 11:277 (1963).
2. J. Chiriboga, Arch. Biochem. Biophys. 116:516 (1966).
3. M. J. Laker, A. F. Hofman, and B. J. D. Meeuse, Clin. Chem. 26:827 (1980).
4. J. E. Buttery, N. Ludvigsen, E. A. Braiotta, and P. R. Pannal, Clin. Chem. 29:700 (1983).
5. C. S. Pundir and R. Nath, Phytochemistry (1984) (in press).
6. R. Bais, N. Potenzy, J. B. Edward, A. M. Rofe, and R. A. J. Conyers, Analyt. Chem. 52:508 (1980).
7. S. K. Shrivastava and P. S. Krishnan, Biochem. J. 85:33 (1962).

DETERMINATION OF URINARY OXALATE BY REVERSED-PHASE

ION-PAIR "HIGH-PERFORMANCE" LIQUID CHROMATOGRAPHY

L. Larsson, B. Libert, and M. Asperud

Dept. of Clinical Chemistry, Linköping University
Linköping, and Dept. of Plant Breeding, Swedish
University of Agricultural Sciences, Uppsala, Sweden

INTRODUCTION

Calcium oxalate is an important constituent of the majority of renal stones. Thus measurement of urinary oxalate has become essential in the basic evaluation of the urolithiasis patient. However, the large number of published methods indicate the presence of considerable methodological difficulties[1]. In this paper we describe our recently developed method for determination of urinary oxalate, based on a reversed-phase ion-pair "high-performance" liquid chromatography (HPLC)[2]. We also describe a comparison performed between our HPLC method, the colorimetric method of Hodgkinson and Williams[3], and a commercial enzymatic method[4].

MATERIALS AND METHODS

Oxalate determinations were performed on urine from 31 consecutive urolithiasis patients from our stone clinic. The urine specimens were obtained as 24-h collections in plastic bottles containing 15 ml of 6 mol/l HCl. The colorimetric procedure was performed according to Hodgkinson and Williams[3]. The enzymatic method was based on degradation of oxalate by oxalate oxidase and performed according to the Sigma instruction manual[4]. For these two methods the urine was acidified to pH < 3.0. The HPLC procedure has been previously described in detail[2]. However, before HPLC analysis, we adjusted the pH of the sample to 2.0 ± 0.1 with orthophosphoric acid. A 2 ml aliquot of urine was injected into an octadecyl-silane bonded-phase packing (Sep-pak C_{18} cartridge; Waters Associates, Milford, MA 01757) that had been pre-treated by successively passing through it 2 ml of methanol and 5 ml of water.

The first 0.5 ml of urine that passed through the cartridge was discarded and the next 1 ml was used for analysis. The standard solutions were treated in the same way. This procedure removes non-polar and semi-polar substances. We then injected a 50 µl aliquot of the "cleaned up" sample into the HPLC system.

RESULTS

Fig. 1 shows a comparison between the results obtained from our HPLC method, and the colorimetric and enzymatic methods. When comparing the HPLC and colorimetric procedures (Fig. 1A) it should be noted that the slope deviated significantly from 1 (t=4.91, df=29, P < 0.001). Higher values were obtained for the colorimetric method above 400 µmol/l although we found no difference between the mean values obtained with these techniques (Sign test 12/31, n.s.). The HPLC method produced significantly higher values than the enzymatic method (Fig. 1B) (Sign test 4/31, P<0.001). We also found significantly higher values for the colorimetric compared with the enzymatic procedure (Fig. 1C) (Sign test 2/31, P < 0.001).

The within-assay standard deviation, calculated from the duplicate determination with analysis of variance[5], was 7.8, 11.8 and 8.0 µmol/l for the HPLC, colorimetric and enzymatic procedures respectively, corresponding to a CV of 3.1, 4.7 and 3.2% at 250 µmol/l. The precision of the HPLC procedure was significantly better than that of the colorimetric (F=2.24, df 30/30, P < 0.01) but not better than that of the enzymatic method (F=1.01, df 30/30, n.s.). The precision of the enzymatic method was also significantly better than that of the colorimetric method (F=2.17, df 30/30, P<0.01). The between-assay precision of the three methods was estimated from duplicate analyses of our internal assay control, a pooled urine. The control was assayed at the beginning of a six-sample series. The mean value was 184 (SD 19) µmol/l (CV 10.3%), 236 (SD 26) µmol/l (CV 11.0%) and 89 (SD 8) µmol/l (CV 9.0%) for the HPLC, colorimetric and enzymatic procedures, respectively.

DISCUSSION

These comparisons were performed on the same urine samples in the same laboratory. Only two comparative studies have previously been presented[6,7] and one of these[6] was performed in 6 different laboratories which means that inter-laboratory differences would affect the evaluation. The HPLC and colorimetric methods did not differ below the 400 µmol/l level. Above 400 µmol/l higher values were obtained by the colorimetric procedure (Fig. 1A). This may partly be explained by the important feature of our HPLC method, i.e. the preparative treatment of urine samples with Sep-pak C_{18} cartridges which eliminate interfering substances.

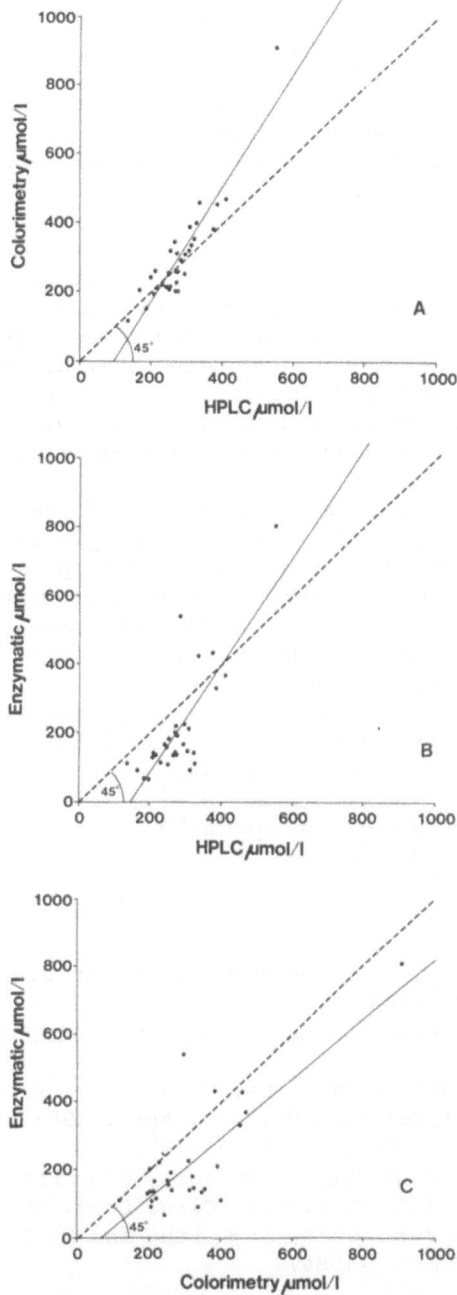

Fig. 1. Correlations between oxalate concentrations determined by HPLC, colorimetry and enzymatic procedures.

We found lower values for the enzymatic procedure than for HPLC (Fig. 1B), which is in contrast to Zerwekh et al[6] who reported overestimation by the enzymatic procedure and underestimation by HPLC. However, the reason for this discrepancy was not reported. In agreement with our lower findings for the enzymatic method, Scurr et al[7] have reported the Sigma enzymatic procedure to underestimate oxalate by 20 to 50%. However, this underestimation was reported to be almost eliminated[7] by a further acidification of the urine to pH 1.0, which is in agreement with our experience from a preliminary experiment.

Our intra-assay coefficients of variation for all methods were lower than reported by Zerwekh, a discrepancy partly explained by the fact that the same personnel performed all our analyses. Our intra-assay figures agree well with those previously reported for individual assays. It should be noted that our HPLC and the enzymatic procedures had the same intra-assay precision but both were significantly better than the colorimetric technique. All our tested methods, however, had an intra-assay variation below 5%.

Unfortunately, we have no experience of the enzymatic procedure on a routine basis, but this method was simple and faster than both the colorimetric and HPLC procedures, and it produced results with the same intra-assay precision as the HPLC procedure. It can also be noted that the equipment needed for the enzymatic procedures was not as expensive as that for HPLC. In our hands HPLC is not significantly faster, but more convenient than the colorimetric procedure of Hodgkinson. As HPLC was more precise than the latter, and thus better for detecting small but significant changes, we chose the HPLC procedure for routine use. The low analytical capacity of the HPLC procedure could also be considerably improved if the injection procedure is automated.

REFERENCES

1. W. G. Robertson and A. Rutherford, Scand. J. Urol. Nephrol. Suppl. 53:85 (1981).
2. L. Larsson, B. Libert, and M. Asperud, Clin. Chem. 28:2274 (1982)
3. A. Hodgkinson and A. Williams, Clin. Chim. Acta 36:127 (1972)
4. Sigma Technical Bulletin No. 590, April 1983.
5. D. Rodbard, Clin. Chem. 20:1265 (1974).
6. J. E. Zerwekh, E. Drake, J. Gregory, D. Griffith, A. F. Hofmann, M. Menon, and C. Y. C. Pak, Clin. Chem. 29:1977 (1983).
7. D. S. Scurr, N. Januzovic, A. Smith, and W. G. Robertson, Urol. Res. 12:90 (1984).

HUMAN PLASMA OXALATE CONCENTRATION RE-EXAMINED

F. E. Cole, K. M. Gladden, D. J. Bennett, and
D. T. Erwin

Division of Research, Alton Ochsner Medical Foundation
New Orleans, La., U.S.A.

INTRODUCTION

There is a discrepancy between the plasma oxalate concentrations measured by in vitro chemical/enzymatic techniques[1,2] (~10 μmol/l) and in vivo isotopic dilution methods (~1 μmol/l) [3,4]. However, recent chemical/enzymatic estimates of plasma oxalate concentration range between 2 and 4 μmol/l[5-7].

ASSAY MODIFICATIONS

To optimize the sensitivity of the radioenzymatic-isotope dilution assay (REIDA) at low substrate concentrations, samples were incubated for 4 min at 37°C, in a sodium citrate buffer (pH 3.2) with an isotope concentration of 100,000 cpm/0.1 ml in a sodium citrate buffer (pH 3.2) with an isotope concentration of 100,000 cpm/0.1 ml[1,8]. For rapid precipitation studies, plasma was ultrafiltered by centrifugation in N_2 for 1 h at 4°C at 1000 x g directly into 2 glass centrifuge tubes containing 0.3 ml 136 mM $CaCl_2$, 12.2 ml 95 % ethanol (v/v), and 1 drop 1 M HCl. The pH of the resulting ultrafiltrate was 7.3. Calcium oxalate (CaOx) was allowed to precipitate for 3 h at room temperature. The precipitate was lyophilized and stored at -20°C. The lyophilized CaOx was dissolved with 1 ml 0.3 M HCl, extracted with ether and dried using a stream of N_2 at room temperature. The dried CaOx was reconstituted with citrate buffer and assayed. The "rapid" precipitation resulted in lower recoveries of the ^{14}C-oxalate internal standard when compared with the former[1] method (70% versus 90%). Sample preparation can be further simplified by limiting the ether extractions from five to three 10 ml extractions.

665

The mean ^{14}C-oxalate recovery was reduced from 83% to 76% using three extractions. Rapid precipitation of plasma oxalate combined with three extractions resulted in recoveries of 56% of ^{14}C-oxalate from plasma. Occasional spuriously high blanks occurred when plain (non-fire-cleaned) glassware was used. Using glassware fired in a self-cleaning oven for 1 h to remove trace organic material, a mean reagent blank value equivalent to 0.24 µmol/l was obtained.

IN VITRO OXALOGENESIS

A fresh plasma pool was divided into samples for: (A) direct precipitation, where ice-cold plasma was ultrafiltered by centrifugation for 1 h directly into a cold (4°C) centrifuge tube containing acidified precipitating solution, (B) delayed precipitation, where the ice-cold plasma was ultrafiltered into a cold, dry centrifuge tube, but the ultrafiltrate was then exposed to room temperature for an additional 55 min before precipitation and (C) delayed ultrafiltration, where the whole plasma was exposed to room temperature for 115 min before ultrafiltration at 4°C directly into a 4°C acidified precipitating solution (Tables 1 and 2). The time between phlebotomy and the initiation of precipitation for (A) was 1 h and 45 min for (B), 4.5 h and for (C), 3 h. It should be noted that samples (A) and (C) were precipitated gradually over the 1 h of centrifugal ultrafiltration, whereas the entire sample (B) was precipitated at one time. The direct precipitation samples (A) yielded significantly lower oxalate levels than the delayed precipitation (B) and delayed ultrafiltration (C) groups, indicating that an in vitro increase in oxalate occurred in both plasma ultrafiltrate and whole plasma. Furthermore, the delayed precipitation samples (B) were significantly higher than the delayed ultrafiltration samples (C).

Table 1. In Vitro Oxalogenesis (µmol/l).

Immediate Ultrafiltration A Direct Precipitation	Immediate Ultrafiltration B Delayed Precipitation	Delayed Ultrafiltration C Direct Precipitation
6.48	17.27	13.07
6.82	15.91	10.00
5.80	17.50	10.34
Mean +SD 6.37 + 0.52	16.89 + 0.86***	11.14 + 1.65***++

Each value represents analyses in triplicate. Statistical analysis was performed using a t-test. **P<0.01 compared with A; ***P<0.001 compared with A; ++P<0.01 compared with B.

666

Table 2. Oxalate Concentrations (μmol/l) using Direct Precipitation (Mean $\pm$ SD).

Rapid Ultrafiltration		Delayed Ultrafiltration	
A	B	C	D
No Inhibitor	With Inhibitor	No Inhibitor	With Inhibitor
4.43	4.66	10.23	11.14
3.86	3.41	8.98	11.48
3.75	2.73	8.75	10.34
-	3.64	7.50	11.48
4.01$\pm$0.37	3.61$\pm$0.80	8.87$\pm$1.12***	11.11$\pm$0.054***++

The individuals studied were apparently healthy white males, aged 22 to 60, taking no medication and with no personal or family history of kidney stones. The samples were drawn after a 12-h overnight fast. ***P<0.001 compared with A or B; ++P<0.01 compared with C.

EFFECT OF INHIBITORS

Plasma oxalate concentrations have been suggested to be erroneously high due to an inhibitable in vitro conversion of glyoxalate[5]. In an attempt to verify this suggestion, 11 paired plasma samples were collected with and without inhibitor and the oxalate was precipitated indirectly[1]. No significant difference was noted between the two groups. Similar studies were done with the direct precipitation technique using "fire-cleaned" glassware. A fresh plasma pool was divided into 4 samples as shown in Table 2, plasma ultrafiltered rapidly in the presence and absence of inhibitors, and plasma ultrafiltered after a 105-min delay at room temperature in the presence and absence of inhibitors. In the samples processed rapidly, no significant difference in oxalate content was found between the plasma samples collected with or without inhibitors. As noted earlier, an in vitro increase in plasma oxalate was demonstrated when ultrafiltration and precipitation were delayed and inhibitors did not prevent it.

ULTRAFILTRATE pH

We noted that plasma ultrafiltrates lay between pH 8 and 9 and investigated whether or not this alkalinity aggravated the observed oxalogenesis. In a single sample, we estimated plasma oxalate concentrations to be 1.40, 1.45, 1.15, 0.70, 0.90 μg/ml in ultrafiltrate collected in HCl to yield pHs of 8.17, 6.92, 5.94, 4.00 and 2.15 respectively. This pH-related reduction of oxalogenesis was confirmed by experiments in two other individuals where estimates of plasma oxalate concentrations from ultrafiltrates at pH 4.0 were 66.% and 56% of those observed at pH 7.0.

DISCUSSION

It has been reported recently that plasma oxalate concentration increases rapidly following phlebotomy and this observation is confirmed in the present report. In one study[5], the increase in oxalate is attributed to the conversion of glyoxylate to oxalate. Our results and those of others[6] do not support this contention but suggest that ascorbate may be the principal source of the nascent in vitro oxalate since (a) oxalate concentration increases more in the more alkaline ultrafiltrates of plasma, a finding consistent with the reported base-catalyzed conversion of ascorbate to oxalate[9],and (b) the process is at least in part non-enzymatic. In 3 individuals, oxalogenesis decreased ($\sim$50%) with the pH of their plasma ultrafiltrate. Thus the discrepancy in estimates of plasma oxalate concentration by in vivo and in vitro assay methods is explainable, at least in part, by a rapid in vitro oxalogenesis which can be minimized using the precautions described in this report. Most importantly, these data suggest that appropriate sample handling may be more important than analytical methodology for accurate measurement of plasma oxalate concentrations less than 2 to 3 μmol/l (as estimated by in vivo isotope dilution measurements)[3,4]. If the in vivo estimates are accurate, they indicate a net renal secretion of oxalate.

ACKNOWLEDGEMENT

This work was supported in part by the Purdue Frederick Co., Norwalk, Connecticut.

REFERENCES

1. D. J. Bennett, F. E. Cole, E. D. Frohlich, and D. T. Erwin, Clin. Chem. 25:1810 (1979).
2. M. Hatch, E. Bourke, and J. Costello, Clin. Chem. 23:76 (1977).
3. H. E. Williams, G. A. Johnson, and L. H. Smith, Clin. Sci. 41:213 (1971).
4. A. Hodgkinson and R. Wilkinson, Clin. Sci. Mol. Med. 46:61 (1974).
5. T. Ackay and G. A. Rose, Clin. Chim. Acta 101:305 (1980).
6. M. Maguire, N. Fituri, B. Keogh, and J. Costello, in:"Urolithiasis:Clinical and Basic Research", L. H. Smith, W. G. Robertson and B. Finlayson, eds., Plenum, New York (1981).
7. B. G. Wolthers and M. Hayer, Clin. Chim. Acta 120:87 (1982).
8. E. A. Newsholme and K. Taylor, Biochim. Biophys. Acta 158:11 (1968).
9. A. Cantarow, B. Schepartz, eds., "Biochemistry", 4th ed. Saunders, Philadelphia (1967).

THE MEASUREMENT OF OXALATE AND GLYCOLATE WITH IMMOBILIZED

ENZYME SYSTEMS

R. Bais, N. Potenzny, A. M. Rofe, and
R. A. J. Conyers

Metabolic Research Group, Division of Clinical
Chemistry, Institute of Medical and Veterinary Science
Adelaide, Australia

INTRODUCTION

Renal stone disease afflicts up to 10% of the male population and calcium oxalate is a major component in over 70% of these stones[1,2]. Diet has traditionally been considered to be the main source of oxalate but, more recently, it has become accepted that the majority of oxalate is derived from endogenous metabolism. Glycolic acid has been identified as a major precursor of oxalate[2,3] and variations in the urinary excretion of this precursor may be important. However, there is little information available regarding its excretion. For the study of the effects of glycolate and oxalate excretion on renal stone formation, specific and sensitive assays for these compounds have been developed in our laboratory.

METHODS

Oxalate oxidase (EC 1.2.3.4) and glycolate oxidase (EC 1.1.3.1) were bound to nylon tubing and used in a continuous-flow system. Conditions for immobilization consist of activating the nylon tubing with triethyloxonium tetrafluoroborate and binding the protein with glutaraldehyde[4,5]. Oxalate oxidase can be bound directly but because commercial preparations of glycolate oxidase are supplied as an enzyme suspension containing ammonium sulphate and flavin mononucleotide (FMN), the enzyme requires pre-treatment. This entails washing the enzyme with ammonium sulphate to remove excess FMN and dissolving the enzyme in 20 mmol/l phosphate buffer (pH 7.3) before immobilization. When not in use the nylon tubing is stored at $4^{O}C$ in a damp bag covered with aluminium foil. Approximately 1.5 m of the immobilized enzyme coil is incorporated into a Technicon Auto-

Analyzer AAII system.   A sampler II operating at 10/h with a 1:2
sample to wash ratio is used.   After contact with the enzyme, the
sample is mixed with the color reagent[5].

Because of the presence of a potent inhibitor of oxalate oxidase in urine, oxalate must be precipitated before assay[5].   There
is also material present in urine that interferes with the glycolate
assay and the samples must be pre-treated using charcoal[6].   Once
immobilized, oxalate oxidase is very stable and in our laboratory
one coil has been used to analyse at least 1200 samples.   However,
immobilized glycolate oxidase is much less stable and the loss of
activity cannot be prevented or reversed by adding albumin,
glycerol, dithiothreitol or high concentrations of FMN ($>$2.0 mmol/l).
We have attempted to prevent inactivation by cross-linking the
enzyme subunits with glutaraldehyde and dimethyl suberimidate before
immobilization but this also has proved unsuccessful.

RESULTS AND DISCUSSION

Previous work showed that partially purified glycolate oxidase
could be stabilized by ammonium sulphate at an ionic strength of 2.0
(0.66 mol/l)[7].   We have repeated this work with the commercial
enzyme preparation (Sigma Chemical Co.) at varying FMN
concentrations and shown that the enzyme loses activity over an 8-
day period, after which it remains stable at 20 to 40% of its
initial activity (Fig. 1).   Because of these results, we chose a
buffer which consists of 20 mmol/l sodium phosphate (pH 7.4),

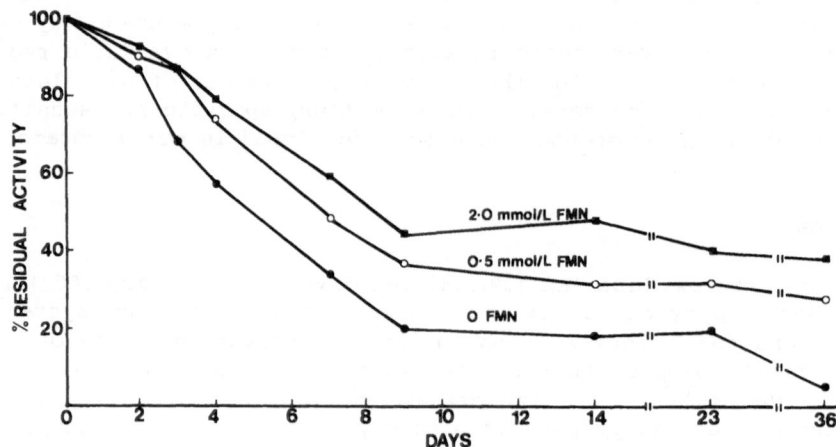

Fig. 1.   The stability of purified glycolate oxidase from spinach.
Samples were removed at the times indicated and assayed at
a glycolate concentration of 5 mmol/l using the system
described for the immobilized enzyme.

0.66 mol/l ammonium sulphate and 0.5 mmol/l FMN.   Although a higher
concentration of FMN was shown to increase the stability of the
enzyme, increasing the FMN concentration in the diluent buffer was
impractical because it interfered with the color reaction.   We have
analyzed more than 300 samples using a single immobilized enzyme
coil.   To compensate for any variation in the enzymic activity,
standards are always assayed in both immobilized systems.

   Fig. 2 shows recordings from both immobilized enzyme systems
and demonstrates the characteristics of continuous flow sampling,

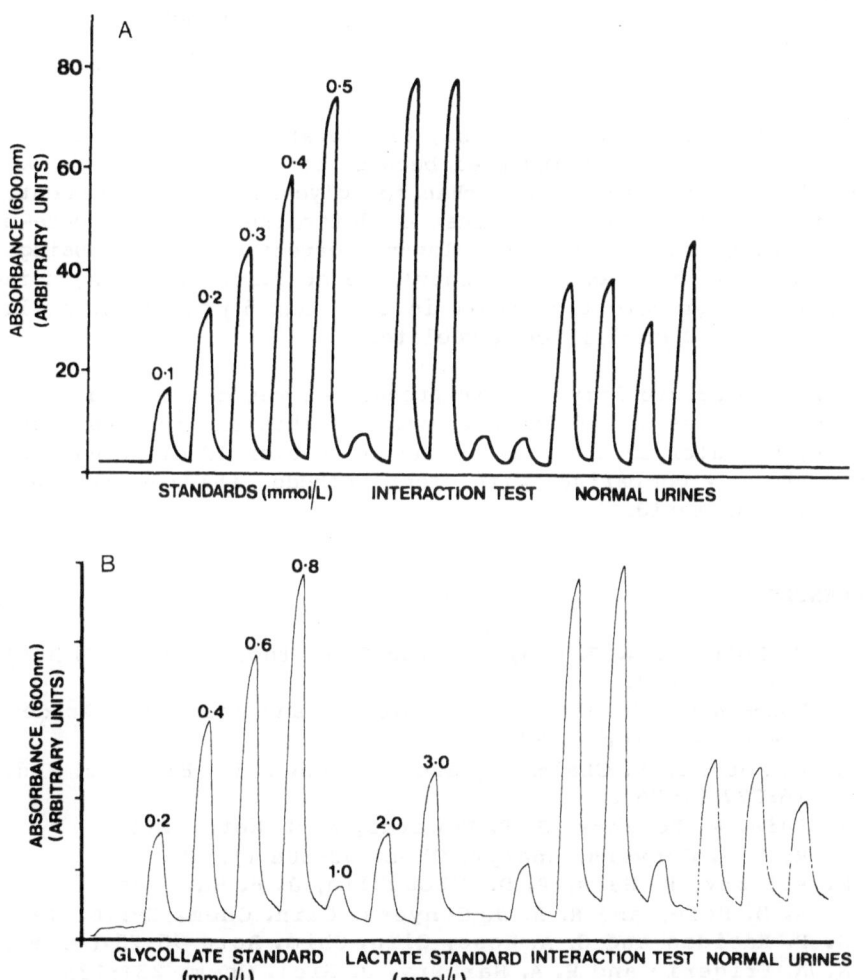

Fig. 2.   The assay of urinary oxalate (A) and glycollate (B) using
         the immobilized enzyme system.   See text for details of
         the sample preparation and the immobilized enzyme system.

Table 1. Precision of Immobilized Oxalate Oxidase and Glycolate
Oxidase Systems.

Oxalate	Within Batch		Between Batch	
No. samples	20	16	12	10
Mean (mmol/l)	0.43	0.56	1.18	0.39
SD (mmol/l)	0.005	0.007	0.012	0.018
CV (%)	1.17	1.21	1.01	4.64

Glycolate	Within Batch		
No. samples	20	20	20
Mean (mmol/l)	0.31	0.45	0.70
SD (mmol/l)	0.011	0.026	0.007
CV (%)	3.5	5.8	0.9

concentration samples. The assay of lactate by the glycolate
oxidase system has been included because this oxidation also occurs,
although at a much lower rate than for glycolate. The concentration of lactate in any sample must be determined, in this case using
lactic dihydrogenase, and the relevant correction made. Using the
criterion that the peak height should be at least twice the noise
level, the lower detection limit is less than 5 μmol/l for oxalate
and less than 20 μmol/l for glycolate.

The reproducibility of both procedures was determined by
multiple analyses of 3 different urines within one run, and for
oxalate, by multiple analyses of one urine over 10 different runs
(Table 1). By comparison with other methods, the are precise,
sensitive and rapid.

REFERENCES

1. A. M. Rofe, R. A. J. Conyers, and D. W. Thomas, Med. J. Aust.
   2:158 (1981).
2. A. Hodgkinson, "Oxalic Acid in Biology and Medicine", Academic
   Press, New York (1977).
3. A. M. Rofe, A. H. Chalmers, and J. B. Edwards, Biochem. Med.
   16:277 (1976).
4. R. Bais, N. Potezny, J. B. Edwards, A. M. Rofe, and
   R. A. J. Conyers, Analyt. Chem. 52:508 (1980).
5. N. Potezny, R. Bais, P. D. O'Loughlin, J. B. Edwards,
   A. M. Rofe, and R. A. J. Conyers, Clin. Chem. 29:16 (1983).
6. G. P. Kasidas and G. A. Rose, Clin. Chim. Acta 96:25 (1979).
7. N. A. Frigerio and H. A. Harbury, J. Biol. Chem. 231:135
   (1958).

THE VALUE OF OXALATE DETERMINATION BY HIGH-PERFORMANCE LIQUID CHROMATOGRAPHY IN CLINICAL PRACTICE

T. Sugimoto, J. Blömer, E. Jungling, F. Recker, Y. Funae, and R. Hautmann

Depts. of Urology and Physiology, RWTH Aachen, FDR and Dept. of Urology and Laboratory of Chemistry University Medical School, Osaka, Japan

INTRODUCTION

Approximately 70% of human urinary calculi contain calcium oxalate. Therefore, measurement of oxalate in urine is important clinically. Various methods for measuring oxalate have been reported, but most are unsuitable for clinical practice. Recently, high-performance liquid chromatography (HPLC) has enabled excellent separation of fatty acids and other low molecular substances to be made from biological fluids. The method is simple and accurate but because the UV detection of fatty acids (at 210 nm or below) is poor in terms of sensitivity and selectivity, they have to be derivatized to produce a stronger absorbance. Some investigators have labeled oxalate with a UV-absorbing compound and with it have assayed oxalate directly in urine. We have used 9-anthryldiazomethane (ADAM) as a labeling reagent for carboxylic acids[1] and found that oxalate reacted smoothly with it to form a fluorescent diester derivative. Aliquots of the reaction mixture were chromatrographed directly on HPLC and analyzed.

MATERIALS AND METHODS

ADAM was purchased from the Funakoshi Chemical Co. Ltd. (Tokyo, Japan). All solvents, oxalate and tri-n-butyl phosphate were of analytical reagent grade. Twenty-four-hour urine samples were collected in bottles containing 5 ml of xylene, and 5 ml aliquots were frozen at -20°C until assayed.

Chromatographic analysis was performed using a Toyo Soda HLC-803B (Tokyo, Japan), Shimadzu RF-530 fluorescence detector (Tokyo,

673

Japan), and a Shimadzu C-RIA data processor. Chromatographic
separation was carried out on a column of 300 x 4mm (Toyo Soda
LS410K, octadecylsilane reverse-phase type).

Urine (0.5 ml) was mixed with 2 N HCl (0.05 ml) in a 10 ml test
tube and tri-n-butyl phosphate (0.5 ml) added. The mixture was
stirred vigorously for 2 min, centrifuged for 10 min at 3000 rpm,
and the organic layer (0.2 ml) transferred to a second 10 ml test
tube. Methanol (0.2 ml) and 0.4 ml of the solution of ADAM in
ethylacetate (2.5 mg/ml) were added and the mixture allowed to stand
for 90 min at room temperature. A 15 µl aliquot was injected onto
the HPLC column and eluted with aqueous acetonitrile ($CH_3,CN:H_2O$,
75:25, v/v) at a rate of 1.7 ml/min at room temperature. The
fluorescence intensity was measured at 410 nm with excitation at 254
nm, and the peak area calculated by a data processor.

RESULTS

Figs. 1 and 2 respectively show the chromatograms of urine from
a non-stone former and urine from which the oxalate had been removed
by the precipitation with calcium sulfate and ethanol. The oxalate
diester was eluted at 15 min. The peaks which were eluted earlier
consisted mainly of the decomposition products of ADAM and the polar
acid ester derivatives. The calibration curve was derived from the
peak area, plotted against the concentration of oxalate. The
linearity was excellent (r = 0.999) over the range 1 to 100 µg/ml.

Oxalate (5, 10, 15, and 20 ug) was added to multiple samples of
a urine with a basal oxalate of 20.8 µg/ml and the assay repeated.
The measured values were 26.1, 31.2, 37.1, and 42.2 µg/ml. The
relationship between peak area and added oxalate was linear
(r = 0.999). The recoveries of added oxalate in the experiments
using two different urine samples ranged between 95 and 105%. Even
at low concentrations, the recovery was adequate. Thus, the
presence of contaminating substances in urine could be ruled out.

The determination of precision was performed using two urine
samples of low (A) and high (B) concentration of oxalate. The mean
($\pm$ SD) values were 10.4 $\pm$ 0.32 and 27.5 $\pm$ 1.02 µg/ml, respectively.
The reproducibility of the method was very high, the coefficient of
variation being 3.0 and 3.7%, respectively.

The correlation between the values obtained by this method and
by the colorimetric method of Hodgkinson and Williams[2] was linear
(r = 0.881). The variation of the values measured by the
colorimetric method was wide at concentrations 5 µg/ml.

The mean ($\pm$ SD) of the daily urinary excretion of oxalate of 20
non-stone formers on a normal diet was 23.8 $\pm$ 9.0 mg, this value

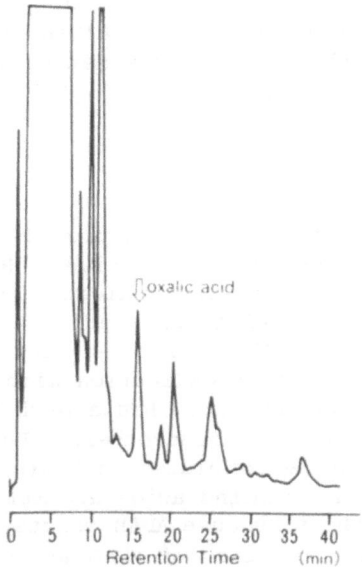

Fig. 1. Chromatogram of a normal urine.

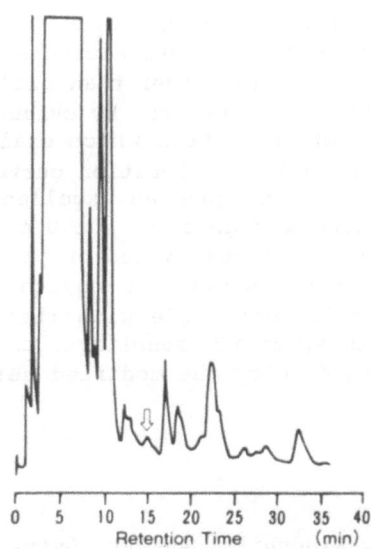

Fig. 2. Chromatogram of urine from which oxalate was removed by precipitation.

being slightly lower than values reported by other workers[2,3]. Good agreement was noted between the values of daily urinary excretion of oxalate obtained by this method and values obtained using the colorimetric method.

DISCUSSION

The reaction of oxalate and ADAM proved to be slow in saline and yielded mainly a monoester derivative. However, oxalate reacted readily with ADAM to form a diester in organic solvents. Therefore, extraction of oxalate from urine using an organic solvent appeared to be feasible. We used tri-n-butyl phosphate for the extraction of oxalate[4] because extraction with ether was time-consuming. Tri-n-butyl phosphate has a much higher partition coefficient with oxalate than does ether. Furthermore, using this solvent, extraction can be completed in 2 min, and basic and water-soluble substances such as amino acids are removed. This method is more specific than others because ADAM reacts with the carboxyl group only. Since the reaction of ADAM and oxalate proceeded smoothly in the preparation containing tri-n-butyl phosphate, this solvent did not have to be evaporated. The reaction mixture containing oxalate diester was injected directly onto the HPLC column and the eluate measured fluorometrically. Fluorometric detection is much more sensitive than UV detection. ADAM and its decomposition products were eluted before the oxalate diester. The other dicarboxylic acids, as well as monocarboxylic acids, were completely separated from oxalate. Hydrophilic carboxylic acids such as malic or hippuric acid were eluted earlier than oxalate. There were no carboxylic acids other than oxalate with the same retention time. This was supported by evidence from the chromatogram (Fig. 2) of urine from which oxalate was removed by precipitation. Because the calibration curve of peak area against the concentration of oxalate gave an excellent linearity (r = 0.999) and the reproducibility was good (CV = 3.0 or 3.7%), we did not use an internal standard. The mean value of the urinary excretion of oxalate by non-stone formers was 23.8 mg/24h with a range of 9.3 to 41.2 mg. This value is compatible with that reported by others[2,3]. This new technique is specific, sensitive, and readily set up. We are now attempting to develop the modified method of assay of oxalate in plasma.

REFERENCES

1. N. Nimura and T. Kinoshita, Analyt. Lett. 13:191 (1980).
2. A. Hodgkinson and A. Williams, Clin. Chim. Acta 36:127 (1972).
3. P. C. Hallson and G. A. Rose, Clin. Chim. Acta 55:29 (1974).
4. P. M. Zarembski and A. Hodgkinson, Biochem. J. 96:717 (1965).

ENZYMATIC DETERMINATION OF OXALATE IN URINE

H. O. Beutler, M. H. Town, J. Ziegenhorn, and
B. Hammer

Boehringer Mannheim GmbH, Biochemical Research Center
D-8132 Tutzing, F.R.G.

INTRODUCTION

Oxalate is a major component of urinary stones and its concentration in urine is important for urolithiasis. Many methods have been described for the determination of oxalate in urine, but so far none has found application in the routine clinical laboratory. The classical chromotropic acid procedure[1] is time-consuming, non-specific, and susceptible to interference. Techniques such as gas-chromatography, HPLC and ion-chromatography involve complex methodology and specialized equipment. We have developed a simple and specific spectrophotometric assay, based on the method of Beutler et al[2], using the enzymes oxalate decarboxylase and formate dehydrogenase. In addition, a method of sample preparation is described which prevents the precipitation of oxalate during storage, resulting in better recovery and precision.

METHODS

The method is based on the fact that oxalate decarboxylase splits oxalate to formate and CO_2 at pH 5.0 and the formate is oxidized to bicarbonate by nicotinamide adenine dinucleotide (NAD) at pH 7.5 by formate dehydrogenase. The increase in NADH, which is stoichiometric with the oxalate destroyed, is determined by means of its absorbance at 334 (Hg) 340 or 365 (Hg) nm.

The oxalic acid kit produced by Boehringer, Mannheim, GmbH was used. It consisted of a phosphate/citrate buffer (pH 5.0), oxalate decarboxylase, phosphate buffer (pH 9.5), β-NAD, and formate dehydrogenase. Dipotassium oxalate (Merck) was used for standards.

677

EDTA was added to urine (500 mg/l) to prevent the formation of insoluble oxalates[3]. Urine samples were analyzed immediately or adjusted to pH 1 for storage. The pH was adjusted to 5 before the determination of oxalate as follows:

Pipette into Cuvettes	Sample Blank (ml)	Sample (ml)	Reagent Blank (ml)	Standard (ml)
Buffer Solution (pH 5)	0.10	0.10	0.10	0.10
Urine Sample (pH 5)	0.20	0.20	–	–
Standard (20 mg/l Oxalic Acid)	–	–	–	0.20
Re-distilled Water	–	–	0.20	–
Oxalate Decarboxylase	–	0.05	–	0.05

Mix and incubate for 30 min at room temperature. Then add:

NAD/Phosphate Buffer	2.00	2.00	2.00	2.00
Re-distilled Water	0.05	–	0.05	–

Mix and read absorbance after approximately 2 min. Then add:

Formate Dehydrogenase	0.05	0.05	0.05	0.05

Mix, incubate for 40 min at room temperature and read absorbances.

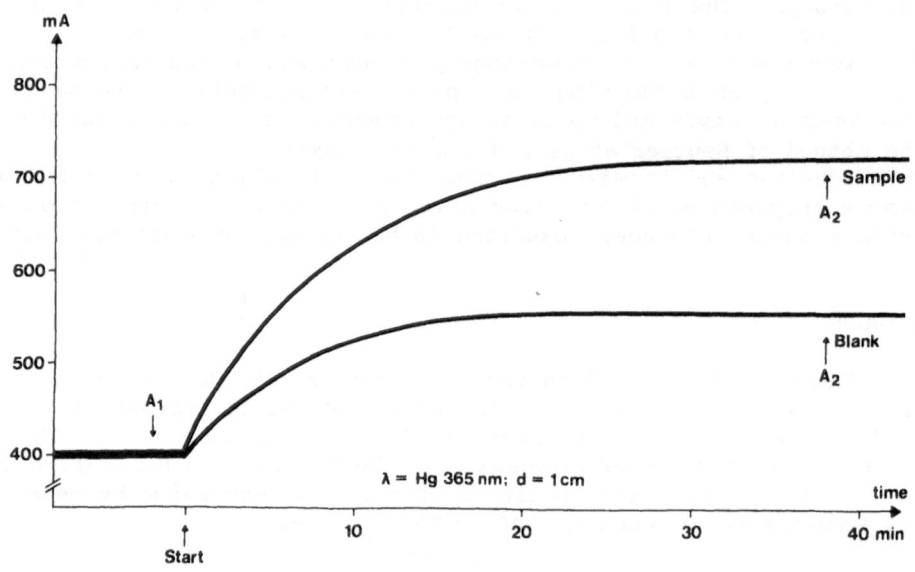

Fig. 1. The reaction time-course of oxalate in urine.

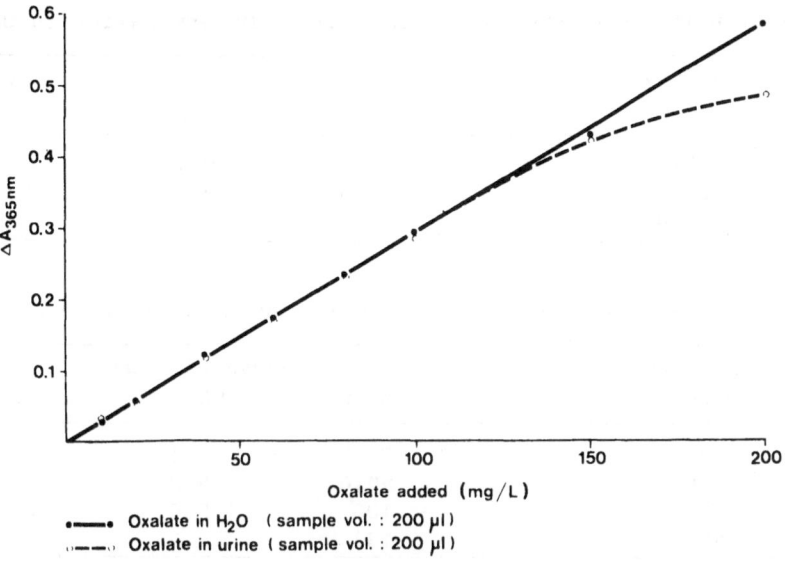

Fig. 2. The effect of urine on the standard curve for oxalate.

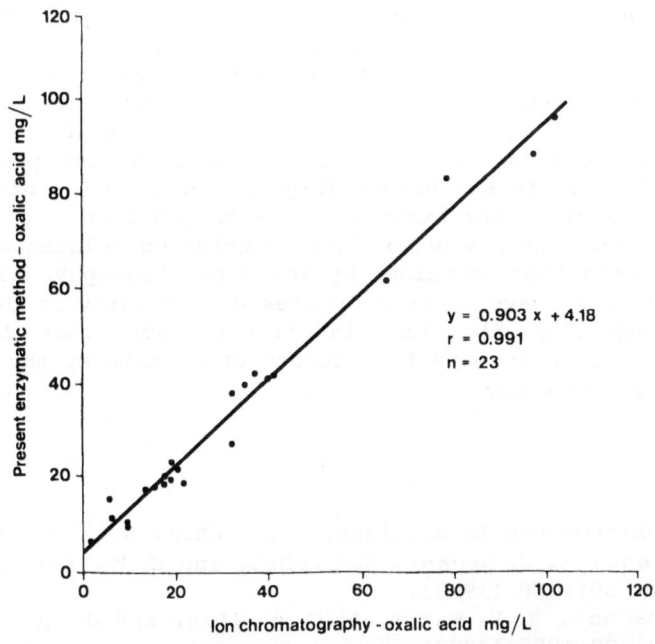

$$y = 0.903 \, x + 4.18$$
$$r = 0.991$$
$$n = 23$$

Fig. 3. Correlation between the present method and the ion-chromatographic method for measuring oxalate in urine.

Table 1. Within-Run Precision for Oxalate Determination in Urine.

Mean (mg/l)	n	SD (mg/l)	CV (%)
15.0	10	0.72	4.8
23.6	10	0.57	2.4
51.9	10	1.71	3.3

Table 2. Analytical Recovery of Oxalate Added to 5 Different Urines.

Oxalate Added (mg/l)	Recovered (mg/l)		
	mean	SD	Percent
20	20.2	2.1	101
50	50.6	5.0	101
100	106	5.6	106
200	183	11.2	91.3

RESULTS AND DISCUSSION

Preliminary experiments showed that the addition of EDTA to urine samples prevented the formation of insoluble Ca oxalate on storage. The incubation time for the formate dehydrogenase step was chosen as 40 min to ensure that an end-point was reached at oxalate concentrations up to 100 mg/l and to overcome inhibition of the reaction by urine (Fig. 1). Under these conditions the standard curve for oxalate added to urine was linear up to 100 mg/l (for aqueous standards up to 200 mg/l) and the recovery was complete when tested in different urines (Fig. 2, Table 1). Intra-assay precision at 3 different oxalate levels ranged from 2 to 5% (Table 2). Estimations of oxalate in urine correlated well ($r = 0.991$) with those obtained by ion-chromatography, although the latter in general gave lower estimates particularly at low oxalate concentrations (Fig. 3). Experiments have shown that this is probably due to an incomplete recovery of oxalate by the ion-chromatographic method.

REFERENCES

1. A. Hodgkinson and A. Williams, Clin. Chim. Acta 36:127 (1972).
2. H. O. Beutler, J. Becker, G. Michal, and E. Walter, Z. Analyt. Chem. 301:186 (1980).
3. G. D. Cannon, R. H. Eaton, A. C. A. Glen, and J. Moncur, Clin. Chem. 29:1855 (1983).

A NEW RAPID SPECTROPHOTOMETRIC METHOD FOR DETECTION

OF XANTHINURIA

J. Costello and E. Al-Dabagh

The Irish Stone Foundation, Meath Hospital, Dublin
and The Renal Research Laboratory, Allegheny General
Hospital, Pittsburgh, Pennsylvania, U.S.A.

INTRODUCTION

The purpose of this study was to develop a rapid procedure for
detecting xanthinuria. In this hereditary defect there is a gross
deficiency of the enzyme xanthine oxidase and the oxypurines,
xanthine and hypoxanthine, replace uric acid in the urine. A number
of enzymic spectrophotometric[1,2] and chromatographic[3,4] methods
have been developed for determining these oxypurines but these
methods are not readily available to most routine laboratories.
The new procedure is based on the absorption maxima of hypoxanthine,
xanthine and uric acid at 250, 270 and 292 nm respectively (Fig. 1).
Because the urines of normal and xanthinuric subjects contain
contrasting concentrations of these compounds, the possibility that
the urinary absorption ratios 250/292 and 270/292 nm would be
significantly different between the two groups was investigated.

METHODS

Urines, 24-h or spot samples, were collected from normal
subjects, three xanthinurics, their parents and siblings. The
urines were titrated to pH 9.3 and 100 μl aliquots were added to 2.0
ml of 0.1 M borate buffer pH 9.3. The samples were then read in
quartz cuvettes (10 mm light-path) on a Zeiss PMQ II
Spectrophotometer at 250, 270 and 292 nm. Urinary xanthine and
hypoxanthine were determined by the method of Chalmers and Watts[2]
and uric acid by that of Praetorius and Poulsen[5].

681

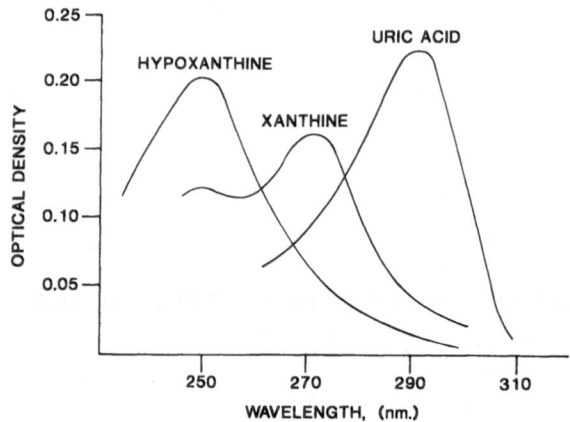

Fig. 1. Absorption spectra for hypoxanthine, xanthine and uric acid at concentration of 20 μmol/l in borate buffer (0.10 M, pH 9.3).

RESULTS

The marked differences in the urinary excretion of xanthine plus hypoxanthine and uric acid by normal and xanthinuric subjects is shown in Table 1. The urinary absorption ratios 250/292 and 270/292 nm obtained for normal and xanthinuric subjects are shown in Tables 2 and 3 respectively. There are significant differences at both ratios ($P<0.001$) between the values obtained for normal and xanthinuric subjects. Ratios for urines of parents and siblings were not significantly different from normal values.

Table 1. Urinary Excretion/24 h of Xanthine plus Hypoxanthine and Uric Acid by Normal Subjects and Three Xanthinurics (mean ± SD).

| | Age | μmol/24h | |
		Xanthine + Hypoxanthine	Uric Acid
Normal Subjects	4-10	57.4 ± 37.4	1044 ± 425
Xanthine Subjects			
M.M.	8	1311	22.5
F.M.	7	1549	15.0
Ma.M	5	1010	25.0

682

Table 2. Absorption Ratios for Urine of Normal Subjects at
          Wavelengths 270/292 and 250/292 nm.

Subject	270/292	250/292
B.B.	0.790	1.330
J.C.	0.778	1.355
M.B.	0.734	1.073
N.F.	0.800	1.560
S.F.	0.676	1.170
N.A.	0.774	1.280
R.W.	0.818	1.480
J.O.	0.728	1.060
H.C.	0.812	1.220
Range	0.676 – 0.818	1.06 – 1.56
Mean ± SD	0.768 ± 0.047	1.28 ± 0.17

DISCUSSION

Cases of xanthinuria are perhaps overlooked or go undetected, we suggest, partly due to lack of a convenient screening method for this defect. The large changes in the urinary excretion of xanthine, hypoxanthine and uric acid by xanthinurics (Table 1) result in significant differences ($P<0.001$) in urinary absorption ratios 250/292 and 270/292 nm compared to those of normal subjects (Tables 2,3). The present procedure, utilizing these differences, makes it possible to screen all urines being sent to clinical laboratories for this metabolic disorder. The method is simple, rapid and inexpensive, buffer being the only reagent required. The entire procedure can be carried out in 5 min. After initial detection of xanthinuria by this technique, confirmation by determining plasma and urinary concentrations of urate, xanthine and hypoxanthine is essential.

Table 3. Absorption Ratio for Urines of Xanthinuric Subjects at
         Wavelengths 270/292 and 250/292 nm.

Subject	270/292	250/292
M.M.	2.41	2.98
F.M.	4.04	4.61
MAJ.M	2.95	3.76
P	<0.001	<0.001

P value compared to normal subjects (Table 2).

REFERENCES

1. J. R. Klinenberg, S. Goldfinger, H. Bradley, and J. E. Seegmiller, Clin. Chem. 13:834 (1967).
2. R. A. Chalmers and R. W. E. Watts, Analyst 94:226 (1969).
3. J. C. Crawhall, K. Itiaba, and S. Katz, Biochem. Med. 30:261 (1983).
4. M. Kito, R. Tawa, S. Takeshima, and S. Hirose, J. Chromatogr. 278:35 (1983).
5. E. Praetorius and H. Poulsen, Scand. J. Clin. Lab. Invest. 5:273 (1953).

COMBINED ENZYMATIC DEGRADATION WITH CHONDROITINASES AND ALCIAN BLUE

PRECIPITATION IN DETERMINATION OF URINARY CHONDROITIN SULPHATES

B. Fellström, B. G. Danielson, S. Ljunghall, and
B. Wikström

Dept. of Internal Medicine, University Hospital
S-751 85 Uppsala, Sweden

INTRODUCTION

It has been claimed that glycosaminoglycans are important
inhibitors of calcium oxalate crystal growth and aggregation[1]. The
mode of action as inhibitors may be through a binding of the glycosaminoglycans to the crystal surface and thereby blocking the growth
sites of the crystals[2]. Chondroitin sulphates can also be
recovered from calcium oxalate crystals after dissolution of
crystals grown in urine[3]. The alcian blue precipitation method[4] is
not specific for urinary glycosaminoglycans, but also precipitates
polyanionic urinary glycoproteins and possibly ribonucleic acid
residues. Using this method it has been shown that stone formers
have a lower urinary excretion of polyanions, that are precipitable
by alcian blue[5]. The purpose of the present study was to measure
glycosaminoglycans specifically in unconcentrated urine.

METHODS AND MATERIALS

We used a modified version of the alcian blue method[4]
to measure the amount of precipitable polyanions in the urine
(ABPP). A 0.4 ml aliquot of urine was mixed with 1.6 ml of the
precipitation buffer containing 50 mM acetate, 50 mM magnesium and
0.06% alcian blue at pH 5.8 and was left overnight. After centrifugation at 3000 g for 15 min the pellet was washed twice in
absolute ethanol and solubilized in 7.5% SDS. The extinction was
read at 620 nm and chondroitin sulphate-A (CS-A) used as a standard.

Prior to incubation with the precipitation buffer, incubations
were also made with chondroitinase-ABC and chondroitinase-AC

(Sigma), respectively. The incubation was performed with 100 µl urine and 300 µl of an incubation buffer containing 0.05 units of enzyme, 60 mM acetate, 140 mM sodium and 170 µg BSA/ml at pH 8. After incubation with the enzyme buffer for 6 h, a total of 40 µl was mixed with 1.6 ml of the precipitation buffer and the procedure carried out as described above. By comparing the amount of precipitated polyanions with or without prior enzymatic digestion, the amount of chondroitin sulphate-A,C (CS-A + CS-C) and chondroitin sulphate-B (CS-B) could be calculated[6]. Nitrous acid oxidation of urine prior to alcian blue precipitation was used in an attempt to determine urinary heparan sulphate[6]. The method was applied to 24-h urines from 15 healthy controls, 25 renal stone patients, 7 patients with acromegaly and 11 children below 7 years of age. The urines had been collected with 0.02% chlorhexidine as a preservative.

RESULTS

The alcian blue precipitation was linear (not shown) for CS-A, CS-B, CS-C, heparin and pentosan polysulphate (SP 54). The relative precipitability of heparin was comparable with the various

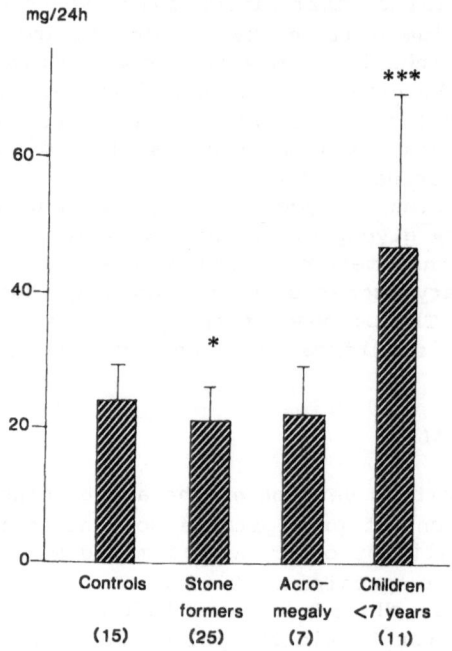

Fig. 1.   24-h urinary excretion of total ABPP in controls, stone formers, and patients with acromegaly. In children urine samples were used. *P < 0.05; ***P<0.001.

686

chondroitin sulphates, but 50% higher for SP 54. The specificity
of the two enzymes for digestion of CS-A, CS-B and CS-C
(chondroitinase-ABC) and CS-A and CS-C (chondroitinase-AC) was
practically 100% (not shown). By calculating the differences
between ABPP with or without the preceding enzymatic digestion, the
urinary content of CS-A + CS-C and CS-B, respectively, could be
calculated. The detection limit of CS-A + CS-C, defined as 2 SD in
10 measurements on blanks, was 1 µg/ml. In the nitrous acid
oxidation procedure only heparin and heparan sulphate (HS) were
chemically degraded, but not the chondroitin sulphates or SP 54.

CS-B (dermatan sulphate) and HS could not be detected in the
urines by the described procedures. The total ABPP was lower in
stone formers than in controls (P<0.06), higher in males than in
females (P<0.05) and substantially higher in the urine samples from
the children (Fig. 1). CS-A + CS-C was not different in stone
formers compared with controls. Patients with acromegaly had a
higher excretion of CS-A + CS-C than the controls (P<0.01). The
highest values were found in urines from the children (Fig. 2).
Males had a higher excretion than females (P<0.05).

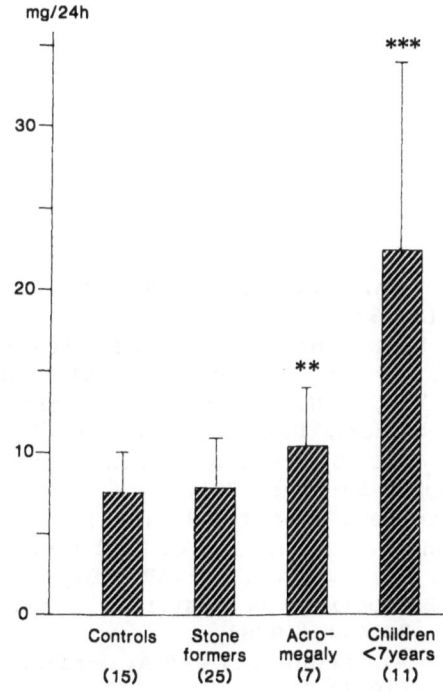

Fig. 2. 24-h urinary excretion of chondroitin sulphates A+C in
controls, stone formers and patients with acromegaly.
In children urine samples were used. **P<0.01; ***P<0.001.

DISCUSSION

The described procedure offers a specific method for measuring CS-A + CS-C (but not CS-B) in small quantities of urine without prior concentration of the urines. The amount of CS found in the urines of healthy controls is in accordance with the results of previous studies[7,8], including the finding of high values in growing children. We do not know of any previous studies of the urinary excretion of chondroitin sulphates in patients with acromegaly. Apparently, these patients have a higher excretion than healthy controls and there also seems to be a relation between the urinary excretion of chondroitin sulphates and the activity of the disease (not shown). Stone patients are reported to have lower levels of ABPP than normals[5]. In the present study, this was also the case but not due to a lower excretion of chondroitin sulphates. In another recent study comparing the urinary excretion of glycosaminoglycans, measured by CPC-precipitation and a subsequent carbazole reaction, no difference was found between stone formers and controls[9]. Whether or not the residual difference in total ABPP in this study was due to heparan sulphate or to some other polyanion in the urine, remains to be elucidated.

ACKNOWLEDGMENTS

This work was supported by the Swedish Medical Research Council (nos. 2329, 6354), the Swedish Society of Medical Sciences and the Tore Nilsson Foundation.

REFERENCES

1. W. G. Robertson, M. Peacock, and B. E. C. Nordin, Clin. Chim. Acta 43:31 (1973).
2. B. Fellström, B. G. Danielson, F. A. Karlsson, and S. Ljunghall, in:"Urolithiasis and Related Clinical Research", P. O. Schwille, L. H. Smith, W. G. Robertson, and W. Vahlensieck,eds., Plenum, New York (1985).
3. J. G. Brockis, R. C. Bowyer, and R. K. McCulloch, Scand. J. Urol. Nephrol. Suppl. 53:67 (1979).
4. P. Whiteman, Biochem. J. 131:343 (1973).
5. W. G. Robertson, M. Peacock, P. J. Heyburn, D. H. Marshall, and P. B. Clark, Br. J. Urol. 50:449 (1978).
6. B. Glimelius, B. Norling, B. Westermark, and Å. Wasteson, Biochem. J. 172:443 (1978).
7. D. P. Varadi, J. A. Cifonelli, and A. Dorfman, Biochim. Biophys. Acta 141:103 (1967).
8. E. Wessler, Biochem. J. 122:373 (1971).
9. R. Caudarella, F. Stefani, E. Rizzoli, N. Malavolta, and G. D. Antuono, J. Urol. 129:665 (1983).

ON THE PRESERVATION OF URINES FOR THE DETERMINATION OF CITRATE

V. Graef, H. Schmidtmann, and K. Jarrar

Institute of Clinical Chemistry and Pathobiochemistry
and Dept. of Urology, University Giessen, F.R.G.

INTRODUCTION

It is known that bacteria use citrate as a source of carbon and many growth media contain citrate. Since many urines contain bacteria, citrate concentration may decrease during the collection of urines or in the time between the collection and the citrate determination. Normal ranges, evaluated by different authors by means of the same method differ from each other. This could be caused by varying degrees of destruction of citrate by different urinary bacteria. In this paper we have studied some preservatives to find the one best suited to protect citrate. This preservative should not interfere with other methods used for the determination of other variables in the urine of stone patients.

METHODS

Citrate determination in urine was performed by the method of Welshman and McCambridge[1] using citrate lyase. Oxalate was measured enzymatically by use of oxalate decarboxylase and formate dehydrogenase[2].

RESULTS AND DISCUSSION

To demonstrate the destruction of citrate this component was determined in 23 urines immediately after the collection and after 48 h at room temperature (20 to 22°C). The mean citrate concentration decreased from 1.42 $\pm$ 0.76 to 0.99 $\pm$ 0.87 mmol/l (Fig. 1A). The citrate concentrations of 26 urines heated for

689

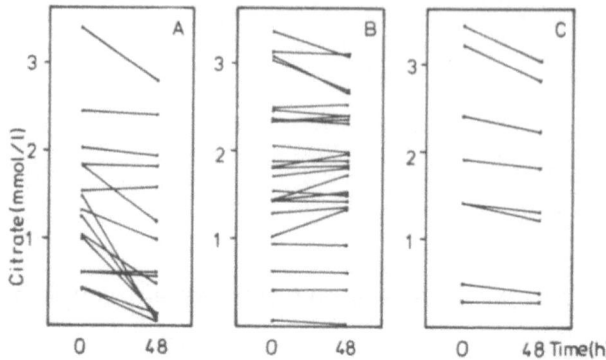

Fig. 1. Citrate concentration of (A) original urines; (B) heated (100°C) urines; (C) urines filtered through a bacteria filter.

10 min at 100°C were determined immediately and after 48 h at 20° to 22°C. There was no decline of citrate concentration during the storage (2.69 ± 1.16 mmol/l at time 0 and 2.67 ± 1.15 mmol/l at 48 h) (Fig. 1B). This demonstrates that bacteria are responsible for the destruction of citrate. Furthermore, 8 urines were filtered through a bacteria filter. Citrate, measured at time 0 and 48 h later, showed only a slight decrease from 1.81 ± 1.06 to 1.62 ± 0.94 mmol/l (Fig. 1C). The same urines, not passed through the filter, exhibited a citrate concentration of 1.18 mmol/l after 48 h. Evidently, enzymes present in urine are not responsible for the loss of citrate.

The preservatives listed in Table 1 were added to 21 urines. Citrate was determined at time 0 and after storage for 48 h at room temperature. The highest recovery was obtained in urines which contained penicillin G/streptomycin sulfate and sodium azide. A further preservative, didecyldimethylammonium chloride, not mentioned in Table 1, was unsuitable because the absorbance produced in the citrate determination was considerably higher in urines which were stored for 2 days than in fresh urines. Since usually oxalate and citrate were determined in the urines of stone patients, the effect of the preservatives was tested on both methods. As shown in Table 2, thymol and sodium azide inhibited the enzymes used for oxalate determination. Therefore, these substances are unsuitable for the preservation of urines. The most suitable preservative is a mixture of penicillin G and streptomycin sulfate (110 + 190 mg/ 24 h urine). Urines of normal subjects and stone patients were collected over penicillin G and streptomycin sulfate. Normal women excreted a higher amount of citrate than normal men, however, the difference was not significant (Table 3). The citrate excretion was significantly higher (P<0.01) in patients with oxalate and urate stones than in normal adults.

Table 1. Effect of Preservatives on Urinary Citrate Concentration.

Preservative	Concentration	Time of storage	Citrate concentration
None	-	0 h	100 %
None	-	48 h	29.1 + 29 %
Benzyltributyl-ammonium chloride	5 mg/ml	48 h	48.1 + 31.6 %
Ethyl mercurithio-salicylate	0.1 mg/ml	48 h	84.2 + 21 %
Thymol	saturated	48 h	85.8 + 15.7 %
Penicillin G +	1000 IU/ml	48 h	95.1 + 8.9 %
Streptomycin sulfate	1000 IU/ml		
Sodium azide	3 mg/ml	48 h	95.5 + 7.7 %

Table 2. Determination of Oxalate and Citrate in Urines with and without Preservatives.

Preservative[*]	Oxalate (mg/l) with preservative	Oxalate (mg/l) without preservative	Citrate (mmol/l) with preservative	Citrate (mmol/l) without preservative
Thymol	6.1	25.6	0.1	1.97
Ethyl mercurithio-salicylate	20.0	20.1	1.40	1.40
Sodium azide	0	27.6	1.19	1.16
Penicillin G + Streptomycin sulfate	16.4	18.1	2.00	1.97

[*]Concentration in urine as in Table 1. The preservatives were added to urine immediately before the assay.

Table 3. Citrate in Urine of Normal Subjects and Stone Patients[*].

Subjects	n	Sex	Citrate (mmol/l)	Citrate (mmol/24 h)
Normal	20	M	1.50 + 0.77	2.20 + 0.76
Normal	19	F	1.82 + 0.86	2.53 + 1.14
Normal	39	M+F	1.66 + 0.82	2.36 + 0.96
Oxalate stone	111	M+F	1.54 + 1.01	3.11 + 1.67
Urate stone	25	M+F	1.58 + 0.90	3.47 + 2.04
Phosphate stone	48	M+F	1.07 + 0.75	2.39 + 1.34

[*]Urines were collected over penicillin G and streptomycin.

In the past some investigators have published a lower citrate excretion in normal subjects than others and it is remarkable that there is a wide normal range of urinary citrate. This may be due to destruction of citrate by urinary bacteria. To avoid such falsely low results we recommend the collection of urines over penicillin G and streptomycin sulfate.

REFERENCES

1. S. G. Welshman and H. McCambridge, Clin. Chim. Acta 46:243 (1973).
2. H.-O. Beutler, J. Becker, G. Michal, and E. Walter, Analytica (Munchen) 1980).

STONE ANALYSIS

A NEW METHOD FOR QUANTITATIVE WET-CHEMICAL ANALYSIS OF URINARY CALCULI AND THE PRINCIPLES FOR CALCULATION OF RESULTS AND MASS RECOVERY BY AN ALGORITHM

L. Larsson, S. Bo, H.-G. Tiselius, and S. Öhman

Depts. of Clinical Chemistry and Urology, Linköping University, S-581 85 Linköping, Sweden

INTRODUCTION

Recently, we described a new method for the quantitative wet-chemical analysis of urinary calculi[1]. This method is capable of analyzing all common constituents even in very small calculi (1 mg). Since algorithmic analysis is a powerful system for monitoring and understanding of information in medical evaluation[2], we wrote an algorithm to facilitate the interpretation of the analytical data. The algorithm transforms the individual analytes to constituents found in renal stones[3] (e.g. calcium oxalate, calcium hydrogen phosphate, apatite). In this paper our wet-chemical analysis and algorithm are presented briefly.

METHODS

The powdered calculus is dried over silica gel and dissolved in nitric acid. After dilution, calcium and magnesium are determined by atomic absorption, phosphate and ammonium by conventional colorimetric methods, and oxalate from its quenching of fluorescence of a zirconium-flavonol complex. Uric acid decomposes in nitric acid to alloxan, which is determined fluorimetrically as its condensation product with 1,2-phenylenediamine. Protein gives the xanthoprotein reaction with nitric acid and is determined spectrophotometrically. Cystine is oxidized by nitric acid to sulfate, which is determined turbidimetrically as its barium salt. The presence of carbonate is shown by effervescence in nitric acid. Internal quality control is performed with specifically designed control samples including all analytes[1,4]. The full description of our wet-chemical method is in press[1].

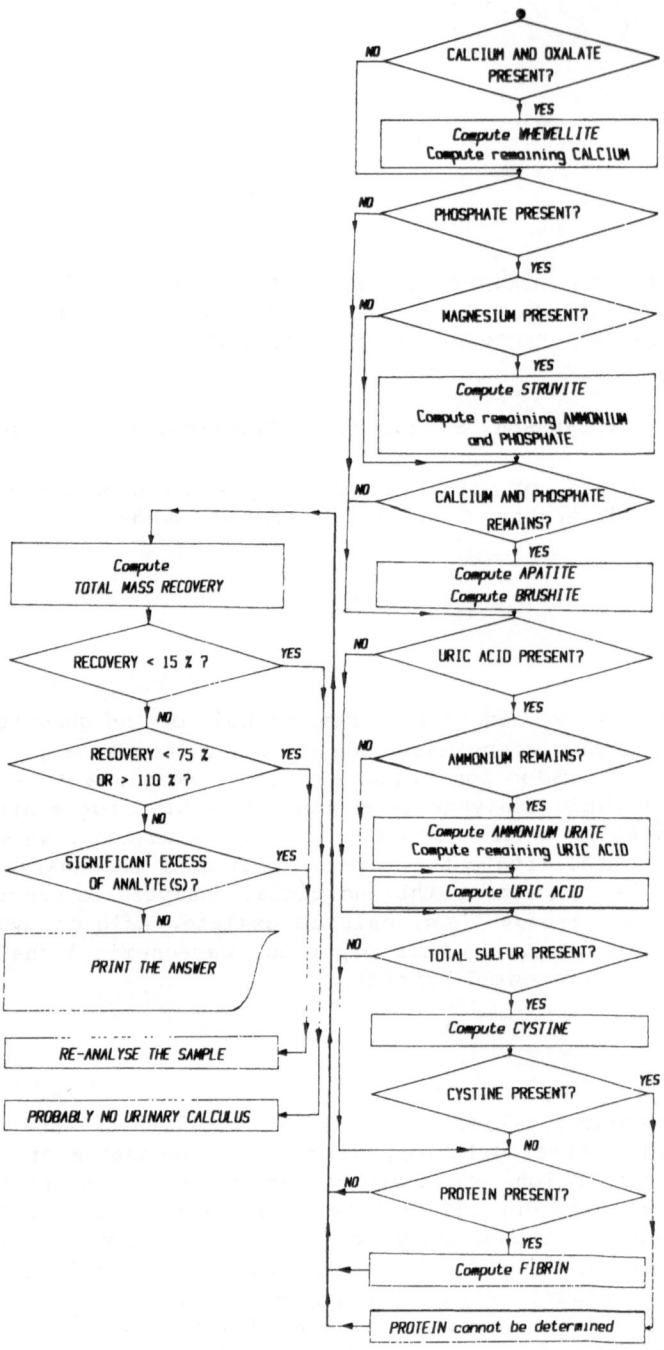

Fig. 1. Flow diagram of the algorithm for computation of the composition of urinary calculi. (See reference 1).

CALCULATION OF STONE COMPOSITION

The findings for the controls are compared with an assigned value stored in the computer. Preliminary limits for acceptance have earlier been presented[4]. The computer program calculates the composition of the original solid material according to the algorithm (Fig.1). This algorithm is based on the following assumptions. (i) All oxalate found in the sample is present as whewellite ($CaC_2O_4.H_2O$). (ii) Phosphate may be present in the following forms: struvite ($MgNH_4PO_4.6\ H_2O$), brushite ($CaHPO_4.H_2O$), or hydroxyapatite ($Ca_{10}(PO_4)_6(OH)_2$). Calcium may be present as the acid itself or as monoammonium urate. All total sulfur comes from cystine. Protein behaves similarly to fibrin in HNO_3.

At the end of the algorithm, the total mass recovery, including crystal water, is calculated. We followed the suggestion of Hodgkinson et al[5], that ionic analytes are present only as the above crystalline compounds. The validity of this procedure was established by NMR determination of crystal water in 15 renal stones[1] where a total mass recovery of 91.5 + 5.0% was found compared with 92.2 + 6.7% obtained in 125 urinary stones with the algorithm. Ideally, the recovery should be 100%, but we suggest, that the deficit is mainly due to presence of other materials, not included in our analysis. A low recovery (<75%) may be caused by an analytical error but very low (<15%) recoveries are found only for artifacts.

DISCUSSION

As the composition of small renal stones may give information as to the initiation of stone formation[5], it is important to analyse these stones with a sensitive and precise method. Routinely we use 5 mg of stone material, but our method allows analysis of a 1 mg stone with respect to all analytes with full precision. If protein and cystine are omitted, 0.5 mg is satisfactory.

One advantage of a wet-chemical method over X-ray diffraction and IR-spectroscopy is, that the sensitivity and analytical precision can be considerably better for certain constituents e.g. the detection limits for oxalate and uric acid correspond to 110 and 60 pmoles respectively. The high sensitivity of our method has revealed the presence of small but significant amounts of minor components (such as magnesium in apatite stones). However, the clinical significance of minor components has not yet been evaluated. Another important feature of our method is that all stones types are completely dissolved by nitric acid before analysis. This is an absolute prerequisite for clinically significant results.

Using our algorithm stone composition was calculated according to previously published assumptions. Firstly, the components containing calcium, magnesium, phosphate, and oxalate were calculated (Fig. 1). Of these analytes only oxalate is found as a single component, whewellite. This component was calculated first and the remaining calcium was assumed to be bound to phosphate. Since phosphate may also be bound to magnesium in the form of struvite this has to be calculated before the calcium phosphate content. Since struvite contains ammonium, an excess of the latter was assumed to be present as ammonium urate. Phosphate not bound to magnesium was assumed to be present as apatite or brushite or both depending on the remaining Ca/P ratio. Usually, mixtures of these components are noted, however, other calcium phosphates, such as octacalcium phosphate have been postulated[6]. The rest of the algorithm includes calculation of uric acid and ammonium urate, cystine, and protein.

Thus we have presented a sensitive and accurate wet-chemical quantitative method for stone analysis and an algorithm that facilitates interpretation of obtained analytical data.

REFERENCES

1. L. Larsson, B. Sörbo, H.-G. Tiselius, and S. Öhman, Clin. Chim.Acta, (1984) in press.
2. C. Z. Margolis, J. Am. Med. Assoc. 249:627 (1983).
3. E. L. Prien and E. L. Prien, Am. J. Med. 45:654 (1968).
4. L. Larsson, B. Sörbo and S. Öhman, in:"Urinary Stone", R. Ryall, J. G. Brockis, V. Marshall, and B. Finlayson, eds., Churchill Livingstone, Melbourne (1984).
5. A. Hodgkinson, M. Peacock, and M. Nicholson, Invest. Urol. 6:549 (1969).
6. P. G. Koutsoukos and G. H. Nancollas, J. Cryst. Growth 53:10 (1981).

ANALYSIS OF URINARY CALCULI BY INDUCTIVELY COUPLED PLASMA

ATOMIC EMISSION SPECTROSCOPY: NEW INSIGHT INTO STONE STRUCTURE

M. A. E. Wandt, M. B. A. Pougnet, and A. L. Rodgers

Depts. of Physical Chemistry and Analytical Science
University of Cape Town, Rondebosch, Cape Town 7700
Republic of South Africa

INTRODUCTION

The constant increase in the incidence of urinary stone disease necessitates intensive endeavours in both scientific and clinical research to gain a deeper understanding of the stone-forming process. In the past 10 to 20 years moderately successful forms of medical treatment have been developed for all types of urinary calculi. An imperative prerequisite for the selection of the appropriate therapy, however, is an accurate knowledge of the stone composition. Stone analysis has become one of the major approaches in the search for a better understanding of the physico-chemical and physiological basis of stone formation and is an essential tool in the formulation of new treatment regimens[1]. While many techniques have been used in the analysis of urinary calculi, all have certain limitations. New procedures are constantly being developed and applied in the hope of identifying compositional and structural features in stones which might otherwise go undetected owing to the shortcomings of the particular technique available. It is for this reason that we decided to investigate the application of Inductively Coupled Plasma Atomic Emission Spectroscopy[2] (ICP-AES) in the analysis of 36 urinary calculi from the Cape Town area. Beneficial aspects of this technique include, amongst others, capability of measuring a large number of elements, high sensitivity and reproducibility, good stability, freedom from inter-element interferences, and linear calibration graphs over several orders of magnitude and speed[3].

METHODS

Powdered stone specimens were first subjected to X-ray powder diffraction (XRD) analysis using both film and goniometer procedures so as to identify qualitatively the crystalline phases present. Microchemical analysis for carbon, hydrogen and nitrogen in each stone was also performed using a method based on the Haraeus universal combustion analyser as described by Monar[4]. For the preparation of solutions for analysis by ICP-AES it was necessary to develop a routine procedure suitable for a wide variety of stones. Crushed stone fragments were pre-digested in Erlenmeyer flasks using concentrated nitric acid and the remaining organic matter was oxidized using a refluxing mixture of concentrated nitric and perchloric acids. To overcome systematic errors in the analysis results the acid contents of the samples and reference standards were matched prior to analysis for calcium, magnesium and phosphorus. Details of sample preparation, experimental conditions and instrumentation are reported elsewhere[5].

RESULTS AND DISCUSSION

Of the 36 stones analysed thus far, 21 belong to the struvite/apatite (STR/APA) group, 11 to the uric acid/calcium oxalate monohydrate (UA/COM) group and 4 to the calcium oxalate (COM/COD) group.

In the STR/APA group the amount of APA ranged between 2 and 56% (w/w). A third component, calcium oxalate, was identified in 5 stones from this group. The relative amounts of each phase in the remaining 16 two-component stones were independently calculated from the Ca and Mg figures and yielded values which agreed within 2 to 3%. It was also possible[6] to calculate the amount of organic matrix present by assuming that the excess nitrogen (i.e. N unaccounted for after stoichiometric calculations involving its presence in STR) was associated with such deposits. This varied but never exceeded 6% in 13 of the calculi. In the remaining stones of this group, the excess N was exceptionally high indicating either an abnormally high matrix content, or, more likely the presence of an additional, undetected organic phase (e.g. ammonium urate).

In the UA/COM group, UA always occurred as the major component. Uric acid dihydrate (UAD) was also detected in 3 stones from this group. With regard to the 4 COM/COD stones, small amounts of phosphorus, corresponding to APA concentrations between 1 and 12% were detected.

Our results illustrate the value of using highly sensitive instrumentation for the detection of very small constituent concentrations which would possibly otherwise go undetected by routine analytical procedures. It is well known that APA is frequently masked by STR in XRD analysis because of its amorphous nature and very small particle size as well as overlapping of important lines[7]. The detection of small amounts of Ca and P in almost all the stones of the present study may indicate the presence of APA in all such samples[8]. It has been shown[9] that STR exists in association with varying amounts of APA, its large crystals often being interspersed with small spherular deposits of the latter. APA has also been reported as constituting the most prevalent second phase in all polymineral calcium oxalate stones[10]. These results, together with our observation of the presence of Ca and P in most calculi, even in minute concentrations, suggest that APA may play the role of a "cementing" agent in stone formation. The fact that APA is always present in microcrystalline form in body fluids and that it precipitates over a wide range lends support to this theory[11].

We have shown that ICP-AES analysis, together with other compound-selective methods, provides a useful tool for the quantitative determination of the crystalline and matrix content of urinary calculi. Matrix is thought to play an architectonic role in calculus formation whereby it acts as a binder, serving to cement an otherwise loose aggregation of crystals into a structurally cohesive unit[12]. Whether this "cementing" mechanism is analogous to that of APA as suggested above remains to be seen. What does emerge, however, is support for an aggregation mechanism as a regular process in urinary calculi formation. On the other hand, the detection of calcium (oxalate) in all uric acid stones again suggests an epitaxial relationship between these two components. Furthermore the repeated association of at least 2 components in all stones indicates that the existence of the so called "pure" stone might be a myth and that a heterogeneous nucleation mechanism might be operative as the primary event in stone formation.

Additional studies involving trace element determination (e.g. Si, Al, Fe, Zn) are currently being investigated by us. The aim is now to develop a method whereby both major and trace elements can be quantitated simultaneously, thereby reducing sample consumption. Many workers believe that trace elements play a role in stone formation[13,14]. By applying ICP-AES to this and other stone problems, we believe that new insight into understanding and controlling the disease can be gained.

ACKNOWLEDGEMENTS

This study was supported by grants from the University of Cape Town, the South African Medical Research Council and the South African Council for Scientific and Industrial Research. We are

grateful to Mr P Abrunhusa of the Teaching Methods Unit of this
University for his assistance in the design and construction of the
Symposium poster.

REFERENCES

1. M. Modlin, S. Afr. Med. J. 59;318 (1981).
2. V. A. Fassel and R. N. Kniseley, Anal. Chem. 46:1110A(1974).
3. S. Greenfield, H. McD. McGeachin, and P. B. Smith, Talanta 22:1
    (1975).
4. I. Monar, Mikrochim. Acta 6:784 (1972).
5. M. A. E. Wandt, M. A. B. Pougnet, and A. L. Rodgers, Analyst
    (in press).
6. A. Hodgkinson, M. Peacock, and M. Nicholson, in: "Proceedings of
    the Renal Stone Research Symposium, A. Hodgkinson,
    B. E. C.Nordin, eds., Churchill, London, (1968).
7. R. H. Morriss and M. F. Beeler, Am. J. Clin. Pathol. 48:413
    (1967).
8. K. Tozuka, T. Konjiki, and T. Sudo, Br. J. Urol. 53:216
    (1981).
9. R. Blaschke, D. B. Leusmann, U.-B. Meyer-Jürgens, and E. Tölle,
    Beitr. elektronenmikroskop. Direktabb. Oberfl. 14:581 (1981).
10. A.-A. Kollwitz, Dtsch. Med. J. 19:22 (1968).
11. C. Lagergren, Acta Radiol. Suppl. 133:1 (1956).
12. L. U. Ogbuji and B. Finlayson, Invest. Urol. 19:182 (1981).
13. J. L. Meyer and E. F. Angino, Invest. Urol. 14:347 ((1977).
14. J. L. Meyer and W. C. Thomas, J. Urol. 128:1372 (1982).

HARDNESS TESTING OF URINARY CALCULI

J. R. Burns, B. E. Shoemaker, J. F. Gauthier, and B. Finlayson

Division of Urology, Dept. of Surgery, Veterans' Administration Hospital, Birmingham, Alabama, and Division of Urology, Dept. of Surgery, University of Florida, Gainesville, Florida, U.S.A.

INTRODUCTION

With the advent of electrohydraulic and extracorporeal shock wave lithotripsy, it is important to document the mechanical properties of urinary calculi. Since the success of both techniques is affected by the compressive and tensile strength of the calculus, we have compared the hardness of a variety of urinary calculi. This information may be important in understanding the limitations of these new techniques.

METHODS AND MATERIALS

Urinary calculi were obtained from Louis C. Herring and Company and the Baylor Urolithiasis Laboratory. Calcium oxalate calculi were composed of at least 85% calcium oxalate monohydrate. Brushite, uric acid, and cystine calculi contained at least 95% of their respective elements. Human infection calculi were a mixture of struvite and carbonate apatite. Struvite calculi obtained from dogs contained at least 95% struvite.

The calculi were placed in a plexiglass mold and embedded with epoxy. After the epoxy had hardened, the mounted calculi were ground to a flat surface using a series of silicon carbide grinding papers (60 to 600 grit). The stone surface was polished on a polishing wheel with a 0.3 μm alumina.

The calculi were tested for hardness with a Tukon micro-hardness tester. This apparatus uses a KNOOP indenter to create indentations in the material being tested. A constant force

703

(2000 g) is applied to the indenter and the length of the indentation measured with a microscope whose eyepiece is etched with a grid. The measured length is expressed in Filar units (1 Filar unit = 0.471 µm) which may be converted to KNOOP hardness numbers from published tables. Each calculus was sectioned at several levels and hardness measurements performed at multiple sites on each level.

The compressive strengths of three infection calculi were tested on an Instrom device. Calculi were cut into cubes with a jeweler's saw and placed in the Instrom device. The compressive strength was calculated from the load and the measured size of the broken surface of the calculus.

RESULTS

The KNOOP hardness number (I) is expressed by the formula:

$$I = L/A_p = L/1^2 C_p$$

where L is the load applied to the identer, A_p the unrecovered projected area of identation (mm^2), 1 the measured length of the long diagonal of the identation (mm), and C_p a constant relating 1 to the projected area. A typical identation created on a calculus is shown in Fig. 1.

The KNOOP hardness values of the calculi tested are summarized in Table 1. Each line is the average of all measurements taken for a single calculus. Each calculus was measured for hardness at 20-30 different sites. Uric acid calculi were subdivided into 2 classes, porous and non-porous. Although all were composed of at least 95% uric acid, a large difference in hardness was noted between the two classes, the porous calculi being softer than the non-porous calculi. Calcium oxalate and brushite were the hardest of the calculi tested. Struvite and the non-porous uric acid calculi were of intermediate hardness. Human infection calculi, cystine, and porous uric acid calculi were the softest. The relative softness of human infection calculi results from the mixture of carbonate apatite and struvite. Pure struvite calculi are much harder than the combination calculi. By Student's T-test, the calcium oxalate and brushite stones are significantly harder than any of the other groups of calculi ($P < 0.001$).

The compressive strengths of the 3 infection calculi were measured on the Instrom device. The calculated compressive strength ranged from 24.9 to 76.2 kg/cm^2.

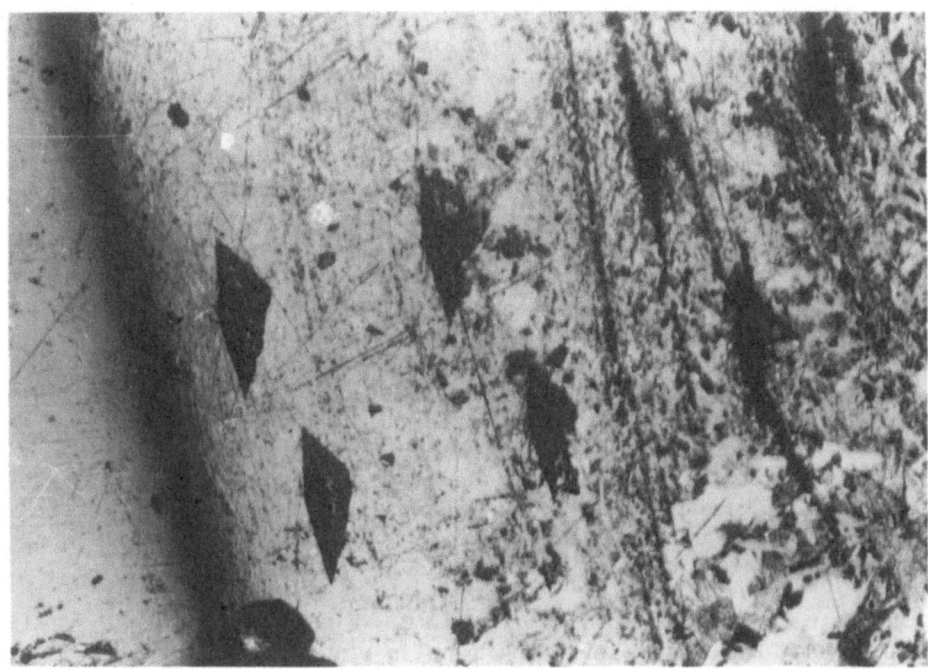

Fig. 1. Identations (light arrow) created on a cystine calculus.

Table 1. Hardness Measurements of Various Urinary Calculi.

Stone type	Number tested	KNOOP Hardness Number (Mean $\pm$ SD)
Calcium Oxalate	7	99.6 $\pm$ 14.8
Brushite	5	90.9 $\pm$ 3.5
Uric Acid (non-porous)	3	47.8 $\pm$ 4.2
Struvite (dogs)	6	39.6 $\pm$ 11.6
Uric Acid (porous)	5	25.8 $\pm$ 2.6
Cystine	4	25.7 $\pm$ 3.3
Infection (Struvite + carbonate apatite)	4	21.3 $\pm$ 2.9

DISCUSSION

Electrohydraulic lithotripsy and more recently, extracorporeal shock wave lithotripsy are now used as a treatment of renal calculi. Both lithotriptors are based on the same principle and depend on the compressive and tensile strength of a calculus.

Although electrohydraulic lithotripsy is an effective means of removing bladder calculi, a small percentage of calculi are unable to be fragmented. The stones which resist fragmentation are reported to be composed of uric acid[2]. A general clinical impression is that uric acid calculi are harder and more difficult to disrupt than other types of calculi. Watanabe, studying compressive and tensile strength of urinary calculi[3,4], found no correlation between the strength of the calculus and its chemical composition. Our study, however, does demonstrate significant differences in the hardness of different types of calculi. In the stones tested, Watanabe found compressive strength to range from 19.2 to 176 kg/cm^2. These values compare favorably with those on the 3 infection calculi in this study. We did not determine the compressive strength of all calculi tested for hardness and although KNOOP values can be converted to tensile strength from standard tables, this conversion would probably not be appropriate for urinary calculi since the published tables are used primarily in carbon steel measurements. In attempting to make the conversions for urinary calculi, the number of approximations used would make the results meaningless.

Urinary calculi do differ in their degree of hardness. It is likely that the compressive and tensile strength of urinary calculi also differ according to composition. Calcium oxalate and brushite were the hardest stones tested. Uric acid calculi were softer and their resistance to electrohydraulic disruption is probably a result of factors other than stone hardness. The difference in the degree of hardness may help to explain why lithotripsy procedures are more effective with certain types of urinary calculi than others. Knowledge of the mechanical properties of urinary calculi will become more important as new techniques of urinary stone removal gain in popularity.

ACKNOWLEDGMENT

The authors wish to thank the Veterans' Administration for financial support.

REFERENCES

1. B. W. Watson, Biomed. Engineer. 5:21 (1970).
2. D. Abrecht, R. Nagel, and C. P. Kölln, Int. Urol. Nephrol. 4:45 (1972).
3. S. Murata, H. Watanabe, T. Takahashi, K. Watanabe, and S.Oinuma, Jap. J.Urol. 68:249 (1977).
4. H. Kaneko, H. Watanabe, T. Takahashi, K. Watanabe, K. Akiyama, K. Kondo, H. Furue, and S. Oinoma Jap. J. Urol. 70:61 (1979).

SCANNING ELECTRON MICROSCOPY STUDIES ON INFECTION-INDUCED

URINARY CONCREMENTS

U.-B. Meyer-Jürgens, D. B. Leusmann, R. Blaschke,
G. Kleinhans, and W. Schmandt

Institut für Medizinische Physik, and Urologische
Abteilung der Chirurgische Universitätsklinik
D-4400 Münster, F.R.G.

INTRODUCTION

The aim of this study was to investigate and identify different
types of bacteria in renal calculi by scanning electron microscopy
(SEM) and with enegery dispersive X-ray microanalysis (EDXA). We
also compared these findings with bacteria cultered from stone
fragments and bacteriological findings of urine, in order to obtain
further information on the role that bacteria may play in the
development of infection-induced urinary concrements. We also
investigated what has been called "bacterial footprints" that are
present in infection stones[1,2].

METHODS

Stones obtained during operation performed in the urological
clinic since April 1983 for presumed infection-induced renal stones,
were divided into 3 parts under sterile conditions. One of these
fragments was cultured for bacteria. The second fragment was fixed
in glutaraldehyde and then critical-point-dried to preserve the
morphology and structure of bacteria to be investigated. The
fragment was analysed by the SEM with EDXA. The third piece was
analysed for crystal content according to the standard method[3].

A second group of renal stones that already had been analysed
according to standard procedures, was re-investigated to look
especially for "bacterial footprints" or for bacteria. The stone
formers all had had bacteria in their urine but no bacterial
cultures had been performed on the stones.

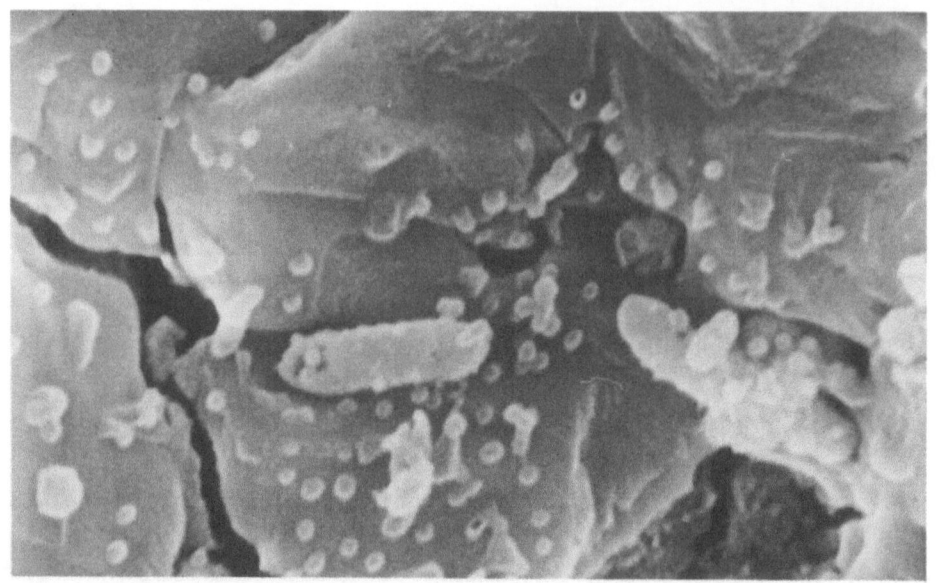

Fig. 1. Klebsiella bacteria in a urinary calculus after fixation
in glutaraldehyde and critical-point-drying (cpd).

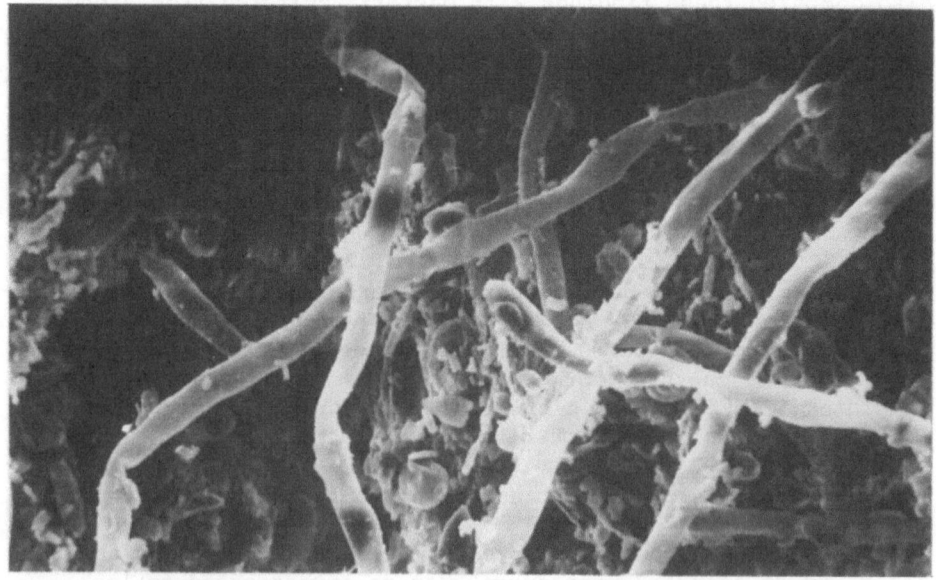

Fig. 2. Candida albicans in a calculus consisting of 90% uric acid
and 10% uric acid dihydrate (after fixation and cpd).

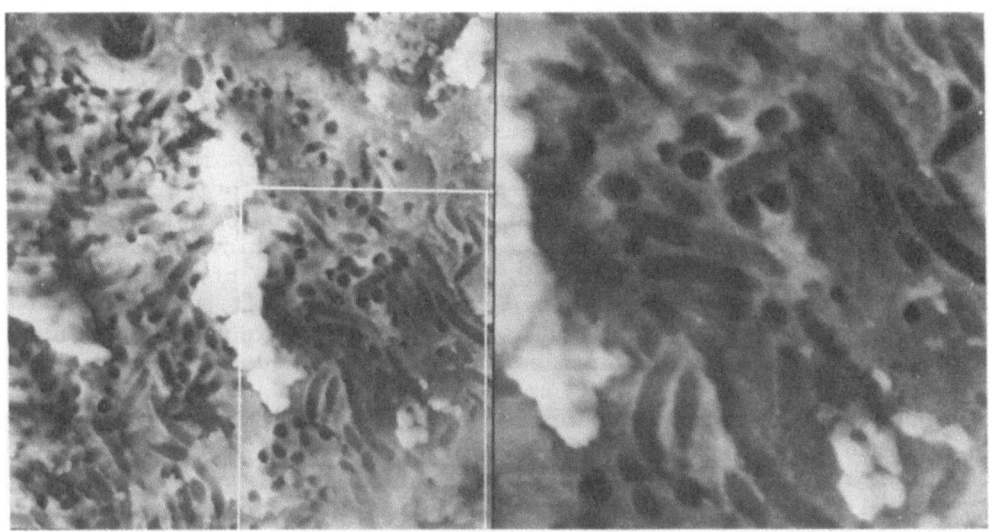

Fig. 3. Bacterial footprints (standard preparation). The round
holes show the diameter of the bacteria. The urine was
infected by E. coli and Proteus.

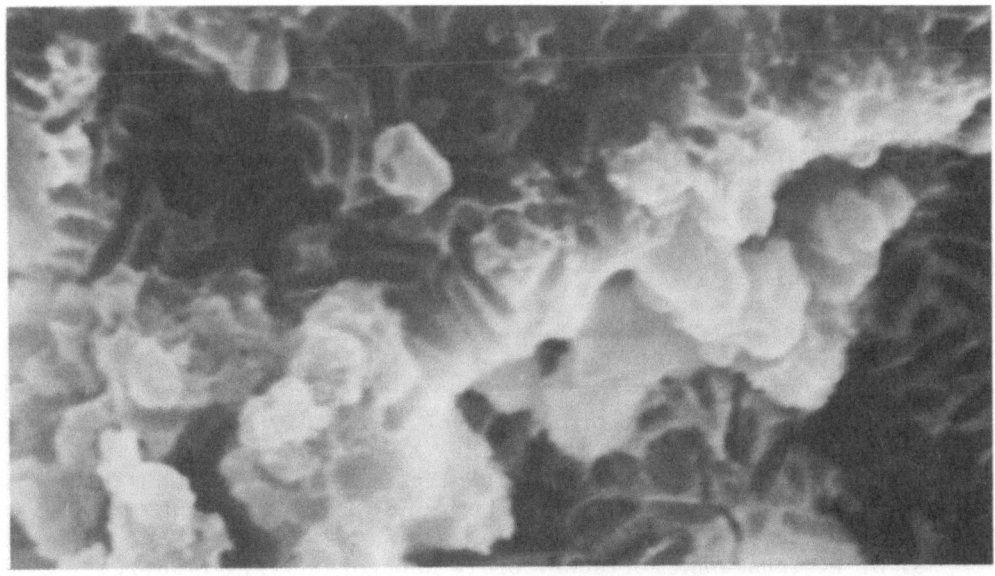

Fig. 4. Bacterial footprints after standard preparation; urine
infected with E. Coli and Enterococcus.

RESULTS

Thirteen renal calculi were investigated by bacteriological culture and SEM. In 4 cases visualization of the bacteria was possible with SEM. These calculi were infected by Escherichia coli, Klebsiella (Fig. 1) and Candida albicans (Fig. 2). In 4 calculi infected by Proteus mirabilis, neither bacterial footprints nor bacteria could be found. In 5 cases bacteriological cultivation did not show any infection, nor were there any prints or bacteria visible. With two exceptions, all the infection stones consisted of apatite and struvite. One, infected by E. coli, was composed of apatite, whewellite and weddelite; the other, infected by Candida albicans, consisted of uric acid and uric acid dihydrate (Fig. 2). All but one patient with E. coli in their urine showed bacterial footprints or bacteria themselves in their calculi. These patients had had infections with E. coli alone or together with Proteus (Fig. 3), Enterococcus (Fig. 4) or E. coli haemolyticum. Other calculi obtained from patients with urine-infections caused by Staphylococcus aureus, Streptococcus, Proteus, Enterococcus and Pseudomonas also showed footprints of the bacteria themselves. In many cases bacteria, especially E. coli, were mineralized by calcium phosphate as already described by Cifuentes-Delatte et al [2] in a TEM-study. Elemental analysis with EDXA showed different ratios of calcium and phosphorus, probably associated with different stages of mineralization.

DISCUSSION

E. coli are often identified in infection-induced urinary calculi. It is generally regarded that E. coli are not urea-splitting and probably cannot cause an increase in urine pH. Therefore a different mechanism for the development of these infection stones should be considered. As has been shown by Keefe[4], bacteria are capable of forming intracellular calcium-containing crystalline deposits. These mineralized bacteria may induce stone formation by acting as a focus for crystallization of renal calculi.

REFERENCES

1. W. Dosch, Fortschr. Urol. Nephrol. 5:67 (1975).
2. L. Cifuentes Delatte, M. Santos, A. Hidalgo, J. Bellanato, and P. F. Gonzalez-Diaz, in:"Urolithiasis Research", H. Fleisch, W. G. Robertson, L. H. Smith, and W. Vahlensieck, eds., Plenum, New York (1976).
3. D. B. Leusmann, Fortschr. Urol. Nephrol. 17:275 (1981).
4. W. E. Keefe and M. J. V. Smith, Invest. Urol. 14:344 (1977).

MATRIX-MINERAL CONFIGURATION IN WHEWELLITE KIDNEY STONES:

ULTRASTRUCTURAL ANALYSIS

L. U. Ogbuji, C. D. Batich, and B. Finlayson

Federal University of Technology, Yola, Nigeria, and
Depts. of Materials Science and Engineering and Surgery
University of Florida, Gainesville, Florida, U.S.A.

INTRODUCTION

Methods of compositional and structural studies of urinary
stones have evolved from visual inspection and bulk chemical
analysis, through light microscopy and X-ray diffraction, to the
present application of sophisticated imaging and analytical
techniques. The newer approaches have provided an increasingly
refined picture of the interactions of the components as a clue to
the causative factors involved in the formation of urinary stones.

One of the causative factors that structure analysis can help
determine is the respective roles of matrix and mineral in the
formation of calculi. In spite of its minute proportion in a
stone, the matrix maintains a pervasive presence throughout the
stone[1,2]; does it bind the mineral crystals together? Conversely,
the mineral is by far the major phase, and often occurs as
aggregates of different but chemically and crystallographically
similar species: is the agency of stone cohesion simply epitaxial
over-growth, or mere sintering (disoriented crystal-to-crystal
fusion)[3], rather than matrix cementation?

In this paper we have focused on the spatial distribution of
matrix and mineral in whewellite kidney stones as a clue to the
architectonic role of those components in the stone's formation.
Whewellite stones consist of a matrix phase of macromolecular
material (mostly proteins) and a mineral phase of calcium oxalate
monohydrate (COM). Allusions exist in the literature to the
pervasive presence of the matrix throughout a whewellite stone.
The techniques reported, however, include polarized and ordinary
light microscopy on stained specimens, scanning electron microscopy

711

(SEM) on stained or unprocessed specimens and demineralization studies. SEM, except in conjunction with energy-dispersive accessories, is not a sensitive tool for phase identification; the other techniques yield only gross impressions at best. So it was never clear to what extent the matrix and mineral interacted. Our investigations were accordingly aimed at this question. In addition to most of the techniques above, we employed transmission electron microscopy (TEM) and electron analytical techniques[4,5]. These yielded reliable evidence of matrix-mineral interaction down to the finest levels of ultrastructure.

TECHNIQUES

Electron Microscopy

Direct imaging of whewellite under the 10 KeV to 300 KeV electron beam of a conventional transmission electron microscope (CTEM) is counter-productive, because of the resulting rapid degradation of the COM. Published CTEM images of COM exhibit a tell-tale rash of blisters, which are actually images of water bubbles liberated by the breakdown of the COM - but which are easily mistaken for structural features of the stone. Similarly, phase identification by diffraction in CTEM is even less reliable or feasible, because of the attendant destruction of the crystal lattice. (By contrast, the less energetic electrons of SEM do negligible damage, but SEM is inappropriate, as we have seen.)

The ionization damage responsible for COM degradation diminishes again at higher voltages, so that reliable images may be obtained by high voltage electron microscopy (HVEM) at electron energies in excess of 1 MeV. Even then the repeated and prolonged irradiation of the same area necessary in diffraction analysis results in unacceptable cumulative damage and diffraction pattern alteration. Thus, HVEM is adequate for imaging (and has been so employed on renal stones[6]) but not easily for direct diffraction studies on COM. Therefore, we employed two indirect diffraction effects in the HVEM to complement direct images. The first is Fresnel fringes that appear in out-of-focus images between two crystals that are not in atomic (sintered) contact across their boundary, and which is capable of revealing any ultrafine gaps between the COM crystals of whewellite. In the other technique, a bright-field picture of the material (obtained by imaging with the central, transmitted electron beam) is compared with a quasi-dark field picture of the same features, imaged with the background stream of electrons inelastically scattered by non-crystalline areas of the material. In the pair of micrographs so obtained, amorphous (matrix) material between crystals is identified by its failure to reverse contrast, bright for dark.

Electron-Analytical Technique

In the absence of direct electron diffraction information, the results obtained by the foregoing methods needed independent confirmation. This was provided by using X-ray photonelectron spectroscopy (XPS) to probe the changes of surface elemental composition upon breaking or crushing the kidney stones in order to expose fresh surface areas. The reasoning was that fracture would occur predominantly <u>between</u> the COM crystals, rather than across them, especially if the spaces between them contained matrix material: inter-phase bonding of the type expected here is inherently weaker than the bonds within the crystals. Such preferentially inter-granular fracture would expose any matrix present between the crystals, and this would be reflected in any apparent increase in the amount of matrix sensed by XPS. The method is able to discriminate between the elements comprising or pre-dominant in the matrix (nitrogen and hydrogenated carbon) and those predominant in the COM (calcium, oxygen and oxygen-bonded carbon). It records that the relative abundance of the elements sensed, from which data relative proportion of matrix and mineral on the exposed surface is determined.

RESULTS AND DISCUSSION

Electron Microscopy (EM)

The data obtained are as follows: (1) COM crystals cluster with their broad faces parallel in all cases. The clusters correspond to the well-known radial striae. Within the clusters all crystals are in coincident crystallographic orientation (hence in identical contrast under crossed polars). To be identically orientated and yet retain their individual identity the crystals must be separated across their broad faces by matrix. (2) Continuous Fresnel fringes separate all crystals in out-of-focus images. Therefore, there is no atomic contact between crystals and matrix or void space must separate them. (3) The spaces between crystals stay bright in both bright- and dark-field images of same features. Therefore, the gaps between crystals contain matrix, rather than void spaces. In summary, all EM results point to matrix cementation of crystals.

X-Ray Photoelectron Spectroscopy

Table 1 summarizes the result of the XPS run on a specimen as indicated, and compares it with the data at the top of the Table computed for a hypothetical surface generated by random fracture through whewellite composed of 95% COM and 5% protein matrix. (The elemental composition of the matrix was also approximated from XPS

Table 1. Atomic Ratios of Elements Determined by XPS for Different Surfaces in Whewellite Kidney Stones Relative to a Value of 1.00 for Oxygen-Bonded Carbon, $C_{(O)}$.

	Ca	O	$C_{(H)}$	N	S
Random-Fracture Surface	0.48	2.45	0.30	0.03	0.00
Outer Surface of Specimen	0.17	1.82	5.25	0.50	0.07
Same Specimen after Washing and Crushing	0.35	1.40	3.27	0.11	0.17

The atomic ratio is proportional to the area under the spectral peak for the element.

runs on the outer surface of the stones, which was assumed to have a coat of matrix material.) Of the 6 chemical species detected in significant quantities (0.01 or higher proportion, and counting carbon bonded to hydrogen and carbon bonded to oxygen as different "species") $C_{(O)}$, Ca and O compose the COM and the other 3 are expected to predominate in the matrix. The sharp boost in signals from the matrix elements and corresponding drop in signals from the COM after fracture means that fracture preferentially exposes the matrix. This is consistent with intergranular fracture, occurring through a matrix phase that separates the crystals.

ACKNOWLEDGMENTS

This work was funded by the National Institute of Health under the University of Florida SCOR program, grant number AM 20586-02.

REFERENCES

1. D. J. Sutor, in:"Urolithiasis: Physical Aspects", B. Finlayson, L. L. Hench, and L. H. Smith, eds., National Academy of Sciences, Washington, D.C. (1972).
2. W. H. Boyce and F. K. Garvey, J. Urol. 76:213 (1956).
3. B. Finlayson, Urol. Clin. North Am. 1:181 (1974).
4. L. U. Ogbuji and B. Finlayson, Invest. Urol. 19:182 (1981).
5. L. U. Ogbuji and C. D. Batich, (submitted for publication).
6. M. Spector and J. C. Lilga, in:"Urolithiasis:Clinical and Basic Research", L. H. Smith, W. G. Robertson, and B. Finlayson, eds., Plenum, New York (1981).

CLINICAL-CHEMICAL STUDY OF URINARY STONES IN SAUDI ARABIA -

I. URIC ACID STONES

R. E. Abdel-Halim, A. O. Baghlaf, and A.-B. B. Farag

Urology Unit, King Abdul Aziz University Hospital, and
Dept. of Chemistry, Faculty of Science, King Abdul
Aziz University, Jeddah, Saudi Arabia

INTRODUCTION

In Saudi Arabia, urolithiasis is the commonest urological
problem. However, there are few reports on this topic and almost
none on the chemical composition of stones. This paper contains
part of an analytical study on 100 stones and the results of
clinical investigations on those patients with uric acid stones.

MATERIALS AND METHODS

One hundred urinary stones were subjected to wet chemical
analysis for the determination of oxalate[1] and phosphate[2] in a
sulphuric acid digest, and urates and xanthine[3] in a lithium
carbonate digest. Ca, Mg, Al, Zn, Pb, Cd, Cu, Fe, Mn, Sr, Co, Ni
and Cr were measured by atomic absorption spectrometry[4]. Ammonia,
carbonate, cystine[3] and cholesterol[5] were analysed qualitatively.
Elemental microanalytical determination of total carbon, hydrogen
and nitrogen in pure organic compounds was carried out using
modifications of the standard methods[6]. Samples as low as 1 mg
could be analysed by this procedure. Uric acid was determined by
infra red spectroscopy[7].

RESULTS

Seventeen percent of the stones were classified as uric acid
calculi[8]. Clinically, there was a preponderance of males with a
peak age of presentation between 26 and 45 years in agreement with
most reports from Western countries. Upper urinary tract stones

were more common than bladder stones (12 out of 17) contrary to the findings in Thailand[8]. Of the bladder stones, one came from a child (10 years old) and four from adults. Unlike the figures quoted in the West[10,11], the incidence of infection stones was very low (1 out of 16). This was a bladder stone in a paraplegic case with a urinary pH of 9 and a Proteus infection. It consisted of amorphous calcium phosphate and triple phosphate. In the rest of the patients, the urine was sterile (pH 5) and in 8 cases contained crystals of uric acid and calcium oxalate, either separately or together. The uric acid crystals were common in groups 3 and 4: calcium oxalate was present in all groups (Table 1). A previous history of stones was reported in 8 cases. Three of them had hyperuricemia and passed stones in groups 3 and 4 (Table 1).

Pure uric acid stones (containing no oxalate or phosphate) were rare. Therefore, the classification proposed in Table 1 on the basis of the phosphate and oxalate content of stones enabled us to cover all the types found in this series. Unlike Category II (an infection stone), Category I contained only traces of phosphate (0 - 1.66%) and variable amounts of oxalate. These were classified into four groups. Group 1 contained more than 30% oxalate, groups 2 and 3 contained oxalate between 20 and 30% and 10 and 20% respectively and group 4 contained up to 10% oxalate[9]. The calcium content was directly related to that of oxalate.

Xanthine was not found in this series. Carbonate was detected in 3 stones and trace amounts of cystine and cholesterol in 10 and 7 stones respectively. Ammonia was present in Category II which contained the highest percentage of Mg and Zn. The high percentage of aluminium in group 1 is unexplainable. Trace elements such as nickel, cadmium and chromium were absent. In Category I, 0.05%

Table 1. Percentage Composition of 17 Uric Acid Stones.

Categories	I				II
Groups	1	2	3	4	1
No. of stones	1	3	4	8	1
Uric Acid	23.7	31.6-49.0	51.6-76.6	84.4-100	26.30
Phosphate	9.3	0 - 1.7	0 - 0.7	0	21.2
Oxalate	38.8	23.7-28.9	13.6-20.8	0 - 6.0	0
Calcium	16	10.1-22.4	6.7- 8.2	0 - 3.8	7.3
Magnesium	0.04	0.02- 0.18	0.03-0.09	0 -0.04	4.1
Zinc	0.01	0.01	0.01-0.02	0 -0.01	0.06
Aluminium	0.05	0 - 0.01	0	0 -0.01	0
Carbon	22.5	24.5-25.8	28.0-31.2	32.8-37.05	10.8
Hydrogen	2.0	2.1- 2.5	2.4- 3.0	2.2-2.8	3.6
Nitrogen	8.2	14 - 17	21.4-23.7	28.2-32.5	11.8

Table 2. The Ranges of Total Nitrogen and Corresponding Uric Acid.

Nitrogen (%)	8 - 14	14 - 21	21 - 28	28 - 32
Urate (%)	24 - 32	32 - 52	52 - 84	84 - 101

Table 3. The Ranges of Total Carbon and Corresponding Oxalate or Phosphate in Uric Acid Stones.

Carbon (%)	23 - 25	25 - 28	28 - 33	33 - 37
Oxalate (%)	30 - 38	30 - 20	20 - 10	10 - 0
Phosphate (%)	←————— Trace of phosphates (1 - 2) ————→			

strontium was present in 2 stones and associated with 0.05% lead in another one. Cobalt (0.30%) was present only in one stone. The ratio of anhydrous uric acid to uric acid dihydrate was 14 : 3 and in these stones, the total nitrogen content was directly proportional to the percentage of uric acid (Table 1).

DISCUSSION

Since the stones in Category I contained 0.01 to 0.02% zinc, the 0.06% Zn in the infection stone (Category II) was considered to be high. Therefore, we may suggest that alkaline urine not only precipitates calcium and magnesium[11] but also zinc with phosphate.

Elemental microanalysis of total organic carbon, hydrogen and nitrogen proved to be an efficient tool for the quick identification of the various types of stones. Unlike oxalate or phosphate stones, uric acid stones have a high percentage of nitrogen ranging from 8 to 32% (Table 2). The percentage of carbon (Table 3) helps to identify the other constituent. Therefore, from the ranges of nitrogen and carbon in Tables 2 and 3, we can categorize uric acid stones according to the classification in Table 1. Although the percentage of carbon found in Category II stones (Table 3) is similar to that of some oxalate stones (unpublished data), the high nitrogen level in the former helps in differentiating between the two types of stones. A nitrogen content below 8% indicates either an oxalate or a phosphate stone. Differentiation of these two types made from the percentage of carbon which ranges mostly between 13 and 23% in oxalate stones and between 3 and 8% in the phosphate stones (unpublished data).

ACKNOWLEDGMENT

This work is supported by a research grant from the Faculty of Science, King Abdul Aziz University, Jeddah, Saudi Arabia.

717

REFERENCES

1. J. D. P. Wooton, "Medical Biochemistry", Churchill Livingstone, London 1954.
2. R. Belcher and A. J. Nutten, "Quantitative Inorganic Analysis", Butterworths, London (1970).
3. C. J. Farrington, M. L. Liddy, and A. H. Chalmers, Am. J. Clin. Path. 73:96 (1980).
4. F. J. Fernandez and H. L. Khan, Clin. Chem. Newsl. 3:34 (1971).
5. H. Varley, "Practical Clinical Biochemistry", 4th Ed. Heinemann, New Delhi (1976).
6. R. F. Culmo, Mikrochim. Acta 175 (1969).
7. A. Hesse and D. Bach, in:"Urinary Stones:Clinical and Laboratory Aspects", G. A. Rose, ed., MTP Press, Lancaster (1982).
8. V. Parasangwatana, P. Sriboonlue, and S. Suntarapa, Br. J. Urol. 55:353 (1983).
9. L. N. Pyrah, "Renal Calculus", Springer-Verlag, Berlin (1979).
10. A. Atsmon, A. DeVries, and M. Frank, "Uric Acid Lithiasis", Elsevier, Amsterdam (1963).
11. M. I. Resnick, Urol. Clin. N. Am. 8:265 (1981).

STRUVITE STONES ANALYSIS BY INFRARED SPECTROPHOTOMETRY IN

ADULTS AND CHILDREN

R. J. Reveillaud and M. Daudon

Dept. of Internal Medicine and Nephrology, and Crystal
Laboratory, Centre Hospitalier, Saint-Cloud, France

INTRODUCTION

The relationship between struvite-containing stones and urinary
infection has been known for a long time, but it has not been
systematically studied. The discrimination between infection-
induced stones and secondarily infected stones is not always clear.
In order to define the proportion and frequency of struvite in renal
stones, we measured the occurrence of this compound in 3,000 stones
analyzed by infra red spectroscopy. Furthermore, we compared the
results with our data on spontaneous struvite crystalluria which are
reported elsewhere[1].

MATERIALS AND METHODS

Every stone was washed and dried at room temperature, and
analyzed by microdissection and infrared spectroscopy. The methods
have been described previously[2,3].

RESULTS

Struvite stones from humans are never pure; they are always
mixed with carbonate-apatite (CA), and often associated with
ammonium urate (Am ur) and/or calcium oxalate (Ca Ox). In adults,
out of 2700 stones analyzed, only 16.6% contained struvite (MAP).
In children, from 300 stones examined, 50% contained struvite;
Am ur was also more frequent in the stones from children (46%)
compared with those from adults (9.7%). The frequency of the
constituents and their main associations are given in Table 1. In

719

Table 1. Frequency of the Constituents and Main Associations (%).

	Children (300)			Adults (2700)		
	Pure	Mixed	Total	Total	Mixed	Pure
Ca ox	6.7	54.3	61.0	82.7	63.2	19.5
Ca ox-Ap	0	20.0	20.0	41.9	41.9	0
Ca pH	0.6	81.0	81.6	75.1	74.7	0.4
MAP	0.3	49.8	50.1	16.6	16.6	0
MAP-CA	0	9.5	9.5	2.9	2.9	0
MAP-CA-Ca ox	0	4.5	4.5	6.1	6.1	0
MAP-CA-Ca ox-AM ur	0	12.8	12.8	2.5	2.5	0
MAP-Ca-Am ur	0	19.6	19.6	2.5	2.5	0
Am ur	0	46.0	46.0	9.7	9.7	0
Na ur	0	0	0	0.5	0.5	0
Ur ac	0	7.0	7.0	16.6	11.2	5.4
Cy	2.3	0	2.3	1.8	0.1	1.7
Miscellaneous			11.0	7.0		
Total	9.9	90.1	100.0	100.0	73.0	27.0

Ca ox = calcium oxalate; Ap = apatites; Ca ph = all calcium
phosphates; MAP = struvite; CA = carbonate-apatites;
Am ur = ammonium urate; Na ur = sodium urate; Ur ac = uric acid;
Cy = cystine; Miscellaneous = various compounds or complex mixtures.

the text below, "struvite stones" are defined as mixed stones
containing MAP and CA with or without other compounds.

Among the adults, 75% were females, of which 70% were between
25 and 55. In children, 75% were boys, of which 60% were under the
age of 5, and 31% between 6 and 13. Urinary infection by urea-
splitting bacteria was present in 60 to 75% of the cases in children
and adults. Proteus was isolated in more than 50%.

Macroscopic and microscopic examination of the stones allowed
us to establish a morphological classification published
previously[3]. With this classification, we recognize 2 or 3 of the
main components in more than 3% of the cases. Stones containing
struvite belong to Type IV (phosphates) with sub-groups a,b,c: Type
IVa: the morphological characteristics are mainly due to the
presence of carbonate-apatites which are predominant; Type IVb: the
struvite is recognizable on certain areas of the surface; Type IVc:
(rare) the struvite is predominant and determines the superficial
and internal morphology. The surface is homogenous, made of large
whitish orthorhombic crystals more or less fused together. On
sectioning, there is a loose radial crystallization round the
nucleus that is not well defined.

720

There are differences in the frequency of the various types between adults and children. In adults, Type IVa represents 18% of all cases and Types IVb and IVc only 4% and 1% respectively. In children, Type IV is more frequent (49%) with 31% Type IVa, 15% Type IVb and 3% Type IVc. Type IVb stones are frequently larger, staghorn and containing a large amount of struvite (in adults, 42% of the staghorn stones belong to Type IVb, and 27% to Type IVa). Struvite is more likely than other components to produce staghorn stones. Within the staghorn group of stones we found 31% struvite-containing stones, 19% ammonium urate stones, 10% CA stones, 7% Ca Ox and less than 5% for Ur ac and Cy. On the whole, staghorn calculi contained struvite in 67% of adults and in more than 80% of children.

From an etiological point of view the analysis of the nucleus is important in order to establish precisely whether or not the infection was present at the time of nucleation of the stone. In adults, struvite was present in the nucleation zone in only 8% of all the stones, but in 48% of the staghorn nuclei. In children, the corresponding frequencies were 31% and 75%. It should also be noted that in terms of ammonium ion content, there was a striking difference between childhood stones (61% contain MAP and/or Am ur) and adult stones (22%).

DISCUSSION

Urine must be supersaturated for crystallization to occur and, with respect to struvite, increased levels of both alkalinity and ammonia are necessary. This occurs in the presence of urease-producing bacteria which split urea and increase urinary pH and the concentrations of ammonium, bicarbonate and carbonate ions. Urinary infection by such organisms is found in 60 to 75% of the cases, children and adults, and Proteus is isolated in 50 to 60%. Theoretically struvite crystallization may occur without urinary infection, and even in slightly acidic urine, when ammonium, phosphate and/or magnesium concentrations are sufficiently elevated. This does not seem to be possible in urine unless alkalinization is present, induced by urea-splitting bacteria.

Recently, Boistelle et al[4] reported struvite crystals in some samples of sterile and acidic urine of stone formers. This could account for some cases of struvite stone formation or growth but this is certainly rare for several reasons: (i) Struvite precipitates easily as large crystals (20 to 50 μm) that have little tendency to aggregate; thus the growth of struvite stones needs repeated periods of high supersaturation which purely metabolic crystallization conditions probably do not permit. If it were so, one can imagine that other clinical or biological abnormalities would be observed in addition to renal lithiasis; (ii) The frequency of struvite stones with urinary infection is higher than the frequency of identified urea-splitting bacteria, such as Proteus, Pseudomonas or Klebsiella; (iii) In routine bacteriological examination, a lower urinary tract infection may mask an upper urinary tract infection due to a different organism. If bacteriological examinations of the surgically removed stone and/or the urine are not performed, the relationship between infection and stone cannot be ascertained; (iv) Some organisms contain urease but are not identified as urea-splitting, for instance, Staphylococcus with negative coagulase (Staphylococcus Saprophyticus); others like Providencia produce ammonia without being urea-splitting. Mycoplasma such as ureaplasma urealyticum produce urease but are not routinely isolated although they may play a role in the genesis of struvite stones in "sterile" urine.

One further point needs to be underlined:differences exist in terms of the frequency of struvite formation according to the age and sex of the patients, since 75% of children with struvite stones were boys and 75% of adult struvite stone formers were females. Although it is recognized that urinary infection is more frequent in women, the infection by the most common urea-splitting bacteria (i.e. Proteus) has more or less the same frequency in males and females. In our experience, in 6100 routine urine examinations of hospitalized non-stone-forming patients, the incidence of Proteus was 17% of infected urine cases for both sexes. Similarly, when crystalluria was present, urine was infected by Proteus in 41% of both sexes[1]. Struvite was found in 30% of crystalluria in males and in 39% of females, whereas struvite was only found in 9% of the stones in males but in 33% of the female stones[1]. Women seem to have a particular suceptibility to struvite stones due to unidentified factors, hence the importance of early diagnosis and treatment of urinary infection by ammonia-producing organisms should be emphasized.

REFERENCES

1. M. Daudon, M. F. Protat, R. J. Reveillaud, and M. Rouchon, Ann. Biol. Clin. 41:199 (1983).
2. M. Daudon, M. F. Protat, and R. J. Reveillaud, Ann. Biol. Clin. 36:475 (1978).
3. R. J. Reveillaud, M. Daudon, M. F. Protat, and G. Ayrole, Eur. Urol. 6:161 (1980).
4. R. Boistelle, F. Abbona, Y. Berland, M. Grandvuillemin, and M. Olmer, Nephrologie (in press).

722

COMPOSITION AND STRUCTURE OF INFECTED STONES

J.-Y. He, G.-D. Liu, and S.-J. Shen

Dept. of Urology, 2nd Affiliated Hospital, Lanzhou
Medical College, Lanzhou, and Institute of Urology
Beijing Medical College, Gansu, People's Republic of
China

INTRODUCTION

Urinary infection is often associated with urinary stones,
owing to the chemical changes in urine resulting from infection. In
this paper, we report on the composition and structure of 18
infected stones using polarized light microscopy, scanning electron
microscopy and energy dispersive X-ray analysis (EDAX).

MATERIALS AND METHODS

Of the 18 infected stones, all were large, 14 were bladder
stones (2 from patients with vesicovaginal fistulas), 1 each came
from the kidney, ureter, and sigmoid conduit respectively, and 1 was
of unknown origin. Urine culture was performed in 5 out of 8 in-
patients. Escherichia coli were found in 4 cases, and one was
sterile. Of the 3 in-patients in whom no urine culture was
performed, 2 were found to have pus cells in their urine.

All the stones were ground to thin sections and their
composition and structure examined by polarized light microscopy.
Four stones were studied by S-550 scanning electron microscopy and
the crystal composition of 3 of these analysed by EDAX.

RESULTS

The composition of the 18 stones is shown in Table 1.
Struvite crystals were of two types, one radiating out like a
feather (Fig. 1), and in the other lump-like (Fig. 2). Ammonium

723

Table 1. Composition of 18 Infected Stones (Number Containing Particular Constituent).

Struvite	Ammonium Urate	Apatite	Whewellite	Uric Acid	Weddelite	Brushite
18	16	14	11	3	1	2

urate took the form of needle-like crystals under polarized light (Fig. 3) and of short columnar crystals (3 um) under SEM. Apatite occurred as spherules between the struvite crystals (Fig. 4). The stones could be divided into two types according to structure. One was infective in origin consisting mainly of struvite, ammonium urate and apatite. There were foreign bodies in the nuclei of one or two stones. All of these stones were oolitic in structure with no radial striations. The other type was associated with infection occurring as a result of stone formation. The composition of the nuclei of these stones was similar to that of sterile stones, namely uric acid and whewellite. Outside the nuclei there were various amounts of struvite and ammonium urate depending on the degree of infection. The first type consisted mainly of radially arranged feathery crystals but in one stone a layer of pure struvite was found (Fig. 1). All except two were oolitic in structure with no radial striations. Sometimes, layers were found consisting of an oolitic band with radial striations.

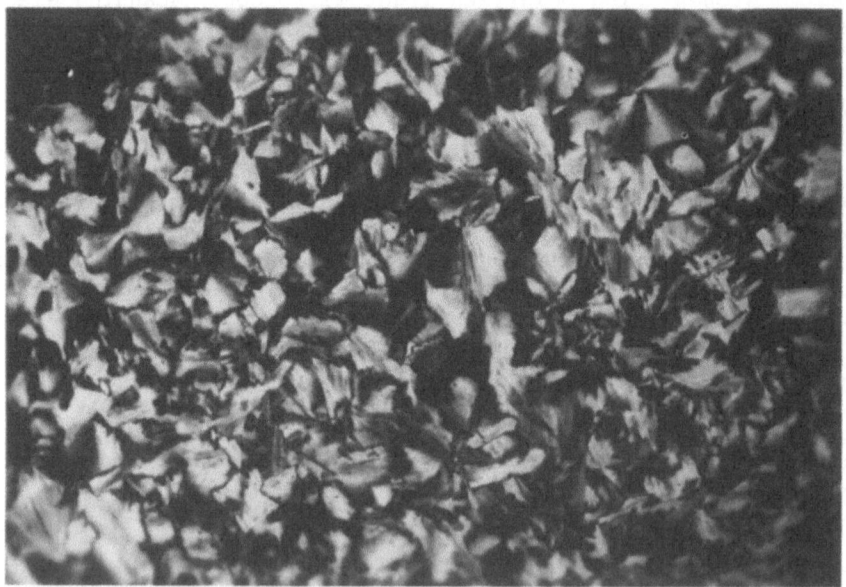

Fig. 1. Radially arranged feathery crystals of struvite (PM).

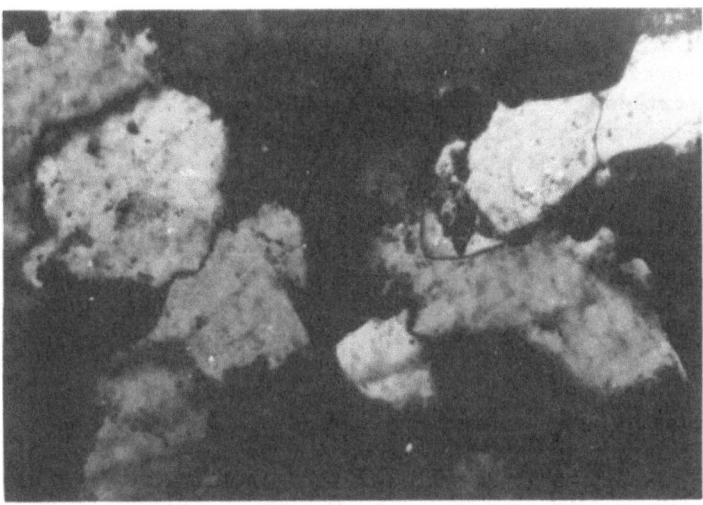

Fig. 2. Lump-like crystals of struvite, with the dark part of ammonium urate microcrystals (PM).

DISCUSSION

The main constituents of infected stones, termed "urease stones"[1], were magnesium ammonium phosphate and calcium phosphate, arising from the high ammonium ion concentrations and alkaline urine produced by urea-splitting organisms.

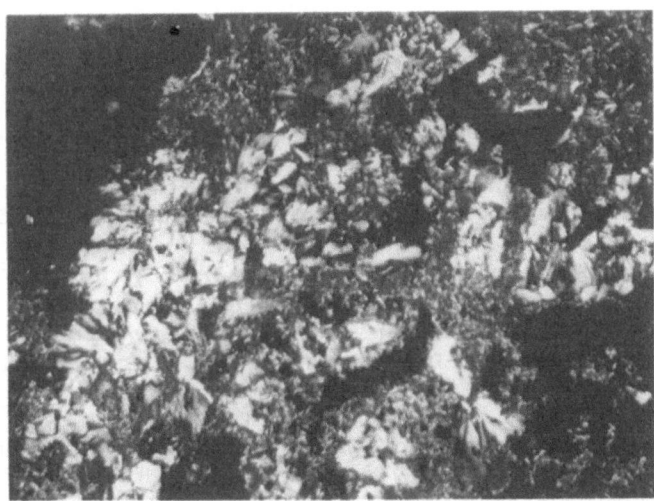

Fig. 3. Radially arranged feathery crystals of struvite between ammonium urate microcrystals (PM).

Some researchers have reported the presence of both ammonium and sodium urate in infection stones but Lagergren has suggested that both urates occur only in bladder stones[2]. In this study ammonium urate was found in 16 stones, and in 10 of these it was the main constituent. Pena et al examined 1100 stones by polarized light microscopy and infrared spectroscopy and found that 235 stones contained ammonium urate. Of these 112 (47.7%) were infected stones containing struvite[3]. Ammonium urate is one of the most common urates in urine. Dantzler studying non-mammalian vertebrates found that the urine of crocodiles was alkaline and contained a great quantity of ammonia, so that ammonium urate was the main salt in urine[4]. Valyasevi et al reported that infants in the villages of Thailand had abnormal crystalluria of calcium oxalate and ammonium urate[5].

In urinary tract infection, urine may become supersaturated with ammonium urate because of the high ammonium ion concentration and alkalinity. Thus both ammonium urate and struvite may be precipitated simultaneously. In the treatment and prevention of infected stones, in addition to using antibiotics to eliminate bacteria in the urinary tract, competitive inhibitors of urease such as acetohydroxamic acid[6] and flurofamide[7] may be used to normalise the urine biochemistry.

ACKNOWLEDGMENT

The authors wish to thank Mr Yu Hen in the Lanzhou Petroleum Machinery Research Institute for his assistance with SEM and EDAX.

REFERENCES

1. D. P. Griffith and D. M. Musher, in:"Colloquium on Renal Lithiasis", B. Finlayson and W. C. Thomas, eds., The University Presses of Florida, Gainesville (1976).
2. C. Lagergren, Acta. Radiol. 133 (Suppl):1 (1956).
3. E. G. Pena, and L. C. Dalatte, in:"Urolithiasis, Clinical and Basic Research", L. H. Smith, W. G. Robertson, and B. Finlayson, eds., Plenum, New York (1981).
4. W. H. Dantzler, in:"Uric Acid", W. N. Kelley and I. M. Weiner, eds., Springer-Verlag, Berlin (1978).
5. A. Valyasevi and S. Dhanamitta, in:"Urinary Calculus", J. G. Brockis and B. Finlayson, eds., PSG Publishing Company, Littleton, Mass. (1981).
6. A. Martelli et al. Urology 17:320 (1981).
7. O. E. Millner, J. A. Andersen, M. E. Appler, J. G. Benjamin, D. T. Edwards, and E. M. Shearer. J. Urol. 127:346 (1982).

URINARY CALCULI IN CHILDREN - EPIDEMIOLOGICAL AND MINERALOGICAL ASPECTS

G. Brien, C. Bothor, W. Berg, C. Schubert, and
P. Schorch

Depts of Urology, Humboldt-University, Berlin
Friedrichshain Hospital, Berlin, and Computing Center
Friedrich-Schiller-University Jena, D.D.R.

INTRODUCTION

In contrast to the accurate epidemiological study on urinary lithiasis in adults carried out by Vahlensieck in the Federal Republic of Germany[1], no such study has been performed on childhood urolithiasis. Most of the published data on this topic refer to selected clinical or out-patient groups of children. This gives rise to an incorrect understanding of the frequency distribution of urolithiasis and certain stone types depending on age, sex and the type of stone removal.

METHODS

A centralized and standardized analysis of all urinary stones has been carried out in the German Democratic Republic since 1970. Data thus obtained have allowed us to draw conclusions on a number of essential factors which play a part in childhood urolithiasis.

RESULTS AND DISCUSSION

Table 1 shows the absolute and relative frequency distribution of the types of urinary calculi in 167,860 analyses out of which 2,134 were performed on stones from children up to 15 years of age. This represents only 1.27% of all the stones. The ratio of male:female stone-formers was 2:1 in the population as a whole and 1.5:1 in children. Significant differences in the frequency distributions of the uric acid, ammonium hydrogen urate, struvite and carbonate apatite concrements and in the whewellite/weddellite

727

Table 1. Distribution of Stone Types in 167,660 Analyses.

Main constituent	Total Number	%	Children Number	%
Uric acid	18,671	11.1	42	2.0
Uric acid dihydrate	4,226	2.5	11	0.5
Ammonium hydrogen urate	610	0.4	31	1.5
Sodium hydrogen urate	30	0.0	2	0.1
Cystine	335	0.2	14	0.7
Protein	784	0.5	25	1.2
Whewellite	100,938	60.2	678	31.8
Wheddellite	22,106	13.1	709	33.2
Octo-calciumphosphate	12	0.0	4	0.2
Apatite	2,489	1.5	54	2.5
Brushite	374	0.2	36	1.7
Carbonate apatite	5,766	3.4	156	7.3
Struvite	7,694	4.6	240	11.3
Artifacts	3,462	2.1	122	6.7
Others	363	0.2	10	0.3
	167,860	100.0	2134	100.0

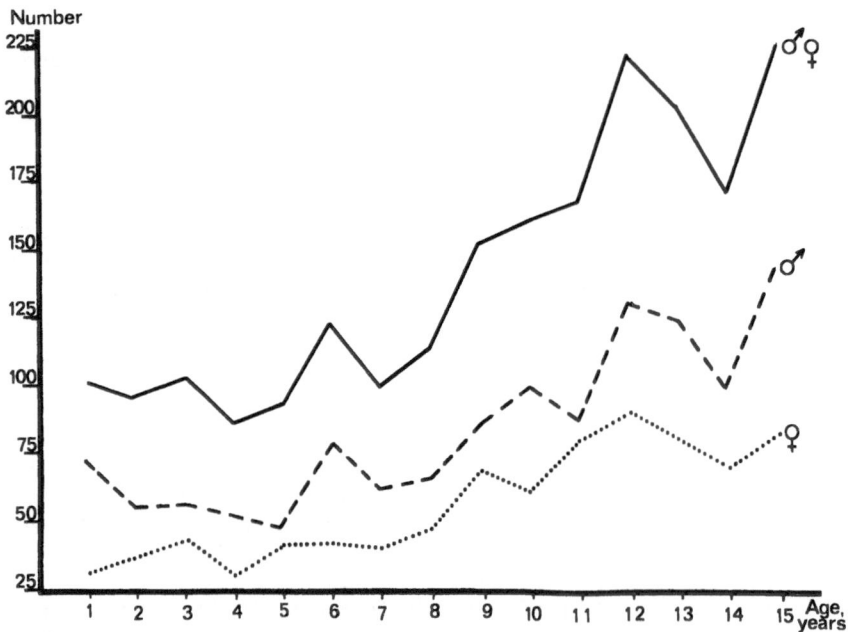

Fig. 1. Frequency of urolithiasis depending on age.

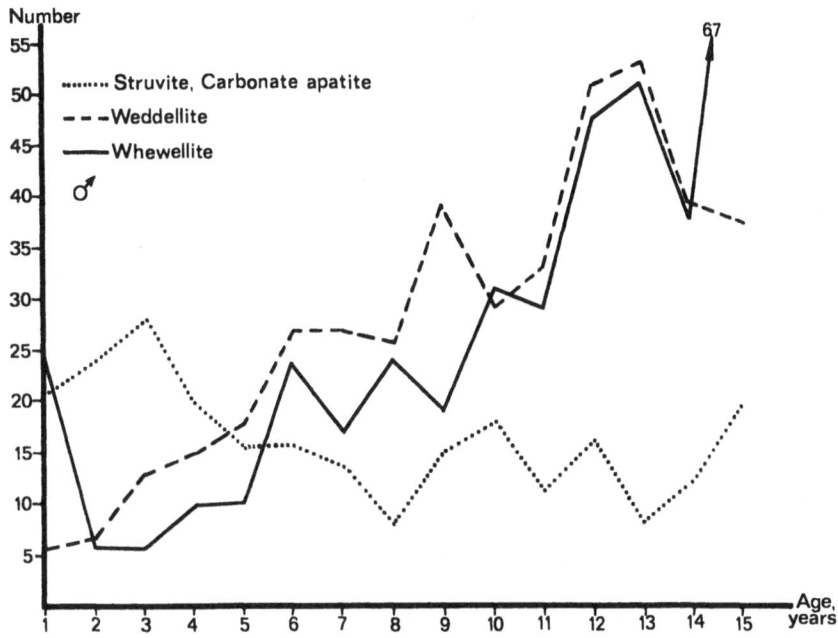

Fig. 2.   Frequency of struvite/carbonate apatite, whewellite
          and weddellite calculi depending on age.

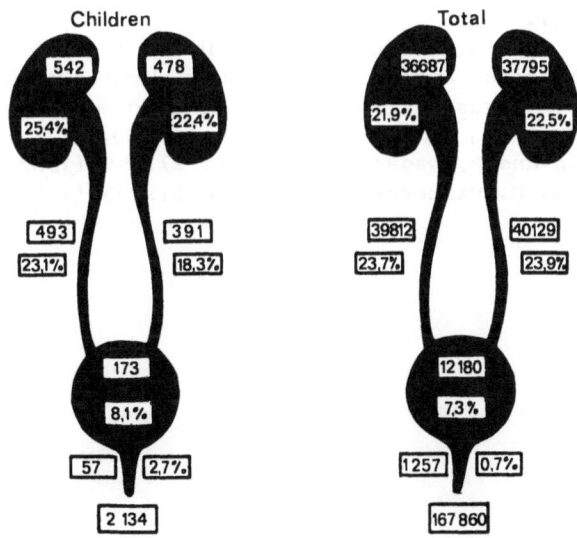

Fig. 3.   Localisation of urinary calculi in children and adults.

729

ratio were found. The proportion of calcium oxalate stones in our children was much higher than that reported by others[2-6].

In the first 7 years of life the frequency of urolithiasis is low, on average, but rises continuously from age 8 onwards (Fig. 1). Differences were found with regard to age distribution and stone type. Fig. 2 shows the age distribution of whewellite, weddellite and struvite/carbonate apatite stones in boys. In the first few years, struvite is found relatively often, its frequency, however, clearly decreases from age 5. Whewellite and weddellite are met more frequently with increasing age except that in the first year of life whewellite is found much more often than weddellite. In girls, the relationships are similar.

In comparison with adults, the site of stone formation in the urinary tract shows no significant differences (Fig. 3). Yet when taking into account the 1- to 5-year-old age group, the share of lower urinary tract calculi is markedly higher than in adults. In boys, 14% of stones were found in the bladder and 5% in the urethral in girls, the corresponding figures were 12% and 2%.

A comparison of the type of stone removal in children and in adults is of some interest. Though the share of spontaneously passed stones in children is lower, it still amounts to 50%. The proportion of girls requiring open surgery is markedly higher than that of boys but it is not as high as that of women (not shown)

REFERENCES

1. E. W. Vahlensieck, D. Bach, and A. Hesse, Urol. Res. 10:161 (1982).
2. R. S. Malek and P. P. Keldalis, J. Urol. 113:545 (1975).
3. E. W. Vahlensieck and H. Bastian, Eur. Urol. 2:129 (1976).
4. V. Zvara, V. Revusova, M. Hornak, L. Landsmannova, J. Payer, and L. Badalik, Urol. Int. 34:36 (1979).
5. V. Borgmann and R. Nagel, Urol. Int. 37:198 (1982).
6. J. Joost and H. Marberger, Urologe A 21:133 (1982).

A SCANNING ELECTRON MICROSCOPY (SEM) STUDY OF THE BLADDER MUCOSA

IN PAEDIATRIC PATIENTS WITH IDIOPATHIC CALCULUS DISEASE

P. Gojaseni, C. Trivitayaratn, and S. Sriurairatha

Section of Urology, Dept. of Surgery, Ramathibodi
Hospital, Bangkok, Thailand

INTRODUCTION

Idiopathic bladder calculus disease, prevalent in Thailand and
many developing countries, has been characterized as a distinct
subgroup of urolithiasis.   It occurs predominantly in children
below 10 years of age and has an uncommon association with renal
calculi[1].   The mechanism by which the vesical calculus is formed is
unclear.   Heavy crystalluria of calcium oxalate, uric acid, and
ammonium acid urate, noted in the children in the endemic areas, is
thought to be associated with the high incidence[2].   Finlayson has
calculated that crystal growth to a critical size is possible in the
bladder[3].   Fixation of the crystals, noted in the kidney tubules
and ducts of Bellini[4], has not been observed on the bladder mucosa.
It is therefore the purpose of this study to evaluate the role of
the bladder mucosa in the genesis of idiopathic vesical calculi.

MATERIALS AND METHODS

Multiple biopsies of the bladders in 9 patients, aged between
6 months and 7 years, were obtained during cystolithotomies.   The
specimens were washed in normal saline and fixed in ice-cold 4.5%
glutaraldehyde in 0.1 M phosphate buffer at pH 7.4 for 2 h.   They
were washed in 0.1M phosphate buffer and dehydrated overnight with
absolute alcohol.   They were gold-coated in an iron splutter and
submitted to scanning electron microscopy (SEM) using an Akashi
Model SEM 4 (Hitachi).

Bladder biopsies from children with other urological diseases
were used as controls.   The crystals were identified by their

morphology and electron microprobe analysis.   The crystalline
particles in the voided and bladder urine obtained intraoperatively
were measured directly by a vernier eye-piece.

RESULTS

        The ultrastructure of a vesicle calculus is shown in Fig. 1.
A specimen of mucosa obtained from a patient with vesico-ureteric
reflux in Fig. 2A reveals microvilli and ridges, the appearance of
which is in marked contrast with the crystalline tile-like
incrustations on the cells in Fig. 2B.   Tiny projections can be
observed on the surface.   Sponge-like crystalline deposits and
exophytic growths are evident in Fig. 2C.   The sponge-like
encrustations conform to the cellular contours, showing multiple

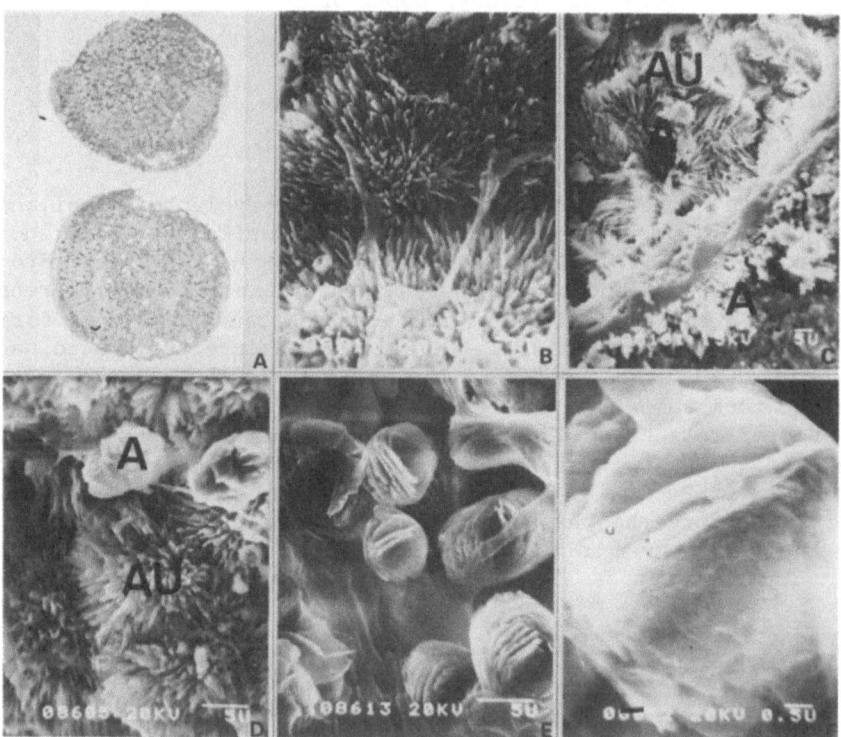

Fig. 1.   A typical vesical calculus:A. The cross-section, showing a
           porous texture; B. Clusters of ammonium acid urate and
           lamellar; C. Ammonium acid urate (AU) and uric acid (A)
           (lower right).   A crystalline boundary; D. A high power
           view of ammonium acid urate (AU) and uric acid (A);
           E. Uric acid crystals; F. A high power view of uric acid.

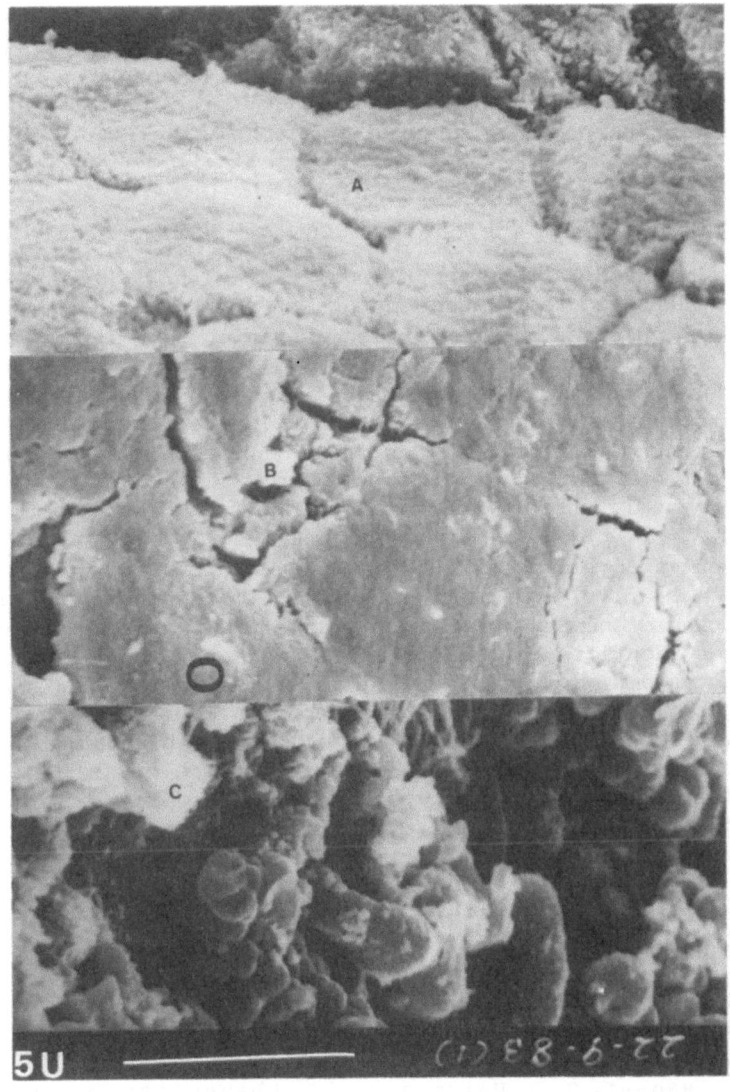

Fig. 2. Microphotographs showing (A) normal transitional epithelium
with micro ridges and villi (X2000); (B) tile-like
crystalline encrustations with visible projections (O)
(X3000); (C) sponge-like polycrystalline deposits
conforming to the cellular contours and exophytes (X5000).

slender projections.   They are probably ammonium acid urate mixed
with uric acid crystals, while the polycrystalline exophytes are
rhombohedral uric acid.   In many areas clusters of bristled
spherulitic ammonium acid urate are abundant.

Calcium oxalate was not found in the deposit but as free crystals in the bladder. Most areas examined by the electron microprobe show strong peaks of calcium and phosphorus, but no definite calcium phosphate crystals. The free crystalline particles in the bladder measured approximately 1 to 100 μm.

DISCUSSION

Halstead and Valyasevi[5] believed that bladder stone nuclei were formed attached to the bladder mucosa in some cases. Lloyd-Davies and Hinman[6] observed micro-globules averaging 3 μm in diameter attached to the bladder epithelium. The globules were increased in amount during infection. Aurora and Gupta[7,8] suggested that injury to the urothelium might cause the efflux of red blood cells and PAS-positive mucopolysaccharide into the potential spaces between the cells. On reaching the luminal surface, these might entrap the urinary crystals thereby initiating stone formation.

In our study, crystalline deposits were observed on the bladder mucosa of children with bladder stones. The predominant crystals were uric acid and ammonium acid urate. The role of calcium phosphates identified in all areas is unclear. Similarly, calcium oxalate crystals, commonly present in the urine of these patients, were not part of these crystalline deposits, but formed free poly-crystalline conglomerates (1 to 100 μm) in the bladder urine. Our preliminary study suggests that fixation of the crystals, chiefly uric and ammonium acid urate, to the urothelium may be significant in vesical calculus formation. The free crystalline particles of calcium oxalate are contributory to further growth by epitaxy.

REFERENCES

1. A. Valyasevi and S. Dhanamitta, in:"Urinary Calculi", J. G. Brockis and B. Finlayson, eds., PSG Publishing Co., Littleton (1981).
2. A. Valyasevi, S. B. Halstead and S. Dhanamitta, Am. J. Clin. Nutr. 20:1362 (1967).
3. B. Finlayson, in:"Idiopathic Urinary Bladder Stone Disease", R. Van Reen, ed., DHEW Publication No. (NIH) 77-1063, Washington (1977).
4. J. Oliver, M. MacDowell, R. Whang, and L. G. Welt, J. Exp. Med. 124:263 (1966).
5. S. B. Halstead, A. Valyasevi, and P. Umpaivit, Am. J. Clin. Nutr. 20:1352 (1967).
6. R. W. Lloyd-Davies and F. Hinman, Br. J. Urol. 43:665 (1971).
7. A. L. Aurora and D. N. Gupta, Indian J. Med. Sci. 24:122 (1970).
8. A. L. Aurora, in:"Idiopathic Urinary Bladder Stone Disease", R. Van Reen, ed., DHEW Publication NIH 77-1063, Washington.

CHILDHOOD UROLITHIASIS IN IRAN: A STUDY OF URINARY CALCULI USING

X-RAY DIFFRACTION, POLARIZING MICROSCOPY AND CHEMICAL ANALYSIS

M. H. Kheradpir and T. Armbruster

Chirurgische Kinderklinik and Laboratorium fur chemische und mineralogische Kristallographie, Bern, Switzerland

INTRODUCTION

The incidence of childhood urolithiasis in the Children's University Hospital of Tehran amounts to one case in 300 admissions. Children admitted to this general hospital originate from all over Iran and cover the full spectrum of social classes. The lack of knowledge about this disease in Iran led us to determine the composition of stones in children in order to compare these results with findings in other countries in the Middle and Far East.

METHODS

Stones were analysed by chemical analysis, optical polarizing microscopy of thin sections and X-ray diffraction.

RESULTS

From a total of 148 patients with urolithiasis undergoing surgery in the Children's University Hospital of Tehran between 1970-1982, 160 calculi originating from 121 children were analysed. Of these children, 98 (65% male) had upper urinary tract stones, 19 (74%) had bladder and urethral stones, and 4 had stones in both the upper and lower tracts. Since there were insufficient metabolic studies in some children, we were able to establish an obvious cause of stone formation, such as metabolic disorders and anatomical abnormalities in only 30% of the cases. The age distribution of children with kidney and ureteric calculi was bimodal with weak maxima at 5 and 11 years.

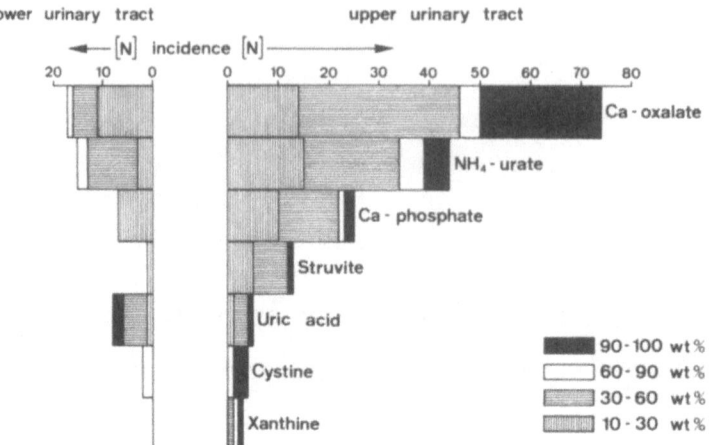

Fig. 1. Incidence of concentrations of salts in calculi from 100 children with upper and 21 children with lower urinary tract stones.

The incidence of the various stone-forming salts, divided into 4 concentration ranges, is shown in Fig. 1. In the cases where we performed X-ray or microscopic phase analysis, an incidence histogram of concrement-forming phases is given in Fig. 2.

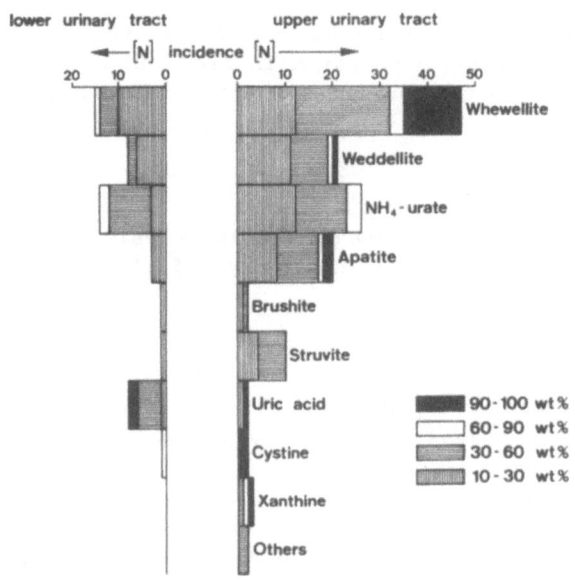

Fig. 2. Incidence of concentrations of phases in 66 children with upper and 19 children with lower urinary tract calculi.

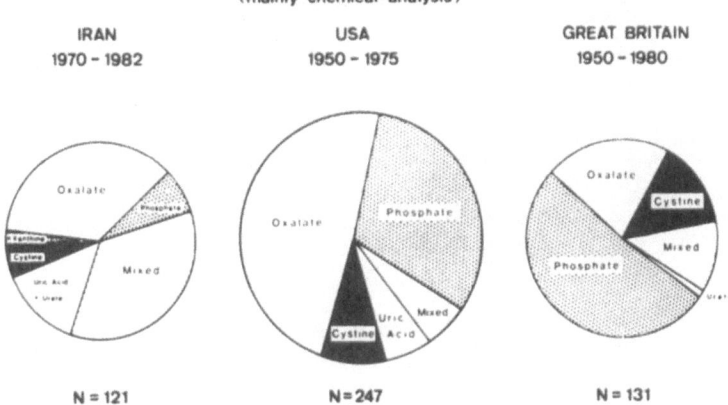

PRECENTAGE OCCURRENCE OF STONE TYPES
(mainly chemical analysis)

IRAN
1970 - 1982

USA
1950 - 1975

GREAT BRITAIN
1950 - 1980

N = 121

N = 247

N = 131

COMPARISON OF THE AETIOLOGY

IRAN
1970 - 1982

USA
1950 - 1975

GREAT BRITAIN
1950 - 1980

N = 121

N = 372

N = 463

Fig. 3. Sector diagrams comparing the characteristics of
urolothiasis in Iran, USA and Great Britain.

Apart from whewellite stones which often occurred in compact
spherulitic and pure forms, the most frequent combination consisted
of whewellite and ammonium acid urate. Microscopic thin sections
showed that urate formed the core of these concrements, with whewellite present in the outer layers. Typical infection stones consisting of apatite and struvite occurred in less than 20% of the cases.
The lower urinary tract calculi more frequently consisted of uric
acid or whewellite plus urate. Pure whewellite concrements were
not found in the bladder or urethra. It was striking that in this
series, 6 stones contained cystine and 3 consisted of xanthine.

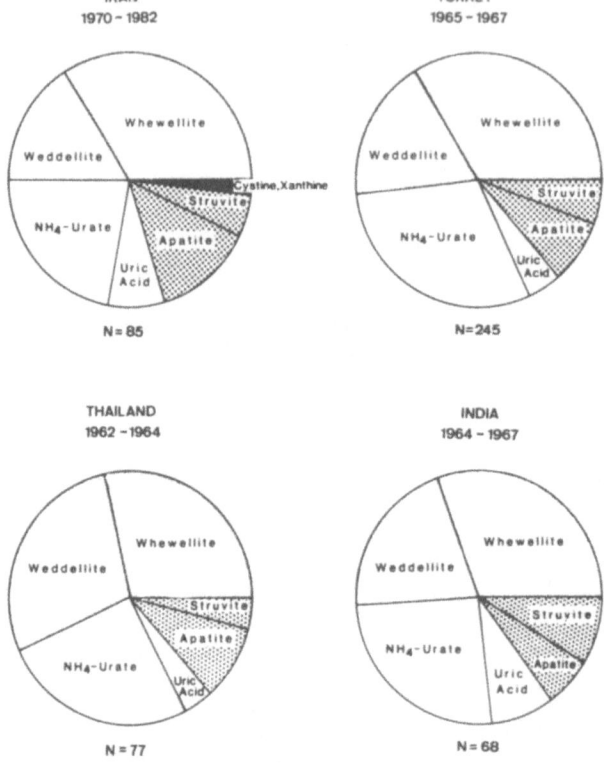

Fig. 4. Sector diagrams showing the percentage occurrence of
components in different countries.

DISCUSSION

In contrast to reports made 12 years ago from other less
developed parts of Iran and from countries such as Thailand, India,
Iraq and Egypt, upper urinary tract calculi were more prevalent than
bladder stones in this study. This might indicate that "endemic
urolithiasis" in Iran is disappearing.

In Fig. 3 the percentage occurrence of stone types in children,
as compiled from recent reports, is compared with our data.   In
Great Britain and the USA calcium-containing stones are the
most common.   In Iran, "mixed stones", composed of whewellite
and ammonium acid urate, predominate.   This stone type is
extremely rare in highly industrialized countries.   If our X-
ray and optical analyses are compared with Lonsdales' findings
for paediatric bladder stones in India, Thailand and Turkey
(Fig. 4), there is a great similarity in stone composition
among those countries.

738

STONE ANALYSIS - IN THE DOCTOR'S OFFICE OR IN A

SPECIALIZED LABORATORY?

H.-J. Schneider, E. W. Rugendorff, and J. Dahlke

Am Ludwigsplatz 11, 6300 Giessen, F.R.G.

INTRODUCTION

Knowledge of the cause of calculus formation is a pre-requisite for an effective treatment programme to prevent recurrence. Often clinical and laboratory investigations do not provide the necessary information, and conclusions can be drawn only retrospectively from the type of stone. Hence, every available urinary stone should be analyzed. There are two competing techniques (Table 1), which differ in cost, effort and precision of analysis and which may be used for assessing further treatment and prophylactic measures. The purpose of this study is to determine which to recommend to urologists and physicians who normally rely on qualitative stone analysis, but who have centralized facilities available for X-ray diffraction, infra red spectroscopy and crystal optics.

MATERIALS AND METHODS

During the period from 1974 to 1983, 355 stone patients were treated. They were divided almost equally between first-time and recurrent calculus patients. The frequency distribution of the various types of calculi was typical of that reported from our country. It was possible to analyze 266 stones from these patients. Eighty were investigated by at least two methods, 35 by three methods:
1. Chemical analysis kit (Temmler Werke, Marburg, Office Laboratory Rugendorff/Schneider, Giessen).
2. X-ray diffraction (Institute for Mineralogy and Petrology, Bonn University).
3. IR Spectroscopy (Clinical Chemical Laboratory, Borstel).

739

Table 1. Advantages and Disadvantages of Various Stone Analysis
Techniques.

Qualitative chemical analysis Temmler Kit Method	Physico-chemical analysis Infrared spectroscopy Crystal optics Thermo
Advantages	
Low investment costs (0.6$) No transport necessary Quick results Can be measured in surgery Test kits available	Precise evidence of the phase type and chemical composition Semi-quantitative analysis is possible
Disadvantages	
Only limited evidence concerning composition of the stone. No phase analysis possible Difficulties with mixed stones	High investment costs (7.8$) Centralization in specialized laboratories necessary Problems with transport and distribution of results

In this way it was possible to make a total of 171 comparisons
between methods. The risk of a sampling error was small. For
multiple analyses the samples were separated by eye into nucleus and
shell, crushed separately in a mortar, mixed, and representative,
equal-sized aliquots analyzed or sent for IR or X-ray investigation.

RESULTS

Assuming that IR spectroscopy is a relatively accurate
technique, chemical analysis performed fairly well with only 4%
completely discrepant results (Fig. 1). Comparing chemical
analysis with X-ray diffraction, however, we found good agreement in
only 60% of cases. The partial agreement in 34% of cases resulted
from the ability of X-ray diffraction to perform separate phase
analysis. The poor agreement obtained between IR spectroscopy and
X-ray diffraction was surprising. This was mainly due to the
varying assignment of the oxalate phases, sometimes resulting in
directly contradictory results (e.g. in one stone, IR gave a
composition of tertiary phosphate with traces of oxalate, whereas
X-ray diffraction gave 80% whewellite and 20% weddellite.
Sometimes the two methods yielded a different value for the
percentages of the components (partial agreement in 15%). In 10
out of 54 comparisons between IR and X-ray analysis, however, the
results were completely discrepant. This was surprising, but one
must keep in mind, that the accuracy of the physico-chemical methods

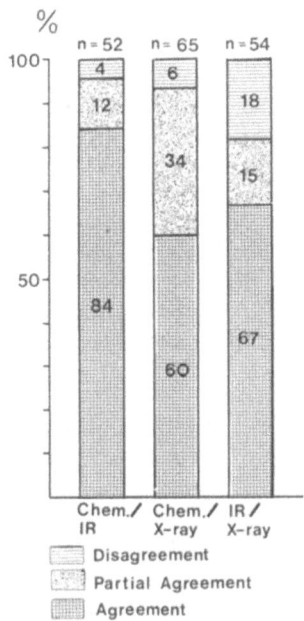

Fig. 1. Bilateral comparisons of all three methods. The amount of
agreement, partial agreement and disagreement is given in
percentages.

is much higher and the mineralogical determination of the material
more precise than with chemical analysis.   Thus, there were some
seemingly poor comparisons between the methods in some cases.

DISCUSSION

    When the analytical results are compared, the agreement is
generally good.   The following points can be made from the study:
(i) the disagreement between the X-ray diffraction and IR
spectroscopic analyses is probably not the fault of the methods
themselves; (ii) the differences between the results of chemical
analysis and those of X-ray diffraction and IR spectroscopic
analysis clearly indicate the limitation of the qualitative chemical
analytical method;   (iii) if the differentiation between the states
of hydration of uric acid and of calcium oxalate, the differences
between the various phosphates (excluding calcium phosphate and
magnesium ammonium phosphate) and the quantitative data on mixed
stones are ignored, then the agreement between the chemical the
other two methods is surprisingly good; (iv) the quality of the
chemical analysis is dependent on its proper execution and the
interpretation of the results.

RECOMMENDATIONS FOR GENERAL PRACTITIONERS

Every calculus should be weighed, and its shape, colour and surface appearance noted and recorded. Large stones should be broken up with a saw and the nucleus separated from the shell. Smaller stones can be crushed completely in a mortar and representative samples of the powder used for analysis.

(2) All primary calculi from adults should be examined by quantitative chemical analysis. If sufficient material is available, a representative sample should be retained for X-ray diffraction or IR spectroscopic analysis if this should become necessary.

(3) Stones from children should be analyzed chemically to identify those which result from a urinary tract infection or from a metabolic disorder.

It is our experience that more than half of all calculi are suitable for chemical analysis within the doctor's surgery. The following categories of calculi should be sent to an analysis center for investigation by X-ray diffraction or IR spectroscopy:(i) stones of suspected metabolic origin in children and uric acid calculi in order to exclude possible confusion with 2,8-dihydroxyadenine concretions; (ii) recurrent calculi for more precise characterization, e.g. to distinguish between whewellite and weddellite; (iii) mixed calculi of uncertain chemical composition; (iv) stones which are too small for chemical analysis. If enough material is available, qualitative chemical analysis should also be carried out in the above cases to obtain information quickly.

COMPUTED TOMOGRAPHIC ANALYSIS OF THE COMPOSITION OF RENAL CALCULI

G. W. Drach, B. J. Hillman, P. Tracey, and J. A. Gaines

Depts. of Surgery and Radiology and Division of
Computer Systems and Biochemistry, University of
Arizona Health Science Center, Tucson, Arizona, U.S.A.

INTRODUCTION

The recent advent of percutaneous removal of renal calculi -
including extraction, dissolution, and ultrasonic or electro-
mechanical destruction of calculi - makes it important to determine
the chemical composition of a patient's calculus prior to deciding
upon the best method of therapy. While blood chemistry, examination of the urine sediment, and review of the patient's clinical
history are helpful in this regard, the true nature of a calculus
often remains in doubt. The experiment detailed in this report
represents an initial, ex vivo evaluation of computed tomography
(CT) as a method of improving the categorization of calculi prior to
deciding upon a treatment plan. Our results indicate that CT may
prove to be a useful adjunct to traditional clinical and laboratory
methods for discriminating among types of renal calculi.

METHODS

The data were derived by ex vivo CT scanning of 63 renal
calculi which were at least 1 cm in their greatest diameter and had
one component which comprised 50% or more of the stone's substance.
Optical crystallography and IR spectroscopy were used to classify
the calculi. For purposes of statistical analysis, we also
classified stones according to purity (i.e. 50%, 74%, 75%, 89%,
and 90% majority constituent) and the character of their minority
constituents. Using these criteria, 23 calcium oxalate, 14 uric
acid, 17 struvite, 2 cystine, 2 ammonium acid urate, 2
hydroxyapatite, 1 tricalcium phosphate, 1 sodium acid urate, and
1 calcium apatite calculi were included.

One of the authors (PT), who was unaware of the stone's chemical composition, scanned all of the calculi with CT and performed region of interest (ROI) measurements. The stones were suspended by a nylon stocking into the center of a two-gallon, round plastic waterbath which approximated the abdominal diameter of a small adult. Overlapping 5 mm-thick scans were performed through the extent of each stone using an upgraded General Electric 8800 CT scanner (100 mA, 120 kV, 2.2 sec). Region of interest measurement was carried out upon the slice in which the stone was seen in its greater diameter. This procedure provided us with the mean $\pm$ SD minimum, and maximum pixel values for each calculus in EMI units (extended scale). Multiple discriminant analysis was used to assess which single or combination of CT parameters best predicted calculus composition. Separate analyses were performed on (i) the 54 calculi representative of the preponderance of stones included in our study (calcium oxalate, struvite, and uric acid) and (ii) an additional 9 calculi of composition other than these three types.

RESULTS

The CT parameters for 54 uric acid, calcium oxalate, and struvite stones permitted good discrimination among these calculi. The mean pixel value was the best single CT parameter for this purpose. Using the mean alone, 13 of the 14 (93%) of uric acid calculi (range: 129-301 EMI units) could be distinguished from struvite and calcium oxalate stones. There was some overlap between the mean pixel values of the 17 struvite (range: 298-743 EMI units) and 23 calcium oxalate (range: 420-830 EMI units) calculi. However, struvite stones were less dense, permitting distinction between the two types of stones in 72% of cases.

Adding the standard deviation of the stone's pixel values to the mean improved discrimination between the stone types (Fig. 1).

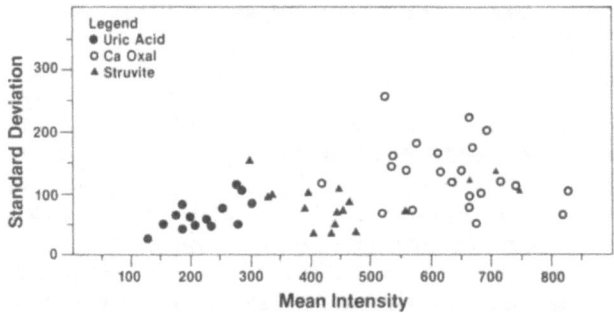

Fig. 1. The mean and standard deviation of pixel values (EMI) units obtained from scanning 54 calculi.

A "map", representative of the distribution of the calculi according to the mean ± SD of their pixel values was then generated by computer. The discrete areas of this "map" (Fig. 1) were generated by describing normal distributions around the mean of the means and the SDs for each of the three types of calculi. The map permits correct classification in 100%, 87%, and 82% of cases for uric acid, calcium oxalate, and struvite calculi respectively. The overall accuracy of categorization for these is 89% (Table 1). The data derived from scanning the other 9 calculi spans a broad range of mean and SD values which make them indistinguishable from struvite and calcium oxalate stones using our best CT parameters. The "map" area described for uric acid calculi was also no longer perfectly discrete, as it encompassed the values of a single cystine and one ammonium acid urate calculus. Neither the minimum nor maximum pixel values of the calculi improved discrimination among the types of calculi in either the limited (54 stones) or inclusive (63 stones) analyses. Similarly, there was no consistent relationship between the purity of a stone or the character of its minority elements and its CT parameters.

DISCUSSION

Because there are now several treatment options for renal calculi, and because selection of the most suitable treatment is dependent upon the nature of the stone, it would be clinically valuable to differentiate accurately the types of renal calculi. Computed tomography - a cross-sectional modality with the ability to quantitate an object's radiation absorption characteristics - would seem an ideal modality for this purpose. Previous investigators have already reported using CT to reliably differentiate lucent calculi from other types of renal collecting system abnormalities[1-7]. Our results indicate that in an ex vivo experimental setting, CT is also quite accurate in differentiating the three most common types of renal calculi - uric acid, calcium oxalate, and struvite - which comprise 90% of calculi encountered in clinical practice[8]. Uric acid calculi are especially well distinguished from other types of calculi by their low mean and SD of CT pixel values. In this study, CT was somewhat less reliable in differentiating those

Table 1. Accuracy of Categorization of 54 Uric Acid, Calcium Oxalate and Struvite Calculi by our Computerized Mapping Program (Based on data in Fig. 1).

Calculus Type	Uric Acid	CaOx	Struvite
Uric Acid	100%	0%	0%
Calcium oxalate	0%	87%	13%
Struvite	0%	18%	82%

calculi with higher mean and SD values. In particular, inaccuracies may be expected with struvite stones, since their mineralization varies considerably and because most of the less frequently encountered calculi scanned fell within the struvite area on our mean-standard deviation distribution "map" (Fig. 1).

The mapping technique is potentially applicable to clinical practice. Once a sufficient number of calculi have been scanned to generate the "map" areas, all successive calculi may be categorized by computer. There are some difficulties, however, in extending the results of our ex vivo experiment to clinical practice. It is evident that small stones will be subject to partial volume inaccuracies in measuring their CT parameters[9]. The location of the calculus relative to the scanner aperture and alterations in radiographic technique may significantly affect the consistency of the numerical values obtained from region of interest measurements[10,11]. Another potential source of error is the non-linearity of CT numbers relative to the radiation absorption of objects over the broad range of values manifest by renal calculi. Our scanner has proved to be quite accurate in this regard[10,12]; however, this may not be the case for all CT scanners. Finally, Levy et al have shown considerable variability in the CT numbers obtained from scanning the same phantom with different equipment[11]. Thus, to employ this method, each institution must first establish mean and standard deviation distributions for the various types of calculi using their own equipment.

REFERENCES

1. H. M. Pollack, P. H. Argler, M. P. Banner, C. B. Mulhern, and B. G. Coleman, Radiology 138:645 (1981).
2. M. P. Federle, J. W. McAninch, J. A. Kaiser, P. C. Goodman, J. Roberts, and J. C. Mall, Am. J. Roentgenol. 136:255 (1981).
3. A. J. Segal, F. Spataro, C. A. Linke, I. N. Frank, and R. Rabinowitz, Radiology 129:447 (1978).
4. R. A. Parienty, R. Ducellier, J. Pradel, J. M. Lubrano, F. Coquille, and F. Richard, Radiology 145:743 (1982).
5. M. Lazica, H. P. Volkmer, and H. J. Treutler, Urologe 21:362 (1982).
6. G. Lemaitre and O. Renouard, J. Radiol. 63:607 (1982).
7. G. W. Drach, in:"Campbell's Urology", J. H. Harrison, R. F. Gitter, E. D. Perlmitter, ed., Saunders, Philadlephia (1978).
8. B. S. Baxter and J. A. Sorensen, Invest. Radiol. 16:337 (1981).
9. T. B. Hunter, G. D. Pond, and O. Medina, Comput. Radiol. 7:199 (1983).
10. C. Levy, J. E. E. Gray, E. C. McCullogh, and R. R. Hattery, Am.J. Roentgenol. 139:443 (1982).
11. B. J. Hillman, S. M. Lee, W. Swindell, and P. Tracey, Invest. Radiol. 17:41 (1982).

VIII. PHYSICAL CHEMISTRY
CRYSTAL FORMATION

URINE SUPERSATURATION: THE NUCLEATION, GROWTH AND

DISSOLUTION OF STONES

G. H. Nancollas

Chemistry Dept. State University of New York
Buffalo, New York, 14214, U.S.A.

INTRODUCTION

It is generally accepted that the formation of stones in the urinary tract involves 4 basic steps: (a) the achievement of solution supersaturation with respect to the mineralizing phase, (b) the formation of stable nidi or nuclei, (c) the development of macrocrystals through crystal growth, aggregation or agglomeration and, (d) the opposing process of dissolution. Elucidation of the controlling mechanisms offers a considerable challenge since the process may result from the failure of natural inhibitors which, in normal subjects, prevent the formation of crystalluria. It is the purpose of this paper to discuss the important factors involved in these processes in relation to an understanding of the mechanisms of stone formation.

URINE SUPERSATURATION

Urine is normally supersaturated with respect to calcium oxalate (CaOx)[1,2] octocalcium phosphate (OCP)[1], hydroxyapatite (HAP)[1], and sometimes dicalcium phosphate dihydrate (DCPD)[3]. However, one of the problems is that of calculating the uncomplexed ion concentrations or activities which control the rates of mineralization of the stone material through the supersaturation S given by:

$$S = \pi^{1/\gamma}/K_{so}^{1/\gamma}$$

where K_{so} is the thermodynamic solubility product of the mineral containing γ ions in the formula unit (for CaOx $\pi = a_{Ca}a_{Ox}$ and $\gamma = 2$).

Although colorimetric methods involving competing chelating reagents have been used for estimating Ca^{2+} concentrations, the more direct specific ion electrode methods are preferable and they have been used in artificial urines[4]. In whole urine, however, macromolecules tend to poison the calcium electrode membranes and hitherto, it has been impossible to verify directly the concentration of Ca^{2+}. The recent application of a protected calcium electrode in our laboratory[5] has enabled the direct measurement of Ca^{2+} activities in whole urine.

A knowledge of the total concentrations of metal ions and anions such as phosphate, oxalate, carbonate, and urate, together with the urine pH enables estimates to be made of the concentrations of free ion species by taking into account as many ion-pairs and complexes as possible. Where experiments are made at low ionic strength, it is necessary to use an iterative computational method in order to correct for changes in the activity coefficients[6-8]. Although it is not possible to include, with confidence, interactions involving larger protein or glycoprotein molecules computational speciation programs have been published by Robertson[4] and by Finlayson[9] by taking into account 22 and 39 ion-pairs and complexes, respectively. Using the program EQUIL proposed by Finlayson[9], it was estimated that about 50% of the total calcium and 40% of the total oxalate are present as free ion species in urines. This has recently been verified in our laboratory[5] using a Ca^{2+} electrode protected by means of a dialysis membrane from the effects of the urinary macromolecules.

NUCLEATION

In biological systems, heterogeneous nucleation may be a more appropriate model than homogeneous nucleation for the formation of renal stones in which precipitation is likely to take place at solid/liquid interfaces. Heterogeneous nucleation is facilitated if the substrate offers good crystal lattice matches to the substance being precipitated. This may lead to epitaxial crystallization and the formation of the mixed mineral phases frequently encountered in vivo. Although it is difficult to establish unequivocally the participation of epitaxial growth in forming the immobile monolayer of regular atomic pattern on which the new phase will crystallize, such a relationship has been demonstrated for the growth of hydrated orthohombic uric acid on crystals of the anhydrous phase[10]. Moreover, crystallization experiments have suggested that CaOx monohydrate (COM) will nucleate on the surface of crystals of DCPD and HAP[11-14]. Secondary nucleation or the production of additional nuclei in the presence of solid phases may also be important in the formation of urinary calculi. The use of mixed suspension mixed product removal crystallizers (MSMPR) was proposed by Finlayson[15] in order to model

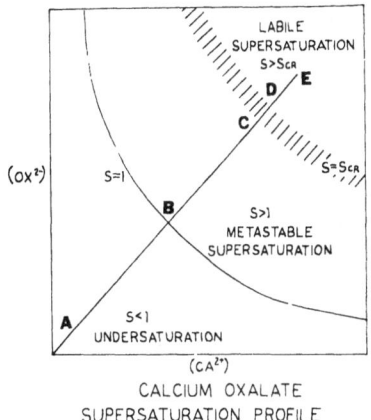

CALCIUM OXALATE
SUPERSATURATION PROFILE

Fig. 1. Calcium oxalate saturation and supersaturation curves.

crystallite formation in vivo and the method has been applied to the measurement of nucleation rates especially in systems where secondary nucleation is important. The outflow from such crystallization cells can be used to estimate both the nucleation and growth rates under urine-like conditions[15,16].

CRYSTAL GROWTH

Although in theory crystallization should take place when S 1, in practice such thermodynamic predictions may be much less important than a knowledge of the rates of nucleation and growth. Typical solubility and critical supersaturation curves for CaOx are shown in Fig. 1. As the concentration of solution containing equivalent calcium and oxalate is increased along the line AE, the concentration product passes through the solubility value at B and from B to C it is possible to prepare supersaturated solutions which are stable for long periods of time and which model in vivo conditions. In region C, nucleation will take place on foreign surfaces present in the solution while along DE, spontaneous precipitation takes place. The position of C clearly depends upon the nature of the solid surfaces and which type of nucleation can take place. Thus for homogeneous nucleation in a clean solution, it may be possible to attain concentrations as high as D before spontaneous precipitation takes place.

In the urinary tract, the mechanism of crystallization of stone minerals may be as important as a knowledge of the degree of supersaturation. In general, crystal growth must involve the bulk diffusion of hydrated lattice ions to the crystal surface, adsorption and dehydration, surface diffusion of these growth units to energetically favourable sites, and incorporation into the crystal lattice. The measured rate of mineralization reflects the slow step or steps in this reaction scheme. In crystallization experiments, it is first necessary to determine whether the growth rates are diffusion- or surface-controlled. For calcium oxalate and phosphates, the rates of crystallization are considerably slower than those calculated for pure diffusion control. This indicates surface-controlled processes which may include spiral growth[17], where the rate of growth (R_g) is: $R_g = k_2 \sigma^2 = k_2(S-1)^2$, following a parabolic dependence on supersaturation, or polynuclear birth and spread models following an exponential rate law[18] according to which $R_g = k_e(\sigma+1)^{7/6} \sigma^{2/3} \ln(1+\sigma)^{1/6} \exp\left(-K_e/\ln(1+\sigma)\right)$. The spiral growth mechanism accounts for the fact that crystals grow at much lower supersaturations than those predicted by surface nucleation models. Singular crystal faces are intersected by screw dislocations (Fig. 2b) which emerge from the ends of steps shown in Fig 2a. Since crystallization takes place at the energetically preferred sites offered by these ledges, growth spirals develop on the crystal surface and offer perpetual steps for crystallization (Fig 2b). Dehydration or partial dehydration must also take place during crystallization and it has recently been shown that in some cases, the removal of a water molecule from the lattice cation may control the rates of crystallization[19,20].

The increase in the relative rate of nucleation with increase in concentration is much greater than that observed for crystal growth. If the formation of a surface nucleus is rapid, therefore, a new layer may start before the development of the underlying layer is complete. This leads to the polynuclear model shown in Fig 2a. The most rapid crystal growth will take place on faces with the greatest number of kinks and steps but it is unlikely that the large number of kinks would persist during crystallization since microscopic examination reveals that imperfect crystals rapidly heal their surfaces in the initial stages of seeded crystal growth. Recent work in our laboratory has demonstrated the importance of taking into account such changes in specific surface area of the crystals during crystallization experiments. In order to study such effects quantitatively, it is necessary to use the constant composition (CC) technique since conventional crystallization experiments provide an insufficient extent of reaction to achieve such crystal perfection under controlled conditions. CC studies of the crystallization of calcium oxalates and phosphates show that in all cases, with the exception of OCP which grows by a predominantly polynuclear mechanism, a spiral growth process predominates, consistent with the Buron, Cabrerra and Frank mechanism[17] The density of steps (Fig 2a) is proportional to lnS and the rate of lateral movement over the surface of the crystal is proportional to (S-1). The total rate of growth will therefore be proportional to (S-1)lnS which, for small values of S, $\approx (S-1)^2$ or σ^2. For CaOx, the parabolic rate law is obeyed outside the supersaturation range

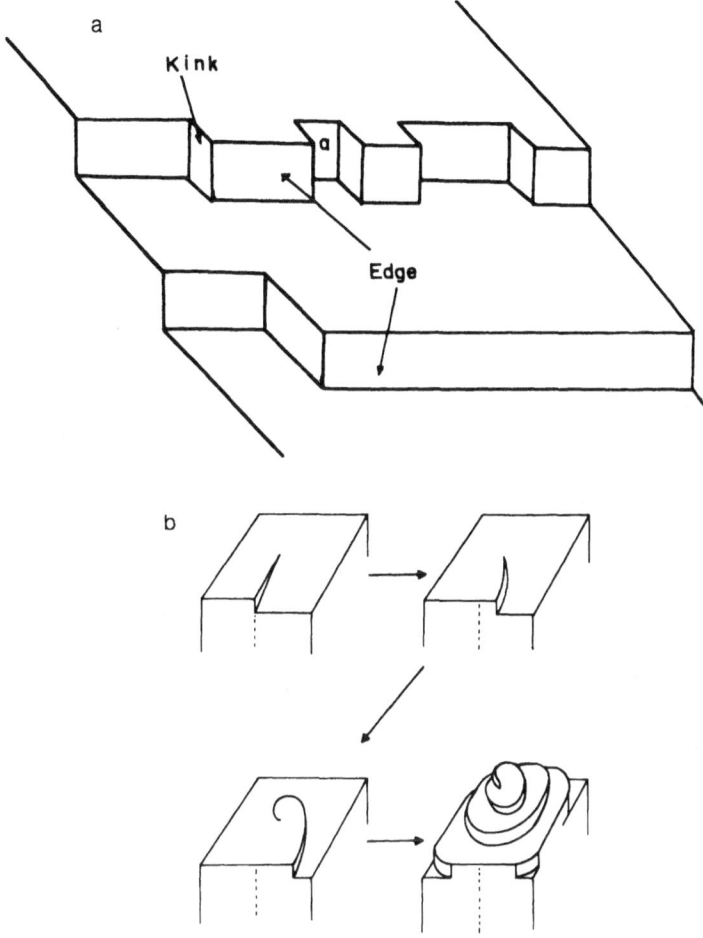

a

Kink

a

Edge

b

Fig. 2. (a) Polynuclear growth model and (b) spiral growth model.

($1 < S < 2$) where these approximations are valid. This suggests that the crystallization is controlled by an integration process rather than by adsorption at the kinks. It is likely that this also involves the dehydration of Ca^{2+} ions at the crystal surface. In vivo, it is important to take into account the possible change in crystallization mechanism in the presence of urinary inhibitors. Not only may this influence the rate of formation of stone minerals but the nature of the phases which form may also be dependent upon the presence of inhibitors. Thus it has been shown[21] that polyphosphate ions have a much large inhibiting effect on the crystallization of COM than on that of the higher hydrates. These less stable precursor phases may therefore be stabilized in vivo. It is interesting to note that urinary calculi frequently consist of mixtures of CaOx dihydrate (COD) along with COM and calcium phosphate phases.

Using the CC technique, it has been possible to stabilize CaOx trihydrate (COT) crystallites sufficiently without transformation to COM in order to establish a spiral growth mechanism. Moreover, the crystallization rate constant for COT, 1.8×10^4 l mol^{-1}min^{-1}m^{-2} was significantly greater than the corresponding value, 3.6×10^3 for COM. This is in accord with the Ostwald-Lussac Law of Stages in which the phase with the highest solubility will be expected to form preferentially in the sequential precipitation reactions. These experiments were extended to urine solutions which were shown to reduce markedly the rate of COM mineralization[22]. Finlayson[23] has drawn attention to the major problems in evaluating urinary inhibiting potentials from the results of such experiments using high dilutions with respect to urine samples. Thus the typically used 100-fold dilution may obscure the inhibitory effect of low molecular weight components such as citrate and pyrophosphate because of the expected differences in adsorption isotherms. Although it has been shown that the degree of inhibition of COM mineralization is approximately proportional to the urinary dilution[22], it is likely that the 100-fold dilution involved may markedly change the distribution of species - especially those with bound calcium - as compared with whole urine. These problems were overcome by the application of the protected Ca^{2+} electrode and typical crystallization experiments are described in this volume[24]. The use of the protected specific ion electrodes in whole urine at constant supersaturations offers excellent opportunities for studying the growth and dissolution of stone minerals.

DISSOLUTION

The attractive possibility of chemolytically dissolving kidney stones directly in the ureter has been the subject of a number of studies[25]. The CC technique has been extended to the study of the dissolution of COM and, striking changes in the mechanism of the reaction at low undersaturation have been revealed. The effective order of reaction appears to approach a value of 2, reflecting a surface-controlled reaction with a parabolic dependence on undersaturation. At higher undersaturations, the process is diffusion controlled, as expected. Moreover, the two regions of undersaturation show markedly different dependencies on changes in temperature, hydrodynamics, and upon the addition of adsorbing molecules. The theory of Burton, Cabrerra, and Frank, as applied to dissolution processes predicts such a change in reaction order from 1 to 2 as the undersaturation is decreased. Studies of the kinetics of dissolution of CaOx kidney stones indicate that in contrast to the diffusion-controlled dissolution of pure synthetic phases, the stones dissolve considerably more slowly by a

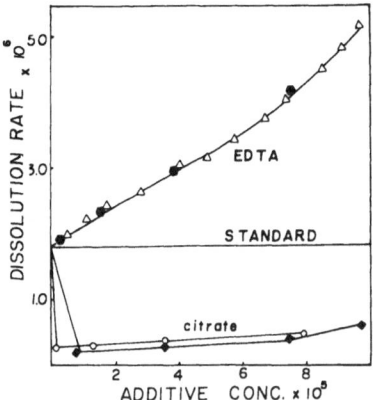

Fig. 3. Dissolution of calcium oxalate monohydrate:influence of citrate and EDTA.

predominantly surface controlled process[26]. As was found for pure COD mineral, the dihydrate stone material transformed into the thermodynamically more stable COM phase upon prolonged exposure to aqueous solution. The CC method has been used to investigate the dissolution of COM in the presence of a variety of synthetic additive molecules. Additives such as EDTA exert their accelerating influence simply through coordination of Ca^{2+} in solution. This is shown in Fig. 3 in which it can be seen that the calculated rates of COM demineralization, corrected for Ca^{2+} sequestration precisely match dissolution rates found experimentally in the absence of EDTA. These results clearly demonstrate that the CC method can be extended to the quantitative evaluation of additive influences on demineralization kinetics provided the proper stability constants for inhibitor Ca^{2+} sequestration are known. In contrast (Fig. 3) citrate ion exerts a specific inhibiting influence on the dissolution of COM. Preliminary studies in our laboratory have revealed the dramatic effect of phosphate ions in reducing the rate of demineralization of COM suggesting that the presence of this ion in stone material may act as an inhibitor of its dissolution. The CC method is ideally suited for studies of the demineralization of urinary components since experiments can be made under conditions close to equilibrium, providing a sensitive measure of the influence of urinary components.

ACKNOWLEDGMENTS

We thank the National Institute of Arthritis, Diabetes, Digestive and Kidney Diseases for a grant (AM19048) in support of this work.

755

REFERENCES

1. W. G. Robertson, M. Peacock, and B. E. C. Nordin, Clin. Sci. 34:579 (1968).
2. W. G. Robertson, M. Peacock, R. W. Marshall, D. H. Marshall, and B. E. C. Nordin, New Engl. J. Med. 294:249 (1976).
3. C. Y. C. Pak, J. Clin. Invest. 48:1914 (1968).
4. W. G. Robertson and R. W. Marshall, C.R.C. Crit. Rev. Clin. Lab. Sci. 15:85 (1981).
5. S. Gaur and G. H. Nancollas, Kidney Int. (in press)
6. I. Tingpo and G. H. Nancollas, Analyt. Chem. 44:1940 (1972)
7. G. H. Nancollas, "Interactions in Electrolyte Solutions", Elsevier, Amsterdam (1966).
8. C. W. Davies, "Ion Association", Butterworths, London (1962).
9. B. Finlayson, in:"Calcium Metabolism, in Renal Failure, and Nephrolithiasis", D. S. David, ed., Wiley, New York (1977).
10. R. Boistelle and C. Rinaudo, J. Cryst. Growth, 53:1 (1981).
11. J. L. Meyer, J. L. Bergert, and L. H. Smith, Clin. Sci. Mol. Med. 52:143 (1977).
12. G. H. Nancollas and G. L. Gardner, J. Cryst. Growth 21:267 (1974).
13. J. L. Meyer, J. H. Bergert, and L. H. Smith, Clin. Sci. Mol. Med. 49:369 (1975).
14. P. G. Koutsoukos, M. E. Sheehan, and G. H. Nancollas, Invest. Urol.18:358 (1981).
15. B. Finlayson, Invest. Urol. 9:528 (1972).
16. J. D. Miller, A. D. Randolph, and G. W. Drach, J. Urol. 117:
17. W. K. Burton, N. Cabrera, and F. C. Frank, Phil. Trans. Roy. Soc. A, 243:299 (1951).
18. A. E. Nielsen and J. Christoffersen, in:"Biological Mineralization and Demineralization", G. H. Nancollas, ed., Springer-Verlag, Berlin (1982).
19. A. E. Nielsen, Pure Appl. Chem. 53:2025 (1981).
20. J. P. Barone and G. H. Nancollas, J. Cryst. Growth (in press)
21. B. B. Tomazic and G. H. Nancollas, in:"Urolithiasis:Clinical and Basic Research", L. H. Smith, W. G. Robertson and B. Finlayson, eds., Plenum, New York (1981).
22. A. C. Lanzalaco, M. E. Sheehan, D. J. White, and G. H. Nancollas, J. Urol. 128:845 (1982).
23. B. Finlayson, Kidney Int. 13:344 (1978).
24. A. Lanzalaco, M. Coyle, S. S. Gaur, T. P. Binette, T. S. Herman, G. Sufrin, and G. H. Nancollas, in:"Urolithiasis and Related Clinical Research", P. O. Schwille, L. H. Smith, W. G. Robertson, and W. Vahlensieck, eds., Plenum, New York (1985).

DISSOLUTION KINETICS OF CALCIUM OXALATE CALCULI

J. R. Burns, J. A. Belcher, and B. Finlayson

Dept of Surgery, University of Alabama, and Veterans'
Administration Hospital, Birmingham, Alabama, and
Dept. of Surgery, University of Florida, Gainesville
Florida, U.S.A.

INTRODUCTION

The solubility of some stone salts (e.g. struvite, uric acid
and cystine) can be increased by altering urinary pH. Calcium
oxalate (CaOx) solubility, however, changes little over the
physiological pH range (4.5 to 7.5) but does increase at pH <4.0.
To assess the feasibility of in vivo dissolution of CaOx by acidic
irrigating solutions, we have determined the dissolution kinetics of
CaOx calculi at low pH.

METHODS AND MATERIALS

All solutions were prepared from reagent grade chemicals
dissolved in doubly distilled water. CaOx calculi were obtained
from Louis C. Herring and Co. and contained at least 80% CaOx. CaOx
dissolution was studied according to the method of Simonelli et al[1].
The apparatus (Fig. 1) provided constant surface for release. Both
stirring speed and the distance from the stir blade to sample
remained fixed. A calculus (1 to 1.5 cm in diameter) was prepared
by placing it in a piece of plexiglass tubing and embedded in liquid
plasic resin. When the resin had hardened, one end of the tubing
was sanded with No. 60 grit sandpaper to expose a cross-section of
the stone. The stone surface was smoothed by wet sanding (No. 240
grit) and polishing (No. 600 grit). The prepared stone was mounted
in a stainless steel die. Before each experimental run, the outline
of the stone surface was traced on acetate paper, the tracing was
enlarged on an overhead projector, and the surface area measured
with a planimeter. Before each run the stone was repolished to
ensure a flat surface.

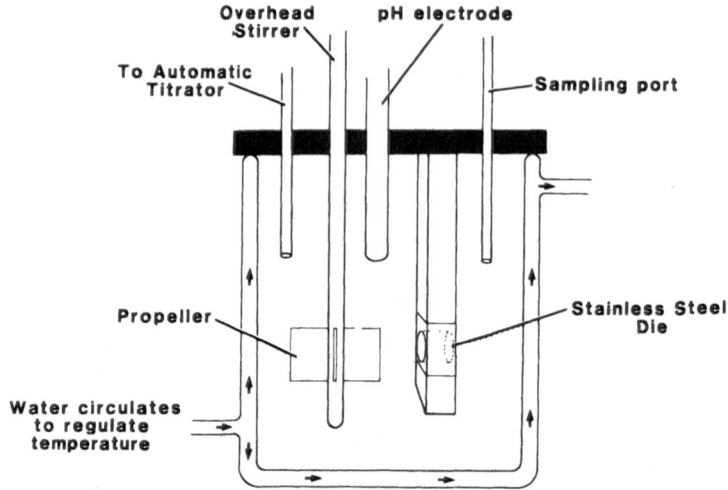

Fig. 1. Dissolution apparatus

All experiments were performed in a double-walled reaction vessel kept at 38°C. The pH was kept constant throughout with a Radiometer RTS-814 titrating system using HCl as titrant. Samples were aspirated through a 0.22 μm Millipore filter at the start of each experiment and at 15 min intervals for 2 h. Ca concentration was analyzed on a Perkin-Elmer 2380 atomic absorption spectrophotometer. Lanthanum oxide was used in all Ca determinations.

Dissolution of CaOx calculi was studied in 0.15 M NaCl. All experimental runs were made at a stir speed of 240 rpm. Duplicate runs with 4 different calculi were made at pH 1, 2, and 3.

RESULTS

The effect of pH on CaOx dissolution in saline is shown in Fig. 2. Each line is a compilation of 4 calculi corrected for surface area. At pH 3 and 2, dissolution appears to be linear with time (r^2 = 0.99). At pH 1, a slight deviation from linearity occurs (r^2 = 0.96). This linear relationship is characteristic of a diffusion-controlled model of dissolution, described by:

$$Q = D_a C_s T/h$$

where D_a is the aqueous diffusion coefficient of CaOx, C_s is the solubility of CaOx, T is the time, h is the diffusion-layer thickness, and Q is the amount of CaOx released per unit surface area[1]. The rate of dissolution at each was analyzed with a linear regression technique and a rate constant calculated (R = Q/time).

758

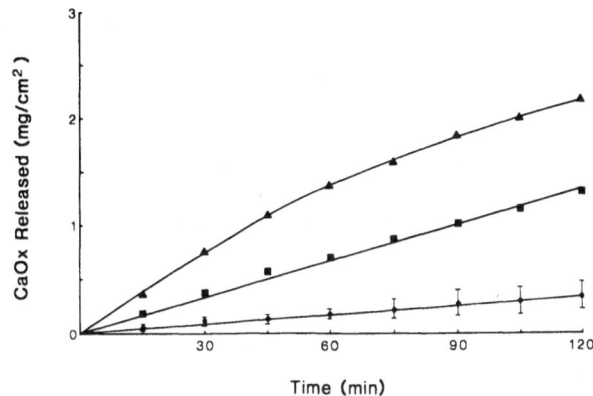

Fig. 2.   Dissolution of calcium oxalate calculi in NaCl solution
at various pHs. ● pH 3.0, R = 0.17 mg/cm^2.h; ■ pH 2.0,
R = 0.67 mg/cm^2.h; ▲ pH 1.0, R = 1.24 mg/cm^2.h.

Table 1. Estimated Time (h) Required to Dissolve CaOx Calculi
at Various pH Values.

	pH		
Stone Diameter (mm)	1	2	3
1	186	47	25
2	388	98	53
4	793	200	108

At pH 3, CaOx dissolved at 0.17 mg/cm^2/h. Using an iterative
computer program that accounts for progressive changes in surface
area, the time required for in vitro dissolution of CaOx calculi of
various sizes at pH 1, 2, and 3 (Table 1) was calculated.   These
calculations assume that the calculus is spherical. A 1 mm diameter
calculus placed in 0.15 M NaCl solution at pH 3 would require almost
8 days to dissolve totally. Stone dissolution occurs more rapidly
at lower pH levels, but, even at pH 1, dissolution of such a
calculus would require 25.3 h.

DISCUSSION

Urinary calculi form because of excessive supersaturation of
urine with respect to a specific stone salt. If the urinary
environment can be changed to one of undersaturation, stone
dissolution becomes possible. The solubilities of uric acid and
cystine increase markedly at alkaline pH and these calculi can thus
be dissolved by either systemic alkalinization or by direct

irrigation of the kidney with alkaline irrigation agents ($NaHCO_3$, THAM, THAM-E). Struvite solubility increases at acidic pH levels. In simple solution, a change in pH from 7.0 to 4.0 increases struvite dissolution in vivo.

The solubility of CaOx, however, changes little over the physiological range of urinary pH. CaOx calculi are therefore resistant to pH-dependent dissolution techniques. CaOx solubility does increase, however, if the pH is $\leqslant 4.0$[3]. These pH levels can be produced by using acidic irrigating agents. At pH 3.0, dissolution was extremely slow (0.17 $mg/cm^2/h$). The in vitro rate of dissolution is known to be affected by the rate of stirring. Our experiments employed a stir rate of 240 rpm. A stir rate of zero (approximating the situation in the kidney) would reduce the rate of dissolution[4]. In NaCl solutions, the mineral content of stones dissolves much faster than the matrix. This results in an ever increasing diffusion barrier to further stone dissolution. Unlike our simple solutions, urine contains a variety of proteolytic enzymes. These may dissolve stone matrix while urine is solubilizing the crystalline CaOx. If the rate of matrix dissolution lags, CaOx dissolution will slow down considerably.

Based on these studies, it is unlikely that CaOx calculi are amenable to dissolution by acidic irrigating solutions. In theory, an irrigating solution at pH 3.0 could be developed that would not produce permanent injury to the urinary mucosa. Even if a safe solution at pH 3 could be developed, however, CaOx stone dissolution would still be impractical based on time considerations. An acidic irrigating solution would be effective only if a powerful chelator of calcium could be incorporated into the solution. This is unlikely since most known calcium chelators act effectively in the alkaline pH range. Although dissolution does proceed more rapidly at pH 2.0 and 1.0, an irrigating solution at these pHs would most likely cause permanent damage to the urinary mucosa.

ACKNOWLEDGMENT

This work was supported by the Veterans' Administration.

REFERENCES

1. A. P. Simonelli, S. C. Mehta, and W. I. Higuchi, J. Pharm. Sci. 58:538 (1969).
2. J. R. Burns and B. Finlayson. J. Urol. 128:426 (1982).
3. G. Hammarsten, Compt. Rend. Trav. Lab, Carlsberg 17:1 (1929).
4. H. I. Suby and F. Albright, New Engl. J. Med. 228:81 (1943).
5. J. R. Burns, J. F. Gauthier, and B. Finlayson, J. Urol. (in press).

A WHOLE URINE SYSTEM FOR STUDYING NUCLEATION, GROWTH AND AGGREGATION OF CALCIUM OXALATE CRYSTALS

R. L. Ryall, C. M. Hibberd, B. C. Mazzachi, and V. R. Marshall

Urology Unit, Dept. of Surgery, and Dept. of Clinical Biochemistry, Flinders, Medical Centre, Bedford Park Australia

INTRODUCTION

Urinary inhibitors have been presumed for many years to be involved in the pathogenesis of renal calculi. Studies on the effects of dilute urines on calcium oxalate crystallisation have contributed greatly to our knowledge of these inhibitors. Nonetheless, the shortcomings of using diluted urines have always been acknowledged[1]. The aim of this study was to develop a system for measuring calcium oxalate crystallisation in whole urine and to determine whether or not undiluted urines from stone formers and normal subjects differ either in their ability to resist precipitation or in their response to a given oxalate load.

MATERIALS AND METHODS

Twenty-four-hour urines were collected without preservative from 32 normal males and 50 men who had passed at least one calcium stone within the previous year. Of these, 24 had experienced at least 2 episodes and 16 at least 3. Almost all of the patients denied any serious effort to modify their diets, but most had attempted to increase their fluid intake. After centrifugation and filtration (0.22 μm), 10 x 20 ml aliquots of each urine sample were titrated with sodium oxalate (200 μl) to give final oxalate concentrations of 0 to 1.5 mM. Rarely, with very dilute urines, these concentrations had to be doubled. The urine samples were incubated in a shaking water bath at 37°C for 30 min and the number of crystals $>$2 μm in each sample determined using a Coulter Counter (Model TAII) fitted with a Population Count Accessory. Crystal

number initially rose linearly in response to increasing oxalate
concentration.   The point at which this line intersected the
abscissa was taken as the minimum amount of oxalate necessary to
induce detectable nucleation.   This amount of oxalate + an
additional 30 μmol was added dropwise to 100 ml samples of the
urine, and the growth of crystals followed for 90 min.   The time
course of crystal growth, as measured by increasing crystal volume,
showed an initial time lag followed by a linear portion, the slope
of which was used as the index of crystal growth.   Urinary calcium
was measured by atomic absorption spectroscopy, oxalate by a GLC
technique and glycosaminoglycans (GAGS) by the technique of
Blumenkrantz and Asboe-Hansen[3].   Statistical comparisons were made
using the Wilcoxon Rank Sum Test.

RESULTS

     Typical "coffin"-shaped calcium oxalate monohydrate (COM)
crystals were the principal crystal type in 19 urine samples.   The
remainder consisted predominantly of classical "envelope" calcium
oxalate dihydrate (COD) crystals, either singly, or in variously
sized aggregates identical to those occurring naturally in urine.
Of the 19 samples which precipitated COM, 16 were from stone
formers.   The frequency of occurrence of COM was significantly
higher in the stone formers (x^2 test, $P<0.02$).   When the occurrence
of COD and COM crystals was compared within the group of stone
formers, crystal morphology was found to be significantly related to
the endogenous concentrations of calcium and oxalate ($P<0.0002$),
with COM crystals tending to precipitate from those urines with the
lower concentrations of these ions.   The stone formers had lower
urinary concentrations of calcium, oxalate and GAGS ($P<0.05$, $P<0.05$,
$P<0.005$ respectively) and higher volumes ($P<0.001$) than normals.

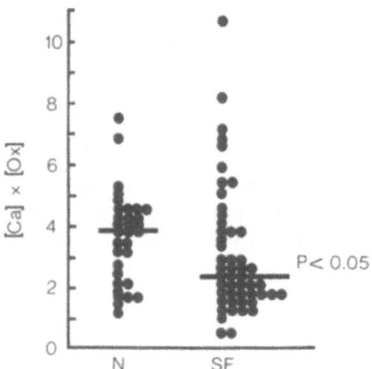

Fig. 1.   Comparison of the [Ca] x [Ox] total product at which
         spontaneous nucleation occurred in the urines from
         normal subjects (N) and stone formers (SF).

The minimum amount of oxalate necessary to induce precipitation was inversely proportional to the urinary calcium concentration ($n = 82$, $r = -0.55$, $P<0.0005$) and to the calcium x endogenous oxalate concentration product ($n = 82$, $r = -0.35$, $P<0.005$), but did not differ significantly between the two groups. On the other hand, the concentration product of calcium and total oxalate (i.e. endogenous + added oxalate) at which spontaneous precipitation occurred was significantly lower ($P<0.05$) in the stone formers than in the normals (Fig. 1). The rate of crystal growth, mean crystal size and total volume of crystals precipitated during the incubation period did not differ between the two groups.

DISCUSSION

In this paper we describe a method for measuring calcium oxalate crystallisation in whole urine. The crystals generated from urine are morphologically identical to those occurring naturally in urine. A significantly higher proportion of stone formers' urines produced COM crystals and this appeared to be related to the lower relative supersaturations. The morphology of calcium oxalate crystals generated from aqueous solutions is known to be a function of relative supersaturation and concentration ratios of the reacting ions[4].

In this system, the inhibitory potential of urine may be classified into two categories: firstly, its ability to tolerate increasing quantities of oxalate before the formation product of calcium oxalate is exceeded (i.e. its relative supersaturation), and secondly, once that point has been reached, its subsequent response to an additional fixed oxalate load. Although the urines from stone formers tended to precipitate at lower levels of added oxalate than those from the normals, the difference was not significant. When, however, the critical limit of metastability was expressed as the product of the urinary Ca concentration and the total (= endogenous + added) oxalate concentration, this product was significantly lower in the urines from the stone formers than those from the normals. Since this was found in whole urine, it is reasonable to conclude that in vivo these urines are more likely to undergo spontaneous precipitation of calcium oxalate than are those from the normal subjects at a given degree of supersaturation.

It may be concluded therefore that stone formers' urines have significantly less inhibitory activity than do the normals'. While this may indeed be so, it cannot be accepted without considering the relative dilutions of the urines. As a group, the stone formers had significantly higher daily urine volumes and correspondingly lower urinary concentrations of calcium, oxalate and GAGS than the normals. Thus the lower limit of metastability of their urines may simply reflect lower urinary inhibitor concentrations. The balance between the relative urinary concentrations of reacting ions and inhibitors may be crucial: it has long been mooted that drinking more water could be self-defeating since it may reduce the concentrations of calcium and oxalate, but also unavoidably lower the inhibitor concentration to ineffective levels, thus allowing precipitation to occur at a lower relative supersaturation.

Once the critical limit of supersaturation had been reached, the urines from stone formers did not differ from those of the normals in their response to a further oxalate load: the rate of growth of the nucleated crystals, their total mass and their size distributions were similar in the two groups. However, it is impossible to conclude that differences would not be found in vivo, since once again, the relative concentrations of inhibitors and ions may be important.

The results of this study suggest that stone formers are deficient in urinary inhibitors compared with normals. Confirmation of this will depend on an examination of urines from stone formers who have not increased their fluid intake above that of the normal controls. The method we describe presents a means of examining the effect of inhibitors on spontaneous CaOx nucleation from undiluted urine. It also has the potential, in combination with a computer model[5], of quantitatively assessing the effects of these inhibitors on crystal growth and aggregation in whole urine.

ACKNOWLEDGMENTS

We wish to thank the Dept. of Clinical Biochemistry, Flinders Medical Centre for performing the calcium measurements. This project was supported by grants from the NH & MRC of Australia and the Flinders Medical Centre Research Foundation.

REFERENCES

1. H. Fleisch, Kidney Int. 13:361 (1978).
2. B. C. Mazzachi, J. K. Teubner, and R. L. Ryall, in:"Urolithiasis and Related Clinical Research", P. O. Schwille, L. H. Smith, W. G. Robertson, and W. Vahlensieck, eds., Plenum, London (1985).
3. N. Blumenkrantz and G. Asboe-Hansen, Analyt. Biochem. 54:484 (1973).
4. J. R. Burns and B. Finlayson, Invest. Urol. 18:174 (1980).
5. R. G. Ryall, R. L. Ryall, and V. R. Marshall, in:"Urinary Stone", R. L. Ryall, J. G. Brockis, V. R. Marshall, and B. Finlayson, eds., Churchill Livingstone, Melbourne (1984).

CRYSTALLIZATION CHARACTERISTICS OF SYNTHETIC URINE

IN A FAST EVAPORATOR

A. L. Rodgers and M. A. E. Wandt

Dept. of Physical Chemistry, University of Cape Town
Rondebosch, Cape Town 7700, Republic of South Africa

INTRODUCTION

Many different approaches to the study of the physico-chemical factors governing urolithiasis have been employed in the past. Several workers have examined diffusion-limited systems in which component ions are permitted to diffuse into a stagnant urine solution causing encrustations to grow on fibers suspended in the medium[1-3]. Others have examined the inhibitory effects of certain ions, again employing static supersaturated systems[4-6]. On the other hand, the urinary tract has been considered as a sequence of continuous crystallizers[7,8] and many studies have been conducted in such mixed suspension mixed product removal (MSMPR)[9-11] systems. Hallson and Rose[12] employed yet another approach in which urine samples were subjected to rapid evaporation at 37°C. They point out that such a process is analogous to that whereby urine is concentrated in the renal tubules by water removal. We decided to carry out a series of crystallization experiments using a fast evaporator system similar to that described by these latter workers in an attempt to gain insight into some of the physico-chemical factors governing crystalluria and urolithiasis.

METHODS

Stock solutions of a standard reference artificial urine (SRAU)[13] were initially refrigerated but were brought to 37°C prior to evaporation. Crystallization experiments were conducted as a function of pH and urine composition. Adjustment of pH was achieved with concentrated NH_4OH or HCl. In all cases a 100 ml aliquot of the SRAU was transferred into a 200 ml evaporation flask connected to a vacuum system. The flask was rotated in a thermostated water bath at 37°C and the SRAU subjected to rapid evaporation until 50 ml distillate had been collected. Precipitates were retrieved by vacuum filtration through Sartorius teflon filters of 0.45 μm pore size and were then washed with distilled water and weighed. Each was analysed qualitatively and semi-quantitatively by X-ray powder diffraction.

RESULTS

In the first set of experiments (Series 1), the pH was varied from 3.0 to 9.5 in steps of 0.5 pH units. The results are presented in Fig. 1. Calcium oxalate monohydrate (COM) was formed in the pH range 3 to 5 together with the trihydrate (COT), the latter being the major constituent. At pH 5.5 brushite (BRU) was detected as well. COT (but not COM) continued to precipitate with BRU (and apatite APA) at higher pH values but finally disappeared in the pH range 6.5 to 7.0. Calcium oxalate dihydrate (COD) was not detected at all. At pH values greater than 7.5, struvite (STR) was identified with BRU and APA. The total mass of precipitate formed in each experiment was relatively low in the pH range 3 to 6 but thereafter increased dramatically reaching a maximum at pH 8. The relative mass of COT within each precipitate decreased with increasing pH while that of COM remained fairly constant; APA and BRU deposits within the particular mixtures were greatest at pH values 6 and 7, respectively.

When the above series of experiments was repeated (Series 2) with an artificial urine that had not been previously refrigerated but had been allowed to stand on the laboratory bench for 4 days prior to evaporation, no COT was formed.

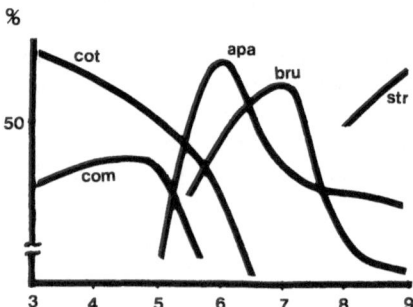

Fig. 1. Qualitative and semi-quantitative results as a function of pH. (Approximate % composition of the precipitate mixtures is plotted along the y-axis).

766

In Series 3 (pH range 5 to 7) the composition of the artificial urine was varied slightly to investigate the role of individual constituents in determining the crystallization characteristics. Appropriate amounts of uric acid (UA), urea (U) and creatinine (C) were each included individually in separate artificial urine samples while in one experiment (C) was added to an artificial urine sample from which the $MgSO_4$ component had been excluded. There were several notable features in this series. Uric acid dihydrate (pH 5 to 6) precipitated in the (UA) run and COD (pH 5) in the (U) run. The (C) experiment yielded an unidentifiable fine amorphous precipitate at pH 5, NaCl at pH 6 and STR at pH 7 while in the experiment from which $MgSO_4$ had been omitted, COM was formed at pH 5 and APA at pH 6 to 7.

DISCUSSION

The precipitation of COT over almost the entire acid range in Series 1 and its absence in Series 2 again suggests that this species might be a thermodynamically unstable precursor of COM[14]. By the same token, BRU (pH 5 to 9) might be regarded as playing some role in APA formation. If these hypotheses are extrapolated to the in vivo situation, it might prove clinically worthwhile to adjust the physico-chemical conditions of stone formers' urine in such a way that formation of these two components is inhibited. Control of pH is an obvious method. Alternatively, based on the observations in Series 3 that the presence of creatinine inhibited precipitation of both COT and BRU, investigation of creatinine levels in the urine of stone- and non-stone-formers might show that it plays an inhibitory role of some sort.

Although it is difficult, at this stage, to place any further interpretation on our results, these preliminary studies suggest that the fast evaporator system provides a simple, yet very useful means for studying the crystallization characteristics of urine solutions. We intend continuing our experimentation in the hope of accurately defining the key physico-chemical factors which are operative in urinary stone disease.

ACKNOWLEDGEMENTS

This work was supported by grants from the South African Medical Research Council and the University of Cape Town. We are grateful to Mr P Abrunhusa of the University's Teaching Method Unit for his assistance in the design and construction of the Symposium poster.

REFERENCES

1. E. S. Lyon and C. W. Vermeulen, Invest. Urol. 3:309 (1965).
2. D. J. Sutor, Br. J. Urol. 41:171 (1969).
3. S. G. Welshman and M. G. McGeown, Br. J. Urol. 44:677 (1972).
4. W. G. Robertson, M. Peacock, and B. E. C. Nordin, Clin. Chim. Acta 43:31 (1973).
5. D. J. Sutor, in:"Urinary Calculi", L. Cifuentes Delatte, A. Rapado, and A. Hodgkinson, eds., Karger, Basel (1973).
6. J. L. Meyer and L. H. Smith, Invest. Urol. 13:31 (1975).
7. B. Finlayson, Invest. Urol. 9:258 (1972).
8. B. Finlayson and L. Dubois, Invest. Urol. 10:429 (1973).
9. G. W. Drach, A. D. Randolph, and J. D. Miller, J. Urol. 119:99 (1978).
10. G. W. Drach, S. Thorson, and A. Randolph, J. Urol. 123:519 (1980).
11. A. L. Rodgers and J. Garside, Invest. Urol. 18:484 (1981).
12. P. C. Hallson and G. A. Rose, Br. J. Urol. 50:442 (1978).
13. J. R. Burns and B. Finlayson, Invest. Urol. 18:167 (1980).
14. B. B. Tomazic and G. H. Nancollas, Invest. Urol. 16:329 (1979).

A COMPARISON OF THE TISELIUS RISK INDEX (RI) AND RELATIVE

SATURATION (RS) OF CALCIUM OXALATE (CaOx) IN STONE FORMERS

D. T. Erwin, D. J. Bennett, M. K. M. Gladden,
and F. E. Cole

Division of Research, Alton Ochsner Medical Foundation
New Orleans, Louisiana, U.S.A.

INTRODUCTION

Recently a simplified estimation of the ion activity product for calcium (AP-CaOx) in urine has been described using a computer program[1]. Subsequently a metabolic risk index, RI, was developed which was posited to be proportional to AP-CaOx at the same urine volume (Fig. 1). The Tiselius Risk Index is given by:
$RI = (Ca/Cr)^{0.71} \times (Ox/Cr)/(Mg/Cr)^{0.14} \times (Cit/Cr)^{0.10}$ where
Ca = calcium, Ox = oxalate, Mg = magnesium, Cit = citrate (all in mmol/l), and Cr = creatinine (in mol/l).

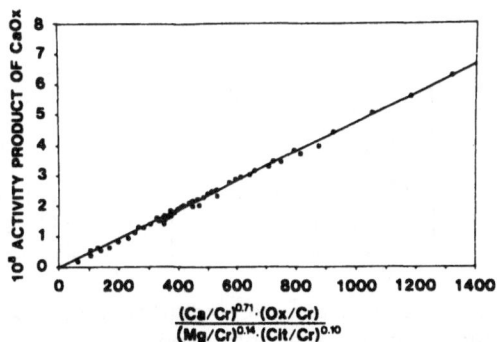

Fig. 1. Calculated relationship between the metabolic risk index
(RI) and the ion-activity product of calcium oxalate
(AP-CaOx) with urine volume and creatinine kept constant at
1500 ml and 0.015 mol/24 h, respectively.

Using different extreme combinations of high and low values for oxalate, calcium, magnesium, and citrate, Tiselius found his activity product index to correlate well with the calculated activity product of CaOx when urine volume and creatinine excretion had a constant numerical relationship (r=0.997).

METHODS

We have examined the relationship between the RI and the CaOx relative saturation ratio (RSR) in 20 stone-forming patients on high and low calcium diets where RSR = (AP-CaOx)/(Ksp-CaOx). The thermodynamic solubility product[2] for calcium oxalate (Ksp-CaOx) is 2.2×10^{-9}.

RESULTS AND DISCUSSION

Patients were grouped using methods similar to those outlined by Pak[3]; hyperabsorptive type I (n=4) with a urinary calcium excretion greater than 200 mg/24 h on a restricted calcium intake (~400 mg/day) which increased on a high calcium intake (~1200 mg/day); hyperabsorptive type II (n=7) excreting less than 200 mg/24 h urine on a restricted calcium but increasing more than 200 mg/24 h urine on a high calcium intake; renal leak (n=4) excreting more than 200 mg/24 h urine on a restricted calcium intake with no change on a high calcium intake, and normocalciuric patients (n=5) who excreted less than 200 mg/24 h urine on both a restricted and a high calcium intake (Fig. 2).

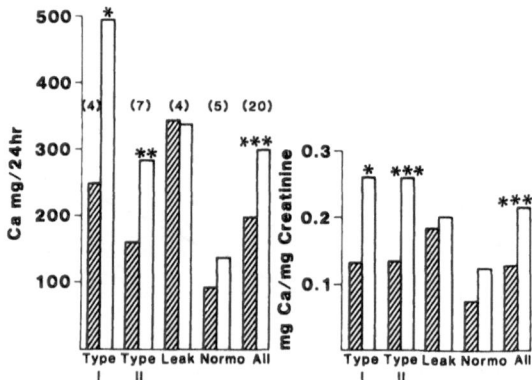

Fig. 2. Calcium and creatinine excretions/24 h. High and low calcium values were compared using a paired t-test. *P<0.05, ** P<0.01, and ***P<0.001.

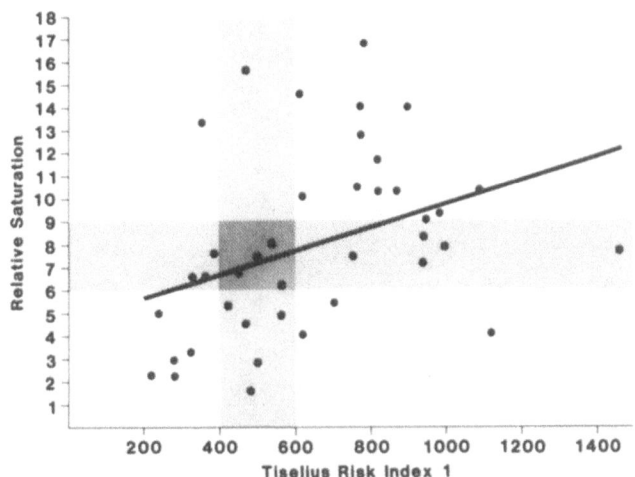

Fig. 3.   The relationship between relative saturation and the
Tiselius risk index on a high and low calcium intake.

Oxalate excretion, as expected, varied inversely with dietary
calcium intake in each group, being significant (P<0.01, n=20) when
the sub-groups were combined.   The mean urine volume (1500 ml) and
creatinine (0.013 mol/day) excretions from the 20 patients were
similar in each group and were near the fixed ratio used in
theoretical calculations[1].   The mean risk index for the group of
patients was 603+61, similar to the 527+17 reported by Tiselius[1] to
be the mean for the stone-forming group (versus 366+14 for normals).
The mean value was significantly higher (726+67, P<0.05) on a high
calcium intake.

Although we obtained a significant (P<0.05) relationship
between RI and RS in stone formers, it was much less precise
(r=0.366) when applied to patients (Fig. 3).   There was a >15-fold
variation in the relative saturation for a small range of risk index
and similarly, a >7-fold range in risk index for a small variation
in relative saturation.

REFERENCES

1. H. G. Tiselius, Clin. Chim. Acta 122:409 (1982).
2. C. Y. C. Pak, Y. Hayashi, B. Finlayson, and S. Chu,
      J. Lab. Clin. Med. 89:891 (1977).
3. C. Y. C. Pak, J. Urol. 128:1157 (1982).

EQUATIONS DEFINING URINARY CRYSTALLIZATION CONDITIONS WITH

RESPECT TO STONE-FORMING CALCIUM SALTS

J. M. Baumann, A. Futterlieb, M. Wacker and
E. Zingg

Dept. of Urology, Regionalspital, 2502 Biel and Clinic
of Urology of the University of Berne, Inselspital
3010 Berne, Switzerland

INTRODUCTION

Most information on the conditions favouring the crystallization of stone-forming salts in urine has been derived indirectly
from computer calculations based on urinary composition[1] or from
experiments performed in saline solutions or in highly diluted
urine[2]. In a comparative study, we measured inhibitory activity
and the state of supersaturation with respect to calcium oxalate and
calcium phosphate directly in the urine from 13 idiopathic calcium
stone formers (ISF), 12 patients with primary hyperparathyroidism
(HPT) and 16 healthy controls (HC)[3]. These results have now been
analyzed mathematically to obtain equations to predict the physico-
chemical behaviour of urine from the chemical composition.

MATERIALS AND METHODS

A detailed description of the methods used is given elsewhere[3].
Samples of 24-h urines collected on a standard diet and after an
oral oxalate load were analyzed for calcium, magnesium, phosphate,
oxalate, (Ox) and pyrophosphate, (PPi). In order to correct for
variations in the concentrations of stone forming substances,
inhibitors, chelators, and ionic strength due to different states of
diuresis, urine used in the test systems mentioned below was always
diluted to a standard excretion of 100 ml/h with bidistilled water.
The solubility of calcium oxalate monohydrate (COM) in urine was
determined by measuring the concentration product of $[Ca] \times [Ox]$
after incubation with 10 mg COM/ml urine at pH 6.0 and the
solubility of brushite by measuring $[Ca] \times [P]$ after incubation with
10 mg brushite/ml urine at pH 6.6. Inhibitory activity was

773

determined by measuring the maximum [Ca] x[Ox] or [Ca] x [P] tolerated in urine without causing secondary nucleation and growth as defined by a decrease in calcium concentration of 0.02 mg/ml COM at pH 6.0 or 0.2 mg/ml hydroxyapatite (HAP) at pH 6.6. The results were plotted using a computer and linear regressions calculated by the method of least squares.

RESULTS AND CONCLUSIONS

The following data obtained from ISF (Δ), HPT ($\square$) and HC (O) showed significant correlations:

Solubility of COM in Urine

The data of Fig. 1 fit best: K_s = Ca x (Ox - k_s).

Multiplication of the average concentration product K_s by the free fraction of calcium (0.55) and of oxalate (0.8) and by the square of the activity coefficient[4] of divalent ions (0.33^2) yields 3.5×10^{-9} $(mol/l)^2$. This value is in the range of the thermodynamic solubility product of COM (3.6×10^{-9} $(mmol/)^2$) obtained in 0.15 molar $NaCl^5$. k_s probably represents a macromolecular oxalate complex[6] which may account for the discrepancy observed between relative supersaturation and activity product ratio calculated for the same urine[7]. The state of urinary saturation valid for a diuresis of 100 ml/h may therefore be estimated from urinary [Ca] and [Ox] in mmol/l, voided volume (V) in litres and the time of urine collection (t) in hours by:

$$(Ca \cdot V/0.1t)(Ox \cdot V/0.1t - k_s) \cdot K_s^{-1}$$

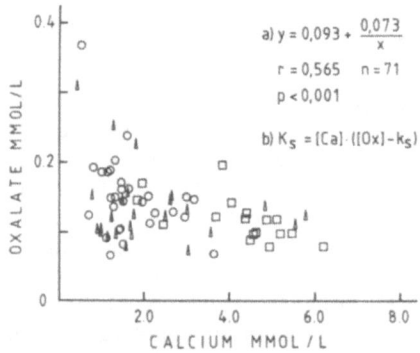

Fig. 1. [Ox] vs [Ca] in urine saturated with respect to COM.

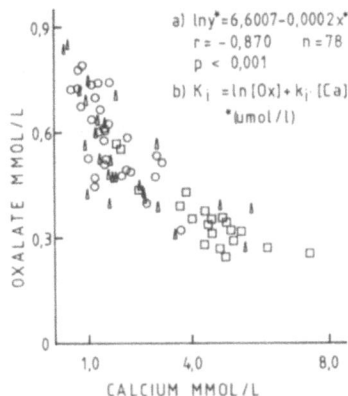

Fig. 2. Maximum [Ox] vs [Ca] tolerated in urine without crystallization of COM.

The State of Urinary Supersaturation with Respect to Brushite

The state of urinary supersaturation with respect to brushite expressed as concentration product ratio showed a linear correlation with [Ca]:

$$y = 0.73 \ x \ (r = 0.95, \ P < 0.001, \ n = 70)$$

which is in agreement with the findings of others[8]. At fixed pH and urine volume the state of saturation can therefore be calculated from [Ca].

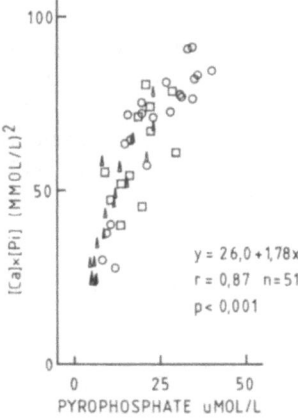

Fig. 3. Maximum [Ca] x [Pi] in urine without crystallization of HAP vs urinary [PPi].

Urinary Inhibitory Activity towards Crystallization of COM

Fig. 2 also shows that hypercalciuria may be important for the formation of calcium oxalate stones since urinary [Ox] required to induce COM-crystallization markedly decreases with an increasing urinary [Ca]. ln of [Ox] reveals a negative linear correlation to Ca shown in equations a and b. The physico-chemical implication of this finding deserves further investigation.

Urinary inhibitory Activity towards Crystallization of HAP

Fig. 3 shows that this inhibitory activity can be predicted from PPi. Urinary PPi, which has been found to be decreased in calcium stone formers with short-term recurrences[9,10], seems to be an important inhibitor of secondary nucleation and growth of small amounts of HAP.

REFERENCES

1. W. G. Robertson, M. Peacock and B. E. C. Nordin, Clin. Sci. 34:579 (1968).
2. B. Finlayson, Kidney Int. 13:344 (1978).
3. J. M. Baumann, K. Lauber, F. X. Lustenberger, M. Wacker, and E. J. Zingg, (in preparation).
4. R. W. Marshall and W. G. Robertson, Clin. Chim. Acta 72:253 (1976).
5. J. L. Meyer and L. H. Smith, Invest. Urol. 13:31 (1975).
6. J. Sheinfeld, B. Finlayson, and F. Reid, Invest. Urol. 15:462 (1978).
7. N. A. Breslau and C. Y. C. Pak, in:"Nephrolithiasis, Contemporary Issues in Nephrology", vol 5, B. M. Brenner and J. H. Stein, eds., Churchill Livingstone, New York (1980).
8. C. Y. C. Pak and K. Holt, Metabolism 25:665 (1976).
9. J. M. Baumann, S. Bisaz, R. Felix, U. Ganz, and R. G. G. Russell, Clin. Sci. 53:141 (1977).
10. B. Wikström, B. G. Danielson, S. Ljunghall, M. McGuire, and R. G. G. Russell, World J. Urol. 1:150 (1983).

CALCULATION OF COMPLEX CHEMICAL EQUILIBRIA IN URINE: ESTIMATION OF

THE RISK OF STONE FORMATION AND DERIVATION OF PROPHYLACTIC MEASURES

W. Achilles and B. Ulshöfer

Urologische Universitätsklinik und Poliklinik Marburg
D-3550 Marburg a.d.Lahn, F.R.G.

INTRODUCTION

The degree of supersaturation of a precipitating system is defined as $G = -RT \ln(AP/K_{sp})$, where AT = the activity product of the precipitating ions and K_{sp} = the corresponding solubility product. In solutions such as urine containing interacting ligands and metal ions, the AP may be governed by multiple equilibrium reactions. This is the case with calcium oxalate, one of the most important constituents of urinary stones. From the corresponding thermodynamic equilibrium constants, AP can be calculated from the total concentrations of all the ions concerned and the pH of the solution[1-4].

In this paper, a computer model has been used to estimate the dependence of supersaturation of calcium oxalate in urine on different concentrations of urinary constituents. From the results of these calculations conclusions may be drawn regarding the treatment of patients with calcium oxalate urolithiasis.

METHODS

A computer program (M-BASIC) has been written which allows the calculation of complex chemical equilibria in a model of human urine, taking into account more than 30 reactions between protons, metal ions and ligands. Equilibrium constants were taken from literature[5-7], and (in the case of organic acids and aminoacids) estimated as mean values from data of analogous compounds. The algorithm of Perrin and Sayce[8] was used for the iteration procedure. The ionic strength of the system was calculated using an additional iteration procedure based on the Davies equation to estimate ion activity coefficients[1]. Calculations were performed by means of an Alphatronic microcomputer 4 (Triumph Adler).

The ratio (Q) on the CaOx activity product (AP) to the solubility product (K_{sp}) was calculated as a function of the normalized total concentrations of urinary constituents. The composition of the 'normal' urine is described below. The mean values were taken from the literature and from our own laboratory data. They are given in mmol/l: Calcium (Ca) = 3.5; magnesium (Mg) = 3.0; sodium (Na) = 130; potassium (K) = 40; ammonium (NH_4) = 20; oxalate (Ox) = 0.30; phosphate (P) = 20; citrate (Cit) = 2.0; sulphate (SO_4) = 15; sum of amino acids (Aa) = 5; sum of organic acids (Pa = 15; uric acid (Ua) = 2.5; pH = 6.0; 24-h urine volume (V_E) = 1400 ml. A value of $3.6\ 10^{-9}$ l/mol (I=0.15 mol/l) was taken for the K_{sp} of CaOx $2H_2O$ [7].

RESULTS AND DISCUSSION

Calculation of the complex chemical equilibria has proved to be useful for determining the activity products (AP) of the ionized components of stone-forming salts[1-4]. In the present paper, similarly to our first study in 1976[4], we carried out a systematic computer simulation in order to determine the effect of varying different urinary constituents on the AP or supersaturation of calcium oxalate. It was the aim of the work to report on these different effects and to deduce rational therapeutic or prophylactic measures from the curves obtained. In order to achieve this, lg Q = lg $(AP/K_{sp})_{CaOx}$ was calculated as a function of the normalized total concentrations and not of the absolute values. This allows the comparison of the influences of all urinary constituents within the same (logarithmic) scale despite their quite different concentrations (e.g., Na_N=130; Ox_N=0.3 mmol/l) and also seems to be reasonable from a physiological point of view.

The results are in Fig. 1 which shows the effect of variation of the various individual constituents, keeping all other variables constant at their normal values. The broken curve indicated by "Volume (24 h)" reflects the simultaneous change of all the constituent concentrations in the system thereby simulating the effect of variation in urine volume or the indirect effect of fluid intake (drinking therapy) on lg Q. The following conclusions may be drawn. Changes in 24-h urine volume or in total oxalate concentration are the most effective for changing lg (AP/K_{sp}). Increasing calcium concentration results in a curve with a maximum which is due to the formation of the Ca_2Ox ion-pair[9] at high CaOx ratios. Thus, a decrease in urine Ca in hypercalciuric patients may have a minimal effect on lg Q depending on the initial conditions.

778

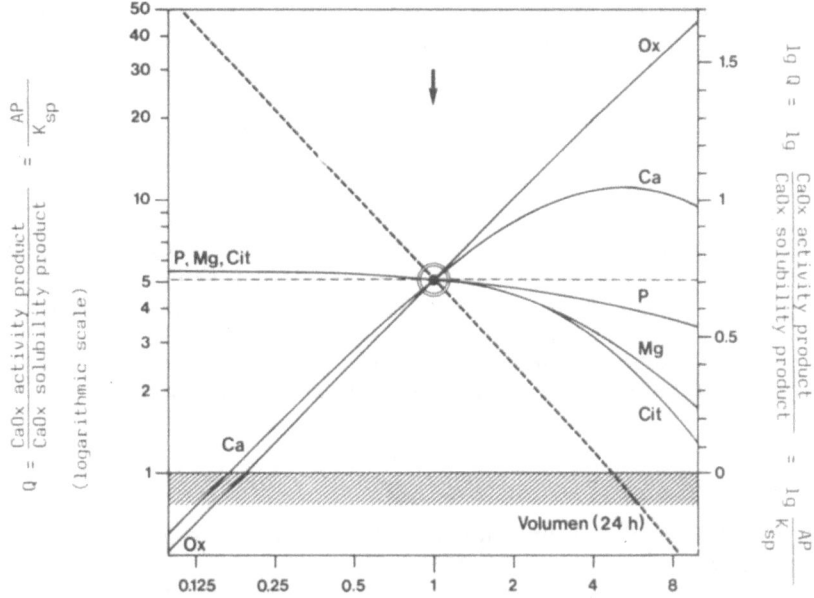

Fig. 1. Supersaturation (expressed as log (AP/K_{sp})) of calcium oxalate in urine as a function of normalized concentrations of various urinary constituents.

Compared with V_e, Ox and Ca, the effects of all other components such as Cit, Mg, P, SO_4 and pH (not shown here) are much less pronounced. For instance, starting from the normal point, an increase of V_E or a decrease of Ox by a factor of 2 results in a decrease in lg Q from about 0.7 to 0.4. To achieve the same effect by varying Mg or Cit requires that the concentrations of these components must be increased 6-fold from their normal values.

Simultaneous changes in normalized Ca and Ox in the same direction result in a drastic change in Q. Simultaneous changes in Ca and Ox in opposite directions may lead to an increase (when Ca↓ and Ox ↑) or decrease in lg Q (when Ca ↑ and Ox ↓).

From a thermodynamic point of view, the following conclusions may be drawn with respect to the prophylaxis of CaOx urolithiasis. A high fluid intake and/or a decrease in oxalate excretion should be the most effective measures for reducing the risk of calcium oxalate stone formation. Because of the shape of the Ca-curve, the effect of Ca variation on lg Q depends on the initial Ca concentration. Decreasing calcium excretion while increasing urinary oxalate to the same extent (in terms of normalized concentrations), e.g., by cation exchange therapy, should be of negligible value for stone prevention and might even increase the risk of stone formation.

779

These considerations say little about crystal growth kinetics except indirectly through the rate-determining CaOx activity product. The kinetic effects of crystal growth inhibitors or promoters and the rate of crystal morphology have not been taken into account. Methods to evaluate those parameters which reflect the overall tendency of a particular urine to form stones are necessary.

Recently, Daniele et al[10] have published a series of stability constants for the interaction of the most important chemical complexes in human urine. The authors have included the dependence of equilibrium constants on ionic strength up to I=0.5 (-0.9). These data are of particular relevance to the calculations presented here and will be taken into account in future studies.

REFERENCES

1. G. H. Nancollas, "Interactions in Electrolyte Solutions", Elsevier, Amsterdam (1966).
2. W. G. Robertson, Clin. Chim. Acta 24:149 (1969).
3. B. Finlayson and F. Reid, Invest. Urol. 15:442 (1978).
4. W. Achilles, G. A. Cumme, and M. Scheffel, in"Urolithiasis Research", H. Fleisch, W. G. Robertson, L. H. Smith, and W. Vahlensieck, eds., Plenum, New York (1976).
5. Stability Constants of Metal-Ion Complexes, Part A:Inorganic Ligands, IUPAC Chemical Data Series No. 21 (1980).
6. Stability Constants of Metal-Ion Complexes, Part B:Organic Ligands, IUPAC Chemical Data Series No. 22 (1979).
7. P. G. Koutsoukos, C. Y. Lam-Erwin, and G. H. Nancollas, Invest. Urol. 18:178 (1980).
8. D. D. Perrin and I. G. Sayce, Talanta 14:833 (1967).
9. B. Finlayson, R. Roth, and L. DuBois, in:"Urinary Calculi", L. Cifuentes Delatte, A. Rapado, and A. Hodgkinson, eds., Karger, Basel (1973).
10. P. G. Daniele and M. Marangella, Ann. Chim. 72:25 (1982).

EPITAXIAL GROWTH OF CALCIUM OXALATE ON URIC ACID

S. Sarig, D. Hirsch, N. Garti, and B. Goldwasser

The Casali Institute of Applied Chemistry, The Hebrew
University, Jerusalem, Israel

INTRODUCTION

In a survey of 10,000 kidney stones, Herring[1] found 944 specimens
containing uric acid. A large proportion of these stones consisted
of a nucleus of uric acid overlaid with calcium oxalate. The
syndrome of calcium oxalate stone formation in normocalciuric-
hyperuricosuric patients is well recognised but it is not yet clear
whether or not treatment aimed at decreasing uric acid excretion
successfully prevents further calcium oxalate stone formation in
these patients.

Crystals form in the urine which is supersaturated with respect
to uric acid. Pak and Arnold attempted to establish a causal
relationship between uric acid crystals formed in this way and
calcium oxalate precipitation. Their studies, along with that of
Coe et al [3], have shown uniquivocally that, whereas sodium urate
induces heterogeneous nucleation, uric acid crystals do not cause
calcium oxalate to precipitate from metastable solutions. These
findings, however, are inconsistent with two aspects of the
relationship between uric acid and calcium oxalate. First, it was
predicted on the basis of convincing crystallographic
considerations[4], that there was a potential for epitaxial growth of
one crystal type on the other. Second, calcium oxalate stones
containing uric acid nuclei are fairly common, while those
containing sodium urate are extremely rare.

The possibility that an additional agent might be involved in
the epitaxial growth of calcium oxalate on uric acid has been
explored in the present study.

Table 1. The Reduction of Calcium Ion Concentration in Metastable Calcium Oxalate Solutions Caused by Seed Crystals in Uric Acid Species.

| Series | Seeds | Number of Tests | pH | Ionic Strength | Range of Concentration | | % Decrease in Calcium Concentration |
					Calcium (10^{-4}M)	Oxalate (10^{-4}M)	
1	Sodium urate	28	7	0.05	4 to 7	4 to 4.5	13.7 ± 4.3
2	Sodium urate	18	7	0.15	5 to 7	5 to 6	13.6 ± 2.2
3	Sodium urate	2	7	0.05	5	-	0
4	Uric acid	2	5.5	0.05	5	5	0
5	Uric acid	2	5.5	0.15	6	3	3
6	Noncompatible seeds (AgCl)	2	7	0.15	6	6	2.5
7	Uric acid +4ppm GA	6	5.5	0.15	6	6	28 ± 8
8	Uric acid +5ppm GA	4	5.5	0.15	6	6	17 ± 3.5

MATERIALS AND METHODS

Metastable solutions of CaC_2O_4 were prepared with ion-products in the range 1.6 to 4.2 x $10^{-7} M^2$ at ionic strengths of 0.05 and 0.15. Seed crystals of uric acid and sodium urate were added. Calcium ion concentration was measured continuously using an Orion calcium-specific electrode mounted on a digital pH/mV voltmeter with a double junction Orion reference electrode (model 90-02). The metastability of the solutions without any additives (blanks) was tested for 15 min duration and the calcium concentration shown not to decrease during this period. The concentration decrease was noted in the presence of seed crystals (0.1 to 0.15 g/200 ml). The seed crystals, after 15 min contact, were quickly filtered off, dried, either gold- or carbon-coated and examined by SEM (Jeol JSM-35) and LINK systems (860) for element identification.

RESULTS AND DISCUSSION

Table 1 shows that seeds of sodium urate induced a decrease in calcium concentration (series 1,2). A control study (series 3) showed that this decrease did not result from the adsorption of calcium ions on the surface of the sodium urate seeds and hence was apparently due to calcium oxalate formation. The introduction of uric acid seeds did not cause a significant decrease in calcium concentration (series 4,5). Also, introduction of neutral seeds at pH = 7, which had no structural fit (series 6), failed to trigger calcium oxalate precipitation. More direct evidence for the preferential occurrence of epitaxy between calcium oxalate and sodium urate was supplied by surface X-ray energy spectrum (SEM-LINK). In the presence of sodium urate this revealed a calcium peak, whereas in the presence of uric acid seeds no calcium peak was detected. This result is in agreement with the electrode determinations in this study and with previously reported results [2,3,5]. We suggest that structural fit and satisfaction of bonding requirements are not sufficient criteria for epitaxial growth to occur within a short period of time. Some factors such as electrostatic attraction, which affects the kinetics of the process, must also be present. This factor must exist in the sodium urate/calcium oxalate system but be absent from that involving neutral uric acid.

Uric acid crystals in urine may acquire a surface charge by adsorption of multifunctional ions are known to affect the crystallization of calcium oxalate in vitro[6] and to participate in kidney stone formation. In the present study, glutamic and aspartic acids were chosen to check this assumption. In fact, a system of uric acid seeds in a metastable calcium oxalate solution containing trace concentrations of amino acids, more closely simulates the conditions in urine than those employed previously[3,5].

The marked effect of glutamic acid on calcium ion depletion is shown in Table 1 (series 7,8). A calcium peak, evidence of calcium oxalate deposition on the seeds of uric acid was detected, when glutamic acid was present in the solution.

The concept of a mediating agent, which is structurally compatible with both members of the epitaxial relationship and which facilitates the start of growth, resolves the inconsistency between the clinical data[1] and the failure to induce epitaxial growth of calcium oxalate on uric acid seeds in pure synthetic experimental systems[3,5]. Moreover, the concept may explain some inconsistencies in the evaluation of the management of hyperuricosuric calcium oxalate stone formers.

Uric acid crystals are formed, especially at low pH by hyper-uricosuric patients. These crystals are thought to be the natural seeds for calcium oxalate stones from theoretical crystallographic considerations[4] and because they are found in the centres of many stones[1]. The natural conclusion is that a drug which reduces uric acid excretion will prevent kidney stone formation. Coe[7] reported that allopurinol, which reduces uric acid levels in urine, actually prevented calcium oxalate stone recurrence. Other reports are less positive[8]. Preliminary clinical investigations which are presently being conducted show that allopurinol may be quite effective for some patients, whereas, for others, the effect is questionable. The connection between the existence of uric acid crystals and the presence of amino acids and related compounds may have some bearing on the success or failure of allopurinol treatment. If this connection is proved clinically, it may help to clarify the conditions under which allopurinol treatment of the uric acid/calcium oxalate syndrome may be beneficial. Furthermore, it may help to identify those cases in whom allopurinol treatment may be insufficient.

REFERENCES

1. L. H. Herring, J. Urol. 88:545 (1962).
2. C. Y. C. Pak and L. H. Arnold, Proc. Soc. Exp. Biol. Med. 149:930 (1975).
3. F. L. Coe, R. L. Lawton, R. B. Goldstein, and V. Tembe, Proc. Soc. Exp. Biol. Med. 149:926 (1975).
4. N. S. Mandel and G. S. Mandel, in:"Urolithiasis, Clinical and Basic Research", L. H. Smith, W. G. Robertson, and B. Finlayson, eds., Plenum, New York (1981).
5. J. L. Meyer, J. L. Berget, and L. H. Smith, Invest. Urol. 14:115 (1976).
6. R. Azoury, A. D. Randolph, G. W. Drach, S. Perlberg, N. Garti, and S. Sarig, J. Cryst. Growth (in press).
7. F. L. Coe and L. Raisen, Lancet i:129 (1973).
8. M. J. V. Smith, J. Urol. 117:690 (1977).

THE CONDITIONS FOR PRECIPITATION OF URIC ACID AND SODIUM

ACID URATE

V. Babić-Ivančić, H. Füredi-Milhofer, O. Milat,
W. E. Brown, and T. M. Gregory

"Ruder Bošković" Institute and Institute for Physics
Zagreb, Yugoslavia, and National Bureau of Standards
Washington, U.S.A.

INTRODUCTION

Anhydrous uric acid (H_2U), uric acid dihydrate ($H_2U.2H_2O$) and
sodium acid urate monohydrate ($NaHU.H_2O$) have been detected in
urinary calculi[1]. A positive relationship between hyperuricosuria
and calcium oxalate stone formation has also been demonstrated[2].
This relationship could be explained by the presence in urine of a
microcrystalline or colloidal form of NaHU which might adsorb the
known inhibitors of crystal growth and aggregation[3] or induce
epitaxial growth of calcium oxalate crystals[4]. Data on the
precipitation of these solid phases from unseeded solutions are
scarce and unsystematic. It would be of considerable interest to
work out phase[5] and precipitation diagrams[6,7] that would show which
solid phase may be expected under given experimental conditions.
In this paper the systems: H_2U-NaOH-HCl-H_2O (I) and H_2U-NaOH-NaCl-
H_2O, at pH = 7.5 (II) are represented by such diagrams.

MATERIALS AND METHODS

Commercial H_2U was dissolved in carbonate-free sodium
hydroxide. H_2UH_2O was precipitated by addition of HCl while sodium
acid urate was obtained by the addition of NaCl at a constant pH of
7.5. After thorough mixing the systems were aged without further
stirring in a $25^{\circ}C$ or $35^{\circ}C$ water bath. Precipitates were
characterized by light or electron microscopy, X-ray or electron
diffraction and thermogravimetric analysis. The boundaries in the
phase diagram and ionic activities were calculated as previously
described[5] using literature values for the dissociation constants of
H_2U[8,9] and the solubility constants of H_2U[8] and $NaHU.H_2O$[9].

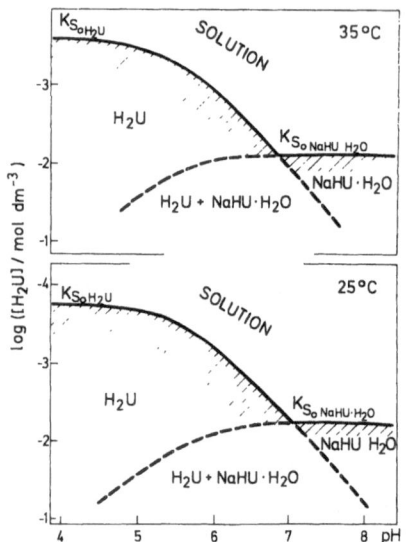

Fig. 1. Computed phase diagram of the system: $H_2U-NaOH-HCl-H_2O$, $25^\circ C$ and $35^\circ C$.

RESULTS AND DISCUSSION

The computed phase diagrams (Fig. 1) pertain to equilibrium conditions. The solubility curves of the thermodynamically stable phases, H_2U and $NaHU.H_2O$ (full lines) intersect at a singular point at which both phases are in equilibrium with the surrounding solution. The precipitation area is divided into concentration regions (broken curves) within which H_2U or $NaHU.H_2O$ are the stable phases. Both compounds are equally probable in the region which lies between the broken curves and transformation of one phase into the other is expected. The precipitation diagram of Systems I and II (Figs. 2 and 3) show the experimental situation at metastable equilibrium, including the thermodynamically metastable phases. In the region of 2 pH 6.5 and total uric acid 3×10^{-4} H_2U 10^{-2} mol dm^{-3} at both temperatures (System I, Fig. 2) $H_2U.2H_2O$ was the first solid phase formed. At $25^\circ C$ this phase was stable for 24 h while at $35^\circ C$ partial transformation into H_2U occurred. In the physiological region the formation of both forms of uric acid is expected. From the data giving the precipitation boundaries mean ion activity products, $(H^+)(HU^-)$, $IP_{25^\circ C} = 1.07 \times 10^{-9}$ $mol^2 dm^{-6}$ and $IP_{35^\circ C} = 1.58 \times 10^{-9}$ dm^{-6} were calculated. Both are in good agreement with published values[8,10].

The precipitation diagram of System II is shown in the lower part of Fig. 3. The upper diagram shows the same data recalculated in terms of ion activity products. At supersaturations S < 80 less

786

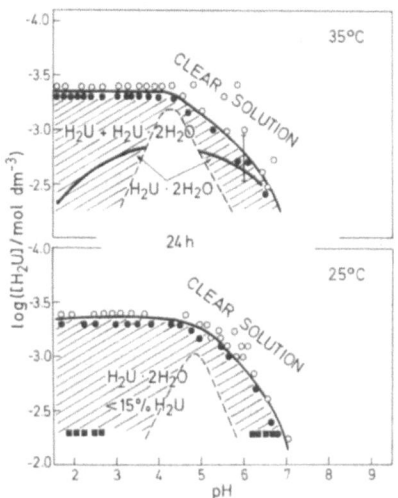

Fig. 2. Precipitation diagrams of the system: $H_2U-NaOH-HCl-H_2O$, 25°C and 35°C. Shaded area indicates precipitation. Bar shows range of urinary concentrations of uric acid.

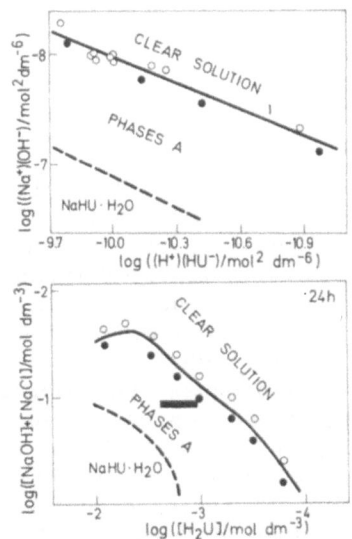

Fig. 3. Precipitation diagram (lower part) and potential plot (upper part) of the system: $H_2U-NaOH-NaCl-H_2O$, at pH = 7.5. The bar indicates urinary concentrations of uric acid and sodium ions.

than 5% of the total uric acid precipitated in the form of at least
two different phases (phases A).   One of them consisted of
particles of needle-like appearance with a diffuse electron
diffraction pattern.   The other phase appeared as aggregates of
microcrystalline material (individual particles <0.02 μm) which
showed several electron diffraction lines characteristic of
$NaHU.H_2O$.   Other intense diffraction lines, characteristic of these
compounds (9.29 A, 7.69 A, 3.18 A, 2.67 A) were consistently
missing.   Phases A are structurally not identical with $NaHU.H_2O$.

If the ionic composition of the solution is known, the slope of
the solid/solution boundary expressed in terms of the logarithms of
ionic activities indicates the molar ratio of the constituent ions
of the precipitate[5,6].   Thus the slope of line 1 in Fig. 3 is 0.91
(r = 0.97) showing that the overall sodium to urate molar ratio of
phases A is approximately 1.   Presumably phases A are more hydrated
and therefore show less crystal order than the thermodynamically
stable $NaHU.H_2O$.   Phases A are formed at urinary sodium and urate
concentrations (bar in Fig. 3) while $NaHU.H_2O$ crystallized at
supersaturations greatly exceeding physiological (S >80).

ACKNOWLEGEMENT

The financial support by the Self-Management Council for
Scientific Research of Croatia (SIZ-V) and the National Bureau of
Standards (Grant No. NBS/G/263) is gratefully acknowledged.

REFERENCES

1. D. J. Sutor and S. Scheidt, Br. J. Urol. 15:22 (1968).
2. F. L. Coe and L. Raisen, Lancet 1:129 (1973).
3. W. G. Robertson, F. Knowles, and M. Peacock, in:"Urolithiasis
   Research", H. Fleisch, W. G. Robertson, L. H. Smith and
   W. Vahlensieck, eds., Plenum, New York (1976).
4. P. G. Koutsoukos, C. Y. Lam-Erwin, and G. H. Nancollas,
   Invest.Urol. 18:178 (1980).
5. W. E. Brown, in:"Environmental Phosphorus Handbook",
   E. J. Griffiths, A. Beston, J. M. Speer and B. T. Mitchell,
   eds.,John Wiley, New York (1973).
6. H. Füredi, in:"The Formation and Properties of Precipitates",
   A. G. Walton, ed., Interscience Publishers, New York (1962).
7. H. Füredi-Milhofer, Croat. Chem. Acta 56:721 (1983).
8. C. Y. Lam, G. H. Nancollas, and S. J. Ko, Invest. Urol. 15:673
   (1978).
9. E. G. Young and F. F. Musgrave, Biochem. J. 26:941 (1932).
10. E. Mentasti, C. Rinaudo, and R. Boistelle, J. Chem. Eng. Data
    28:247 (1983).

THE OXALATE-TOLERANCE-VALUE: A DIAGNOSTIC TOOL FOR THE RECOGNITION OF STONE FORMING PATIENTS

T. Briellmann, H. Seiler, F. Hering, and G. Rutishauser

Institut für Anorganische Chemie, Universität Basel and
Urologische Klinik, Abt. Chirurgie, Kantonsspital Basel
Switzerland.

INTRODUCTION

The thermodynamic parameters involved in the formation of calcium oxalate crystals are the concentrations of Ca^{2+} and C_2O_4, the total ionic strength of the solution and the presence of inhibitors. The kinetics of the growth of particles is governed by temperature, the presence of nuclei and inhibitors, the diffusion properties of the participating substances, (influenced by the concentration of all substances present), the agitation of the surrounding liquid and the possibility of coprecipitation[1-5]. Since the composition of urine with respect to some of the thermodynamic and kinetic parameters differs from one person to another and from one voiding to another, the aim of the present work was to find a method which allows comparison of the formation of crystals in different urines without disturbing the original composition of the urine.

METHODS

Aliquots of individual whole urines were titrated at $37^{\circ}C$ with $Na_2C_2O_4$ at a constant rate of addition using a motor-driven micro-burette and constant agitation. The onset of precipitation was detected by turbidimetry. pH was followed during the whole experiment (Fig. 1). In another aliquot of the same urine the total calcium-concentration was determined by FAAS (using acetylene and nitrous oxide). The standard curve for oxalate-tolerance was established by measuring the oxalate-tolerance of a synthetic mixture containing the main constituents - both organic and inorganic - of human urine but varying the calcium concentration

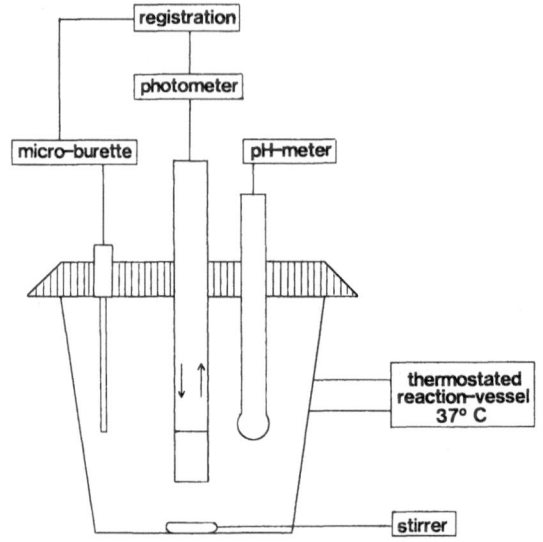

Fig. 1. Measuring equipment

over a wide range.   These measurements were made under the
conditions described above.

RESULTS

     Using the method described above, the urines of first-time
stone-formers, of recurrent stone-formers (both groups forming
oxalate and/or phosphate stones) and of a group of probands without
oxalate stones were compared. The results are given in % of
oxalate-tolerance values above and below the standard curve
(Table 1, Figs. 2 and 3).

Table 1. Comparison of Oxalate-Tolerance Values Above and Below
         the Standard Curve.

	Above Standard Curve	Below Standard Curve	n
First-time Stone-formers	38.5	61.5	13
Recurrent Stone-formers	57.7	42.3	26
Others	67.6	32.4	34

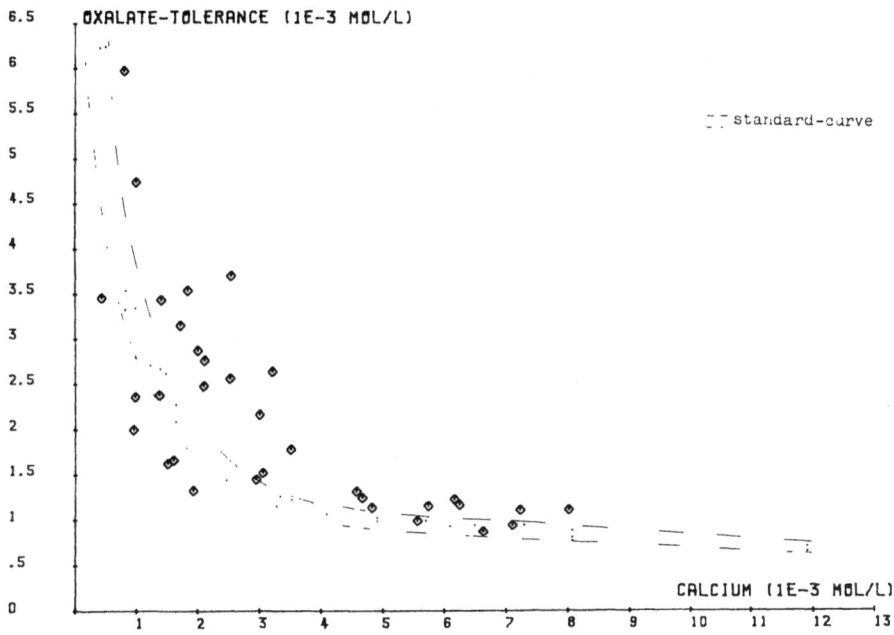

Fig. 2. Oxalate-tolerance values of oxalate stone-formers.

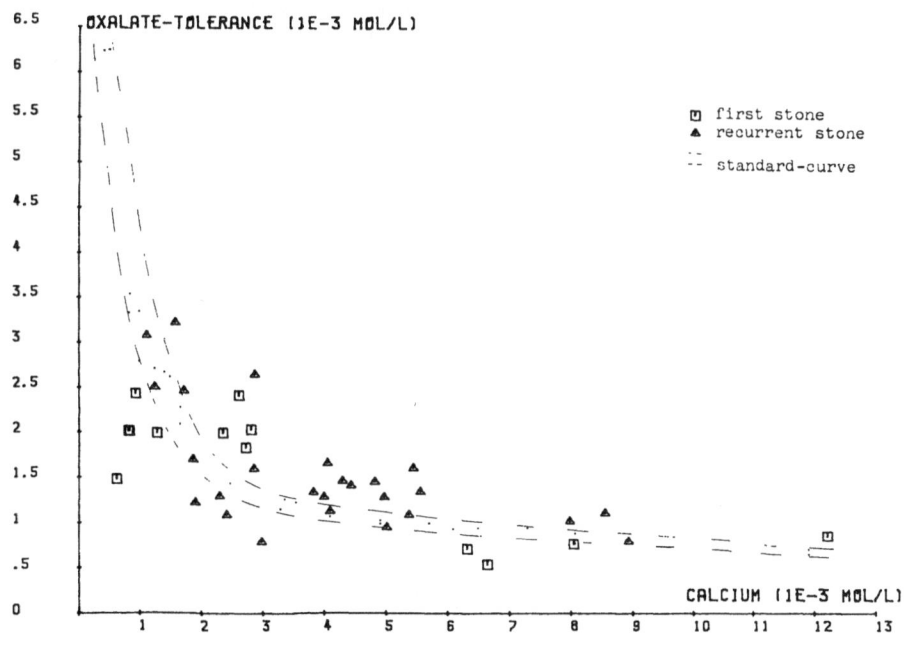

Fig. 3. Oxalate-tolerance values of others.

DISCUSSION

   The anticipated result that urines from all oxalate stone-formers would have oxalate-tolerance values below the standard curve whereas all other values would be above it was not obtained, although Table 2 shows that there is a tendency towards that situation. The reason for the uncertainty as to whether a urine will have a value above or below the standard curve arises not only from the presence or absence of inhibitors in the urine, but also from the total concentrations of all the other ions in that urine. The results obtained using spontaneous urine samples led us to conclude that valid information concerning the stone forming tendency of an individual patient can only be obtained by repetitive determination of the oxalate-tolerance value in different urines over a period of time. Further studies will be made to elucidate these effects and to find a practicable method for defining the stone-forming potential of a given urine.

REFERENCES

1. J. L. Meyer and L. H. Smith, Invest. Urol. 13:31 (1975).
2. S. Sarig, N. Garti, R. Azoury, Y. Wax, and S. Perlberg, J. Urol. 128:645 (1982).
3. W. G. Robertson, D. S. Scurr, and C. M. Bridge, J. Cryst. Growth 53:182 (1981).
4. J. L. Meyer and L. H. Smith, Invest. Urol. 13:36 (1975).
5. J. M. Baumann and M. Wacker, Urol. Res. 8:171 (1980).

THE CRYSTALLIZATION OF MAGNESIUM AMMONIUM PHOSPHATE

(STRUVITE) IN ACIDIC STERILE URINE

R. Boistelle, F. Abbona, Y. Berland, M. Grandvuillemin, and M. Olmer

Centre de Recherche sur les Mécanismes de la Croissance Cristalline, Campus Luminy, and Service de Nephrologie Hôpital de la Conception, Marseille, France

INTRODUCTION

It is usually accepted[1,2] that magnesium ammonium phosphate ($MgNH_4PO_4 \cdot 6H_2O$) nucleates and grows only from infected alkaline urines. However, crystal growth experiments carried out in pure aqueous solutions[3,4] show that nucleation, growth and also phase transition of struvite into newberyite ($MgHPO_4 \cdot 3H_2O$) occur easily within the acid pH range. The aim of the present study is to check whether or not alkaline infected urines are really required for the crystallization of struvite.

METHODS

Freshly voided urines from non-stone-formers were centrifuged, after addition of small quantities of hibitane to prevent infection, and divided into two aliquots, A and B. Magnesium was added to A and ammonia and/or phosphate to B in the form of aqueous solutions of $MgSO_4 \cdot 7H_2O$, $NH_4H_2PO_4$, NH_4Cl and NaH_2PO_4. The pH was adjusted by addition of NH_4OH or NaOH. After mixture of A and B, the dilution of urine was always less than 10%. With this method the effects of pH, magnesium, ammonia and phosphate up to 250 mM could be investigated individually. The effect of varying pH was examined over the range 5.0 to 9.6. The initial and final concentrations of urine were measured by spectrophotometry. Finally, the urinary sediments of 47 stone-formers were collected and identified. In the voidings of 8 of these patients struvite crystals were found and compared with those grown in vitro.

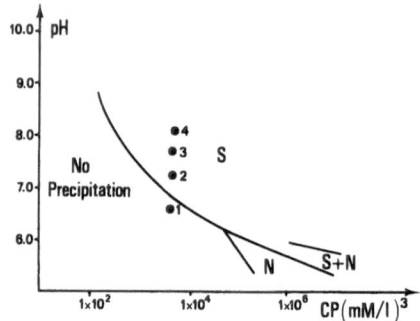

Fig. 1. The nucleation fields of struvite and newberyite in urine
as a function of pH and concentration product, CP
(where CP = [magnesium] x [ammonia] x [phosphate]).

RESULTS

    In Fig. 1, crystallization is shown as a function of pH and the
concentration product CP = [total magnesium] x [total ammonia] x
[total phosphate] . The two main areas represent the crystallization range of struvite and a region where no precipitation occurs
within 5 days. At high CP and low pH there are two small domains
where newberyite can nucleate as the first phase. It is noteworthy
that struvite can form very close to the normal range. In the
neighbourhood of this range, the crystallization of struvite may be
achieved by increasing either pH or CP, or both at the same time.
Another point of interest is that no nucleation of struvite occurs
when CP < 200 $(mM)^3$, except in a few cases where the concentration of
Mg is greater than 3mM.

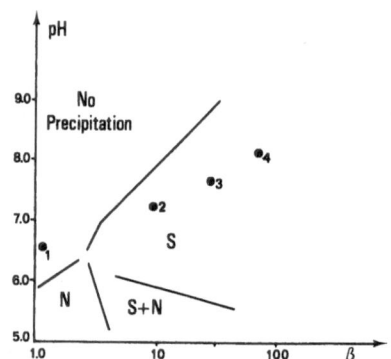

Fig. 2. The nucleation fields of struvite and newberyite in urine
as a function of pH and supersaturation with respect to
struvite.

794

However, the question remained as to whether or not urines with a low CP but a very high pH were under- or supersaturated with respect to struvite. The supersaturations were therefore computed using an iterative method taking into account the most important ionic species and the ionic strength of urine. The results are given in Fig. 2 where the CPs of Fig. 1 have been replaced by the corresponding supersaturations $\beta = \underline{a}(Mg^{2+}) \times \underline{a}(NH_3) \times \underline{a}(HPO_4^{2-})/K_{sp}$, where $\underline{a}$ refers to activities and K_{sp} is the solubility product of struvite. Nucleation should occur when $\beta > 1$. The most striking fact in Fig. 2 is that the upper left part corresponds to urines definitely supersaturated with respect to struvite but which deposit no crystals. It is also noteworthy that only ammonia and/or phosphate has been added to these urines which remain in a metastable state for more than 5 days. Also the influence of pH can be seen on Fig. 2 by considering the 4 points with the same CP values shown on Fig. 1. For this given CP, there is a difference of almost two orders of magnitude in the supersaturation when the pH increases from about 6.6 (point 1) to 8.1 (point 4).

DISCUSSION

When there is enough ammonia in urine, the addition of sodium hydroxide to increase pH does not significantly change the precipitation regions shown in Fig. 1. However, in this situation, there is also rapid precipitation of an amorphous phase which precedes the crystalline phase. Another point is that the crystallization of struvite reduces not only the concentrations but also pH. If the pH decreases too much, the struvite crystals become unstable due to their higher solubility in an acidic environment. They dissolve and undergo a solution-mediated phase transition into newberyite. The process has been described in detail for aqueous solutions[4] but it is also valid for urine. Only the kinetics are different. Finally, struvite crystals exhibit the same habits whether they are grown from pure aqueous solutions, or from urine in vitro, or collected in the urines of stone formers.

In conclusion, it must be emphasized that magnesium ammonium phosphate can also nucleate and grow in acidic sterile urine. This is clearly demonstrated by the experiments carried out in vitro. In these experiments both the initial growth conditions and the final equilibrium conditions are known. On the contrary, it is likely that urine which stays in the bladder and contains struvite crystals does not have the same composition as that in which the crystals nucleated and grew. Certainly, both the initial concentrations and pH are altered as a result of crystallization and dilution. The composition of voided urine corresponds more to a final state than to an initial one. However, for comparison with the in vitro experiments, it is noteworthy that, of the 8 patients who passed struvite crystals, only 2 suffered infection and had a urinary pH in the alkaline range. Te urine of the 6 others were sterile and acidic (7 < pH < 5.63). In view of the pH and of the ionic concentrations it appeared that 4 urines were undersaturated with respect to urine at the moment where they were voided. Only the adsorption of the natural impurities temporarily prevented the crystals from dissolving. Anyhow, the present study show that struvite crystals can form and sometimes survive in acidic sterile urine.

Returning to the crystallization process, it appears that for each pH there is a critical concentration product above which nucleation occurs spontaneously. Magnesium seems to play an essential role especially in the range of low concentration products. This can be partially attributed to the fact that magnesium competes with calcium for the precipitation of phosphates. In the low CP range an increase in magnesium from 2 to 3 mM is more effective for nucleating struvite than an increase in ammonia from 10 to 50 mM.

Finally, from Fig. 1, it is possible to predict the risk of struvite nucleation without making any assumptions, since it is derived from experimental data. It is only necessary to measure the urinary pH and the concentrations of total magnesium, ammonia and phosphate. Obviously the data in Fig. 1 can also help to establish a computed nomogram.

Concerning crystal habit, it is important to bear in mind that crystals are very sensitive to supersaturation. These habits which are skeletal, dendritic, flat rectangular, short prismatic etc. with decreasing supersaturation are therefore good indicators of the initial growth conditions.

REFERENCES

1. D. P. Griffith, Kidney Int. 13:372 (1978).
2. D. P. Griffith, Kidney Int. 21:422 (1982).
3. F. Abbona, H. E. Lundager Madsen, and R. Boistelle, J. Crystal Growth 57:6 (1982).
4. R. Boistelle, F. Abbona, and H. E. Lundager Madsen, Phys. Chem. Minerals 9:216 (1983).

IN VITRO INVESTIGATIONS OF STONE GROWTH INHIBITION AND DISSOLUTION

H. P. Bastian and M. A. H. Gebhardt

St. Josef-Hospital, D-5210 Troisdorf and Mineral-
ogisch-Petrologisches Institut, D-5300 Bonn, F.R.G.

METHODS

Using the stone forming simulator[1], we treated sections of whewellite stones with various urines. It was necessary to prevent bacterial contamination and growth which might otherwise alter the pH of the system. This could be controlled by adding a disinfectant (Betaisodona). Into each 4 filter crucibles two parts of a whewellite stone were suspended. The weight of the stone fragments was measured directly using microscales. Each was bathed with urine of various compositions. During the experiment the weight of the stones and the pH of the bathing solution were measured every 12 h. Since a new 24-h urine was collected daily samples were taken before, at 12 h and at 24 h for the analysis of Na, K, Ca, Mg and Cl. At the end of the experiment the two fragments of the whewellite stone were dried. One was used for scanning electron microscopy (SEM) and energy dispersive element analysis and the other for X-ray diffraction analysis.

RESULTS AND DISCUSSION

The first whewellite stone was treated with urine (2 litres) to which 346 mg of $CaCl_2$ had been added. SEM showed a partly schisted texture, and recent formation of uric acid dihydrate was observed on the stone surface in the form of fine grained, spherical aggregates. X-ray diffraction analysis of the second fragment showed 5% uric acid dihydrate corresponding to 200 mg stone weight. A parallel experiment confirmed the formation of uric acid dihydrate (Fig. 1). The increase in weight in both cases was 10 mg after 4 days.

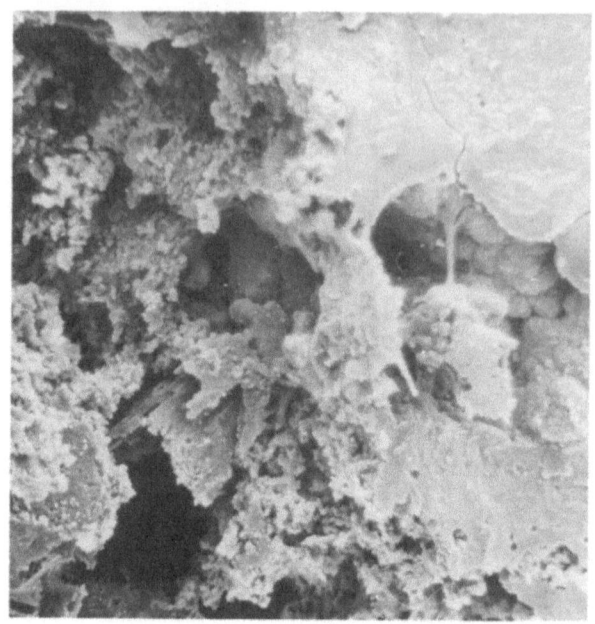

Fig. 1.   Uric acid texture

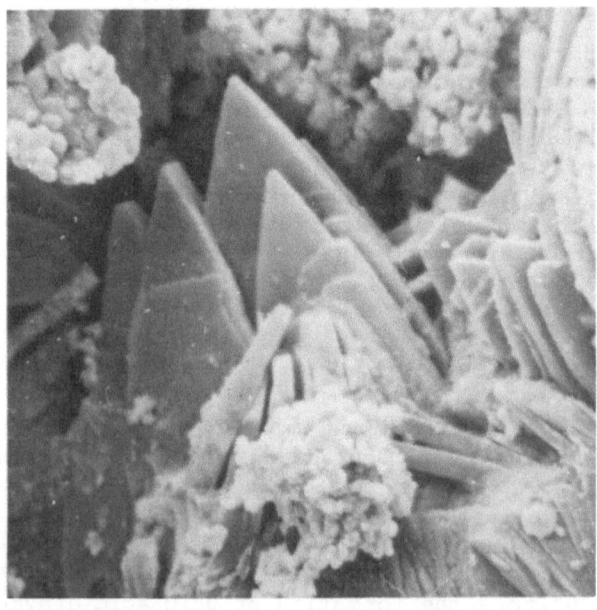

Fig. 2.   Whewellite stone

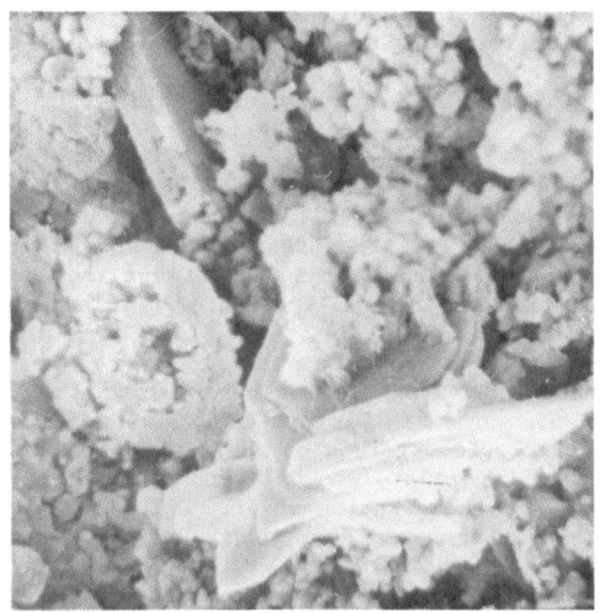

Fig. 3. Whewellite crystals with uric acid.

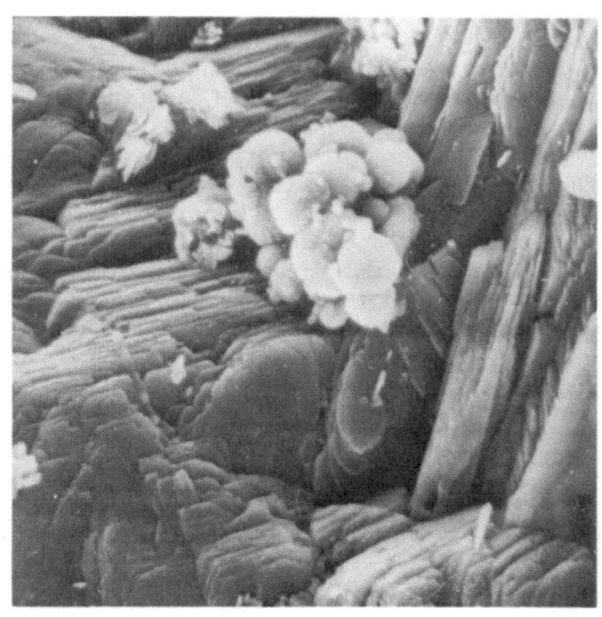

Fig. 4. Newly formed apatite crystals.

It is thought that this new formation is due to the fact that the added calcium has a higher affinity for protein thereby displacing uric acid into the surrounding solution. This increases the supersaturation with respect to uric acid. The pH-value was betwen 5.3 and 5.7 in these experiments.

The second experimental series was made by adding 250 mg uric acid to 2 litres of urine. The whewellite stones were rinsed again for 4 days (Fig. 2). The SEM investigation showed uric acid dihydrate deposition. During this experiment the equilibrium between dissolution and crystallization of uric acid and Ca oxalate was reached after one day.

In further experiments 22.2 mg pyrophosphate were added to 1000 ml urine (Fig. 3). The SEM picture showed whewellite crystals with newly formed uric acid crystals on their surfaces. No increase in the solubility of Ca oxalate was detected by addition of pyrophosphate. Crystallization of uric acid took place as a result of the acidifying effect of the pyrophosphate.

In further experiments 37.76 mg Ca oxalate was added to 2 litres of urine. The SEM-pictures showed a heteroblastic texture of scaly whewellite crystals with distinct indications of dissolution. In the space between the whewellite crystals, fine-grained spherical apatite aggregates were observed. In other parts of the stone a second generation of whewellite crystals was found. No change in weight could be measured. The analysis of the electrolytes showed in a decrease of the Ca concentration with time.

In the next experiment 125 mg of citric acid monohydrate was added to 2 litres of urine. The whewellite crystals were scaly with a parallel texture and distinct indications of dissolution. Through a larger fissure the fine grained texture of whewellite crystals could be observed. Only sporadically micro-grained newly formed newberyite crystallites were found. In the cavities of the dissolving whewellite crystals needle-like newberyite crystals were seen. The flaky, fine whewellite texture showed rounded edges caused by dissolution. In the spaces between the whewellite crystals grape-like aggregations of small apatite crystals were found (Fig. 4). The weight decreased by 10 mg and the pH of 5.1 was lower than that in the original urine. Dissolution was confirmed by the increase in the Ca concentration in the bathing urine.

REFERENCE

1. H. P. Bastian and M. A. H. Gebhardt, Akt. Urol. 7:275 (1976).

INHIBITORS AND PROMOTERS

INHIBITORS OF THE PRECIPITATION OF STONE-FORMING URINARY
CONSTITUENTS: ARE THE ESTABLISHED INHIBITORS EFFECTIVE IN
PREVENTING STONE FORMATION AND GROWTH OR IS A MOSS-COVERED
STONE INEVITABLE?

J. D. Sallis

Dept. of Biochemistry, University of Tasmania
Hobart, Tasmania 7001, Australia

There is no concensus on the controversy concerning the nature,
function or effectiveness of either natural or synthetic inhibitors
in relation to urinary stone formation. Since the pioneering work
of the Fleisch group in recognizing the inhibitory potential of the
urinary constituent, pyrophosphate[1], the search has been escalated
to find a constituent which might effectively control the
development of a stone. Today, a number of natural compounds have
been presented as possible candidates. Simultaneously, knowledge is
advancing on inhibitor mechanisms prompting the development of
synthetic compounds as hopeful therapeutic agents.

Both small molecules and ions (Mg^{2+}, citrate, pyrophosphate,
aminoacids, nucleotides etc) and macromolecules (acidic peptides,
glycoproteins, glycosaminoglycans, RNA etc) are considered to have
inhibitory effects on the crystallization of calcium phosphate
and/or calcium oxalate. The true extent of their contribution,
however, is difficult to determine as there are many weaknesses in
the gathering and interpretation of the data. This becomes evident
when we ask the questions: Was inhibitory potential measured in a
purely physiochemical system or were the compounds assessed in the
presence of fresh urine? Was the urine undiluted and were the
constituents known and quantitatively assessed? Has the possible
synergism of inhibitors been reconciled or has the inhibitory power
been weakened by an anti-inhibitor substance? The list of
questions grows and the uncertainties magnify. What progress has
been made then to elucidate the importance of these inhibitors?

Pyrophosphate, the first identified urinary inhibitor, has to
some extent fallen from favour because of estimated variable
concentrations in urine and the likely effect of pyrophosphatases.

Nevertheless, it could still contribute up to 10% of the urine's inhibitory activity[2]. Its action appears to be directed more against apatite formation than against calcium oxalate crystallization. As an overall controller of biological calcification processes, of course, it should be noted that there are many reactions which generate pyrophosphate in tissues which could well temporarily increase the concentration of the compound at important selected sites. It is possible to raise the pyrophosphate concentration in urine by oral orthophosphate supplements[3], or by thiazides[4]. An added advantage of this type of treatment is a reduction of urinary calcium, but not all investigators agree as to the overall success of such treatment for idiopathic calcium stone disease.

Other small ions such as Mg^{2+} and citrate must have an important influence. In the case of Mg^{2+}, although its actual inhibitory potential may be less than some urinary constituents, there does appear to be an important inverse relationship between Mg^{2+} concentration and calcium oxalate crystal formation[5]. Clearly, the Mg^{2+}/Ca^{2+} ratio is important as Mg^{2+} can compete with the calcium ion to form the more soluble magnesium oxalate. As an inhibitor, Mg^{2+} may act through stabilization of the dihydrate phase of calcium oxalate formation[6]. While there seems to be strong evidence that a Mg^{2+} deficiency will accelerate deposition of calcium oxalate crystals in the kidney[7], data on the efficacy of magnesium salts given to stone patients suggests that as a controlling agent, magnesium may be rather poor[8].

The role of the citrate ion is also very much disputed. Levels of urinary citrate can fluctuate quite widely under varying conditions. It has been suggested that the apparently low observed excretion and concentration of citrate in stone forming patients may well be responsible for a lowered urinary inhibitor potential[10]. Citrate in its own right is a powerful chelator substance but as an inhibitor of in vitro crystallization, it is weak compared with many others. In vivo, however, as much as 50% of urinary inhibitor activity could derive from citrate[2]. In order to improve the usefulness of citrate as a biological inhibitor, Meyer and Thomas[11] have been investigating trace metal-citrate complexes. Of interest in this regard is the apparent selectivity of an iron-citrate complex in inhibiting calcium phosphate crystallization rather than calcium oxalate crystallization. Although the data have been gathered from in vitro studies, the possibility exists that under suitable urinary conditions of citrate and trace metal concentrations, such complexes might function as effective inhibitors of urolithiasis.

Turning to recent information available on macromolecular inhibitors, urinary glycopeptides, glycosaminoglycans (GAGs), and RNA have all been implicated. The most powerful seem to be the GAGs class. It should be emphasised however, that an analysis of their involvement needs to be carefully delineated. Today, more attention is being paid to the phase of crystal formation in which an inhibitor might be involved and whether it affects only calcium phosphate, calcium oxalate or both. In the case of the GAGs, their effect is on crystal aggregation rather than nucleation and growth[12,13].

Whilst the early studies of Robertson et al [14] demonstrated the ability of commercially available GAGs to be effective inhibitors in vitro, doubt has been expressed that the major natural urinary GAGs, in particular, chondroitin sulphate is all that effective. Some years ago, we attempted to isolate natural GAG compounds from human urine and assess the contribution of inhibitory power from each type of GAG isolated[15]. Using a glass fibre nucleating calcium oxalate growth test system, we concluded that the major urinary GAGs were not as inhibitory as one might have anticipated from the in vitro studies with the commercial preparations. The test system of course did not differentiate the various phases of calcium oxalate crystallization. Nevertheless, the data obtained did raise a query as to whether the recognised GAGs did have the ability to regulate strongly calcium oxalate crystal growth. The investigations also suggested that there was an unidentified compound more powerful than any of the other GAG compounds.

These interesting leads were not pursued further at the time but other investigators have now reported the presence of urinary constituents with carbohydrate components which do display strong inhibitory power. Coe, for example, has isolated acidic glycopeptides with interesting properties [16] and Pak has also reported on the isolation and characterization of some glycoproteins in urine [17]. The findings of these latter researchers suggest that low molecular weight glycoproteins are potent inhibitors and that they appear to be in lesser amounts in the urine of stone formers. Uromucoids which are present in much larger amounts than glycoproteins do not appear to be inhibitory. In fact, the contrary action has been assigned to them, namely as promoters of crystal growth[18].

Another interesting aspect which needs consideration relates to the degree of sulfation of the GAGs and the effect that this might have on inhibition[19,20]. A recent suggestion concerning the possibility that urinary GAGs have their origin in the endothelium of the bladder rather than the kidneys is also interesting and needs further clarification[21]. Evaluating the true contribution from GAGs is another problem due to an association from urate. Sodium urate is an important factor in the control of calcium oxalate nucleation and aggregation. Not only can sodium urate directly promote calcium oxalate crystallisation by inducing heterogenous nucleation but it seems that sodium urate can bind organic macromolecules thus

reducing the inhibition of aggregation that might take place[22].
From this brief survey, it is clear that much more extensive
investigations are required to ascertain the true potential of the
various carbohydrate compounds.

While research continues to try and unravel the complexities
surrounding the control of crystal formation and growth in the
natural environment, renewed efforts have been made to develop
synthetic compounds with two objectives in mind: (a) as useful
therapeutic agents and (b) to accrue information regarding the
structureactivity relationship which might hopefully lead to the
development of better drugs.

The background of the diphosphonates does not need an
introduction as it is well documented[23]. These enzyme-resistant
analogues of pyrophosphate are recognized as powerful inhibitors of
calcification and their only restriction for widespread use against
many calcium disorders is their known undesirable secondary side-
effects. Ethane-1-hydroxy-1,1-diphosphonate (EHDP) given orally is
not well absorbed[24] and in the large dosages required to be
effective, EHDP does have adverse effects on bone turnover and
mineralization[25]. Not all of the diphosphonates, of course, have
identical properties. In an attempt to produce a more ideal
diphosphonate, Shinoda et al[26] have investigated the structure-
activity relationship of a wide range of substituted diphosphonates.
Some correlation was found to exist between in vitro inhibition of
calcium phosphate precipitation and in vivo mineralization, but no
correlation could be found in relation to parameters connected with
bone resorption. Nevertheless, the studies did indicate that the
aliphatic side-chain should be at least 5 carbons in length to
improve its intestinal absorption and its ability to inhibit bone
resorption. The overall picture, however, is confused regarding the
most useful diphosphonate for general therapeutic purposes but the
investigations do highlight significant progress and the need for
further research along these lines.

In our own studies, we have continued to explore the tremendous
potential of a natural, anticalcifying compound, namely
phosphocitrate[27-29]. Although not yet assessed clinically in
comparison with the diphosphonates, from in vitro studies, we know
that phosphocitrate is more powerful than EHDP in preventing the
transformation of amorphous calcium phosphate to hydroxyapatite[30,31]. With respect to preventing calcium oxalate
crystallization, phosphocitrate is again inhibitory but less so than
other recognised inhibitors[29]. If phosphocitrate is a more
specific inhibitor of hydroxyapatite than of calcium oxalate
crystallization this could be a useful attribute.

The recognition of phosphocitrate as an anticalcifying agent
led us to reappraise the structure-activity relationship for

806

inhibitors of hydroxyapatite formation. The most desirous of structural requirements appears to be a phosphate group at one site and another phosphate, or more preferably a carboxylic acid moiety, at a second position. However, a close examination of the potential arising from altered structures suggests that any overall theoretical evaluation of a compound's potential must take into account numerous secondary factors such as the number and proximity of active groups, their stereochemistry, steric factors and lipophilic nature[31]. With this knowledge, it should be possible to synthesize even more potent anticalcifying compounds. Although we now have evidence that phosphocitrate can prevent ectopic calcification in such tissues as kidneys[32] and arteries[33], we are not yet convinced that the compound is stable enough for therapeutic purposes. Studies in vitro demonstrate that phosphocitrate can be inactivated through phosphohydrolase activity (albeit slowly and with a large excess of enzyme). Furthermore, radiolabelled phosphocitrate studies in vivo suggest that at least in the kidney, phosphocitrate is rapidly destroyed[29].

With these data in mind, our recent studies have been directed toward producing analogues of phosphocitrate. Initially we sought to prepare a PNC compound but technical difficulties, which have only now been overcome, have not yet enabled us to characterize fully this analogue. Instead, we prepared a sulfamate analogue (an SNC compound) recognising the resilience of the sulfamate bond to enzyme attack[34]. Neither sulfatases nor sulfaminidases hydrolyse the analogue sulfoaminotricarballylate, either in vivo or in vitro.

As for its inhibitory action, the compound can prevent hydroxyapatite or calcium oxalate crystallization but it does not appear to be as powerful as phosphocitrate or EHDP. Sulfoaminotricarballylate can inhibit in vivo calcification of aortic segments[33] and can also reduce the formation of calcium oxalate crystals in the kidneys of rats given a sodium oxalate challenge. Whilst we would have hoped for, but not necessarily predicted, a more powerful inhibitory response, a pleasing feature is the excellent absorptive properties of the compound and the apparent better performance against calcium oxalate crystallization. If, as we suspect, there is a rapid clearance and prolonged residence time in urine, then the disadvantage of a reduced potency may be more than made up for by the specificity and other characteristics of the molecule. Of course, more extensive studies are still required to evaluate any possible longterm toxic effects on cells and tissues. Irrespective of the final outcome, valuable information regarding structure-activity relationships of such analogues should be derived from future studies.

If suitable agents cannot be developed which will safely and selectively control calcium deposition and crystal formation and growth, what alternatives may be envisaged in the future? Perhaps folklore medicine may provide some insights. In a Mediterranean region, it is well known among the inhabitants that, at the first sign of renal colic, the treatment is to prepare a root extract from a local species of lichen, referred to as "the stonesplitter". The infusion, which is taken at night, relieves the renal colic and the next morning many stone fragments appear in the urine.

Whilst evidence relating to this phenomenon is difficult to obtain to satisfy scientific scrutiny, experiments relating to plant extracts have been described[35,36]. Such extracts can apparently prevent urinary calculi recurrence in experimental animals. There is a suggestion that the active principle might be related to anthraquinones. The reference in the title of this paper then to a "moss-covered stone" takes on an added meaning. It is said that "a rolling stone gathers no moss" and obviously if a stone is small enough, it can be passed and would not need splitting. However, a stone lodged and growing in a sequence of events that cannot be controlled by natural or synthetic inhibitors may need to be covered by a moss extract to break it to a size small enough to be passed. Is this a possible future aspect for urolithiasis research?

REFERENCES

1. H. Fleisch and S. Bisaz, Am. J. Physiol. 203:671 (1962)
2. S. Bisaz, R, Felix, W. F. Neuman, and H. Fleisch, Min. Electr. Metab. 1:74 (1978).
3. H. Fleisch, S. Bisaz, and A. D. Care, Lancet 1:1065 (1964).
4. A. Woefel, R. A. Kaplan, and C. Y. C. Pak, Metabolism 26:201 (1977).
5. P. C. Hallson, G. A. Rose, and S. Sulaiman, Clin. Sci. 62:17 (1982).
6. B. B. Tomazic and G. H. Nancollas, J. Urol. 128:205 (1982).
7. H. G. Rushton, M. Spector, A. L. Rodgers, M. Hughson, and C. E. Magura, Invest. Urol. 19:52 (1981).
8. C. D. Fetner, D. E. Barilla, J. Townsend, and C. Y. C. Pak, J. Urol. 120:399 (1978).
9. H. G. Tiselius, C. Ahlstrand, and L. Larsson, Urol. Res. 8:197 (1980).
10. P. O. Schwille, D. Scholz, M. Paulus, W. Engelhardt, and Sigel, Invest. Urol. 16:457 (1979).
11. J. L. Meyer and W. C. Thomas, J. Urol 128:1376 (1982).
12. H. Fleisch, Scand J. Urol. Nephrol. (Suppl) 53:53 (1980).
13. R. L. Ryall, R. M. Harnett, and V. R. Marshall, Clin Chim Acta, 112:349 (1981).
14. W. G. Robertson, M. Peacock, and B. E. C. Nordin, Clin Chim. Acta 43:31 (1973).
15. J. D. Sallis and M. F. Lumley, Invest. Urol. 16:296 (1979).
16. Y. Nakagawa, H. C. Margolis, S. Yokoyama, F. J. Kezdy, E. T. Kaiser, and F. L. Coe, J. Biol. Chem 256:3936 (1981).

17. T. Kitamura, J. E. Zerwekh, and C. Y. C. Pak, Kidney Int. 21:379 (1982).
18. P. C. Hallson and G. A. Rose, Lancet i:1000 (1979).
19. W. O. Foye, H. S. Hong, C. M. Kim, and E. L. Prien, Invest. Urol. 14:33 (1976).
20. H.Itatani, H. Itoh, T. Yoshioka, M. Namiki, T. Koide, A. Okuyama, and T. Sonoda, Invest. Urol. 19:119 (1981).
21. K. A. Edyvane, R. L. Ryall, and V. R. Marshall, in"Urinary Stone", R. Ryall, J. G. Brockis, V. Marshall, and B. Finlayson, eds., Churchill Livingstone, Melbourne (1984).
22. J. E. Zerwekh, K. Holt, and C. Y. C. Pak, Kidney Int. 23:838 (1983).
23. H. Fleisch, Met. Bone Dis. Rel. Res. 4&5:279 (1981).
24. R. R. Recker and P. D. Saville, Tox. Appl. Pharm. 24:580 (1973).
25. H. G. Bone, J. E. Werwekh, F. Britton, and C. Y. C. Pak, J. Urol. 121:568 (1979).
26. H. Shimoda, G. Adamek, R. Felix, H. Fleisch, R. Schenk, and P. Hagan, Calc. Tiss. Int. 35:87 (1983).
27. G. Williams and J. D. Sallis, Anal. Biochem. 102:365 (1980).
28. W. P. Tew, C. Mahle, and A. L. Lehninger, Biochemistry 19:1983 (1980).
29. G. Williams and J. D. Sallis, in"Urolithiasis, Clinical and Basic Research, L. H. Smith, W. G. Robertson, and B. Finlayson, eds., Plenum, New York (1981).
30. G. Williams and J. D. Sallis, Biochem. J. 184:181 (1979).
31. G. Williams and J. D. Sallis, Calc. Tiss. Int. 34:169 (1983).
32. M. R. Brown and J. D. Sallis, in:"Urolithiasis and Related Clinical Research", P. O. Schwille, W. G. Robertson, L. H. Smith, W. Vahlensieck, eds., Plenum, London (1985).
33. R. Shankar, S. Crowden, and J. D. Sallis, Atherosclerosis (1984) (in press).
34. M. R. Brown and J. D. Sallis, Anal. Biochem. 132:115 (1983).
35. W. Berg, A. Hesse, K Hensel, G. Unger, U. Hartmann, and H. J. Schneider, Urologie, 15:188 (1976).
36. H. J. Schneider, G. Unger, D. Rossle, C. Bothor, W. Berg, and G. Ernst, Z. Urol. Nephrol.72:237 (1979).

THE RELATIVE IMPORTANCE OF CALCIUM PHOSPHATE URINARY INHIBITORS

J. L. Meyer

Mineralized Tissue Research Branch, N.I.D.R.
National Institutes of Health, Bethesda
Maryland 20205, U.S.A.

INTRODUCTION

Crystal growth inhibitors may play an important role in the regulation of urinary stone formation. The major inhibitors of calcium phosphate precipitation in urine have been shown to consist of Mg, citrate and pyrophosphate (PP_i) ions as well as at least one unknown low molecular weight component. Studies using diluted urines have suggested that PP_i and the unknown component are the most important calcium phosphate inhibitors[1] whereas an investigation of inhibitory activity at physiological concentrations have shown that citrate and Mg are most important[2]. Each of these investigations, however, used an initial single addition of inhibitor and no attempt was made to maintain the fixed, steady-state concentrations of inhibiting species which are expected to exist in a system under biological control. In this study, the inhibition of calcium phosphate crystal growth is investigated at constant inhibitor concentrations so that a more realistic assessment of the relative importance of the three known calcium phosphate urinary inhibitors, Mg, citrate, and PP_i can be made.

METHODS

Stable supersaturated solutions were prepared by carefully increasing the pH of solutions containing 1.5 mM Ca and 1.0 mM phosphate from 5.0 to 7.4 with 0.1 N KOH at 37°C and an ionic strength of 0.15 (NaCl). Crystal growth was initiated by the addition of an aliquot of hydroxyapatite (HAP) seed slurry to the metastable solution. The rate of crystal growth was monitored by withdrawing aliquots at various time intervals, filtering off the

811

crystalline phase with a 0.22 μm membrane and analyzing the filtrate for Ca (Perkin-Elmer Model 603 atomic absorption spectrometer) and phosphate[3]. Crystal growth inhibitors were added to the super-saturated solution before the seed crystals were introduced.

The concentrations of PP_i and citrate in the solution phase were estimated by the amount of ^{32}P and ^{14}C radioactivity, respectively, which remained in solution after the addition of known amounts of labeled compounds. The concentration of Mg remaining in solution was determined by atomic absorption. Relatively constant concentrations of PP_i, citrate, and Mg were maintained in certain experiments by determining their concentrations in the solution phase, as described above, and adding sufficient additional inhibitor ion, when necessary, to increase the solution concentration to that present initially in solution.

RESULTS

The effect of an initial concentration of 2 μM PP_i on the rate of calcium phosphate crystal growth is shown in Fig. 1. Also shown is the actual PP_i concentration remaining in solution at various stages of the experiment. It is clear that HAP crystals rapidly adsorb PP_i from solution and that this adsorption of inhibitor ion results in the complete inhibition of crystal growth. Only when

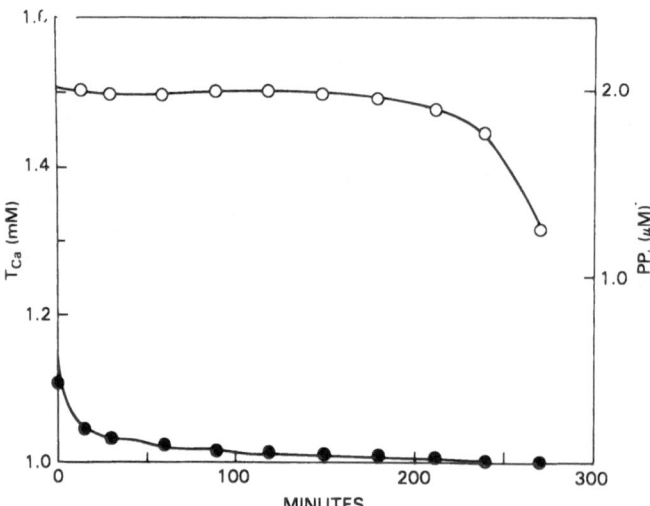

Fig. 1. The effect of 2 μM initial addition of PP_i on the rate of crystal growth of calcium phosphate as shown by the decrease in total Ca concentration, T_{Ca}, (O) and PP_i concentration (●) with time of reaction. Seed crystals of HAP are added at time zero.

PP$_i$ has been completely removed from solution does crystal growth begin to occur. Experiments in which the PP$_i$ concentration was maintained at approximately constant levels were performed and representative results are shown in Fig. 2 for 1 μM PP$_i$. Also given for comparison are the results of experiments involving approximately constant compositions of citrate (0.5 mM) and magnesium (0.8 mM).

The results indicate that, although citrate and Mg ions slow the rate of calcium phosphate crystal growth, they do not completely inhibit the growth process. In contrast a constant concentration of 1 μM PP$_i$ completely prevents crystal growth for an apparently indefinite period of time. The apparent increase in calcium concentration after 48 h results from the slight evaporation of the reaction solution. An initial addition of 1 μM PP$_i$, however, resulted in an inhibition of only 1 h duration followed by a rate of calcium phosphate crystal growth comparable to that of a control experiment.

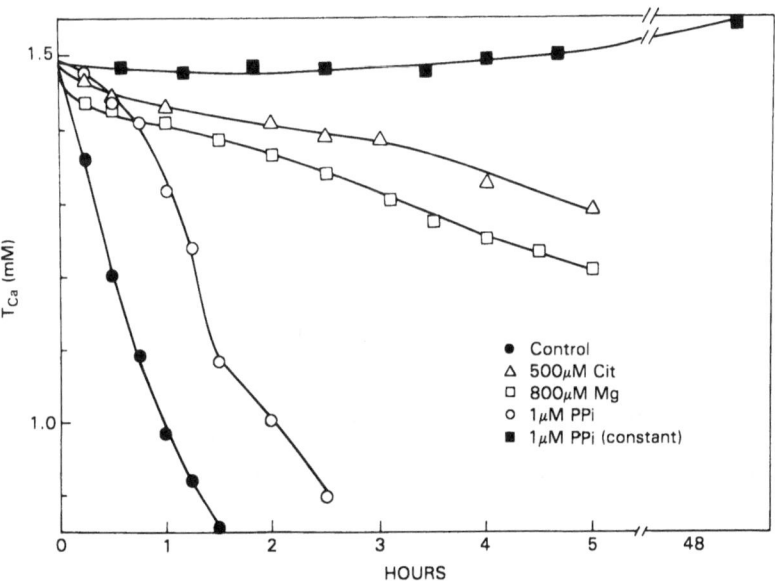

Fig. 2. The effect of constant, physiological concentrations of the inhibitors PP$_i$, magnesium (Mg), and citrate (Cit) on the rate of crystal growth of calcium phosphate. Shown for comparison are a control experiment in which no inhibitors have been added and an experiment in which only an initial 1 μM PP$_i$ was present in solution. Seed crystals of HAP were added at time zero.

DISCUSSION

The inhibition of calcium phosphate crystal growth by an initial, physiological concentration of PP_i was characterized by an induction period in which no crystallization occurred followed by crystal growth which occurred at a rate comparable to that of control experiments. Analysis of the solution phase showed that the crystal growth process occurred only after PP_i was depleted from solution. Biological systems tend to maintain homeostasis, however, and similar experiments were performed to assess the ability of constant concentrations of PP_i to inhibit crystal growth. A constant 1 μM PP_i concentration, which is approximately 1/10 that reported in human urine[4], was shown to inhibit crystal growth completely for an extended period of time. Constant, physiological concentrations of Mg and citrate ions, however, merely slowed down the crystal growth of calcium phosphate. Previous studies involving only initial concentrations of inhibitors have indicated that citrate and Mg are more important than PP_i in physiological solutions[2,5]. It is clear, however, that if these inhibitors were compared at fixed equilibrium concentrations, PP_i would be the most important. This study suggest, therefore, that the means of assessing the relative importance of urinary calcification inhibitors should be reviewed. If homeostasis of the various crystallization inhibitors is assumed to occur in the urinary system, then it would appear that the strongly adsorbed, highly specific inhibitors, such as PP_i, would be most important in controlling urolithiasis.

REFERENCES

1. L. H. Smith and J. L. Meyer, in:"Colloquium on Renal Lithiasis", B. Finlayson and W. C. Thomas, eds., Gainesville University Presses, Florida (1976).
2. S. Bisaz, R. Felix, W. F. Neuman, and H. Fleisch, Min. Electr. Metab. 1:74 (1978).
3. J. Murphy and J. P. Riley, Anal. Chim. Acta 27:31 (1962).
4. H. Fleisch and S. Bisaz, Am. J. Physiol. 203:671 (1962).
5. J. L. Meyer and H. Fleisch, Min. Electr. Metab. (in press).

NATURAL INHIBITORS OF FORMATION AND DISSOLUTION OF STONE MINERALS

A. Lanzalaco, M. Coyle, S. Gaur, T. P. Binette,
T. S. Herman, G. Sufrin, and G. H. Nancollas

Depts. of Chemistry and Urology, State University of
New York at Buffalo, and Veterans Administration Medical
Center, Buffalo, New York 14214, U.S.A.

INTRODUCTION

In assessing the inhibitory activity of urine, seeded COM mineralization experiments are usually made in the presence of high urine dilutions (typically 100-fold) but there is some question as to whether these results can be extrapolated to in vivo conditions[1,2]. In our laboratory, by using a calcium-specific ion electrode protected from the poisoning effects of urinary macromolecules by means of a dialysis membrane, it is now possible to measure rates of mineralization and demineralization of stone components in whole urines with a precision hitherto unattainable.

MATERIALS AND METHODS

Crystallization experiments were made as described previously[3]. In the urine experiments the protected calcium electrode was used to adjust the free calcium ion activity to the value required for a particular supersaturation. Separations of macromolecular components were made on Biogel columns and these samples were added to the supersaturated solutions prior to inoculation with seed substrates.

RESULTS AND DISCUSSION

A typical crystallization experiment is shown in Fig. 1 in which the moles of calcium oxalate grown on COM seed crystals is plotted as a function of time. It can be seen that the rates, corrected for the increase in surface area, assuming the seeds to be

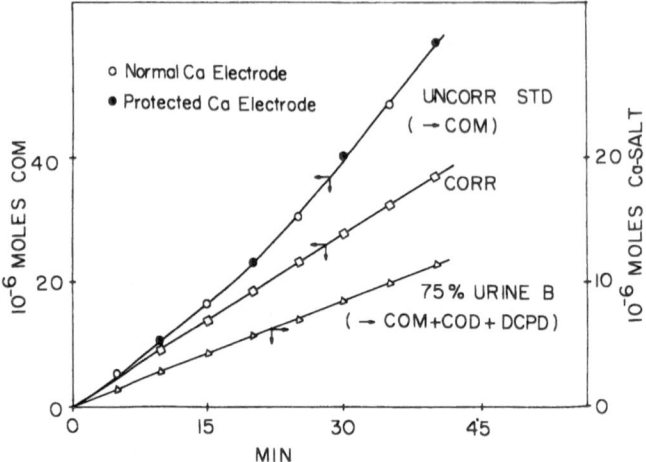

Fig. 1. Calcium oxalate seeded growth. Influence of urine.

perfect spheres or cubes, are strikingly linear. Moreoever, it can
be seen in Fig. 1 that the protected calcium specific ion electrode
yields the same rate of mineralization as that of the unprotected
electrode. Experiments in the presence of high concentrations of
urine (Fig. 1) indicate that marked changes in solid phase
composition may accompany the mineralization reactions. Thus,
seeding urine B with COM seed crystals produced COM, COD, together
with the acidic calcium phosphate phase, DCPD, even though the pH of
the urine was 6.9. It is interesting to note that the
concentration of free calcium ions in most urine samples was about
50% of the total calcium concentration as measured by atomic
absorption spectrophotometry, a value close to that predicted by
speciation programs. For another urine containing molar calcium
and phosphate concentrations of 7.8 x 10^{-3} and 3.8 x 10^{-2} mol/l
respectively, only about 40% of the calcium ion was free at pH =
5.0. Subsequent seeding of this urine with COM showed no
precipitation. Clearly, the free ionic concentration of calcium is
an important parameter for deciding whether a urine will
spontaneously form stone minerals or whether it will remain stable.

The results of experiments designed to test the inhibiting
effects of molecular weight fractions of urines, separated on Bio-
Gel chromatographic columns are summarized in Table 1. Molecular
weight fractions >50,000 at a dilution of only 1.2% by volume,
provided little mineralization retardation (Experiment 79a). In
contrast, however, (Experiment 90a) molecular weights above 10,000
showed strong (76.4%) inhibition with an appreciable retardation
also seen below 10,000 (Experiment 94a). The results indicate an
important urine inhibitor molecular weight fraction lying between
about 5,000 and 50,000 daltons. Experiments with serum (Table 1)
are especially interesting since marked inhibition is observed with

Table 1. Inhibition of Calcium Oxalate Crystal Growth.

Sample	Fraction	Rate (µmol/min)	Inhibition (%)	Dilution (%)
Urine	MW >50,000	1.60	3.0	2.0
	MW >10,000	0.39	76.4	1.96
	MW <10,000	0.69	58.2	1.98
Serum	whole	0.67	59.4	0.010
	whole	0.84	49.1	0.005
	dialyzed	0.86	47.8	0.010
	MW >10,000	1.20	30.3	0.005
Urine	pre-bladder	0.63	62.1	1.20
	pre-bladder	0.86	47.9	1.10

dilutions as high as 1:1,000 (Experiment 81a). Dialysis of the
serum prior to inhibition testing reduced the inhibition (Experiments 97a,96a) by only 12 to 19%. One source of macromolecular
inhibitors in urine could be from the glomerular filtrate as opposed
to epithelial secretion. Serum components filtered at the glomeru-
las may be responsible for an important part of the mineralization
in vivo. For pre-bladder urines (Experiment 73a,86a), it can be
seen (Table 1) that before passage through the bladder, the urine
has an appreciable inhibiting capacity for COM mineralization.

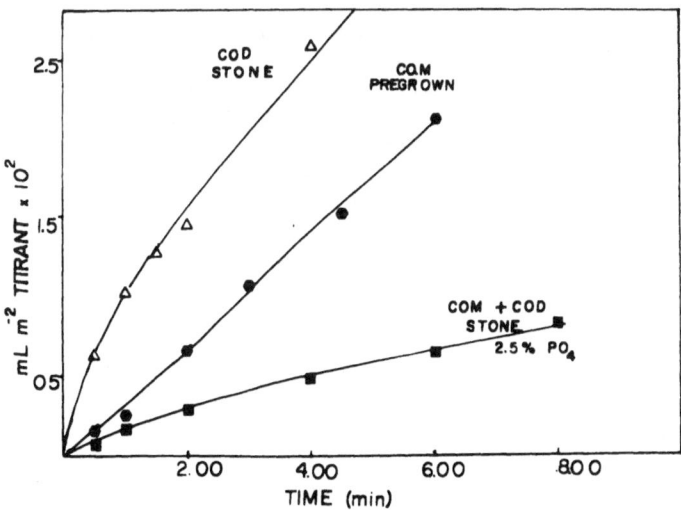

Fig. 2. Dissolution of calcium oxalate stones. Kinetic plots.

In the CC demineralization experiments, the titrant solution consisted of background electrolyte (0.15 mol/l sodium chloride) with the titrant addition controlled potentiostatically using a calcium-specific ion electrode. The influence of released organic matrix upon the specific ion electrode could be avoided by using the protected probe. For COM/COD mixed stones, the rates of dissolution increase with the amount of COD in the stones. Moreover, kidney stones consisting of calcium oxalate phases may dissolve more than ten times faster than similar stone materials containing orthophosphate (Fig. 2). Not only are the rates of stone dissolution lower than synthetic samples, but in contrast to the diffusion-controlled dissolution of pure synthetic phases, it appears that kidney stones dissolve predominantly by a surface-controlled process[4]. Low molecular weight urine components may also have a significant effect on the rates of dissolution. Thus a complexing anion such as citrate specifically inhibits dissolution at low levels while at high concentrations, complexing with calcium increases the rate of reaction. The results of these studies demonstrate the importance of understanding the mechanism of mineralization and demineralization of stones and stone-forming salts.

ACKNOWLEDGMENTS

We thank the National Institute of ARthritis, Diabetes, Digestive and Kidney Diseases for a grant (#AM 19948) in support of this work.

REFERENCES

1. M. B. Rose, Invest. Urol. 12:428 (1975).
2. B. Finlayson, in:"Calcium Metabolism in Renal Failure and Nephrolithiasis", D. S. David, ed., Wiley, New York (1977).
3. D. J. White, J. Christoffersen, T. S. Herman, A. C. Lanzalaco, and G. H. Nancollas, J. Urol. 129:175 (1983).
4. B. B. Tomazic and G. H. Nancollas, J. Urol. 128:205 (1982).

URINARY INHIBITORS OF HYDROXYAPATITE CRYSTAL GROWTH:

A CONSTANT COMPOSITION APPROACH

J. W. L. Wilson, P. G. Werness, and L. H. Smith

Nephrology Research Unit, Mayo Clinic and Foundation
Rochester, MN 55905, USA, and Dept. of Urology, Queen's
University, Kingston, Ontario, Canada K7L 2V7

INTRODUCTION

Howard and Thomas first proposed the existence of inhibitors of crystallization in urine and postulated that patients with urolithiasis had a deficiency of these inhibitors[1,2]. This was based on the observation that urine from patients with renal calculi tended to calcify rachitic rat cartilage (so called "evil urine"), whereas urine from normal subjects did not ("good urine"). Since then, considerable effort has been expended on the isolation and characterization of these inhibitors.

It is known that there is a pH-dependence of the inhibitors of calcium oxalate crystal growth. Pyrophosphate increases inhibitor activity 100-fold, from pH 5 to pH 7, in the seeded crystal growth system[3]. Similarly, there is also an increase in the inhibitory activity of urine on calcium oxalate crystal growth[4] from pH 5.5 to pH 7.

For hydroxyapatite crystal growth, known inhibitors include pyrophosphate, citrate and magnesium[5]. Attempts to determine the pH-dependence of hydroxyapatite crystal growth inhibitors in the solution depletion seeded crystal growth system, are complicated by the induction of other calcium phosphate phases. As the reaction proceeds, and calcium and phosphate are incorporated into the growing crystal, the specific ion activities of calcium and phosphate phases decrease, thereby decreasing the supersaturation. Thus, as the reaction proceeds, the solution may be metastable to more than one calcium phosphate phase and complex formation and dissolution characteristics may preclude data analysis.

METHODS

We used the constant composition technique[6,7] to overcome this problem. For hydroxyapatite, calcium and phosphate are added in stoichiometrically equivalent amounts with the pH-regulated addition of base, allowing for growth at constant supersaturation. Standard rates were determined and with the addition of varying amounts of inhibitor these rates could be compared with Langmuir adsorption isotherm was used to analyze rates. The amount of material required to produce a 50% reduction in crystal growth rate was defined as one inhibitor unit.

The computer program EQUIL[8] was used to model test solutions to maintain the same supersaturation of hydroxyapatite at different inhibitor concentrations to take into account complexation, ion-pairing and pH.

RESULTS AND DISCUSSION

The results showed that pyrophosphate increased inhibitor activity slightly with a pH change from 7.40 to 5.80. The change, a factor of 2, compares to the situation in the calcium oxalate system where there was a 100-fold decrease in inhibitor activity over the pH range from pH 7.00 to 5.00. Similarly citrate increased inhibitor activity with a decrease in pH, whereas magnesium decreased inhibitor activity over this pH range.

We examined three separate pooled urine collections, and observed that inhibitor activity decreased with decreasing pH, from a range of 143 to 169 inhibitor units per litre at pH 7.40 to 55 to 69 inhibitor units per litre at pH 5.80.

We conclude that pyrophosphate is the most significant inhibitor of hydroxyapatite crystal growth at present in urine. The pH-dependence of pyrophosphate inhibition is much less than that seen in the calcium oxalate system. Citrate and magnesium are also active inhibitors of hydroxyapatite crystal growth present in urine in significant concentrations and the pH dependence of these inhibitors is relatively small. Undetermined promoters or inhibitors of hydroxyapatite crystal growth are active in urine over this pH range.

REFERENCES

1. J. E. Howard, and W. C. Thomas, Trans. Am. Clin. Chem. Assoc. 70:99 (1958).
2. W. C. Thomas and J. E. Howard, Trans. Assoc. Am. Physcns. 72:181 (1959).

820

3. L. H. Smith, in:"Urolithiasis Research", H. Fleisch,
   W. G. Robertson, L. H. Smith, and W. Vahlensieck, eds.,
   Plenum, New York (1976).

4. H. G. Tiselius, Br. J. Urol. 53:470 (1981).

5. L. H. Smith, J. L. Meyer, and J. T. McCall, in:"Urinary
   Calculi", L. Cifuentes-Delatte, A. Rapado, and A. Hodgkinson,
   eds., Karger, Basel (1973).

6. M. B. Tomson and G. H. Nancollas, Science 200:1059 (1978).

7. P. Koutsoukos, Z. Amjad, M. B. Tomson, and G. H. Nancollas,
   J. Am. Chem. Soc. 102:1553 (1980).

8. B. Finlayson, in:Calcium Metabolism in Renal Failure and
   Nephrolithiasis", D. S. David, ed., J. Wiley, New York
   (1976).

GEL FILTRATION OF CONCENTRATED URINE: THE RELATION BETWEEN
CALCIUM OXALATE CRYSTAL GROWTH INHIBITION AND GLYCOSAMINOGLYCAN
CHROMATOGRAMS

B. Fellström, B. G. Danielson, S. Ljunghall, and
B. Wikström

Dept. of Internal Medicine, University Hospital
751 85 Uppsala, Sweden

INTRODUCTION

Macromolecular urinary constituents have been suggested to be
important inhibitors of calcium oxalate crystal growth and aggregation. Glycosaminoglycans have been most widely investigated and
shown to inhibit both crystal growth[1] and aggregation[2]. Acidic
polypeptides[3] and polyribonucleotides[4] have also been claimed to be
important as inhibitors. Low molecular weight glycoproteins have
been proposed to be more important inhibitors than glycosaminoglycans[5]. Uromucoid or Tamm-Horsfall glycoprotein has recently been
shown to exert some inhibitory activity[1,6] on calcium oxalate precipitation and crystal growth. The present investigation was undertaken in order to investigate further the relation between macromolecular components in the urine and the inhibition of calcium
oxalate crystal growth.

METHODS

Pooled urine from 5 healthy members of the staff was concentrated using an ultrafilter with a cut-off at 10,000 daltons
(Amicon). The concentrate was redissolved in 300 mM NaCl and
reconcentrated with ultrafiltration 5 times. The urine was concentrated to 3% of the original volume and applied to a Sephadex G-200
column (1.5 x 90 cm). The column had been equilibrated and was
eluted with 300 mM NaCl at a flow-rate of 4 ml/h. Five ml of the
urinary concentrate was applied to the column and 4 ml fractions
collected at 4°C.

The absorbance at 280 nm was measured directly in all fractions. The total alcian blue precipitable polyanions (ABPP) and the content of chondroitin sulphate (CS) were measured with a combined enzymatic and precipitation procedure[7]. The inhibitory activity of calcium oxalate crystal growth was measured with a seeded crystal procedure[8].

RESULTS

The ABPP-chromatogram contained two distinct peaks. One coincided with the void volume but contained no chondroitin sulphate. The other consisted mainly of chondroitin sulphate and a small residue of precipitable polyanions, apart from chondroitin sulphate (Fig. 1). The absorbance at 280 nm contained 3 distinct peaks. The first and highest was in the void volume. The second coincided with the albumin marker and the third immediately after (Fig. 2). Near V_t there were also two small peaks in the A_{280}-chromatogram. The inhibition of calcium oxalate crystal growth was positive throughout all fractions, but with two distinct peaks (Fig. 2). The most prominent peak coincided with that of chondroitin sulphate. The second peak of crystal inhibition did not correspond to any ABPP-peak, but was near V_t and coincided with a minor A_{280}-peak.

DISCUSSION

A great number of macromolecular urinary components have been claimed to exert inhibitory activity of calcium oxalate crystal growth and aggregation, including glycosaminoglycans[1,2], polypeptides[3] and polyribonucleotides[4]. It is believed that some of these macromolecular inhibitors may act by being adsorbed to the crystal surface[9,10] and thereby blocking the growth sites of the crystals and preventing continued crystal growth and particularly aggregation. The interrelationship between the various urinary macromolecular constituents regarding inhibitory activity is not clear. Glycosaminoglycans have been claimed to be the most important inhibitors[2] of aggregation. Other investigators, however, claim that polyribonucleotides[4] or low molecular weight glycoproteins[5], are the most important.

In this study we examined the inhibitory activity of urinary constituents >10,000 daltons. The most prominent inhibitory activity was found to coincide with the maximum ABPP and the maximum chondroitin sulphate peaks. It is suggested, therefore, that the main macromolecular inhibitors in urine may consist of glycosaminoglycans. The second peak of inhibition was found near V_t and coincided with a small A_{280}-peak, possibly consisting of low molecular weight glycoproteins, as suggested previously[5]. The highest absorbance at 280 nm was found in the void volume where also

824

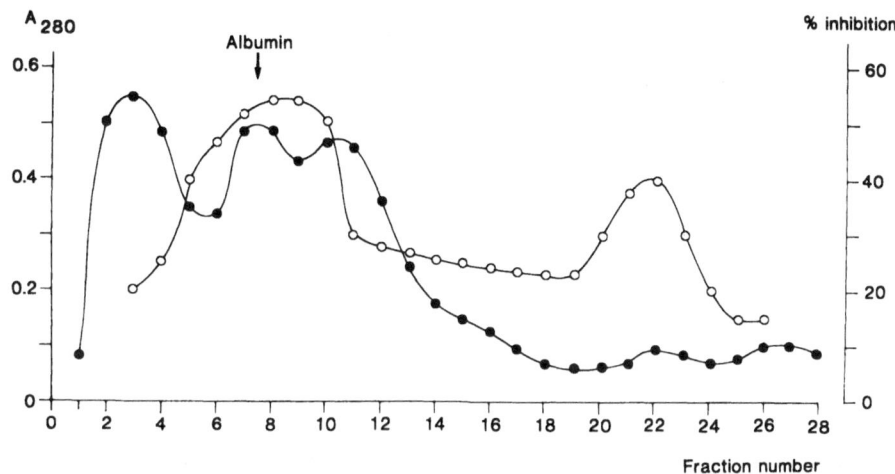

Fig. 1. Gel filtration of concentrated urine by Sephadex G-200
(1.5 x 90 cm). Total alcian blue precipitable polyanions
(ABPP) (●); residual ABPP after enzymatic degradation with
chondroitinase-AC (o); chondroitin-sulphate A and C (■).

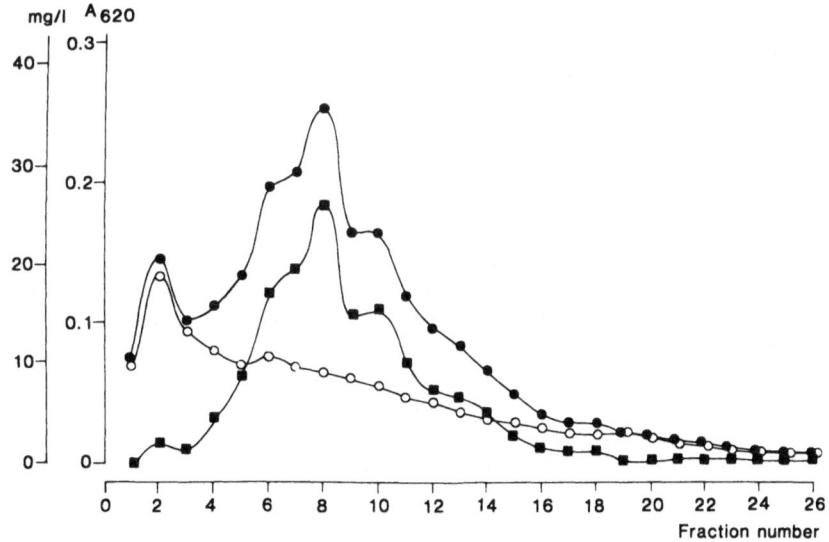

Fig. 2. Gel filtration of concentrated urine. Inhibition of
calcium oxalate crystal growth (o); absorbance at
280 nm (●).

a slight ABPP-peak was detected. This was possibly due to the content of high molecular weight glycoprotein polymers, such as Tamm-Horsfall glycoprotein. The void volume probably also contained excreted immunoglobulins such as Ig-G and Ig-A[11], both of which are glycoproteins.

ACKNOWLEDGEMENTS

This work was supported by the Swedish Medical Research Council (nos. 2329, 6354), the Swedish Society of Medical Sciences and the Tore Nilsson Foundation.

REFERENCES

1. B. Fellström, B. G. Danielson, S. Ljunghall, and B. Wikström, in:"Urolithiasis and Related Clinical Research", P. O. Schwille, L. H. Smith, W. G. Robertson, and W. Vahlensieck, eds., Plenum, New York (1985).
2. W. G. Robertson, M. Peacock, and B. E. C. Nordin, Clin. Chim. Acta 43:31 (1973).
3. H. Ito and F. L. Coe, Am. J. Physiol. 233:F455 (1977).
4. E. E. Schrier, K. E. Lee, J. L. Rubin, P. G. Werness, and L. H. Smith, in:"Oxalate in Human Biochemistry and Clinical Pathology", G. A. Rose, W. G. Robertson, and R. W. E. Watts, eds., Wellcome Foundation, London (1979).
5. T. Kitamura, J. E. Zerwekh, and C. Y. C. Pak, Kidney Int. 21:379 (1982).
6. T. Kitamura and C. Y. C. Pak, J. Urol. 127:1024 (1982).
7. B. Fellström, B. G. Danielson, S. Ljunghall, and B. Wikström, in:"Urolithiasis and Related Clinical Research", P. O. Schwille, L. H. Smith, W. G. Robertson, and W. Vahlensieck,eds., Plenum, New York (1985).
8. B. Fellström, U. Backman, B. G. Danielson, K. Holmgren, S. Ljunghall, and B. Wikström, Clin. Sci. 62:509 (1982).
9. B. Finlayson and L. DuBois, Clin. Chim. Acta 84:203 (1978).
10. B. Fellström, B. G. Danielson, F. A. Karlsson, and S. Ljunghall, in:"Urolithiasis and Related Clinical Research", P. O. Schwille, L. H. Smith, W. G. Robertson, and W. Vahlensieck, eds., Plenum, New York (1985).
11. I. Berggard, in:"Proteins in Normal and Pathological Urine", Y. Manuel, J. P. Revillard, and H. Betuel, eds., Karger, Basel (1970).

EFFECT OF ADDITIVES AND WHOLE URINE ON

CALCIUM OXALATE DIHYDRATE FORMATION

X. Martin, L. H. Smith, and P. G. Werness

Nephrology Research Unit, Mayo Clinic, Rochester
Minnesota, USA, and Service d'Urologie et de Chirurgie
de la Transplantation, Hôpital E. Herriot, Lyon, France

INTRODUCTION

Calcium oxalate occurs as two different crystal phases in
urine, calcium oxalate monohydrate (COM) and dihydrate (COD). The
less stable COD may be a transitional form to COM[1]. Unlike COM,
COD is difficult to obtain in vitro from simple supersaturated
solutions of CaOx. However, COD crystals are obtained almost
exclusively from precipitation of a mixture of whole urine and
ammonium oxalate[2]. This suggests that urine contains specific
substances that promote the formation of COD over COM. The effect
of additives, including some inhibitors of CaOx crystal growth on
the formation of COD were investigated. Mixtures of CaOx crystal
growth inhibitors, and human urine were studied for their ability to
form COD. Finally, the effect of pH on the formation of COD in the
presence of additives was investigated.

MATERIALS AND METHODS

Synthetic solutions used in these experiments were supersaturated solutions of 8.3 mM $CaCl_2$, 1.3 mM Na_2Ox, and 0.1 M NaCl.
For each experiment 25 ml portions of the test solution was mixed
with 1 ml 0.05 M ammonium oxalate, and incubated for 7 min. The
solutions were vacuum filtered (0.2 μm Nuclepore filters), and the
resulting crystals collected on the filter. One mg of the
collected crystals was used for infra-red spectrophometric analysis
to determine the fractional content of COD. Using reference
spectra of mixtures of known proportion of COM (reagent grade) and
COD (from a pure stone) it was possible to determine quantitatively
the fractional content of COD over COM in the samples[3].

The additives tested in the synthetic CaOx solution were pyrophosphate (1 to 8×10^{-5}M), sodium citrate (10^{-4} to 2×10^{-3}M), magnesium chloride (10^{-4} to 10^{-2}M), chondroitin sulfate from shark cartilage (1×10^{-6} to 1.6×10^{-4}M), RNA from yeast (5×10^{-9} to 5×10^{-7}M) and heparin (2×10^{-9} to 2×10^{-7}M). Experiments were performed at pH 6.5. The effects of pyrophosphate (5×10^{-5}M) citrate (1.25×10^{-3}M), and RNA (1.6×10^{-7} and 4.2×10^{-7}M) were studied from pH 4.5 to 7.5. The additivity of the effects of CaOx crystal growth inhibitors was tested at pH 6.5 for citrate-pyrophosphate and RNA-pyrophosphate mixtures.

Pooled human urine from normal subjects was studied after filtration to remove particles. Undiluted urine, and mixtures of urine and synthetic CaOx solution (25%, 50%, 75%) were tested at pH 6.5. The effect of varying pH between 4.5 and 7 was studied with undiluted urine. Fresh individual urine samples were collected from healthy male subjects. Urines were centrifuged (2000 rpm for 10 min), and the fractional content of COD determined at pH 5.6 after the addition of 1.5 ml (instead of 1 ml) 0.05M ammonium oxalate. Results were compared with the values of CaOx crystal growth inhibitors measured in a seeded crystal growth system[4].

RESULTS

A strong linear relationship was found between the fractional content of COD in the samples and the molar concentrations of pyrophosphate (slope = 90.9×10^5; r = 0.98; P<0.01), citrate (slope = 3.03×10^4; r = 0.92; P<0.01), RNA (slope = 5.72×10^7; r = 0.94; P < 0.01), and heparin (slope 2.4×10^8; r = 0.96; P<0.01). Magnesium and chondroitin sulfate had no effect. This relationship with the concentration of inhibitor was linear until the inhibitor concentrations reached a value, above which a plateau was observed (6×10^5M for pyrophosphate; 1.5×10^{-3} M for citrate; 1.4×10^{-7} M for heparin; 5×10^{-7} M for RNA).

Table 1. Effect of pH on the COD Fractional Content of Samples of Inorganic Solutions Containing Various Inhibitors.

Inhibitor	COD Fractional Content (%) (Mean $\pm$ SEM)			
	pH 4.5	pH 5.5	pH 6.5	pH 7.5
Pyrophosphate (5×10^{-5}M)	5.6 ± 1.8	32.5 ± 0.5	50.5 ± 0.5	64.0 ± 3.0
Citrate (1.25×10^{-3}M)	4.5 ± 2	31.6 ± 2.8	41.6 ± 2.4	49.1 ± 0.5
RNA (50 mg/l)	5 ± 2.5	26.8 ± 1.5	33.0 ± 2.5	47.0 ± 1.5

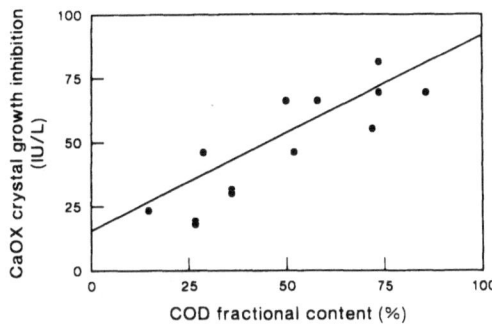

Fig. 1. Correlation between COD fractional content (in %) and CaOx crystal growth inhibition (IU/l) in urine from normals.

Variations in pH resulted in parallel variations of the COD fractional content in the samples with pyrophosphate and citrate. A different pattern was obtained with RNA (Table 1). In urine, increase of pH was correlated with an increase in the COD fractional content observed (slope = 11.5; r = 0.81; P<0.01). When inhibitor mixtures were tested, the fractional content (in %) of COD obtained was not different from the sum of the values measured when each inhibitor was tested separately, respectively 43.1 $\pm$ 3.8 versus 45.1 $\pm$ 3.8 for the citrate-pyrophosphate mixture and 46.7 $\pm$ 7.9 versus 51.7 $\pm$ 4.1 for the pyrophosphate-RNA mixture. The experiments involving human urine, added in various proportions (v/v to the synthetic solutions) showed that a linear relationship existed (slope = 0.92; r = 0.98; P<0.01) between the effect observed and the dilution of urine. When individual urines were tested, a mean value of 49.8 $\pm$ 5.6 COD fractional content was obtained. When the data obtained were examined in the linear regression system, a correlation of 0.87 (P < 0.01) was obtained between COD fractional content and CaOx crystal growth inhibition in urine (Fig. 1).

DISCUSSION

An assay is described to measure the effect of different additives on the formation of COD. Several substances that are known CaOx crystal growth inhibitors were potent in promoting the formation of COD. The preferential formation of COD over COM in the presence of CaOx crystal growth inhibitors may be the result of (1) the inhibition of the phase transformation of the COD into the more thermodynamically stable COM[5], or (ii) the preferential inhibition of COM crystal growth. Surface adsorption of inhibitors is higher for COM than COD, a situation that could allow the preferential adsorption of the inhibitors on the COM phase[1]. Therefore, the effect observed in this study may be regarded as a phase-stabilization of COD produced by inhibitors of CaOx crystal growth. At pH 7, urine induced maximal COD formation, but only part of the effect observed can be explained by the substances tested. Citrate and pyrophosphate at the concentration present in urine would account for 45% of the effect observed. RNA, at a concentration of 20 mg/l, would account for only 16% and chondroitin sulfate would have no effect. However, the RNA from yeast used in our experiments, as well as chondroitin sulfate of shark cartilage, may not have the same properties as the RNA-like material and glycosaminoglycans present in urine. Acidic glycopeptides[6], known to be present in urine, or inhibitors not yet demonstrated in urine (citrate-metal complexes[7] or phosphocitrate[8]) may have an effect on COD formation in our system, but they were not tested in this study.

In the assay described, pyrophosphate, citrate, RNA and heparin have been shown to have a phase-stabilizing effect of COD. Thèse substances are known inhibitors of CaOx crystal growth. Additivity of the effect of inhibitors on CaOx crystal growth[9] and the change in the potency of inhibitors with pH change[10] have been described. Similar observations on the effect of inhibitors and urine on phase stabilization are reported in this study. In fresh urine samples from normal subjects, CaOx crystal growth inhibition correlates with the phase-stabilizing effect. The assay is able to study the effect of inhibitors on phase stabilization at concentrations present in whole urine. The phase-stabilizing effect may reflect factors involved in crystal formation and crystal growth inhibition in simple solutions as well as in undiluted urine.

ACKNOWLEDGMENTS

This work was supported in part by the research grant AM 20605 from the National Institutes of Health, Bethesda, and by Fondation pour la Recherche Médicale, Paris.

REFERENCES

1. B. Tomazic and G. H. Nancollas, J. Cryst. Growth 46:355 (1979).
2. H. Philipsborn, Protoplasma 41:415 (1952).
3. J. Bellanato, L. Cifuentes-Delatte, A. Hidalgo, and M. Santos, in:"Urinary Calculi", L. Cifuentes Delatte, A. Rapado, and A. Hodgkinson, eds., Karger, Basel (1973).
4. J. L. Meyer and L. H. Smith, Invest. Urol. 13:31 (1975).
5. B. B. Tomazic and G. H. Nancollas, Invest. Urol. 16:329 (1979).
6. H. Ito and F. L. Coe, Am. J. Physiol. 233:F455 (1977).
7. J. E. Howard, Johns Hopk. Med. J. 139:239 (1976).
8. J. L. Meyer and W. C. Thomas, J. Urol. 128:1372 (1982).
9. P. G. Werness, J. H. Bergert, and K. E. Lee, Clin. Sci. 61:487 (1981).
10. H. G. Tiselius, Br. J. Urol. 53:470 (1981).

830

CRYSTAL INHIBITION:BINDING OF HEPARIN AND CHONDROITIN SULPHATE

TO CALCIUM OXALATE, SODIUM URATE AND URIC ACID CRYSTALS

B. Fellström, B. D. Danielson, F. A. Karlsson, and
S. Ljunghall

Dept. of Internal Medicine, University Hospital
S-751 85 Uppsala, Sweden

INTRODUCTION

Urinary glycosaminoglycans may be important inhibitors of calcium oxalate crystal growth and aggregation[1]. These inhibitors may act by blocking the growth sites of the crystals and thereby prevent or delay crystal development. Calcium oxalate crystals, that had grown in human urine, have been found to contain chondroitin sulphate[2]. Furthermore, a solid phase of sodium urate in urine has been suggested to act as an anti-inhibitor by binding urinary glycosaminoglycans and thereby reduce its inhibitory activity against calcium oxalate crystallisation[3,4]. The binding of heparin to sodium urate crystals was also shown to be enhanced in the presence of divalent cations, such as calcium or magnesium[5]. We applied the principles used in receptor studies to examine the affinity of two potential inhibitors, heparin and chondroitin sulphate, to calcium oxalate, sodium urate and uric acid crystals.

METHODS

[3]H-heparin (New England Nuclear) and ^{3}H-chondroitin sulphate-A (prepared from de-acetylated chondroitin sulphate) were added separately in trace amounts to crystal suspensions of calcium oxalate, sodium urate and uric acid (30 mg/ml, 0 to 1000 µl). The radioactive tracers were homogeneous, as judged by Sephadex G-100 chromatography. The crystals were prepared as described previously[6]. The tracers were incubated with the crystals[6] for 1 h at 37°C in 140 mM NaCl, with a 10 mM sodium cacodylate buffer, pH=6.0. Using calcium oxalate crystals, the incubations were also made at pH=2, 4, 6, 8 and 10 in 140 mM NaCl and at pH=6 in 0, 140 or

1000 mM NaCl.   Using sodium urate or uric acid crystals the
incubations were also made under the standard conditions with the
addition of 3.4 mM CaCl$_2$ or 0.22 mM sodium oxalate or in a
metastable calcium oxalate solution (relative super-saturation,
R.S.=0.6).

Following incubation, the crystals were separated by
centrifugation at 20,000 g for 20 min and the amounts of tracer in
the crystal pellet and in the supernatant measured by liquid
scintillation and compared with the original amount of tracer.   The
amount of tracer bound to the crystals could thereby be calculated.

In competition experiments, addition of increasing amounts of
non-radioactive heparin, chondroitin sulphate or pentosan polysulphate (SP 54) were made and the procedure carried out as
described above.

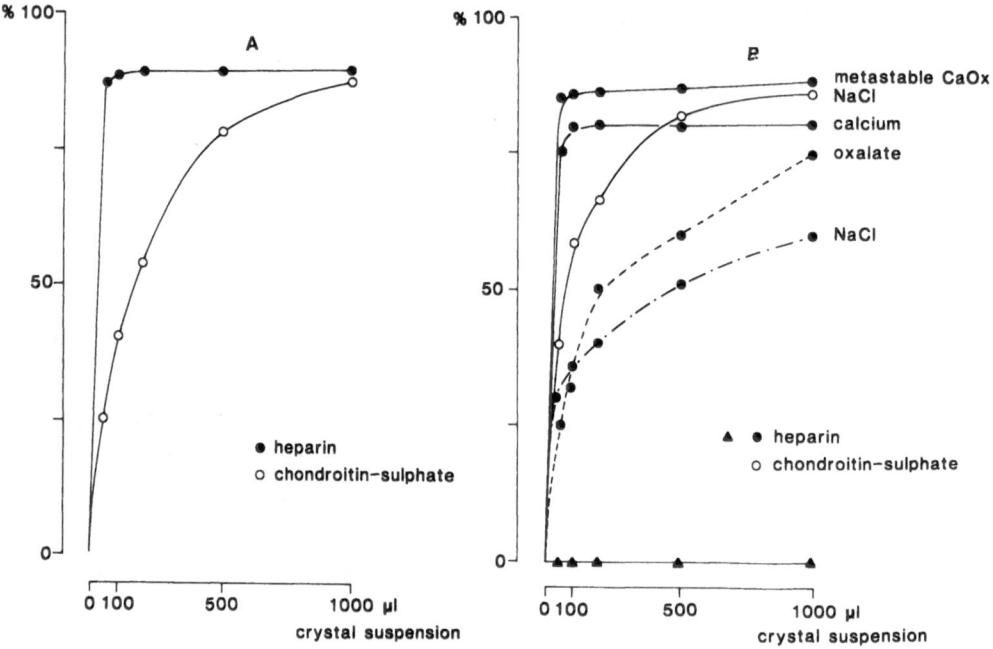

Fig. 1a. The binding (%) of ^{3}H-Heparin (●) and of ^{3}H-chondroitin
sulphate (o) to calcium oxalate crystals in 140 mM NaCl.

1b. The binding of ^{3}H-heparin to sodium urate crystals in
140 mM NaCl (·-o-·), 0.22 mM sodium oxalate (--●--), 3.4 mM
CaCl$_2$ (- ● -), in a metastable calcium oxalate solution
(-●-) and to uric acid crystals in 140 mM NaCl or in calcium
oxalate solution (▲).   The binding of ^{3}H-chondroitin
sulphate to sodium urate crystals in 140 mM NaCl (o).

832

RESULTS

When identical amounts of heparin and chondroitin sulphate
tracers were incubated with calcium oxalate crystals a marked
difference in binding was observed. Heparin bound much more
efficiently to the crystals. As little as 50 µl crystal suspension
caused maximal binding, whereas 1000 µl crystal suspension was
needed to cause similar binding of chondroitin sulphate (Fig. 1).
This approximately 20-fold binding difference was further investigated in competition experiments. In experiments with similar
extent of tracers bound to crystals, increasing amounts of unlabeled
glycosaminoglycans were added. The concentration of heparin needed
to cause about half-maximal displacement of tracer was around 10
times lower than the corresponding amount of chondroitin sulphate.
These data indicate that calcium oxalate crystals bind heparin with
a higher affinity than chondroitin sulphate. The difference in
binding observed in Fig. 1 appears mainly to reflect a difference in
affinity and to a smaller extent binding capacity. SP 54 competed
with ^{3}H-heparin bound to the calcium oxalate crystals, but a higher
concentration was required than in the case of heparin.

The influence of ionic strength on the binding of heparin
to calcium oxalate crystals was studied. Addition of NaCl to
the binding solutions caused a shift to the left of the binding
curves, indicating increased binding affinity. The binding
was not influenced by changes in pH.

Binding studies of ^{3}H-heparin and ^{3}H-chondroitin sulphate to
sodium urate and uric acid crystals showed that heparin did bind to
sodium urate crystals and the binding increased substantially in a
metastable calcium oxalate solution compared with buffered saline
(Fig. 2). This effect was dependent on the presence of calcium but
not oxalate. Chondroitin sulphate also bound to sodium urate
crystals and the binding was higher in the presence of calcium ions.
Uric acid crystals did not bind heparin at all, even in a metastable
calcium oxalate solution.

DISCUSSION

It has previously been shown that glycosaminoglycans appear to
be important inhibitors of calcium oxalate crystal growth and
aggregation[1,7]. In human urine, the highest macromolecular
inhibitory component after gel filtration coincided with urinary
chondroitin sulphate[8]. We have previously shown that urinary
macromolecular inhibitors bind to calcium oxalate crystals[6]. In
the present study, using a different technique, it has been shown
that both heparin and chondroitin sulphate bind to calcium oxalate
crystals, heparin having a higher affinity than chondroitin sulphate
and being more firmly bound at low than at high ionic strengths.

Sodium urate crystals may interfere with urinary macromolecular inhibitors of calcium oxalate crystal growth[6,9], and cause an attenuation of the inhibition. It has been shown that heparin becomes bound to sodium urate crystals[5], facilitated by the presence of calcium and magnesium ions. In this study, the binding of heparin to sodium urate crystals was greatly enhanced in the presence of calcium in the solution. Chondroitin sulphate also bound to sodium urate crystals, with an affinity that increased with the calcium concentration. Uric acid crystals on the other hand did not bind heparin under any of the tested conditions.

It is suggested that glycosaminoglycans may act as inhibitors of calcium oxalate crystal growth by blocking the growth sites of the crystals. A solid phase of sodium urate, but not of uric acid, may also bind these calcium oxalate crystallisation inhibitors. The importance of these observations depends on whether or not such a solid phase exists in human urine.

ACKNOWLEDGEMENTS

This work was supported by the Swedish Medical Research Council (nos. 2329, 6354), the Swedish Society of Medical Sciences and the Tore Nilsson Foundation.

REFERENCES

1. W. G. Robertson, M. Peacock, and B. E. C. Nordin, Clin. Chim. Acta 43:31 (1973).
2. R. C. Bowyer, J. G. Brockis, and R. K. McCulloch, Clin. Chim. Acta 95:23 (1979).
3. W. G. Robertson, F. Knowles, and M. Peacock, in":Urolithiasis Research", H. Fleisch, W. G. Robertson, L. H. Smith, and W.Vahlensieck, eds., Plenum, New York (1976).
4. C. Y. C. Pak, K. Holt, and J. E. Zerwekh, Invest. Urol. 17:138 (1979).
5. B. Finlayson and L. DuBois, Clin. Chim. Acta 84:203 (1978).
6. B. Fellström, U. Backman, B. G. Danielson, K. Holmgren, S. Ljunghall, and B. Wikström, Clin. Sci. 62:509 (1982).
7. B. Fellström, B. G. Danielson, S. Ljunghall, and B. Wikström, in"Urolithiasis and Related Clinical Research", P. O. Schwille, L. H. Smith, W. G. Robertson, and W. Vahlensieck, eds., Plenum, New York (1985).
8. B. Fellström, B. G. Danielson, S. Ljunghall, and B. Wikström, in"Urolithiasis and Related Clinical Research", P. O. Schwille, L. H. Smith, W. G. Robertson, and W. Vahlensieck, eds., Plenum, New York (1985).
9. J. E. Zerwekh, K. Holt, and C. Y. C. Pak, Kidney Int. 23:838 (1983).

STUDIES ON THE MODE OF ACTION OF POLYANIONIC INHIBITORS OF

CALCIUM OXALATE CRYSTALLIZATION IN URINE

D. S. Scurr and W. G. Robertson

MRC Mineral Metabolism Unit, The General Infirmary
Leeds LS1 3EX, U.K.

INTRODUCTION

Many studies have been carried out on the identification and role of inhibitors of calcium oxalate crystallization in urine[1-5]. The main inhibitors of agglomeration appear to be polyanions such as glycosaminoglycans[1,2,4,6], RNA-like material[3] and acidic glycoproteins[5] including non-polymerised Tamm-Horsfall mucoprotein (THM)[7]. The main inhibitors of crystal growth are RNA, citrate and an acidic glycoprotein[5]. The object of this paper is to study the effects of some of these molecules on the surface properties of calcium oxalate crystals in vitro.

MATERIALS AND METHODS

The surface properties of characterized calcium oxalate monohydrate (COM) crystals were assessed by measuring the zeta potential (ZP) on the crystal surface[7]. From a stock suspension of COM in water (0.35 g/l), 27 ml was mixed and equilibrated with 3 ml artificial urine[8] but containing no oxalate and only 2.96 mmol/l magnesium. The basal ZP of COM crystals in this 10% artificial urine was -5 mV.

The effect of adding various polyanionic inhibitors to 10% artificial urine on the ZP of the COM crystals was measured and compared with the effect of adding the same inhibitors to 10% natural urine. Finally, the effects of adding THM to artificial urine and of increasing the concentration of natural urine to nearly whole urine were investigated.

835

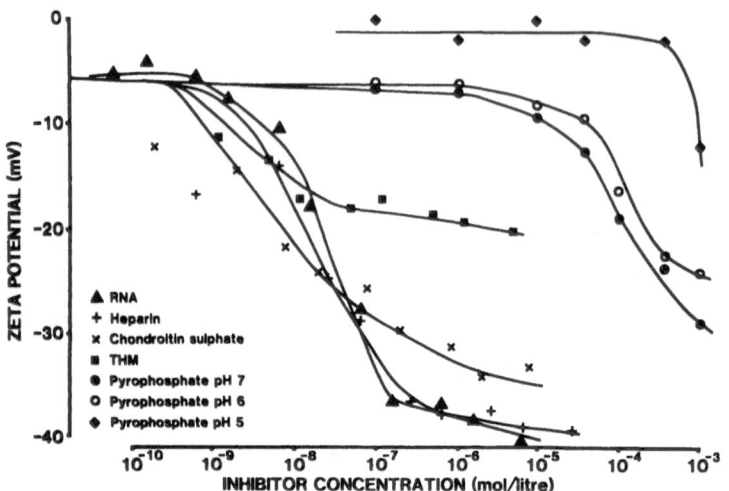

Fig. 1. The zeta potential produced on COM crystals by inhibitors.

RESULTS AND DISCUSSION

Fig. 1 shows the effect of increasing concentrations of various polyanionic inhibitors on the ZP on the surface of COM crystals in 10% artificial urine. This shows that RNA, heparin and chondroitin-4-sulphate (CSA) all caused the ZP to become more

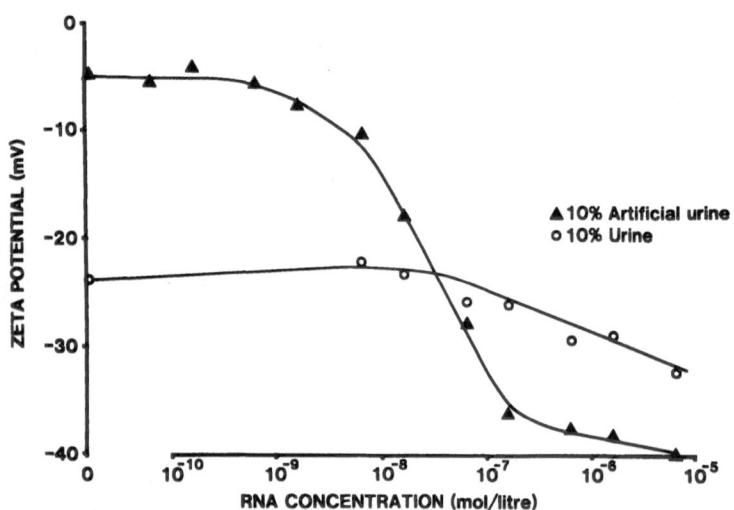

Fig. 2. The effect of urine on the ZP on COM produced by RNA.

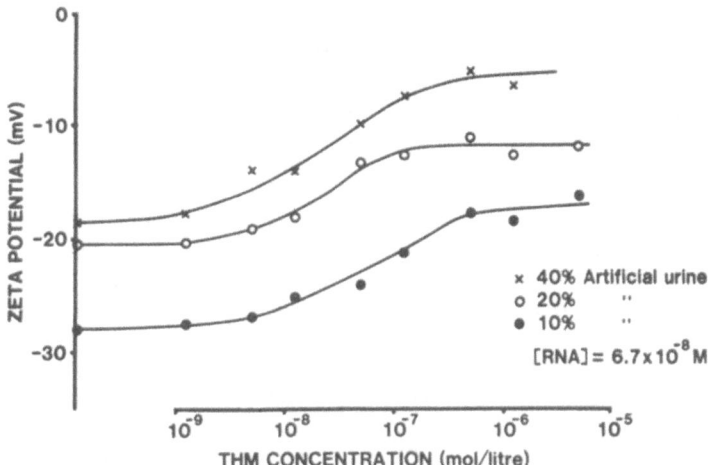

Fig. 3. The effect of THM on the ZP on COM produced by RNA.

negative, reaching a maximum negativity of about -40 mV.
Pyrophosphate also caused the ZP to become more negative but at much
higher molar concentrations than the macromolecular polyanions.
THM, at concentrations between 10^{-10} and 10^{-8}M, acted like the other
macromolecular polyanions but at higher concentrations the ZP curve
flattened off at about -20 mV. Fig. 2 compares the relative effects
of increasing the concentration of RNA in 10% artificial urine and
10% natural urine on the ZP. This suggests that the ability of RNA
to adsorb to the surface of COM is impaired by some constituent of
urine, a finding confirmed with CSA and heparin (not shown). Since

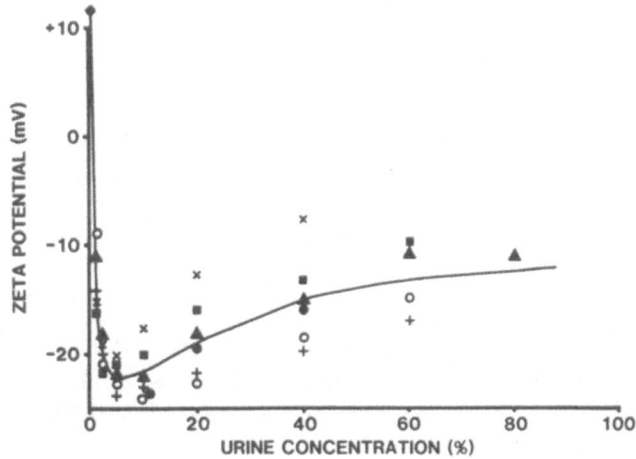

Fig. 4. The effect of urine concentration on the ZP of COM.

the ZP curves in the presence of 10% natural urine all flattened off roughly at the same level of ZP as produced by THM (Fig. 1), we suspected that THM might be the culprit. We therefore measured the effect of increasing concentrations of THM on the ZP produced by 6.7 x 10^{-8}M RNA. Fig. 3 shows that in 10% artificial urine 6.7 x 10^{-8} RNA produced a CP of -28 mV as also shown in Fig. 1. Addition of THM, however, produced a less negative ZP, presumably because THM competed with RNA for surface binding sites. This effect was accentuated by increasing the % of artificial urine to 20% and further to 40%. This would cause compression of the double layer and influence the binding of polyanions to the crystal surface.

The net effect of these phenomena is seen in Fig. 4 which shows the ZP on COM crystals equilibrated with increasing concentrations of urine from 6 normal men. Up to between 5 and 10% urine the increasing negativity in the ZP is due to the increasing concentration of inhibitors contained in the urine. Above 10% urine, the effects of increasing ionic strength and THM concentration combine to reverse the trend in negativity so that the final ZP in the presence of nearly whole urine is close to -10 mV. This is within the range (-15 to +15 mV) over which crystal agglomeration is known to occur. Clearly the actual ZP on the crystal surfaces of COM in whole urine is highly dependent on the relative concentrations of the polyanionic inhibitors and THM and on the ionic strength of the urine concerned. THM is particularly interesting since at low concentrations ($<10^{-8}$M) it inhibits agglomeration, whereas at higher concentrations it interferes with the adsorption of inhibitors and creates a situation where agglomeration of COM is likely to occur.

REFERENCES

1. W. G. Robertson, M. Peacock, and B. E. C. Nordin, Clin. Chim. Acta 43:31 (1973).
2. J. D. Sallis and M. F. Lumley, Invest. Urol. 16:296 (1979).
3. H. Ito and F. L. Coe, Am. J. Physiol. 235:F455 (1977).
4. R. L. Ryall, R. M. Harnett, and V. R. Marshall, Clin. Chim. Acta, 112:349 (1981).
5. Y. Nakagawa, V. Abram, F. J. Kezdy, E. T. Kaiser, and F. L. Coe, J. Biol. Chem. 258:12594 (1983).
6. W. G. Robertson, D. S. Scurr, and C. M. Bridge, J. Crystal Growth 53:182 (1981).
7. W. G. Robertson, A. B. Latif, D. S. Scurr, A. M. Caswell, G. W. Drach, and A. D. Randolph, in:"Urinary Stone", R. Ryall, J. G. Brockis, V. Marshall, and B. Finlayson, eds., Churchill Livingstone, Melbourne (1984).
8. A. D. Randolph and G. W. Drach, J. Crystal Growth 53:195 (1981).

THE RELATIVE INHIBITORY POTENTIAL OF URINARY MACROMOLECULAR

FRACTIONS ON CaOx PRECIPITATION

R. Azoury, B. Goldwasser, S. Perlberg, Y. Wax,
N. Garti, and S. Sarig

Casali Institute of Applied Chemistry, The Hebrew
University of Jerusalem, Jerusalem 91904, Israel

INTRODUCTION

One promising approach to increasing the understanding of
crystallization inhibitors is to separate the inhibitors and
potential promoters from normal healthy urines[1]. These substances
have been found either to promote[2] or inhibit CaOx precipitation.
In most of the reported studies the accepted approach has been to
isolate macromolecular fractions from healthy normal urine and to
compare their inhibitory potential with that of similar fractions
separated from stone formers' (SF) urine. The main conclusions
from these studies have been: (a) there are no significant
differences in the urinary content of inhibitors in SF and normals,
(b) some of the fractions isolated from urine may have been damaged
by the preparative procedures, and (c) the inhibitory potential in
normal urine could not be explained by the inhibition potential of
the isolated inhibitors. Thus the inhibitory potential must be due
to unknown compounds.

The present study uses a different approach. Using the Discriminating Index (DI) test of Sarig et al[3], we examined the
residual inhibitory potential in the urines of SF and normals after
ultrafiltration with different membranes.

MATERIALS AND METHODS

First morning voided urine specimens were collected from a
group of 17 healthy volunteers and 7 CaOx SF. The individual
samples were filtered through 0.2 μm filter. Subsequently the urine
was ultrafiltered through Diaflo membranes with molecular weight

839

cut-offs at 10,000, 1,000 and 500 daltons at 5°C and under 25 psi
nitrogen pressure. At the termination of each filtration the
overall inhibitory potential in the filtrates was determined using
the DI test[3]. The differences, in each of the studied groups, with
respect to the rates of the change in the DI values, after
consecutive removal of inhibitory substances, were examined
graphically and analytically. The residues remaining on the
membrane surfaces were analyzed qualitatively for phosphates,
sulphates, sugars and amino acids. Statistical analysis was
performed using the Student t-test.

RESULTS

In all urine samples a general trend of decrease in the urinary
inhibitory potential as the pore size decreases was evident. The
sharpest decrease in the inhibition power (in DI value) was achieved
after the 500 dalton filtration. The overall trend in the SF
urines is very similar to that found in the normal urines, though
the actual modification values are smaller in this group. Fig. 1
shows a bar diagram of the average change of DI values produced by
the 4 filtrations according to membrane pore sizes and divided into
the response of SF population, the intermediate group and the
healthy normals. In most of the analyzed urines two major changes
in DI values were found after the consecutive filtration. The
steepest change was caused by the removal of 500 to 1,000 dalton
fraction but the differences in the DI values between SF and normal
populations did not reach statistical significance (the corresponding P value for pairwise multiple comparison test = 0.13). Removal
of macromolecules >10,000 daltons from normal urine reduced the
inhibitory potential (DI values) more significantly (the corresponding P value for the paired multiple comparison test = 0.05) than
removal of the same fraction from SF urine. Fig. 2 shows the
differences between SF, intermediate and normal populations. It

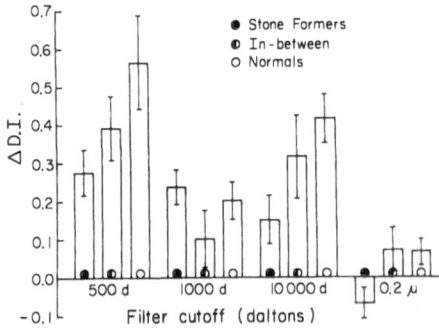

Fig. 1. Bar diagram of the average change of DI produced by
consecutive filtration.

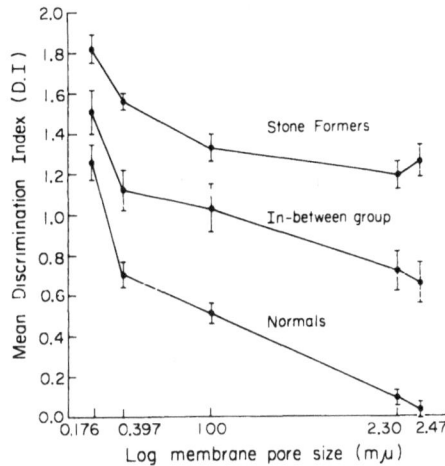

Fig. 2. The estimated mean values of DI as a function of log
membrane pore size in various groups of subjects.

describes the estimated mean of DI values computed on the basis of
all subjects as a function of the continuous log membrane pore size
(r). The equations of the lines can be expressed as:

$$DI = a + b \log (r)$$

Fig. 2 shows the relatively high contribution and importance of the
500 to 1,000 dalton fraction to the urinary inhibitory potential.

DISCUSSION

The present study focused on the relative contribution of
macromolecular fractions to the urinary inhibitory potential.   A
non-continuous gradation of molecular weight with at least two
distinct groups of macromolecular inhibitors exists in the urine of
the non-SF population (Fig. 2).   The molecular weight of the first
group of inhibitors is >10,000 daltons while that of the second
group is >500 but <1000 daltons.   Our results suggest that while
the inhibitors of >10,000 daltons are nearly absent or inactivated
in the urine of SF, inhibitors of the second group are nevertheless
present in their urine.   It is generally accepted that evaluation
of the relative contribution of the different known inhibitors is
very difficult.   It appears that the known inhibitors represent
only a small part of the total urinary inhibitory power[4] and a large
part of it was ascribed to unknown macromolecules[1].   Using the DI
test[3] enabled us to show the relative importance of the
macromolecular inhibitors present in urine.   The removal of this

fraction from the urine caused the sharpest decrease in the inhibitory potential of both normal and SF urine.

On the other hand, removal of macromolecules >10,000 daltons caused a significant decrease in the inhibitory potential of normal urines.   Fig. 2 shows that the residual inhibitory activity after 500 dalton filtration in the healthy group was significantly higher (one-tailed P value <0.001) than that in SF urines.   This could indicate a deficiency of inhibitors <500 daltons in SF urines.

The present results are in good agreement with the hypothesis that there exist several kinds of inhibitors in urine.   The results suggest that the difference between SF and normals may be ascribed to the urinary activity of inhibitors if not to their content.   The activity of the 500 to 1,000 dalton fraction is evident in SF and normal urine but SF have almost no activity in the >10,000 dalton fraction of organic macromolecules and almost no inorganic inhibitory activity.

REFERENCES

1. W. B. Gill, J. W. Karesh, L. Garsin, and M. J. Roma, Invest. Urol. 15:95 (1977).
2. P. Hallson and G. A. Rose, Lancet 12:1000 (1979).
3. S. Sarig, N. Garti, R. Azoury, Y. Wax, and S. Perlberg, J. Urol. 128:645 (1982).
4. J. L. Meyer and L. H. Smith, Invest. Urol. 13:36 (1975).

ADSORPTION OF RNA ONTO AGED CALCIUM OXALATE MONOHYDRATE (COM)

C. M. Brown, P. Senior, H. Charest, and B. Finlayson

Division of Urology, Dept. of Surgery, University of
Florida, Gainesville, Florida 32610, U.S.A.

INTRODUCTION

We studied the interaction of COM and ribonucleic acid (RNA), by
adsorbing RNA onto the COM surface and inhibiting crystal growth.
The choice of RNA as an adsorbate was two-fold: (i) it is of
interest in urolithiasis, and (ii) it is a useful model for the
study of adsorption of linear polyelectrolytes because of the
existing detailed understanding of its physical chemistry.

METHODS AND MATERIALS

RNA (35,000 daltons) was adsorbed onto the COM surface in
flasks of increasing [RNA] using a solution depletion method. The
experiments were conducted at 3 pHs and 4 [Ca] in the range of 30 to
4800 µM.   COM was prepared by mixing equal volumes of 0.5 M $CaCl_2$
and 0.5 M KC_2O_4.   Lyophilization of the precipitate produced a fine
powder which was stored under vacuum.   Powder surface area by
electronic particle counting (epc) was 3.02 m^2/dl^1 and by gas
adsorption (BET) was 26.3 m^2/dl^{-1}.   The powder gave a COM X-ray
diffraction pattern.   Each adsorption system contained 2.5g of COM
in 50 ml of buffer solution (0.1 M NaCl and 0.01 M HEPES buffer).
The RNA ranged from 0.2 to 50 mg/dl. Adsorption systems were
equilibrated at 37^OC for 2 h and then filtered.   The filtrate was
analyzed for Ca, Na, K, pH, and RNA.   Slurry particle size
distribution was routinely determined by epc.   Electrophoretic
mobility (EM) of the particles was measured by optical tracking.

Inhibition of COM crystal growth was studied in a water-
thermostatted 4 x 4 array of 2 ml seeded crystallizers.   The

843

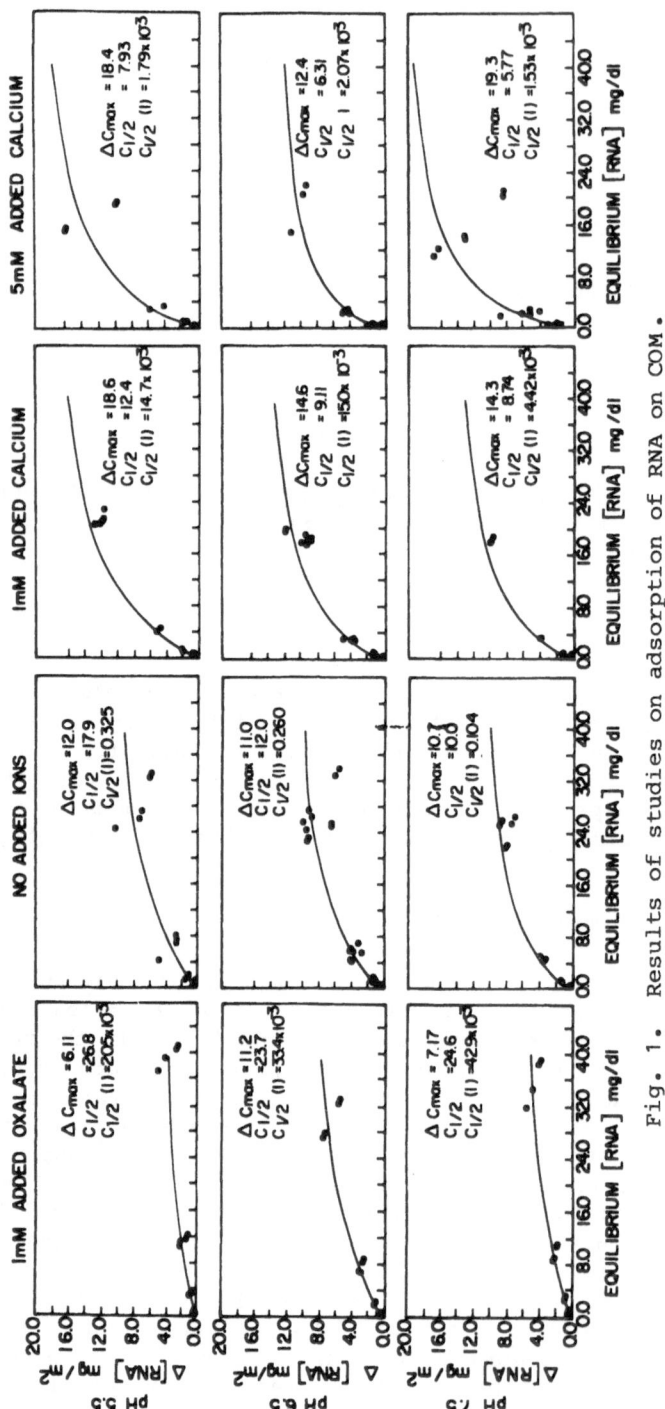

Fig. 1. Results of studies on adsorption of RNA on COM.

initial COM relative supersaturation (RS_0) was 10.0 $\pm$ 0.1. A seed slurry of 50 µg/ml was established immediately after loading each well, crystal growth proceeded for 20 min, and the contents of each well were filtered and analyzed for $[^{14}C\text{-}C_2O_4]$ and [Ca] .

The difference (ΔC) between initial and final solution RNA (C) is the amount adsorbed. Using a nonlinear least squares fitting program with C and C, parameters were fitted to the Langmuir adsorption isotherm, $\Delta C/C_{max} = C/(C + C_{1/2})$. This yielded estimates of ΔC_{max}, the maximum possible adsorbate accommodated in a monolayer on the surface, and $C_{1/2}$, the final [RNA] at which $\Delta C = \Delta C_{max} \cdot (C_{1/2})^{-1}$ is proportional to the affinity of RNA for the surface. Independent estimates of $C_{1/2}$ were made with crystal growth inhibition studies ($C_{1/2}$ (I)). Values of [Ca] , [Ox] , [Na], [Cl] and pH were used in the solution speciation program, EQUIL, to determine the COM relative supersaturation at 20 min (RS_{20}) in the crystallizer wells. RS_{20} and RS_0 permitted the estimation of a growth rate constant using the parabolic rate law. $C_{1/2}$ (I) was estimated with nonlinear least squares parameter fitting, assuming Langmuir adsorption.

RESULTS

Fig. 1 shows the relationships between $C_{1/2}$ and ΔC_{max}, and the Langmuir adsorption isotherms implied by these data. ΔC_{max} was sensitive to changes in both [Ca] and pH. It increased 3-fold over the range of [Ca] , but showed an inconsistent tendency to decrease with pH. The extremes occurred at the lowest [Ca] , lowest pH and at the highest [Ca] , highest pH. The largest ΔC_{max} indicated a maximum coverage of 19.3 mg/m^2. $C_{1/2}$ decreased with increasing [Ca] at all pHs, with the greatest effect at the highest pH. Generally, there was a small decrease in $C_{1/2}$ with increasing pH. The greatest pH effect was seen in the "no-added-ions" column. The $C_{1/2}$(I) showed the same qualitative response to changes in [Ca] and pH found by solution depletion, but was several orders of magnitude smaller than $C_{1/2}$ (Fig. 1). The change in $C_{1/2}$(I) with increasing [Ca] was a factor of almost 200. There was a clear tendency for the $C_{1/2}$(I) to decrease with increasing pH, except at the highest added calcium level.

Fig. 2 shows a pseudo-3-D plot of particle volume-frequency histograms in relation to [RNA] . The area under the curves passes through a minimum; as [RNA] was increased to 5 mg/dl, the total particle count decreased, the distribution broadened, and the peak tended to move to higher particle volumes, indicating aggregation of slurry particles; as [RNA] was increased beyond 5 mg/dl, these trends were reversed, indicating a reduction in aggregation. EM of COM was positive at the lowest [RNA], it decreased as [RNA] increased and became negative before 16 mg/dl RNA.

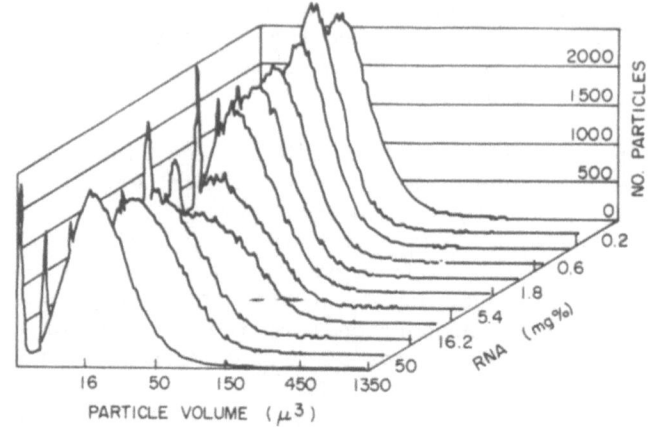

Fig. 2.   Evolution of volume-frequency histograms.

DISCUSSION

The evolution of the COM particle size distributions followed expected behavior.   Polymeric bridging occurring at low [RNA] results in aggregation, but the denser polymer layer at the surface prevents aggregation at higher [RNA] by steric repulsion.   The change in sign of EM with increasing [RNA] indicates adsorption.

The increase in ΔC_{max} due to added Ca is greatest at pH 7.5 where the value in the 1 mM-added-oxalate column, 7.17 mg/m^2(epc), is almost tripled at 5 mM-added-calcium, 19.3 mg/m^2 (epc). Based on the maximum ΔC_{max}, the minimum area occupied by an RNA molecule is 800 Å^2 (BET), which is consistent with a radius for RNA of 28 Å. The Ca effect on ΔC_{max} results from Ca binding by RNA, which reduces its net charge and steric repulsion.   Ca also increases the COM surface charge (as predicted by the Nernst equation and confirmed by EM measurements).   These effects all permit a higher density of molecules on the crystal surface.   The consistent decrease in $C_{1/2}$ with increasing Ca at all pHs can be explained the same way.   The correlation of pH with $C_{1/2}$ is consistently negative, the greater the surface charge, the stronger the attraction for negatively charged RNA molecules.

The surface properties of the growth sites differ from those of the bulk COM surface.   The effect of Ca on $C_{1/2}(I)$ is 200 times that on $C_{1/2}$. We conclude that anionic polyelectrolytes may be useful probes of the surface properties of growth sites.

THE ADDITIVE EFFECTS OF MAGNESIUM AND TARTRATE UPON INHIBITION

OF CALCIUM OXALATE CRYSTAL FORMATION IN WHOLE URINE

P. C. Hallson and G. A. Rose

St Paul's Hospital and Institute of Urology
Endell Street, London, U.K.

INTRODUCTION

Stone formation in southern India is said to be much rarer than in the north[1], perhaps due to tamarind fruit consumption which is eaten only in the south[2]. Tamarind is rich in tartaric acid, a substance known to complex Ca^{2+} ions. Sur et al [2] demonstrated the inhibitory effect of tartrate in diluted urine upon calcium oxalate crystal formation. The inhibition tests described here, however, have been carried out using concentrated whole urine from which urinary crystals arise naturally, and the tests extended to cover calcium phosphate crystalluria. Since magnesium is effective in reducing calcium oxalate crystal formation[3], it seemed worthwhile to establish whether or not magnesium together with tartrate would either enhance the inhibitory action of tartrate or diminish it owing to magnesium tartrate complexing.

METHODS

The quantitative crystal methods have been described elsewhere[4]. Fresh urine samples from normal individuals were adjusted to pH 5.3, 6.0 or 6.8 with hydrochloric acid or sodium hydroxide. Each urine sample was divided into 4 aliquots, 2 being untreated control samples and 2 test samples containing added tartrate, magnesium or both,. Sodium tartrate was added to test aliquots to give a concentration after evaporation of 5 mmol/l and magnesium chloride to raise urinary magnesium post-evaporation by 4 mmol/l. Also sodium oxalate was added to all samples to raise the final oxalate concentration by 0.22 mmol/l. All additives were adjusted to the pH of the urine under test.

Each sample was evaporated in a rotary evaporator[5] to 1250 mosmol/kg (for calcium oxalate tests) or 1050 mosmol/kg (for calcium phosphate tests). In calcium oxalate experiments, ^{14}C-oxalate in the precipitate was measured by scintillation counting. Calcium phosphate deposits were assessed from calcium determination by atomic absorption spectroscopy.

Duplicate crystal determinations were made in all experiments. Where ^{14}C-oxalic acid was used 145 tests were carried out, but only 81 included in which the difference between each duplicate and the mean value of the duplicates was less than 12%. When crystal masses were determined in the calcium phosphate study, the results of all experiments are included since the difference between duplicates and their mean ($\pm$ SD) value was 7.4 $\pm$ 5.8%.

RESULTS

Tartaric Acid

The effects upon calcium oxalate crystalluria of addition of L(+), D(-) and meso-tartrate are shown in Fig. 1. For urines at pH 5.3 the mean ($\pm$ SEM) precipitated calcium oxalate, as a percentage of the control values, was 70 $\pm$ 5.8%, 77.6 $\pm$ 7.4%, and 84.8 $\pm$ 6.0% for the L(+), D(-), and meso-isomers respectively. Similar results were found when a further 30 experiments were repeated at pH 6.0. Here the mean recoveries of precipitated calcium oxalate were 51.2 +6.5%, 82.7 $\pm$ 6.2%, and 90.8 $\pm$ 7.6% for the L(+), D(-) and meso-forms respectively. The addition of L(+) tartrate to urine at pH 6.8 (Fig. 2) produced a drop in calcium phosphate crystals in 18/20 cases. Recoveries ranged from 33 to 127% (mean 75.3 $\pm$ 4.4%).

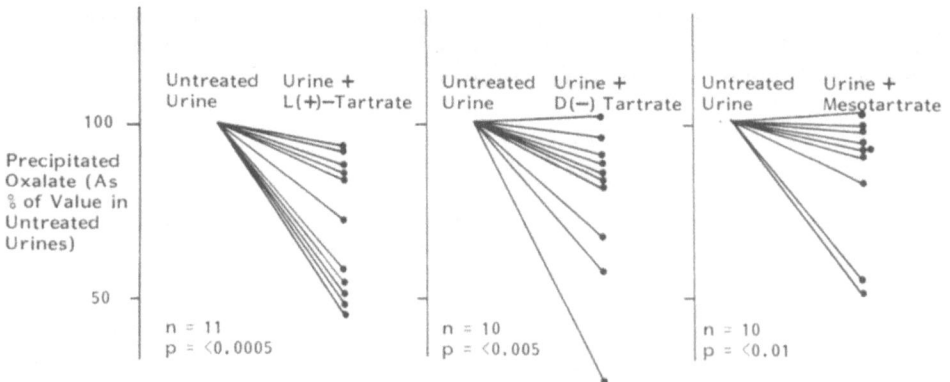

Fig. 1. The effect of L(+), D(-) and meso-tartrate (5 mmol/l) upon calcium oxalate crystalluria in whole urine at pH 5.3.

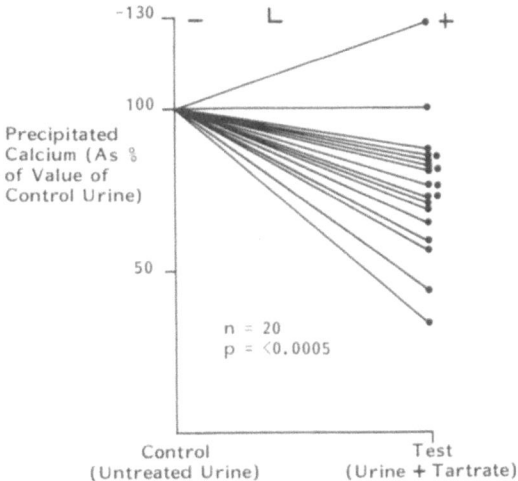

Fig. 2. The effect of (L+) tartrate (5 mmol/l) upon calcium
phosphate crystalluria in whole urine at pH 6.8.

Magnesium with Tartrate

    Counts from aliquots at pH 5.3 containing both magnesium and
tartrate were compared with samples containing one of these
substances alone (Fig. 3). Precipitated calcium oxalate decreased
in all 10 tests in which L(+) tartrate was added to urine with
raised magnesium.   (Range 53 to 98%, mean 75.0 $\pm$ 4.7%). Similarly
calcium oxalate precipitates decreased in 10/10 tests where
magnesium was added to urine with raised tartrate.   The range of
observed precipitates was 16 to 78% (mean 50.0 $\pm$ 6.6%).

DISCUSSION

    Our tests show that all stereo-isomers of tartaric acid are
effective in inhibiting calcium oxalate crystallisation in
concentrated whole urine, the important point being that this is the
medium from which urinary crystals arise naturally.   Calcium
phosphate is similarly inhibited by L(+) tartrate.   When magnesium
is combined with tartaric acid the inhibitory effects are additive
suggesting that magnesium tartrate complex formation or ion-pairing
are not significant factors.   Tartaric acid is known to be safe for
oral administration being present in fruits, wines, confectionery,
soft drinks and culinary preparations.   A combination of tartaric
acid with magnesium could be included in an effervescent drink or
confectionery which would be cheap, pleasant to take and therefore
unlikely to be overlooked, and entirely safe.

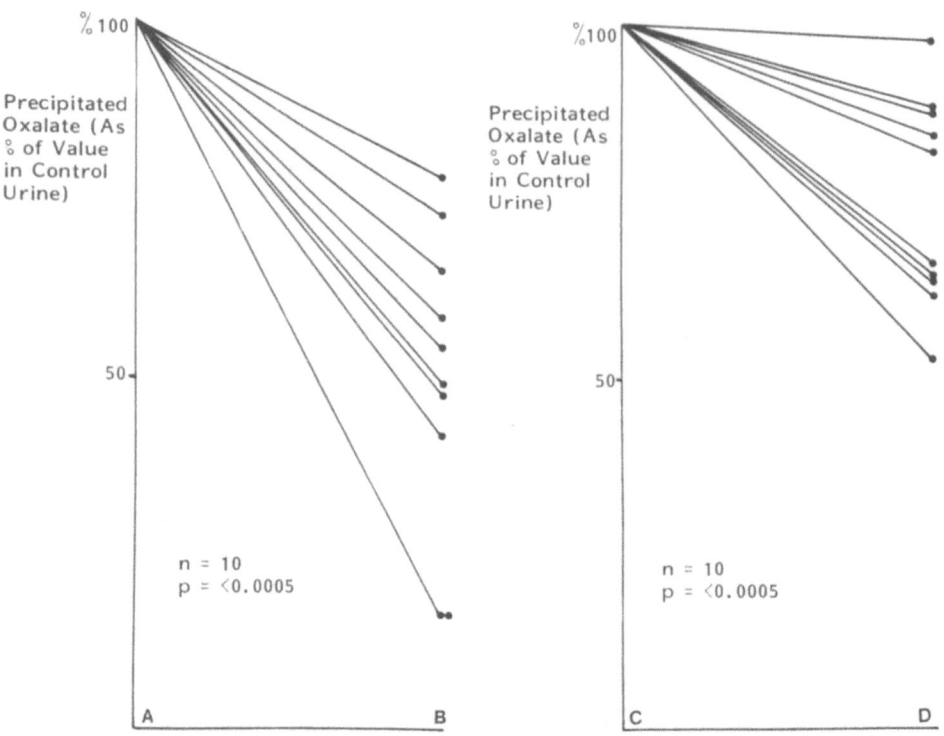

Fig. 3. Crystal recoveries from urines containing magnesium
(4 mmol/l) with L(+) tartrate (5 mmol/l) (B and D)
compared with control urines containing either
magnesium (C) or tartrate (A) alone at pH 5.3.

REFERENCES

1. B. N. Colabawalla, Presentation to I.C.M.R. study group on
   urolithiasis (1970).
2. B. K. Sur, H. N. Pandey, S. Deshpande, R. Pahwa, R. K. Singh,
   and Tarachandra, in:"Urolithiasis: Clinical and Basic
   Research", L. H. Smith, W. G. Robertson, and B. Finlayson,
   eds., Plenum, New York (1981).
3. P. C. Hallson, G. A. Rose, and S. Sulaiman, Clin. Sci. 62:17
   (1982).
4. G. A. Rose and S. Sulaiman, J. Urol. 127:177 (1982).
5. P. C. Hallson and G. A. Rose, Br. J. Urol. 50:442 (1978).

CALCIUM OXALATE CRYSTAL GROWTH: INVESTIGATIONS ON INHIBITORY

ACTIVITY OF MODEL COMPOUNDS AND URINE SAMPLES

J. Joost, M. Lusser, and K. Kleboth

Dept. of Urology and Institute of Inorganic and
Analytical Chemistry, University of Innsbruck
Austria

INTRODUCTION

Seventy per cent of all kidney stones contain calcium oxalate.
Urine is ordinarily supersaturated with respect to this salt and the
question is why only some people form stones and why others only
have crystalluria. In addition to particle retention in the upper
urinary tract, lack of urinary inhibitors of crystallization may
also be important. One of the best techniques to study the
inhibitory activity of synthetic substances and of urine with
respect to crystal growth is the constant composition approach of
Sheehan and Nancollas[1]. Using this method the following problems
have been investigated: (a) the influence of different seed crystals
on the kinetics of crystal growth; (b) the inhibitory activity of
different substances on crystal growth; and (c) the inhibitory
potential of urine from recurrent calcium oxalate stone formers and
from normal controls.

MATERIALS AND METHODS

The supersaturation of the crystallization system is maintained
constant by the addition of solutions containing the crystal lattice
ions. This addition is controlled potentiometrically by means of a
calcium-ion selective electrode. Calcium oxalate monohydrate (COM)
seed crystals were prepared in two different ways: (a) sodium
oxalate (1 mol) was dissolved in conductivity water (2 litre)
maintained at 60°. A $CaCl_2$ solution (1 mol $CaCl_2$ in 4 litre water)
was added dropwise over 17 h, while the reaction mixture was stirred
continuously. The seed crystals were washed twice in 1 litre (60°)
and were aged for 3 weeks at 37°; (b) $CaCl_2$ (0.25 mol) was

851

dissolved in water (1 litre) and added dropwise to a sodium oxalate solution (0.25 mol in 1 litre water) within 1 h at 70°C. The crystals were washed in 0.5 litre water (60°) and treated as above. The solubility product was in agreement with that in the literature. The reactant solutions contained 4.5×10^{-4} mol/1 $CaCl_2$ and $Na_2C_2O_4$ at an ionic strength of 0.150 with NaCl. The starting volume was 270 ml at 37°C and pH 6.0 to 6.2.

Urine (fasting morning sample) was centrifuged and stored at 4° before use. One or 2 ml of urine were added to 270 ml of COM supersaturated solutions. The Ca^{2+} activity was restored by addition of $CaCl_2$, $Na_2C_2O_4$ or 0.15 molar NaCl solution.

The substances investigated included polyacrylic acid (PAA 2000), polyaspartic acid (PAsA 26000, PAsA 14000), polyglutamic acid (PGA 21000), polyvinylpyrrolidone (PVP 40000, PVP 10000), citrate, γ-carboxyglutamic acid (Gla), and silicic acid.

RESULTS

Seed crystals prepared by various methods and different batches prepared by the same method exhibited linear relationships between crystal growth rate and seed crystal concentration (Fig. 1). The amount or concentration of COM crystals was chosen to give a pre-determined growth rate in the absence of inhibitors under standard conditions. The additives that produced inhibition are listed below in order of decreasing potency (Fig. 2). PVP, citrate, Gla and silicic acid had no observable inhibitory effect. Dilute samples of urine from stone formers and normal controls with widely differing total calcium contents were investigated. Normal urine inhibited COM growth (Fig. 3) but the urines of calcium oxalate stone formers retarded crystal growth to a lesser degree than those of normal controls (Fig. 4).

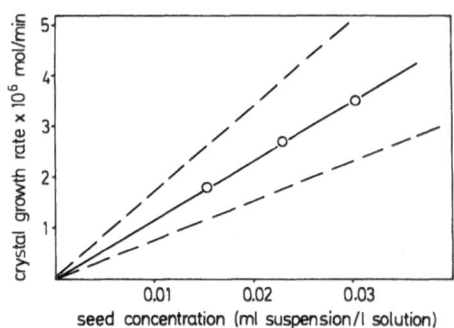

Fig. 1. Plot of crystal growth rate versus seed concentration for different seed suspensions.

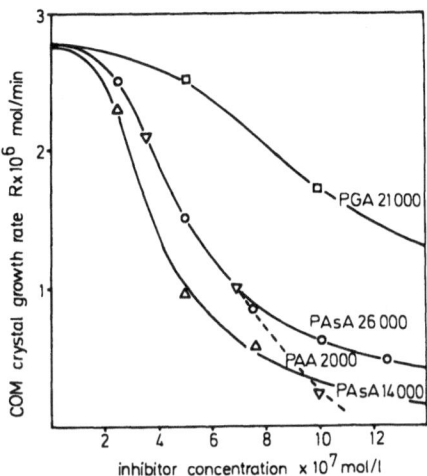

Fig. 2. Plot of COM crystal growth rate versus inhibitor concentration.

DISCUSSION

The results indicate that COM seed crystals of different size can be used if a constant, predetermined growth rate is attained in pure calcium oxalate solutions. It is not necessary to know the actual concentration of the active surface of the crystals. The method of COM crystal preparation does not influence the experiments.

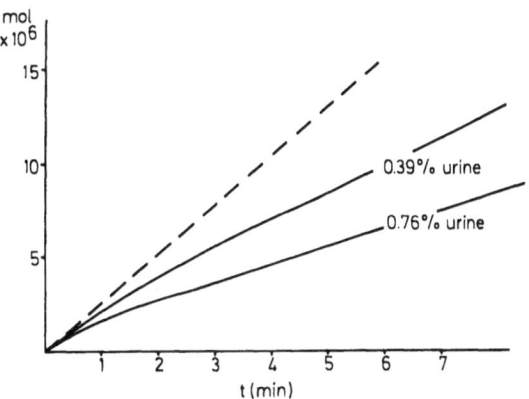

Fig. 3. Rate plots of COM growth. Dashed line: $R_O = 2.7 \times 10^{-6}$ mol/min. Continuous line: inhibition of crystal growth by urine.

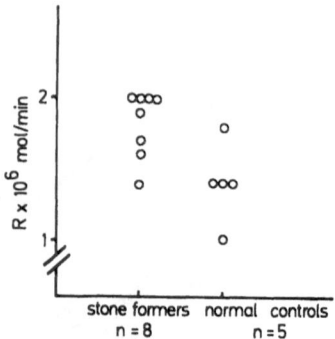

Fig. 4. Inhibition of COM growth by urine (0.37%) of calcium
oxalate stone formers and normal controls.

Only polymeric substances with negatively charged end-groups
(COO^-, $SO_3^=$) exhibited inhibitory activity at low concentrations. If
the experiments were performed with the same Ca^{2+} activity no
inhibitory effect was observed with polymers such as PVP or with
Ca^{2+}-complexing agents. The shape of the curves (Fig. 2) suggests
that the polymeric inhibitors are precipitated on the crystal
surface. Polymers with a lower molecular weight show greater
inhibitory activity. This may be explained by the faster diffusion
of small ions on to the crystal surface.

Despite the limited number of urine samples investigated, a
difference with respect to the inhibitory potential between the
urines of calcium oxalate stone formers and normal controls was
detected at the 95% confidence level.

REFERENCE

1. M. E. Sheehan and G. H. Nancollas, Invest. Urol. 17:446 (1980).

THE EFFECT OF URIC ACID ON THE INHIBITORY ACTIVITY OF

GLYCOSAMINOGLYCANS AND URINE

R. L. Ryall, R. M. Harnett, and V. R. Marshall

Urology Unit, Dept. of Surgery, Flinders Medical
Centre, Bedford Park, Australia

INTRODUCTION

One theory advanced to explain the apparent influence of urate
on calcium oxalate (CaOx) stone formation proposes that the binding
of colloidal urate to urinary glycosaminoglycans (GAGS) reduces
their inhibitory potency and thereby indirectly increases the risk
of CaOx stone formation in vivo[1]. In this study normal human
urine, chondroitin sulphate and heparin were preincubated with uric
acid to determine whether or not this altered their inhibitory
effect on CaOx crystal growth and aggregation.

MATERIALS AND METHODS

Spot urine samples were collected and Millipore -filtered[2]
(0.22 µm) from 10 healthy males with no history of kidney stone
disease. Pre-incubations containing no urate were used as controls.
The standard pre-incubation solution contained Ca and NaCl buffered
at pH 6.00 with MES. After pre-incubation, the solutions were
Millipore-filtered (0.22 µm) to remove the uric acid and filtered
oxalate solution added dropwise to give final concentrations of 0.20
mM oxalate, 1.0 mM Ca, 0.15M NaCl and 10 mM MES. A seed crystal
suspension of CaOx monohydrate was added and growth and aggregation
measured using a Coulter Counter[2]. Crystal growth was expressed as
the cumulative increase in crystal diameter (ΔD) and aggregation as
the percentage decrease in crystal number (N %) by using a computer
model[3]. $1/\Delta D$ and $1/N$ were plotted against $1/T$ (where T = time) and
the slopes of the regression lines gave estimates of the rates of
crystal growth and aggregation respectively. Results represent the
mean of at least 6 determinations.

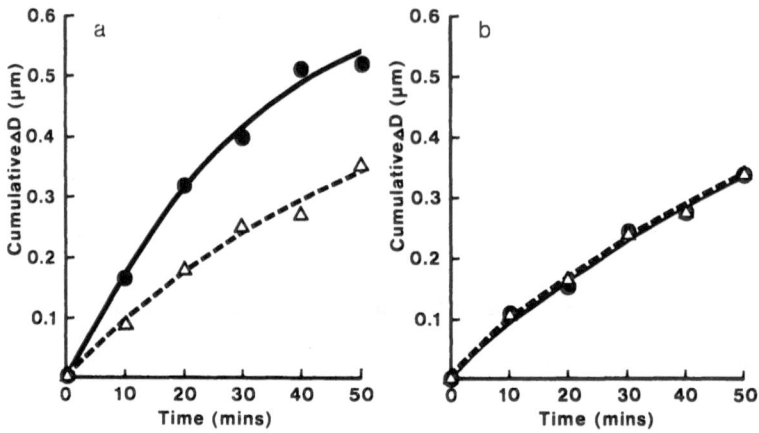

Fig. 1. Crystal growth in the presence of (a) heparin (5 x 10^{-4}g/l) and (b) chondroitin sulphate (5 x 10^{-3}g/l) after pre-incubation with (●) and without (△) sodium urate.

RESULTS

Fig. 1a shows the time course of crystal growth in the presence of heparin (5 x 10^{-4}g/l). Since heparin retards CaOx crystal growth[2], the higher growth rate occurring after pre-incubation with uric acid must reflect a decline in the inhibitory effect of heparin on crystal growth. The difference between the rates of crystal growth calculated from these curves is significant (P<0.0001). Fig. 1b shows the corresponding results for chondroitin sulphate (5 x 10^{-3}g/l). There was no significant difference between the rates of crystal growth calculated from the curves.

Fig. 2a shows the time course of crystal aggregation in the presence of heparin (5 x 10^{-5}g/l). The % decrease in crystal number after pre-incubation with uric acid is significantly (P<0.0001) greater than that occurring after the control pre-incubation, again indicating a decline in the ability of heparin to inhibit crystal aggregation. The corresponding results for chondroitin sulphate (5 x 10^{-5}g/l) are shown in Fig. 2b. The rates of aggregation were not significantly different.

A comparison of the rates of crystal growth obtained in the presence of 1% urine showed that the presence of uric acid in the pre-incubation solution had an inconsistent effect on the final measured crystal growth rates and there was no significant difference between the rates of crystal growth measured in the two groups. In contrast, in all cases pre-incubation of the urine specimens with uric acid resulted in a greater rate of aggregation than was obtained after the control incubations (P = 0.029).

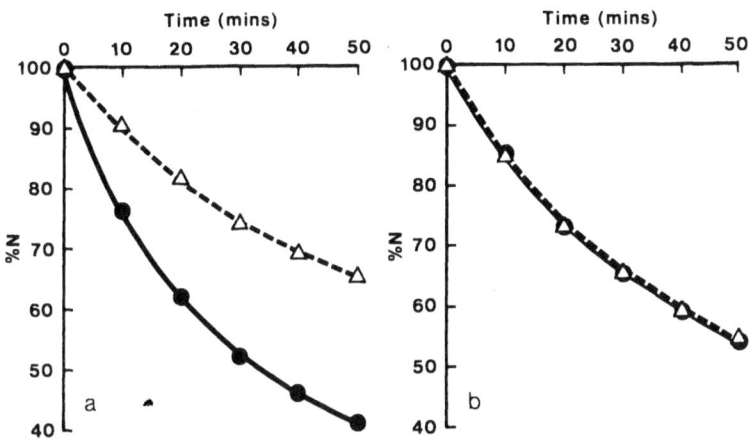

Fig. 2. Crystal aggregation in the presence of (a) heparin
(5 x 10^{-5}g/l) and (b) chondroitin sulphate (5 x 10^{-5}g/l)
after pre-incubation with (●) and without (Δ) urate.

DISCUSSION

Few studies have attempted to test directly the hypothesis that
colloidal urate can decrease the inhibitory activity of urine by
binding to endogenous GAG molecules[1]. Pak et al[4] found that the
inhibitory potency of heparin on CaOx crystal nucleation was
significantly reduced after pretreatment with sodium urate. We
have observed a similar effect with uric acid. However, heparin
does not occur naturally in human urine[5]. Of more physiological
relevance are the studies involving chondroitin sulphate. In
accord with Pak et al[4] who studied crystal nucleation, we were
unable to demonstrate any effect of pre-incubation with uric acid on
the rates of crystal growth and aggregation occurring in the
presence of chondroitin sulphate.

Only one other study has examined the influence of pre-
incubation with sodium urate on the inhibitory effect of human urine
on crystal growth. Fellstrom et al[6] found only a very slight
reduction in the inhibitory activity of the ultrafiltrate, but the
inhibitory potency of the macromolecular fraction was reduced by
80%. Our failure to demonstrate the same effect may be due to our
use of (i) unfractionated urine samples, which might mask any
separate responses of macromolecular or ultrafiltrable fractions,
(ii) a lower urine concentration (1% as opposed to the 9%), and
(iii) a larger number of single urine samples rather than one pooled
specimen which might iron out the responses of individual urines to
uric acid pre-treatment. On the other hand, all urine samples
showed a fall in their inhibitory effect on crystal aggregation
after uric acid treatment. Since pre-incubation had no effect on

chondroitin sulphate, the principal urinary GAG[5], it is most
unlikely that this reduction is caused by the binding of urate to
glycosaminoglycan molecules. However, various proteins, including
human albumin and immunoglobulin G, have been shown to bind to
crystalline sodium urate[7] and it is possible that similar binding to
uric acid may occur. Since proteins are known to contribute to the
inhibitory activity of urine[8], it is feasible that the reduction in
the inhibitory effect of urine on crystal aggregation may have been
caused by binding of urinary protein to the uric acid.

The plausibility of both current theories relating uricosuria
and CaOx stone disease relies on the presence in urine of
particulate urate or uric acid. However, crystalline sodium urate
and uric acid are so rarely found in urine or stones that it is
unlikely to bind to urinary components or induce heterogeneous
nucleation of CaOx in vivo. Nonetheless, the apparent beneficial
effect of allopurinol in reducing CaOx stone recurrence must have
some basis. Perhaps future work should investigate more fully the
possibility that allopurinol modifies the excretion of urinary
metabolites other than urate, or that dissolved urate may reduce the
potency of urinary inhibitors by molecular interaction.

ACKNOWLEDGMENTS

This work was supported in part by grant no. G21/82 from the
Australian Kidney Foundation and a grant from the Flinders Medical
Centre Research Foundation.

REFERENCES

1. W. G. Robertson, F. Knowles, and M. Peacock, in:"Urolithiasis
   Research", H. Fleisch, W. G. Robertson, L. H. Smith, and
   W. Vahlensieck, eds., Plenum, New York (1976).
2. R. L. Ryall, R. M. Harnett, and V. R. Marshall, Clin. Chim.
   Acta, 112:349 (1981).
3. R. G. Ryall, R. L. Ryall, and V. R. Marshall, in:"Urinary
   Stone", R. L. Ryall, J. G. Brockis, V. R. Marshall, and
   B. Finlayson, eds., Churchill Livingstone, Melbourne (1984).
4. C. Y. C. Pak, K. Holt, and J. E. Zerwekh, Invest. Urol. 17:138
   (1979).
5. J. M. Goldberg and E. Cotlier, Clin. Chim. Acta 41:19 (1972).
6. B. Fellström, U. Backman, B. G. Danielson, K. Holmgren,
   S.Ljunghall, and B. Wikström, Clin. Sci. 62:509 (1982).
7. F. Kozin and D. J. McCarty, J. Lab. Clin. Med. 89:1314 (1977).
8. T. Koide, M. Takemoto, H. Itatani, M. Takaha, and T. Sonoda,
   Invest. Urol. 18:382 (1981).

HYPERURICOSURIA AND CALCIUM OXALATE STONE FORMATION

B. Goldwasser, S. Sarig, R. Azoury, Y. Wax, and M. Many

Dept. of Urology, Chaim Sheba Medical Center, Sackler School of Medicine, Tel-Aviv University, Israel

INTRODUCTION

Uric acid is implicated in calcium oxalate (CaOx) kidney stone formation. Crystallographic considerations suggest that uric acid might trigger off calcium oxalate crystallisation by epitaxy[1]. In vitro experiments on uric acid, however, show negative results, although CaOx growth does occur on sodium urate crystals[2]. Sodium urate crystals have not been detected in fresh urine and are uncommon in stones and so Robertson suggested that a colloidal gel of urate may be formed that removes natural inhibitors of calcium oxalate aggregation[3].

The present study examines the effect of uric acid on the ability of urine to retard the in vitro precipitation of calcium oxalate using the Discriminating Index (D.I.) test[4].

PATIENTS AND METHODS

The study included 37 hyperuricosuric patients, 25 of whom had a history of calcium oxalate stone formation. They were screened to exclude other metabolic derangements so as to eliminate the possible effect of other abnormalities on calcium oxalate crystallization. Hyperuricosuria was defined as urinary uric acid excretion of over 800 mg/24 h in a female and 850 mg/24 h in a male. All patients were on a free diet and none was receiving medication known to affect uric acid metabolism.

The Discrimination Index (D.I.)[4] was determined on a first morning urine sample at least twice, in all 37 hyperuricosuric

859

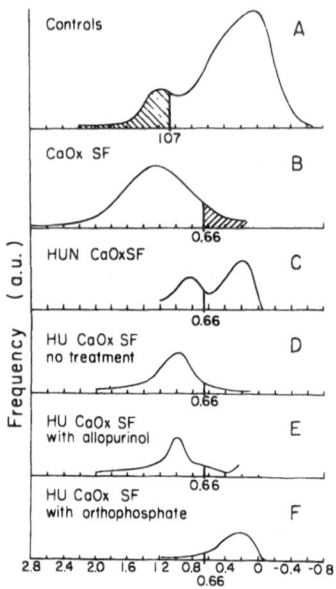

Fig. 1. DI values in (A) 146 normal controls; (B) 84 idiopathic
CaOx stone formers; (C) 12 hyperuricosuric non-CaOx
stone formers; (D) 25 hyperuricosuric CaOx stone formers;
(E) 22 hyperuricosuric CaOx stone formers treated with
allopurinol; (F) 14 hyperuricosuric CaOx stone formers
treated with orthophosphate.

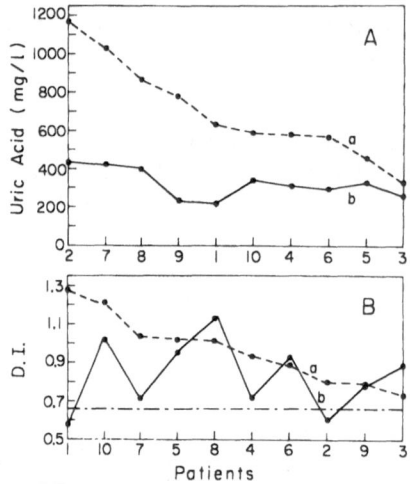

Fig. 2. Change in uric acid levels (A) and D.I. (B) before (broken
line) and after (solid line) incubation of urine sample
with sodium urate crystals.

860

patients. D.I. values above 1.07 are associated with stone formers while values below 0.66 are characteristic of normal subjects. The distribution of D.I. values of 26 hyperuricosuric calcium oxalate stone formers (HCaOxSF) was compared with that of 11 hyperuricosuric non-calcium oxalate stone formers (HNCaOxSF), 84 idiopathic CaOxSF and 146 normals.

The influence of the reduction of uric acid concentration on the D.I. value of HCaOxSF was examined. Samples of first morning urines of 10 stone formers were incubated with sodium urate crystals by the procedure of Pak et al[5]. The incubation caused a reduction in uric acid concentration to the saturation level. The D.I., uric acid, and sodium urate concentrations were determined in each sample before and after incubation. Allopurinol 200 to 300 mg/day was administered to 22 HCaOxSF. This dose reduced uric acid excretion to normal levels in all these patients. The D.I. was determined following 2 to 6 weeks of treatment.

Orthophosphate supplements at a daily dose of 600 to 900 mg of elemental phosphorus was administered to 14 HCaOxSF. In all patients it was initiated following the failure of allopurinol to reduce the D.I.; for 3 patients it was the initial form of treatment. The D.I. was determined after 2 to 6 weeks.

RESULTS AND DISCUSSION

The distribution of the D.I. values in the hyperuricosuric population was compared to that of the general population by the x^2 test. The hyperuricosuric and idiopathic CaOxSFs showed similar (P >0.7) distributions of D.I. values (Fig. 1). The distributions of D.I. values in non-SFs of both populations were very similar (P> 0.9). The difference within the hyperuricosuric group, between SFs and non-SFs was significant (P<0.01).

The effect of uric acid on the inhibitory potential was tested more directly in vitro by incubating urines of HCOxSFs with seed crystals of sodium urate thus causing a reduction of uric acid to the saturation level[5]. The relationship between the values of D.I. before and after incubation was assessed through a Kendall-Rank correlation coefficient. The relationship was insignificant (P < 0.10). This indicates that the removal of uric acid did not release any inhibitors of CaOx crystallization (Fig. 2).

Treatment of patients with allopurinol prevented uric acid crystals forming during the process of urine formation by bringing the uric acid concentration to normal. The comparison of the distributions of D.I. values before and after treatment was performed by Wilcoxon matched pair test. There was no significant change in D.I. values in 22 CaOxSFs (P>0.5). Thus it seems that uric acid is not the main factor in the HCaOxSF urines' inability to retard calcium oxalate precipitation.

In a recent report on the follow-up of idiopathic calcium oxalate stone formers treated with orthophosphate a significant decrease was noted in the D.I. values that correlated significantly with the reduced recurrence of CaOx stone formation[6]. In the 14 HCaOxSF treated with orthophosphate there was a significant (P < 0.001) reduction in D.I. values.

The D.I. value of urine is affected by all inhibitory and promoting substances present in urine. It could be expected that the removal of uric acid either by the in vivo or in vitro techniques would change the D.I. of uric acid interacted with any of the inhibitors. In both instances no change occurred. However, the D.I. values of hyperuricosuric CaOxSFs were significantly (P < 0.001) reduced by orthophosphate treatment.

These findings and the distribution of D.I. values in the different patient populations described would seem to suggest that HCaOxSFs suffer from the same yet undefined etiology as other CaOxSFs.

REFERENCES

1. N. S. Mandel and G. S. Mandel, in:"Urolithiasis:Clinical and Basic Research", L. H. Smith, W. G. Robertson, and B.Finlayson, eds., Plenum, New York (1981).
2. F. L. Coe, R. L. Lawton, R. B. Goldstein, and V. Tembe, Proc. Soc. Exp. Biol. Med. 149:926 (1975).
3. W. G. Robertson, F. Knowles, and M. Peacock, in:"Urolithiasis Research", H. Fleisch, W. G. Robertson, L. H. Smith, and W.Vahlensieck, eds., Plenum, London (1976).
4. S. Sarig, N. Garti, R. Azoury, Y. Wax, and S. Perlberg, J. Urol. 128:645 (1982).
5. C. Y. C. Pak, Y. Hayashi, and L. H. Arnold, Proc. Soc. Exp. Biol. Med. 153:83 (1976).
6. S. Sarig, N. Garti, R. Azoury, S. Perlberg, and Y. Wax, J. Urol. 129:1258 (1983).

FURTHER STUDIES ON THE POSSIBLE LITHOGENETIC ROLE OF URIC

ACID IN CALCIUM OXALATE STONE DISEASE

B. Baggio, G. Bambaro, E. Cicerello, F. Marchini,
and A. Borsatti

Institute of Internal Medicine, Postgraduate School of
Nephrology, University Hospital, University of Padova
35100 Padova, Italy

INTRODUCTION

The possible role of uric acid in aggravating recurrent
"idiopathic" calcium oxalate (CaOx) nephrolithiasis is still a
matter of discussion. Substantially, two hypotheses have been
advanced; the first proposes direct induction of CaOx precipitation
by uric acid crystals or colloidal uric acid[1,2], while the second
suggests that uric acid interferes with the glycosaminoglycan (GAGS)
inhibitors of CaOx stone formation[3-5]. Since the urine of CaOx
stone formers is generally free from uric acid crystals[6,7], theories
assigning a primary role to uric acid crystals seem untenable; that
there is binding between uric acid and GAGS which reduces GAGS
inhibitory activity on CaOx crystal formation seems more feasible,
as does the direct action of molecular or colloidal uric acid on
CaOx precipitation. The possible existence of a direct bond
between uric acid and GAGS is investigated in this study; in
addition the likelihood that uric acid directly promotes CaOx
precipitation has been evaluated.

MATERIALS, METHODS AND PATIENTS

A study was carried out to test the effect of uric acid on CaOx
crystallization by the direct addition of uric acid (up to 600 mg/l)
to a metastable solution of CaOx. After each uric acid addition,
the solution was passed through an Amicon UM2 membrane to check for
the formation of colloidal uric acid. The inhibitory effect was
evaluated according to the method of Ligabue et al[8].

Studies on the binding affinity of uric acid with GAGS were carried out in two ways. The <u>in vitro</u> studies consisted of adding to a 1.2 mM solution of uric acid in 0.5 M Tris-HCl buffer (pH 7.8) containing 1.2 mM NaCl, various concentrations of chondroitin sulphate (CS) or heparan sulphate (HS), together with 1 μC of ^{14}C-uric acid. After incubation for 24 h at room temperature, the solution was dialyzed overnight against the same buffer. The concentration of uric acid bound to GAGS was obtained from the ratio of ^{14}C-urate counts pre- and post-dialysis.

<u>In vivo</u> studies to verify the existence of binding between uric acid and GAGS in whole urine, consisted of measuring urinary excretion of both uric acid and GAGS in 4 groups of subjects with different urinary uric acid levels. The groups consisted of 22 normal subjects, 24 "idiopathic" CaOx renal stone formers, selected as previously described[9], 21 patients with biopsy-proven glomerulo-nephritis, and 15 proteinuric-free insulin-dependent diabetics. Urine was collected from 07.00 to 09.00 and filtered through a 0.22 μm Millipore filter, pH, uric acid before (U) and after filtration (UF) through a UM2 Amicon membrane, GAGS, and creatinine were measured. Uric acid and GAGS excretion were corrected per g of creatinine. The quantity of non-ultrafiltrable uric acid was obtained from the ratio U/UF.

RESULTS AND DISCUSSION

The effect of uric acid on CaOx crystallization is illustrated in Fig. 1, which shows that concentrations of uric acid up to 600 mg/l are incapable of modifying either nucleation or crystal growth. It is worth stressing that at concentrations over 300 mg/l, uric

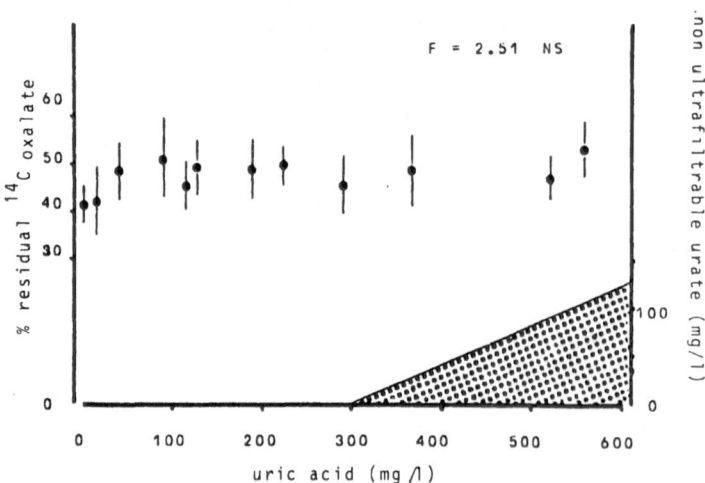

Fig. 1. Effect of uric acid on CaOx crystallization in vitro.

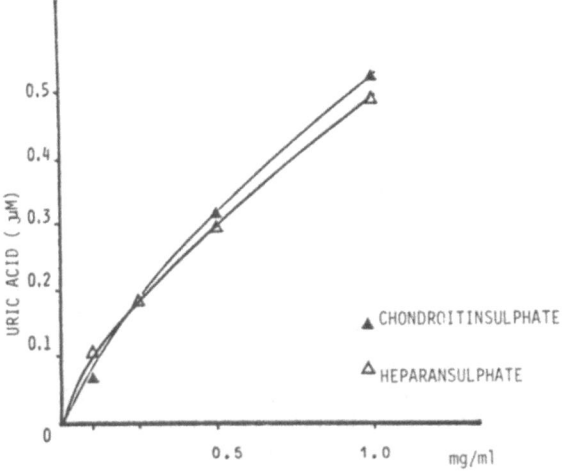

Fig. 2. Binding of uric acid with GAGS in vitro.

acid is present as a colloid as demonstrated by the appearance of quantities of uric acid which cannot be filtered through an Amicon UM2 membrane. This experiment, together with other similar observations[6,7] rules out the possibility that uric acid (molecular or colloidal) is able to promote CaOx crystallization directly.

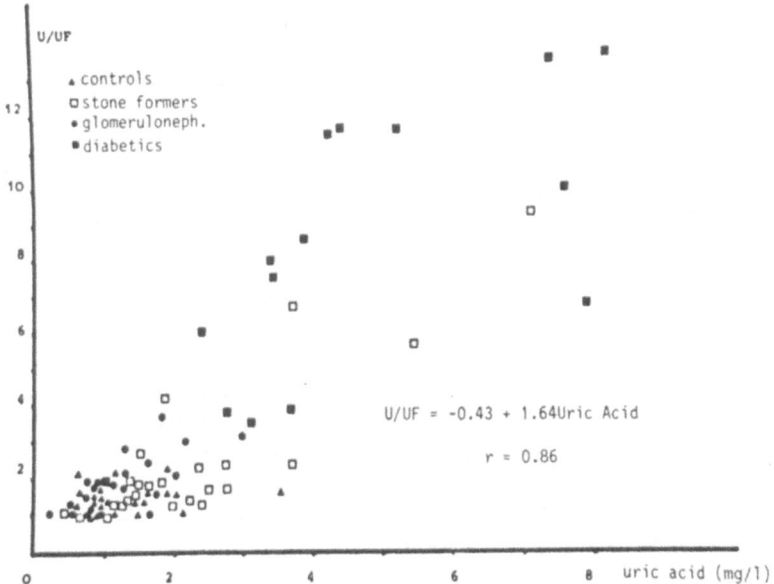

Fig. 3. Correlation between non-ultrafiltrable and total uric acid in urine.

Fig. 2 shows the binding of CS and HS to uric acid. The maximum binding capacity seems to be about 250 nmol/mg GAGS. Since the daily excretion of GAGS is about 100 mg, the total binding capacity can be estimated in 25 μmol of uric acid, which represent no more than 0.6% of a 24-h uric acid excretion. This low figure denies the possibility that uric acid plays a significant pathogenetic role in CaOx stone disease by reducing GAGS concentration.

No relationship was found between non-ultrafiltrable uric acid and GAGS concentrations, (not shown) whereas a fairly good correlation was observed between non-ultrafiltrable and total uric acid (Fig. 3). In our opinion, if non-ultrafiltrable uric acid were able to bind with GAGS, we should have found a direct relationship between non-ultrafiltrable uric acid and GAGS. On the other hand, the direct relationship observed between non-ultrafiltrable and total uric acid seems to support the existence of uric acid in a colloidal form.

Taken together our data seem to rule out the hypothesis that uric acid, either in molecular or in colloidal form, can promote CaOx stone formation by binding to GAGS. Furthermore, the hypothesis that molecular or colloidal uric acid directly promotes CaOx precipitation is not supported by our study.

REFERENCES

1. F. L. Coe, R. L. Lawton, R. B. Goldstein, and V. Tembe, Proc. Soc. Exp. Biol. Med. 149:926 (1975).
2. C. Y. C. Pak and L. H. Arnold. Proc. Soc. Exp. Biol. Med. 149:930 (1975).
3. W. G. Robertson, in:"Urolithiasis Research", H. Fleisch, W. G. Robertson, L. H. Smith and W. Vahlensieck, eds., Plenum, New York (1976).
4. B. Finlayson and L. Du Bois, Clin. Chem. Acta 84:203 (1978).
5. C. Y. C. Pak, K. Holt, and J. E. Zerwekh, Invest. Urol. 17:138 (1979).
6. C. Y. C. Pak, D. E. Barilla, K. Holt, L. Brinkley, R. Tolentino, and J. E. Zerwekh, Am. J. Med. 65:593 (1978).
7. J. G. Brockis and R. C. Bowyer, in:"Urolithiasis, Clinical and Basic Research", L. H. Smith, W. G. Robertson and B. Finlayson, eds., Plenum, New York (1981).
8. A. Ligabue, M. Fini, and W. G. Robertson, Clin. Chim. Acta 98:36 (1979).
9. B. Baggio, G. Gambaro, E. Ossi, S. Favaro, and A. Borsatti, J. Urol. 129:1161 (1983).

DOES THE BLADDER MUCOSA CONTRIBUTE TO URINARY INHIBITORY ACTIVITY?

K. A. Edyvane, R. L. Ryall and V. R. Marshall

Urology Unit, Dept. of Surgery, Flinders Medical Centre
Bedford Park, Australia

INTRODUCTION

Glycosaminoglycans and mucosubstances in the mucosal layer of
the bladder appear to have a bacterial anti-adherence function[1].
The washing of these macromolecules off the bladder wall may
contribute to the inhibitory activity of urine. The aim of this
study was to determine whether or not the bladder contributes to
urinary inhibitory activity.

MATERIALS AND METHODS

Saline bladder washings were obtained from 21 patients undergoing routine cystoscopy. Care was taken to exclude any who had
bladder infection or neoplasm. An initial urine sample was
collected via the cystoscope and the bladder rinsed of any residual
urine by filling and emptying twice with sterile normal saline. The
bladder was then filled and lavaged via the cystoscope for 30
seconds using a 50 ml syringe and the washout collected. In the
first 9 patients, washout and urine samples were checked visually
for blood contamination; in the remaining 12, the presence of blood
was excluded using Multistix test strips. The concentration of
creatinine in the washout and urine samples were determined. To
account for urinary contamination in the washout, a urine control
was prepared by diluting the urine sample with saline, to the same
creatinine concentration as the washout. After centrifugation and
filtration both the urine control and the washout were brought to a
final concentration of 1.00 mM Ca and 0.2 mM (COONa)2 by the
addition of calcium and oxalate. The inhibitory effect on calcium
oxalate crystal growth and aggregation was then measured[2].

RESULTS

In 8 of the 9 subjects in whom blood contamination was excluded by visual examination only, the percentage inhibition of crystal growth caused by the washout was significantly greater (P<0.05) than that caused by the diluted urine. Similarly, the bladder washouts consistently produced greater inhibition of aggregation compared with the urine controls (P 0.01). To determine whether or not this observation was real and not due to some minor trauma resulting from the lavaging technique, the effect of blood in this sytem was examined. Inhibitory activity was measured at concentrations <0.01% blood, at which blood cannot be detected visually.

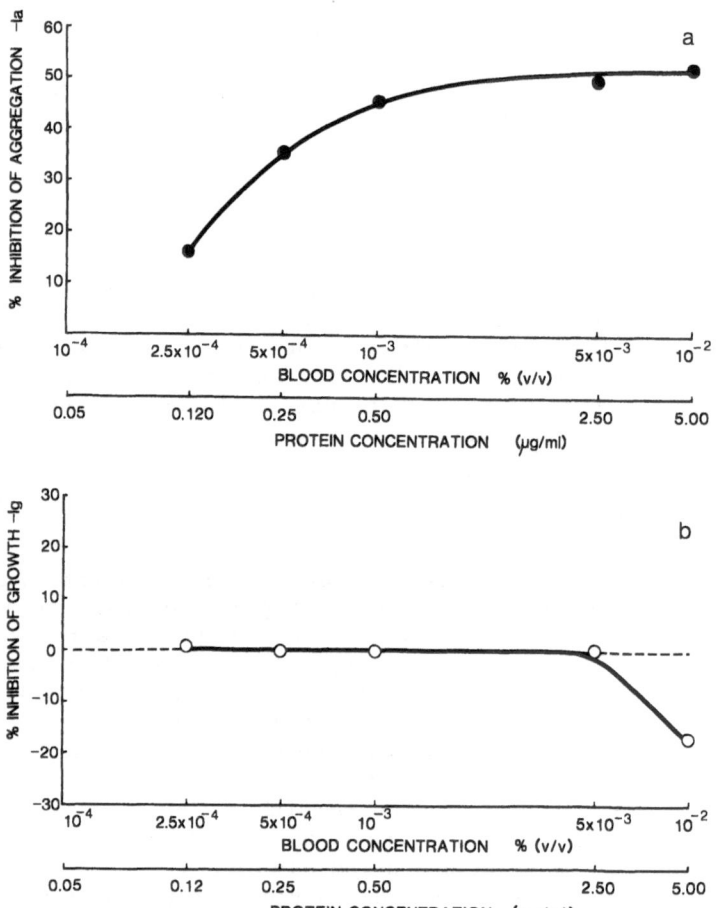

Fig. 1. The relationship between inhibition of calcium oxalate (a) crystal aggregation and (b) crystal growth and blood and protein concentration.

Figs. 1a and 1b show that crystal aggregation is more sensitive to blood contamination than is crystal growth. Aggregation was inhibited by 45% at a final blood concentration of 0.001% (= 0.5 µg/ml protein, Fig. 1a). However, at this concentration there was no effect on crystal growth (Fig. 1b). No effect on crystal growth was detected until a blood concentration of 0.01% was reached at which precipitated protein promoted crystal growth.

Figs. 2a and 2b show results for 12 more washouts and urines in which microscopic blood contamination was excluded. In contrast to our earlier observation, no increase in activity was found in the washout with regard to inhibition of aggregation (Fig. 2b).

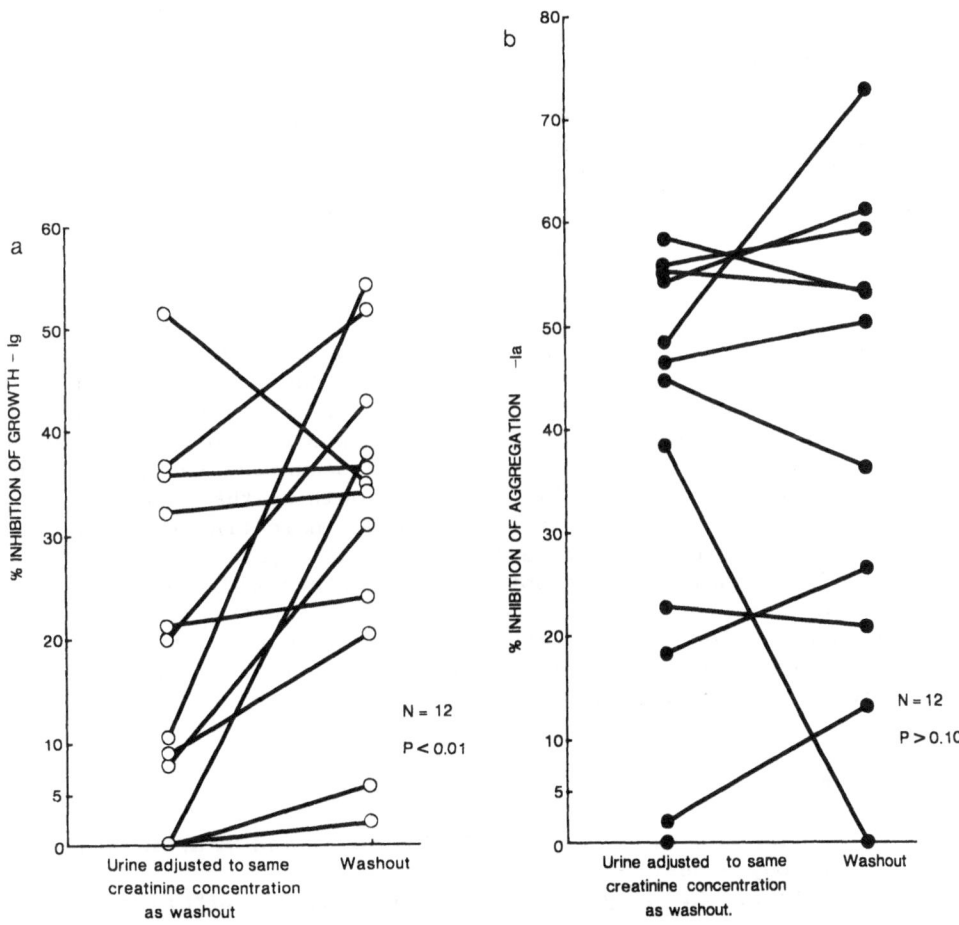

Fig. 2. Inhibition of calcium oxalate (a) crystal growth and (b) crystal aggregation in bladder washouts and urines adjusted to the same creatinine concentrations as the washouts.

Fig. 2a confirms that there is an increase in inhibitory activity with regard to growth in the washout compared to the urine controls (P<0.01). Protein analysis[3] of the washouts and urine controls indicated that all the protein in the washout could be attributed to urinary contamination.

DISCUSSION

The initial approach in this study was to assume that the kidney urine was the only source of inhibitors. If this were the case then, when bladder urine was diluted to the same creatinine concentration as that of the bladder washout, it would have been expected that the inhibitory activities would have been the same. However, our earlier set of results showed that the washouts consistently inhibited both growth and aggregation more strongly than did the urine controls. This indicates that the bladder is a source of substances that are inhibitors of calcium oxalate crystal growth and aggregation in vitro. Although the activity detected was far less than that in whole bladder urine, the washout fluid was only in contact with the bladder mucosa for 30 seconds. Under normal circumstances urine is in contact with the mucosa for many hours and in that time would be expected to contain more of these substances.

The finding that microscopic levels of blood could influence crystal aggregation led to the collection of 12 more washouts where we excluded contamination by the use of the Multistix. The absence of any significant increase in inhibition of aggregation in the washout suggested that our earlier result was probably due to micro-scopic amounts of blood. However, even accounting for the presence of blood, an increase in inhibition of growth in the washout compared with the urine control was found, indicating that the bladder is contributing some inhibitor(s) of crystal growth. The nature of the inhibitor has not yet been determined, but it does not appear to be a protein. Our results have shown that trace levels of blood can affect crystal aggregation. Therefore, studies measuring urinary inhibitory activity must take into account the effects of even microscopic amounts of blood.

REFERENCES

1. C. L. Parsons, C. Greenspan, S. W. Moore, and S. G. Mulholland, Urology 9:48 (1977).
2. R. G. Ryall, R. L. Ryall, and V. R. Marshall, in:"Urinary Stone", R. L. Ryall, G. Brockis, V. R. Marshall, and B. Finlayson, eds., Churchill Livingstone, Melbourne (1984).
3. A. Bensadoun and D. Weinstein, Analyt. Biochem. 70:241 (1976).

THE CONTRIBUTION OF THE BLADDER TO CALCIUM OXALATE CRYSTAL

GROWTH INHIBITION IN VOIDED URINE

X. Martin, T. J. Opgenorth, P. G. Werness,
R. T. Rundquist, J. C. Romero, and L. H. Smith

Nephrology Research Unit, Mayo Clinic and Mayo
Foundation, Rochester, Minnesota, U.S.A. and Service
d'Urologie et de Chirurgie de la Transplantation
Hôpital E. Herriot, Lyon, France

INTRODUCTION

Large molecular weight inhibitors of calcium oxalate crystal growth and aggregation have been partially characterized in human urine[1]. These inhibitors include glycosaminoglycans, RNA-like substances, and acidic glycoproteins, and are thought to represent the most important part of the inhibition of calcium oxalate crystal formation in urine. The uroepithelium of the bladder is covered with the glycocalyx, a mucous coat containing glycosaminoglycans[2]. The existence of glycosaminoglycans at the level of the bladder opens the possibility that part of the mucous substance covering the bladder may be discharged in urine, thus modifying its composition with respect to glycosaminoglycans, and its ability to inhibit calcium oxalate crystal growth.

The purpose of this study was to compare the amount and chemical nature of the inhibitors of calcium oxalate crystal growth present in kidney urine, with that present in voided, bladder urine.

MATERIALS AND METHODS

Nine female dogs (weighing 13.8 $\pm$ 2 kg) fed the same standard diet were used in these experiments. Urine collections were performed before and after bilateral ureterostomies in order to obtain bladder and kidney urine. All urine collections corresponded to a 6-h period, and were performed at the same time of the day. Bladder urine was collected in a metabolic cage, and also by direct suprapubic puncture. For kidney urine collection, the dogs were semi-immobilized in a harness in order to prevent leakage

871

from the collecting device. Normal renal function, pre- and post-operatively, was assured by the absence of changes of plasma creatinine, creatinine clearance and the absence of dilatation of the upper urinary tract post-operatively on intravenous pyelography.

The inhibition of calcium oxalate crystal growth was measured using a seeded crystal growth system[3]. The alcian blue precipitable material (ABPM) was determined in urine samples by the method of Whiteman[4]. The ABPM is believed to correspond in urine mainly to glycosaminoglycans but also RNA-like material, and other glycoproteins.

RESULTS

Calcium oxalate crystal growth inhibition concentration increased from kidney to bladder urine (0.07 ± 0.01 IU/mg creatinine and 0.14 ± 0.03 IU/mg creatinine, respectively); mean change $+ 0.07 \pm 0.02$ IU/mg creatinine; $P<0.02$). Alcian blue precipitable material showed a parallel increase from kidney to bladder urine (0.08 ± 0.02 mg ABPM/mg creatinine and 0.14 ± 0.02 mg/mg creatinine, respectively; $P<0.02$). A correlation ($r = 0.85$; $P<0.01$) was found between the individual kidney-bladder changes in calcium oxalate crystal growth inhibition and alcian blue precipitable material concentration.

DISCUSSION

The measured inhibition of calcium oxalate crystal growth present in urine increases as the urine moves from kidney to bladder. The parallel increase of the alcian blue precipitable material observed in bladder urine suggests that this fraction is responsible for the observed increase in calcium oxalate crystal growth inhibition. The presence of glycosaminoglycans at the level of the glycocalyx make them a likely source of the increased inhibition observed in bladder urine, but other more potent inhibitors such as RNA-like substances or other acidic polyanions may be involved.

The increase in calcium oxalate crystal growth inhibition observed in bladder urine, as compared to the values of kidney urine lead to several observations and speculations: (1) the measurement of calcium oxalate crystal growth inhibition in voided urine may be an inaccurate estimation of the inhibition present at the level of the kidney. The addition by the bladder of calcium oxalate crystal growth inhibition in urine might mask possible decreased levels of inhibition that may be expected from stone formers; (ii) citrate, pyrophosphate, as well as other inhibitors of renal origin may represent a larger proportion of the calcium oxalate crystal growth inhibition than previously thought; (iii) characterization and

872

separation of calcium oxalate crystal inhibitors may be more
fruitful from kidney urine.

ACKNOWLEDGEMENT

This work was supported in part by research grant AM 20605 from
the National Institutes of Health, and by the Fondation pour la
Recherche Médicale, Paris, France.

REFERENCES

1. W. G. Robertson, D. S. Scurr, and C. M. Bridge, J. Cryst. Growth
   53:182 (1981).
2. C. L. Parson, C. Stauffer, and J. D. Schmidt, Science 208:605
   (1980).
3. J. L. Meyer and L. H. Smith, Invest. Urol.13:31(1975)
4. P. Whiteman, Biochem. J. 131:351 (1973).

EFFECTS OF HUMAN URINE ON THE AGGREGATION OF CALCIUM OXALATE CRYSTALS: NORMAL PERSONS VERSUS STONE-FORMERS

G. W. Drach, K. Springman, B. Gottung, and
A. Randolph

Depts. of Surgery and Chemical Engineering, University
of Arizona, Tucson, Arizona 85724, U.S.A.

INTRODUCTION

During the last 10 years we have carried out experiments on the continuous crystallization of calcium oxalate (CaOx)[1-4]. These have shown a surprising lack of difference between normal and stone-forming urine (diluted to 5%) when it is added to our synthetic urine[3]. In addition, we have had technical problems with our MSMPR system which resulted in a crystal product which represented only 30% of that expected[4]. Recently this has been increased to 90% or more[5]. Although there was no significant difference in the nucleation rate between stone-forming and normal urine, there was a trend towards increased nucleation in the presence of stone-forming urine which led us to suspect that aggregation was playing a part in the process of stone-formation[5-7]. Others have studied CaOx crystal aggregation in one form or another[8-11] but they have not applied continuous flow techniques to their studies. We have now used our continuous flow (mixed suspension-mixed product removal) (MSMPR) system in series with a Couette agglomerator to analyze further the effects of addition of human urine to synthetic urine.

METHODS

Crystallization was carried out in a continously stirred vessel of about 450 ml total capacity. Sixty-six 3 mm glass beads were added to the slurry, which was bottom-stirred with a Teflon-coated magnetic bar. Input consisted of an artificial urine described previously[4], with or without addition of 5% human urine (v/v), containing $[Ca] = 6$ mmol and $[Ox] = 0.6$ mmol[5]. Tau (duration of average crystal in crystallizer) was set at 10 mins. Crystallizer output was instantly analyzed on a PDI zone-sensing particle counting analyzer, with data reduction on a PDP8 computer to yield values for the nucleation rate (B^O) linear crystal growth rate (G) and total crystal mass produced (M_T) (Table 1). Alternatively, output from the crystallizer was diverted to the agglomerator, and subsequently analyzed. For this study, an agglomerator rotation of 80 rpm was used as our standard as faster rotation (near 150 rpm) resulted in significant disaggregation[5]. The values chosen for comparison of agglomeration were: $\Delta \bar{L}_{4,3(A-C)}$ = difference in mass-weighted average size between crystallizer (C) and aggregator (A) and ΔN_{A-C} = difference in number of particles $>$15 μm (or $>$24 μm) between A and C. Initial experiments by Gottung[5] at 150 rpm compared 5 each normal and stone-forming persons. For the current experiments, we have compared 10 normal persons with 8 stone forming persons. Within the latter group, none was on specific therapy. Data analyses were by one-way anova tests between control (no urine addition), normal or stone-forming groups.

RESULTS

Table 1 shows the basic crystallization of the 3 groups. Addition of human urine resulted in a slightly increased growth rate and decreased nucleation rate when compared to control experiments. Only the control nucleation rate differed significantly, however, from the urine addition experiments[3]. Table 2 shows the changes that occurred when the crystallizer output passed through the aggregator. Addition of any urine markedly inhibited the aggregation, which occurred rapidly and extensively in the control experiments. There was a tendency for stone-formers' urines to allow larger crystal aggregates, but only the mean particle size of stone formers was significantly greater than in normals. The numbers of larger particles were not significantly different. Since, however, aggregator function is dependent on the particle number and size of the input from the crystallizer, and these values differed in the different experiments, the observations in Table 2 were normalized using the crystallizer output of all particles in the range 5 um to infinity. After normalization, the stone-formers showed significantly larger numbers of large particles than did the normals (Table 3). Nevertheless, urine from either group strongly inhibited aggregation when compared to non-urine controls.

DISCUSSION

After addition of 5% (v/v) human urine to synthetic urine supersaturated with calcium oxalate, crystal growth and total mass did not differ significantly between the control, normal or stone-former studies. The values for B^O were significantly higher in the control experiments than for either human group. This contrasts

876

Table 1. Crystallization Observations

Variable	Control	Normals	Stone-formers
(G) (um/min)	0.33 ± 0.02[*]	0.36 ± 0.03	0.35 ± 0.03
(B^O) (n/ml/min)	15208 ± 2171[*]	11669 ± 15909	11256 ± 1678
(M_T) (mg/l)	35.8 ± 4.5	37.7 ± 7.2	33.6 ± 5.9

[*] Differs from normals and stone-formers (P<0.02).

Table 2. Aggregation Observations

Variable	Control	Normals	Stone-formers
$\Delta \bar{L}_{4,3}$ (μm)	3.89[*]	1.46	1.72[**]
$>15_{A-C}$(n)	1360[*]	658	916
$>24_{A-C}$(n)	438[*]	13	22

[*] Control > stone-formers (P<0.01); stone-formers > normal (P=0.05).

Table 3. Normalized Aggregation Observations

	Control	Normals	Stone-formers
$\Delta \bar{L}_{4,3}$N	5.6×10^{-4}	2.1×10^{-5}	2.5×10^{-4}[**]
>15N	4.1×10^{-2}[*]	1.1×10^{-2}	1.8×10^{-2}[**]
>24N	1.3×10^{-2}[*]	2.2×10^{-4}	4.8×10^{-4}[***]

[*] Control different from normals and stone-formers (P<0.001);
[**] stone-formers > normals (P<0.05); [***] stone-formers > normals (P=0.05).

with the earlier observations[3,4] which were reproduced using only the high molecular weight fractions from urine[6]. Significant technical modifications have occurred since our earlier studies[5]. It seems likely, then, that these different observations in our present experiments are results of improvements in methodology.

Kraljevich also produced changes in aggregation of calcium oxalate crystals with addition of high molecular weight urinary extracts. Using SEM she reported only qualitative results[6]. Gottung established that one can measure calcium oxalate crystallization and aggregation utilizing the MSMPR crystallizer and Couette agglomerator serially attached to a particle analyzer[5]. Her human urine experiments, which were done as in this study, failed to show significant differences between normal and stone-forming persons. Theoretical analysis of her aggregation system revealed that this was owing to use of too great an rpm in the aggregator, with resulting disaggregation of the particles. Adjustment of our present aggregator rpm to 80 has overcome this problem.

We are now certain that urine contains an inhibitor of growth and aggregation of CaOx crystals, in agreement with previous investigators. Our serial analysis system allows us to hypothesize that the major difference in CaOx crystallization between normal and stone-forming persons rests in a deficiency in aggregation inhibition in stone-formers, so that they are capable of generating larger particle masses. Presence of a bi-modal particle size distribution for crystals from urine of stone formers with a second mode of large particles has been noted by ourselves and others[12,13], and we believe, is the result of aggregation inhibitor deficiency. It seems likely that the high molecular weight fractions of urine account for this deficiency[4,6,14-16].

REFERENCES

1. J. D. Miller, A. D. Randolph, and G. W. Drach, J. Urol. 117:342 (1977).
2. G. W. Drach, A. D. Randolph, and J. D. Miller, J. Urol. 119:99 (1978).
3. G. W. Drach, S. Thorson, and A. D. Randolph, J. Urol. 123:519 (1980).
4. G. W. Drach, Z. Kraljevich, and A. D. Randolph, J. Urol. 127:805 (1982).
5. B. Gottung "Calcium Oxalate Agglomeration in Urine-like Mother Liquors", Ph.D. Thesis, University of Arizona (1983).
6. Z. Kraljevich, "Effect of Urinary Macromolecules on Crystallization of Calcium Oxalate in Synthetic Urine Solutions", Ph.D. Thesis, University of Arizona (1981).
7. A. D. Randolph and G. W. Drach, J. Crystal Growth 53:195 (1981).
8. T. Koide, M. Takemoto, H. Itatani, M. Takaha, and T. Sonoda, Invest. Urol. 18:382 (1981).
9. R. L. Ryall, C. J. Gagley, and V. R. Marshall, Invest. Urol. 18:401 (1981).
10. D. N. Adamthwaite, Br. J. Urol. 55:95 (1983).
11. W. G. Robertson, M. Peacock, and B. E. C. Nordin, Clin. Chim. Acta 43:31 (1973).
12. J. D. Miller, "Crystallization Kinetics of Calcium Oxalate in Simulated Urine", Ph.D. Thesis, University of Arizona (1976).
13. W. G. Robertson, Clin. Chim. Acta 26:105 (1969).
14. D. J. White, T. Christofferson, T. S. Herman, A. C. Lanzalaco, and G. H. Nancollas, J. Urol. 129:175 (1983).
15. R. L. Ryall, R. M. Harnet, and V. R. Marshall, Clin. Chim. Acta 112:349 (1981).
16. W. G. Robertson, D. S. Scurr, and C. M. Bridge, J. Crystal Growth 53:182 (1981).

DETERMINATION OF STONE FORMING RISK BY MEASURING CRYSTALLIZATION INHIBITOR ACTIVITY IN URINE WITH A GEL MODEL

C. Röhrborn, H.-J. Schneider, and E. W. Rugendorff

1st Urological Dept., Falkeneck Hospital Braunfels
F.R.G.

INTRODUCTION

To study the risk of crystal formation in urine[1], we developed
a gel model to measure the crystallization inhibitor activity and to
investigate the mode of action of various inhibitors[2,3].

MATERIALS AND METHODS

Our gel model[2,3] is based on previous reports of calcium
oxalate crystallization in gel systems[4,5]. With it we tested the
inhibitory activity of citrate and $MgCl_2$ solutions (1.0 to to 200
mM). That of urine was measured in spontaneously voided samples
and 24-h samples to which thymol crystals were added to prevent the
growth of bacteria. Buffering of the gel was achieved with
cacodylate at pH 6. To examine the effect of oral treatment with
magnesium and alkali, 10 healthy persons collected 24-h urines after
loading with 10 g K_6Na_6 pentacitrate hydrate (Uralyt-U[R]) and 60 mmol
Mg^{++} (Biomagnesin[R]). At the same time in vitro tests were performed
by enrichment of spontaneous urine samples with $MgCl_2$ and citrate
solutions. Finally, the inhibitory activity in the urine of
recurrent stone formers and healthy controls was compared.

RESULTS

The correlation between the inhibitor index (I) and the concentration of citrate or $MgCl_2$ added is shown in Fig. 1. Inhibition
begins within the physiological range.

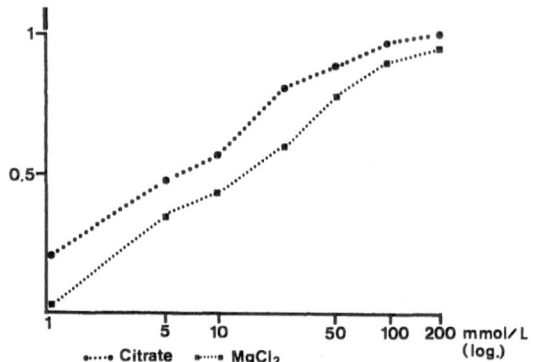

Fig. 1. Diagram showing the correlation between inhibitor index and
corresponding molarity of citrate and $MgCl_2$ solutions
(semi-logarithmic).

Spontaneous urine samples were supplemented with citrate, $MgCl_2$
and $CaCl_2$ and the inhibitory index determined before and after
addition of these ions (Fig. 2). After addition of 3 to 5 mmol/l,
a rise in the inhibitory activity can be clearly seen for citrate
and $MgCl_2$ (not shown). After intersecting the curve of the pure
inhibitor solution, which is dependent upon the index of the native
urine, the indices correspond to the respective concentrations of
pure inhibitor. Addition of $CaCl_2$ results in a decrease in
inhibitory activity (Fig. 2).

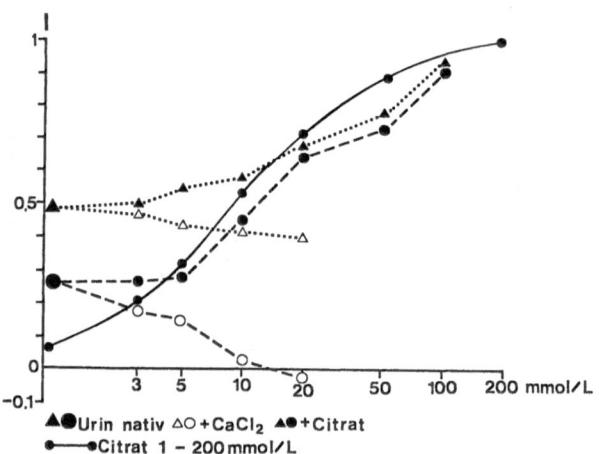

Fig. 2. Inhibitor index of native urine samples before and after
enrichment with citrate and $CaCl_2$ solutions. The
correlation between I and molarity of pure inhibitor
solution is drawn for comparison.

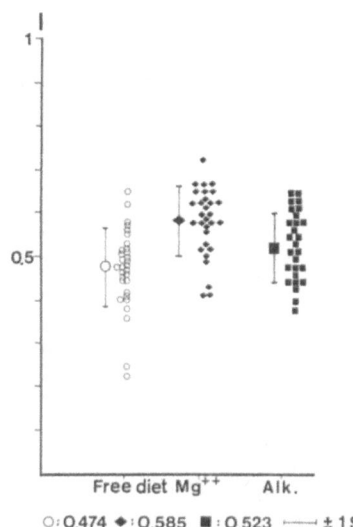

Fig. 3. Inhibitor indices of all 24-h urine samples (n = 30) on an unrestricted diet, plus magnesium and alkalinizing agents. Mean indices are characterized by larger symbols.

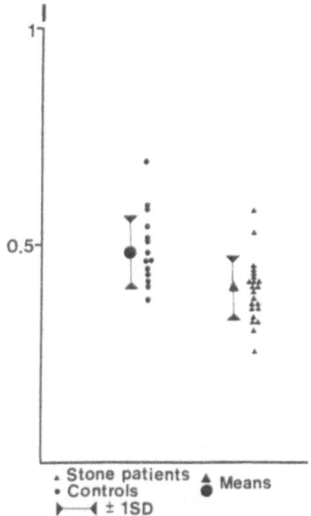

Fig. 4. Inhibitor indices of pooled 24-h urines of recurrent stone formers (n = 22) and healthy controls (n = 14). The difference between the means is significant (0.01>P>0.001).

Ten healthy persons received an oral load of magnesium or alkali. Three pooled 24-h urines collected on an unrestricted diet and during each loading period were collected and analyzed for volume, pH, specific gravity, calcium, magnesium, citrate, oxalate and creatinine and the inhibitor index determined. The following changes were statistically significant: (i) an increase in pH with both types of load (P<0.001); (ii) an increase of magnesium level with Biomagnesin[R] from 3.18 to 7.76 mmol/l (P<0.001); (iii) an increase of citrate level from 2.16 to 3.3 with Biomagnesin[R] and to 3.65 mmol/l with Uralyt-U[R] (P<0.001); and (iv) a decrease of calcium from 4.02 to 2.28 mmol/l with Uralyt-U[R] (P<0.01). As expected, the inhibitor indices of the urine samples rose in proportion to the increase in the magnesium and citrate levels and the decrease in the calcium level (Fig. 3). The mean value for all persons was 0.474 on the unrestricted diet, 0.585 with Biomagnesin[R] and 0.523 with Uralyt-U[R] (P<0.05).

Finally the inhibitor indices of 22 recurrent calcium stone formers (mean value 0.404) and that of 14 healthy controls (mean value 0.497), were significantly different (P<0.024) (Fig. 4).

DISCUSSION

This study demonstrates that changes in the composition of the urine which influence the formation of calcium oxalate crystals can be measured and reproduced by means of a gel model. The gel model is simple and inexpensive, providing a means to determine the need for treatment and the response to treatment with oral preparations containing magnesium and citrate. It also should facilitate the long-term follow-up of stone-formers.

ACKNOWLEDGEMENTS

This work was supported by a grant from Temmler Werke, Marburg, and Madaus & Co., Köln. We wish to thank Mr R Mees for technical advice and Prof. Kienholz and his assistants for carrying out the chemical analyses.

REFERENCES

1. P. Leskovar, R. Hartung, and J. Riedel, Med. Welt 30:937 (1979).
2. H.-J. Schneider, C. Rohrborn, and E. W. Rugendorff, World J. Urol. 1:155 (1983).
3. H.-J. Schneider, C. Rohrborn, and E. W. Rugendorff, Fortschr. Urol. Nephrol. 22:365 (1984).
4. S. Bisaillon and R. Tawashi, J. Pharm. Sci. 64:958 (1975).
5. R. Phaneuf-Mimeault and R. Tawashi, Eur. Urol. 3:171 (1977).

MACROMOLECULES IN WHOLE URINE THAT PROMOTE CALCIUM OXALATE

AND PHOSPHATE CRYSTAL FORMATION

G. A. Rose and S. Sulaiman

St. Peter's Hospital and the Institute of Urology
London, U.K.

INTRODUCTION

Qualitative studies[1] have shown that Tamm-Horsfall mucoprotein
(T-H) increases both calcium oxalate and calcium phosphate crystals
formed when dilute whole urine is rapidly evaporated.   This was
confirmed quantitatively for calcium oxalate[2] but on addition of T-H
to urinary ultrafiltrates the recovery of both crystal types formed
was incomplete suggesting that there might be in urine a second
macromolecule crystal promoter.   This possibility is explored.

METHODS

The methods have been described fully elsewhere[1-5]. Crystal-
free urine samples were evaporated at 37^0C on a rotary evaporator to
1250 mosmol/kg at pH 5.3 or 6.8 for calcium oxalate and calcium
phosphate studies respectively.   For oxalate precipitation studies
^{14}C-oxalate was added to urine and the recovered radio-activity in
the precipitate taken as a measure of crystal formation.   For the
larger calcium phosphate precipitates, calcium was measured by
atomic absorption flame spectrophotometry.   Sodium dodecyl sulphate
(SDS; 0.3% or more) was added to whole urine prior to evaporation to
reduce aggregation of T-H.   The effect of this upon crystal
formation after evaporation was studied.   Urine samples were
ultrafiltered with molecular weight cut off of 10,000 daltons and
the ultrafiltrates and urine combined in various ratios, all the
mixtures evaporated to the same osmolarity and crystal formation
assessed.   Fractions that trigger crystal formation were studied by
double ultrafiltration using molecular weight cut-offs at 10,000,
100,000, and 300,000 daltons before evaporation.

883

RESULTS

For the quantitative studies of promotion of calcium phosphate crystal formation by T-H mucoprotein at pH 6.8, twenty urine samples were treated with T-H sufficient to give a final concentration after evaporation of 35 mg/l . Whole urine and the ultrafiltrates with and without added T-H were evaporated to 1250 mosmol/kg. ^{14}C-oxalate was counted in the dissolved precipitates. The results are summarised in Table 1 (section A) but are available in full elsewhere[3]. Both the fall in precipitation on ultrafiltration and the rise on adding T-H were statistically significant.

The effect of T-H mucoprotein on the clumping of calcium phosphate crystals was studied as described above in 20 samples of urine. The precipitates were sieved through a nylon mesh of 10 μm pore size. Both sieved and whole precipitates were measured and the results are shown in brief in Table 1 (section B and C) but are reported in full elsewhere[3]. There was a statistically significant fall in the percentage of precipitate retained on the sieve following ultrafiltration and this was largely restored on adding T-H to the ultrafiltrates.

Table 1. Effect of Ultrafiltration on Whole Urine at pH 6.8 and of Addition of T-H Mucoprotein to Ultrafiltrates on Calcium Precipitates after Evaporation.

Calcium precipitated (mmol/l)	Whole urine Mean (range)	Ultrafiltrate (U/F) Mean (range)	U/F + T-H Mean (range)
A. Whole precipitate	20.89 (1.1 - 46.5)	4.82 (0.63 - 15.2)	14.38 (1.2 - 30.3)
B. Precipitate retained	9.27 (0.21 - 25.3)	0.75 (0.05 - 2.2)	7.32 (0.31 - 21.5)
C. %Precipitate retained	44.2	15.6	50.9

These results on the relation between the concentration of macromolecules to the triggering of crystal formation are shown briefly in Table 2 and in full elsewhere[3]. It can be seen that there are direct relationships between the concentrations of macromolecules and sizes of precipitates of both calcium oxalate and calcium phosphate.

In the differential ultrafiltration studies, samples of urine were ultrafiltered first with a molecular weight cut-off of 300,000

Table 2. Effect of Concentration of Macromolecules upon Crystal Formation Relative to Whole Urine (Means $\pm$ SEM).

% Whole urine mixed with U/F	0	10	25	50	75
^{14}C-oxalate precipitated at pH 5.3	10.0$\pm$1.9	16.1$\pm$2.0	28.9$\pm$1.9	55.2$\pm$3.5	83.8$\pm$5.2
Calcium precipitated at pH 6.8	15.2$\pm$1.5	27.9$\pm$1.7	44.4$\pm$1.7	67.1$\pm$2.3	84.7$\pm$1.9

Table 3. Means ($\pm$ SEM) of ^{14}C-Oxalate or Calcium Precipitated Following Evaporation of Ultrafiltrates. Results are Expressed as % of Those from Corresponding Whole Urines.

Measurement	n	Molecular weight cut-off		
		300,000	100,000	10,000
^{14}C-Oxalate	14	33.0 $\pm$ 5.1		21.4 $\pm$ 5.2
^{14}C-Oxalate	10	–	34.0 $\pm$ 11.0	25.5 $\pm$ 9.1
Calcium	14	23.3 $\pm$ 5.0	–	10.4 $\pm$ 3.3

or 100,000 daltons and secondly with a molecular weight cut-off of 10,000 daltons. It was shown that the first ultrafiltration removed all the measurable T-H. All samples (urines and ultrafiltrates) were evaporated to 1250 mosmol/kg and the precipitates examined for ^{14}C-oxalate or calcium. The results are shown in brief in Table 3 and in full elsewhere[5]. Ultrafiltration with a 300,000 dalton cut-off reduced the precipitates formed by 33% of the value for whole urine but there was a further reduction with ultrafiltration using a 10,000 dalton cut-off. However, when the first ultrafiltration employed a 100,000 dalton cut-off, there was only a small reduction after the second ultrafiltration.

The effect of addition of SDS to urine was studied on 15 samples of urine at pH 5.3 and another 15 at pH 6.8 were evaporated to 1250 mosmol/kg with and without added SDS. The precipitated ^{14}C-oxalate or calcium were measured. The results are given in full elsewhere[4]. Briefly 0.3, 0.6, and 1.2% SDS reduced ^{14}C-oxalate precipitated to 61.1, 53.0, and 66.9% of control values. Corresponding results for calcium precipitated at pH 6.8, were 52.6, 46.5, and 46.8% respectively.

DISCUSSION

These findings confirmed quantitatively three points previously found qualitatively[1]. First, removal of macromolecules clearly reduces the calcium phosphate precipitate formed in urine after rapid evaporation to 1250 mosmol/kg. Second, this reduction is largely, but not entirely, abolished by addition of physiological quantities of T-H to the ultrafiltrates. The lack of completion of this restoration might indicate that insufficient T-H had been added or that there is a second promoter of calcium phosphate precipitation removed on ultrafiltration. Third, clumping of calcium phosphate crystals is reduced on removal of macromolecules and restored by addition of T-H.

The promotion of both calcium oxalate and phosphate crystals in the urine is proportional to the concentration of macromolecules, and therefore had more T-H been added to the ultrafiltrates restoration of total crystals precipitated could have been complete. However, the differential ultrafiltration studies show that there may be a second promoter of calcium phosphate precipitation with a molecular weight less than 300,000 daltons.

Aggregation of T-H is dependent upon ionic strength and for this reason an effect upon crystal formation is only seen in concentrated urine. Studies performed under artificial conditions at low ionic strength will clearly not show the effect[6]. Addition of SDS dissociates T-H[7] and it can be shown that when SDS is added to urine it also reduces calcium oxalate and phosphate precipitation, again suggesting that it is the aggregated T-H which is active in promoting crystal formation.

ACKNOWLEDGMENTS

S. Sulaiman received a grant from the Government of Iraq.

REFERENCES

1. P. C. Hallson and G. A. Rose, Lancet (i):1000 (1979).
2. G. A. Rose and S. Sulaiman, J. Urol. 127:177 (1982).
3. G. A. Rose and S. Sulaiman, Urol. Res. (in pres).
4. G. A. Rose and S. Sulaiman, Urol. Int. 39:68 (1984).
5. G. A. Rose and S. Sulaiman, Urol Int. 39:144 (1984).
6. T. Kitamura and C. Y. C. Pak, J. Urol. 127:1024 (1982).
7. K. H. Bichler, H. Haupt, G. Uhlemann, and H. G. Schwick, Urol. Res. 1:50 (1973).

THE INHIBITION OF CALCIUM OXALATE CRYSTAL GROWTH BY CHONDROITIN
SULPHATES, HEPARIN, PENTOSAN POLYSULPHATE AND TAMM-HORSFALL
GLYCOPROTEIN

B. Fellström, B. G. Danielson, S. Ljunghall, and
B. Wikström

Dept. of Internal Medicine, University Hospital
S-751 85 Uppsala, Sweden

INTRODUCTION

A large number of the urinary constituents have been reported
to inhibit calcium oxalate crystal growth and aggregation.
Pyrophosphate, for example, is a potent inhibitor of crystal growth[1]
and glycosaminoglycans potent inhibitors of crystal aggregation[2].
Regarding urinary macromolecular inhibitors of calcium oxalate
crystallization, a number of substances such as glycosaminoglycans[2],
polypeptides[3], polyribonucleotides[4] and glycoproteins[5] have been
claimed to be of importance. There has also been a debate as to
whether uromucoid or Tamm-Horsfall glycoprotein is a promoter or an
inhibitor of the crystallization process[6]. The purpose of the
present study is to compare the inhibition of calcium oxalate
crystal growth by pyrophosphate, polyanionic glycosaminoglycans and
Tamm-Horsfall glycoprotein. This comparison has also been extended
to include two drugs with a structure similar to pyrophosphate and
heparin respectively.

METHODS

The inhibition of calcium oxalate crystal growth was measured
by a seeded crystal procedure, whereby seed crystals of calcium
oxalate were added to a metastable calcium oxalate solution together
with the inhibitor to be tested[7]. Crystal growth was monitored by
measuring ^{14}C-oxalate remaining in solution. The crystal growth
experiments were performed at pH 6 in 140 mM NaCl. A simplified
procedure for estimating the degree of inhibition was adopted and is
described in Fig. 1.

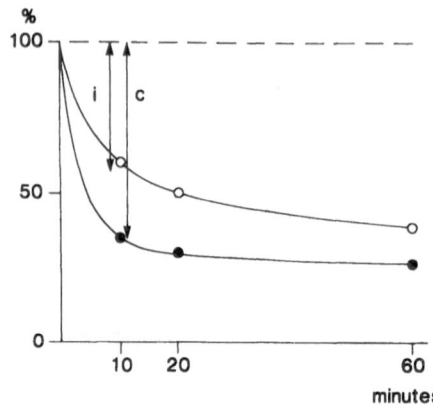

Fig. 1. Principle for calculation of inhibitory activity of calcium
oxalate crystal growth. Crystal growth was monitored by
^{14}C-oxalate remaining in solution (%) 10, 20 and 60 min
after the addition of seed crystals to the inhibited (o)
and the uninhibited systems (●).
Inhibition = 100 (c-i)/c(%).

Tamm-Horsfall glycoprotein was prepared according to the
original procedure[8]. Chondroitin sulphates A, B, C (CS-A, CS-B,
CS-C), heparin and pyrophosphate were obtained from Sigma. The
trisodium-phosphone-formate (Foscarnet[R]) and the semisynthetic low
molecular weight heparin analogue, pentosan polysulphate (SP 54),
were kindly provided by Astra and Pharmacia, respectively.

In order to evaluate the relative importance of these
inhibitors in vivo, a comparison was made of their inhibitory
activity at concentrations normally found in urine. It was assumed
that the concentration of pyrophosphate was 4 mg/l, the
concentration of chondroitin sulphates 7.5 mg/l. Tamm-Horsfall
glycoprotein was tested in the concentration received in the above
preparation from urine. The urinary concentration of SP 54 was
assumed to be 25 mg/l after an oral dose of 400 mg.

RESULTS

Among the polyanions, heparin was the most efficient inhibitor
(Table 1). The chondroitin sulphates exerted about 40% of the
inhibitory activity of heparin. There was no significant
difference in inhibition between the various chondroitin sulphates.
SP 54 inhibited crystal growth, which was 80% of activity found from
heparin. Pyrophosphate was, however, the most efficient inhibitor
tested. Phosphone-formate exerted about 40% of the inhibition of
pyrophosphate.

888

Table 1. Calcium Oxalate Crystal Growth Inhibition (%) by
          Expected Concentrations of Potential Inhibitors in Urine.

Tamm-Horsfall glycoprotein	17%
Chondroitin sulphate A (7.5 mg/l)	16%
Chondroitin sulphate C (7.5 mg/l)	19%
Pentosan polysulphate (25 mg/l)	40%
Pyrophosphate (4 mg/l)	70%

DISCUSSION

Our study showed that pyrophosphate is an important inhibitor
of crystal growth as has been described previously[1]. In the concentration normally found in urine, pyrophosphate seems to be a more
efficient inhibitor of calcium oxalate crystal growth than either
CS-A or CS-C[9]. Phosphone-formate also strongly inhibited crystal
growth, but unfortunately it is not known what concentrations might
be expected in urine after oral administration of the drug.

Among the glycosaminoglycans, heparin was the most potent
inhibitor of crystal growth. Heparin is not usually found in urine
but instead heparan sulphate[10], which occurs in lower concentrations
than do the chondroitin sulphates. The reason why chondroitin
sulphate was a less efficient inhibitor than heparin is probably due
to its lower charge density and affinity for calcium oxalate
crystals[11].

The low molecular weight analogue of heparin, SP 54, can be
given orally. About 10% is absorbed in the gastrointestinal tract
and excreted in the urine. This substance was a very efficient
inhibitor, probably due to the presence of 2-3 sulphate groups per
disaccharide unit. It may turn out to be a useful drug for the
treatment of calcium stone disease.

Tamm-Horsfall glycoprotein, in the concentration normally found
in urine, inhibited within the same range as the chondroitin
sulphates. Tamm-Horsfall glycoprotein has recently been shown in
another study to cause a slight inhibition of both spontaneous
precipitation and of crystal growth of calcium oxalate[6]. The present
results would support the view that this glycoprotein is an
inhibitor rather than a promoter of calcium oxalate crystallization.

ACKNOWLEDGEMENTS

This work was supported by the Swedish Medical Research Council
(nos. 2329, 6354), the Swedish Society of Medical Sciences and the
Tore Nilsson Foundation.

REFERENCES

1. L. H. Smith, J. L. Meyer and J. T. McCall, in:"Urinary Calculi",
   L. Cifuentes Delatte, A. Rapado, and A. Hodgkinson, eds.,
   Karger, Basel (1973).
2. W. G. Robertson, M. Peacock, and B. E. C. Nordin, Clin. Chim.
   Acta 43:31 (1973).
3. H. Ito and F. L. Coe, Am. J. Physiol. 233:F455 (1977).
4. E. E. Schrier, K. E. Lee, J. L. Rubin, P. G. Werness, and
   L. H. Smith, in:"Oxalate in Human Biochemistry and
   Clinical Pathology", G. A. Rose, W. G. Robertson, and
   R. W. E. Watts, eds., Wellcome Foundation, London (1979).
5. T. Kitamura, J. E. Zerwekh, and C. Y. C. Pak, Kidney Int. 21:379
   (1982).
6. T. Kitamura and C. Y. C. Pak, J. Urol. 127:1024 (1982).
7. B. Fellström, U. Backman, B. G. Danielson, K. Holmgren,
   S. Ljunghall, and B. Wikström, Clin. Sci. 62:509 (1982).
8. I. Tamm and F. L. Horsfall, J. Exp. Med. 95:71 (1952).
9. B. Fellström, B. G. Danielson, S. Ljunghall, and B. Wikström,
   in:"Urolithiasis and Related Clinical Research",
   P. O. Schwille, L. H. Smith, W. G. Robertson, and
   W.Vahlensieck, eds., Plenum, New York (1985).
10. W. D. Comper and T. C. Laurent, Physiol. Rev. 58:255 (1978).
11. B. Fellström, B. G. Danielson, F. A. Karlsson, and S. Ljunghall,
    in:"Urolithiasis and Related Clinical Research",
    P. O. Schwille, L. H. Smith, W. G. Robertson, and
    W. Vahlensieck, eds., Plenum, New York (1985).

N-SULFO-2-AMINO TRICARBALLYLATE, A NEW ANALOG OF PHOSPHOCITRATE:

METABOLISM AND INHIBITORY EFFECTS ON RENAL CALCIFICATION

M. R. Brown and J. D. Sallis

Biochemistry Dept., University of Tasmania, Australia

INTRODUCTION

Although the mechanism of action of urinary inhibitors has not been fully elucidated, most authors agree that measures which increase endogenous or exogenous inhibitors prevent kidney stone disease. As a therapeutic agent, an inhibitor should be well absorbed when given orally, potently effective with minimal side-effects, target specific and rapidly cleared. Few compounds meet these criteria. Phosphocitrate (PC), a naturally occurring, inhibitor of calcification in vitro appears to be promising but is susceptible to enzyme hydrolysis. This led us to develop a more stable PC analog, N-sulfo-2-amino tricarballylate (SAT) (Fig. 1).

MATERIALS AND METHODS

SAT and PC were prepared as described previously[1,2]. ^{35}S-SAT was synthesized in a similar fashion. Ethane-1-hydroxy-1,1-diphosphonate (EHDP) was a generous gift from Procter and Gamble.

The stablility of SAT in vivo was determined following the intravenous administration of ^{35}S-SAT (10 μmol, specific activity 0.24 mCi/mmol) to rats (200 g). The ureters were ligated and at predetermined times the rats sacrificed. Liver, kidneys and bladder plus contents were removed, as well as samples from blood and bone. Total counts in the tissue were measured following the oxidation of samples by a $HClO_4/H_2O_2$ mixture. Counts attributable to ^{35}S-SAT were determined separately after the preparation of an acid extract from tissues and removal of contaminating ions from radiolabeled products by ion-exchange chromatography. The eluant

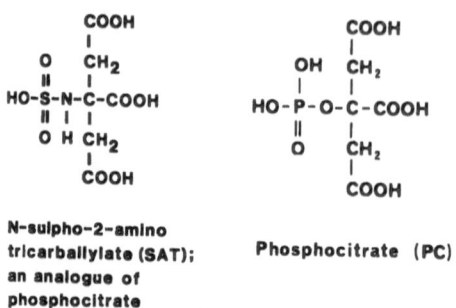

Fig. 1. Structures of N-sulfo-2-amino tricarballylate (SAT) and
phosphocitrate (PC).

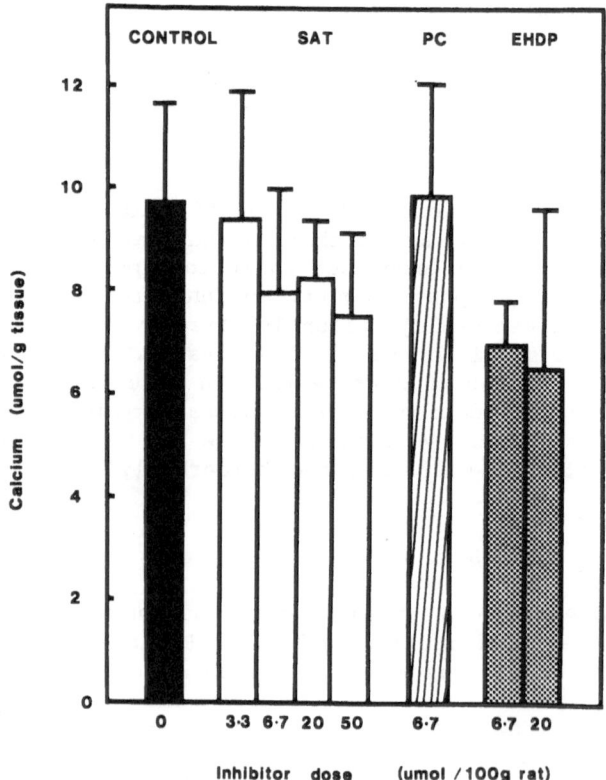

Fig. 2. Effect of inhibitors on the deposition of calcium oxalate
in kidney tissue.   Rats received an intraperitoneal dose
of inhibitor 1 h prior to an intraperitoneal challenge of
sodium oxalate (7 mg).   The rats were sacrificed 4 h
later and kidney calcium determined.

was desalted, lyophilized, redissolved in a minimum volume and the radio-labeled products analysed by paper electrophoresis.

The absorption of SAT following oral administration was established using a similar dose of ^{35}S-SAT given to rats (200 g) in metabolic cages. Urine and faeces were collected after 1, 2 and 3 days and treated as above following acid extraction.

The two effects of SAT on calcification in vivo was studied using two different models: (i) Rats (100 g) were given an intraperitoneal dose of inhibitor (3.3 to 50 μmol) 1 h prior to an intraperitoneal challenge of sodium oxalate (7 mg). In the absence of inhibitor this model has been shown to result in the massive deposition of CaOx crystals within the kidney[3]. The rats were sacrificed 4 h later and the extent of CaOx deposition in renal tissue determined by Ca analysis after tissue digestion. (ii) Rats (50 g) were given an intraperitoneal dose of inhibitor (3 μmol) 1 h prior to an intraperitoneal dose of calcium gluconate (1.0 ml; 10%) daily for 9 days. This results in the massive deposition of hydroxyapatite (HA) within the kidney[4]. Kidneys were removed 24 h after the final injection and Ca determined by methods previously described.

RESULTS

The distribution of radioactivity following the intravenous administration of ^{35}S-SAT showed that, following the initial uptake of counts by tissues from blood, radioactivity was cleared rapidly into the urine. Few counts were present in tissues after 24 h with the exception of bone which retained 1% of the initial dose for at least 3 days. Electrophoretic analysis proved that SAT was resistant to enzymic degradation in all of the tissues and body fluids studied. When SAT was given orally, there was 70% absorption with 80% of this was cleared in the urine within 24 h.

In relation to the studies on the effects of PC and SAT on calcification in vivo, the inhibitors had differing effects depending on the particular model studied. With the model involving CaOx deposition, SAT (6.7 μmol) reduced by 25% kidney Ca relative to the control whereas PC at this level had no effect. The degree of inhibition was only slightly increased by higher concentrations of SAT; 50 μmol of SAT resulted in only a 30% reduction (Fig. 2). Oxalate analyses also confirmed these trends. With the other model, phosphocitrate was very effective in preventing HA formation, reducing kidney Ca by 50% relative to control confirming the results produced by other authors[4]. SAT however, failed to cause any reduction at the same concentration (Table 1). EHDP was used as a reference inhibitor in these studies and with both models proved more potent than either PC or SAT.

Table 1. The Deposition of Calcium Within Renal Tissue Following
the Daily Administration of Calcium Gluconate (1.0 ml; 10%)
with Inhibitor (3 μmol/day) to Rats for 9 Days.

Inhibitor	Number of Rats/Group	Kidney Calcium[*] (μmol/g tissue)
None (control)	10	45 ± 12
SAT	5	52 ± 4
PC	3	25 ± 10

[*] Left and right kidney were analyzed separately.

DISCUSSION

Previous studies have shown that SAT is capable of inhibiting
both CaOx crystallization and HA formation in vitro. Although not
as good as PC, its activity is comparable to that of pyrophosphate[1].
In this study, SAT was found to be well absorbed, resistant to
enzymic degradation, and rapidly cleared into the urine. In the
short term, there was no evidence of toxicity in rats given large
doses. The data suggest that SAT may be more effective in
preventing CaOx nephrolithiasis than PC, whereas with the deposition
of HA, the reverse action of inhibitors seemed to occur. This
difference may be related to the sites of crystallization and
distribution of inhibitors within tissues, metabolism of inhibitors,
mechanism of action of the inhibitors in relation to the different
crystal types or various other factors.

ACKNOWLEDGEMENTS

This work was supported by a grant from the National Health and
Medical Research Council.

REFERENCES

1. M. R. Brown and J. D. Sallis, Analyt. Biochem. 132:115 (1983).
2. G. Williams and J. D. Sallis, Analyt. Biochem. 102:169 (1980).
3. S. R. Khan, B. Finlayson, and R. L. Hackett, Invest. Urol.
    17:199 (1979).
4. W. P. Tew, C. D. Malis, J. E. Howard, and A. L. Lehninger,
    Proc. Nat. Acad. Sci. 78:5528 (1981).

THE EFFECT OF SODIUM SULFOPENTOSAN ON THE CRYSTALLIZATION

OF CALCIUM OXALATE

H.-G. Tiselius

Dept. of Urology, University Hospital, Linköping, Sweden

INTRODUCTION

Several authors have demonstrated a lower inhibition of calcium oxalate (CaOx) crystallization in the urine of patients with CaOx stone disease when compared with that of normal subjects[1-6]. Various substances have been ascribed inhibiting properties, e.g. citrate, pyrophosphate, and macromolecular polyanions[7]. In this respect glycosaminoglycans are of particular interest[8,9] inasmuch as they apparently inhibit both crystal growth and aggregation. Thus heparin was shown to reduce considerably the rate of CaOx crystallization[8].

Although several forms of treatment have been described to reduce the level of CaOx supersaturation, few methods are available to increase the inhibition of CaOx crystallization. Sodium sulfopentosan (SPS; Elmiron; kindly supplied by Pharmacia AB, Uppsala) is a glycosaminoglycan-like substance thought to be excreted in urine following oral administration. This investigation was undertaken in order to study the effect of SPS on CaOx crystallization in vitro.

METHODS

One ml of solutions containing SPS in concentrations from 0.1 to 100 mg/l, was added to 50 ml of a crystallization system metastable with respect to CaOx. Crystallization was followed by measuring the concentration of ^{14}C-oxalate remaining in solution at different times after addition of seed crystals.

In a second study, the crystallization of CaOx was followed in
solutions of SPS which were made highly supersaturated with CaOx by
addition of sodium oxalate and calcium chloride.

In a third study, SPS was added to pooled urine which was
subsequently supersaturated by addition of sodium oxalate. The
crystallization rate was determined from the change in ^{14}C-oxalate
concentration. The crystal size distribution was measured in a
Coulter Counter after 2 h. A crystal size ratio was calculated by
dividing the number of crystals with diameters in the range 6.5 to
11 µm by those with diameters in the range 11 to 27.5 µm.

RESULTS

In the metastable crystallization system (Fig. 1) the rate of
crystal growth was retarded by SPS in concentrations of 10 to 100
mg/l. Fig. 2 shows that concentrations of SPS as low as 39 µg/l
caused obvious inhibition. From the measurements in the highly
supersaturated crystallization system (Fig. 3), it was evident that
SPS decreased the rate of crystallization. When urine was
supersaturated with sodium oxalate the rate of crystallization was
slightly reduced by SPS at concentrations >5 mg/l. A more
pronounced effect was observed in the crystal size ratio, which
increased with increasing concentrations of SPS (Fig. 4). Thus
SPS might influence CaOx crystal aggregation.

DISCUSSION

These preliminary results show that SPS decreases CaOx crystal
formation. Inhibition effects were observed in salt solutions and
urine, and although an effect on crystal aggregation is possible,

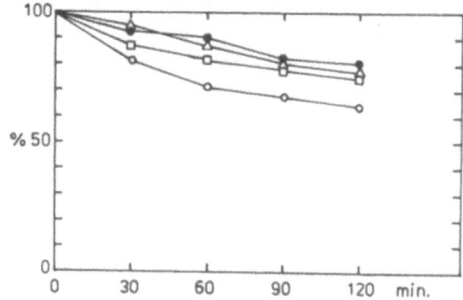

Fig. 1. Per cent ^{14}C-oxalate remaining in a metastable, seeded
crystallization system. One ml of solutions containing 10
(□), 50 (Δ) and 100 (●) mg/l of SPS was added to 50 ml of
the system. (O) A control without SPS.

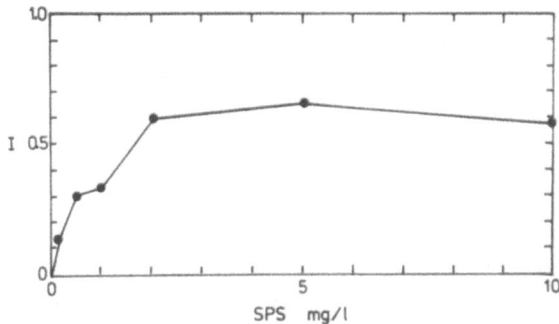

Fig. 2. The inhibition index as determined in the metastable
crystallization system when 1 ml of the various SPS
solutions was added to 50 ml of the crystallization system.

the methods used did not distinguish between inhibition of crystal
growth and crystal aggregation.   The importance of these results
are difficult to evaluate, and further studies are essential.
However, if excreted in urine following oral administration SPS
might provide a possible alternative form of treatment for the
prevention of recurrent renal stone formation.

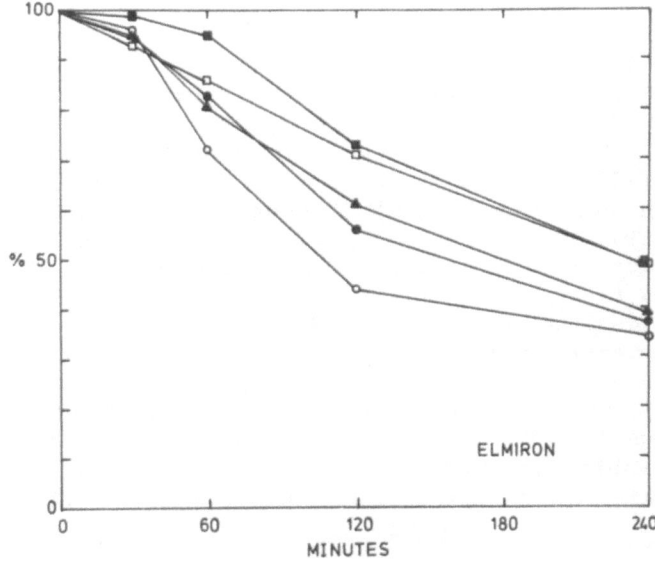

Fig. 3. Per cent ^{14}C-oxalate remaining in solutions of SPS with
concentrations of 2 (●), 5 (▲), 10 (◻), and 100 (◼)
mg/l, following supersaturation with calcium chloride and
sodium oxalate.   (O) A control with physiological saline.

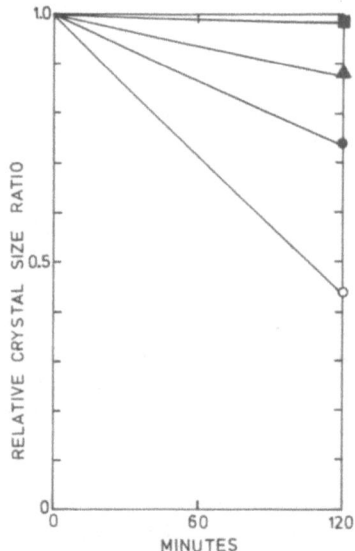

Fig. 4. The relative change in the crystal size ratio in urine which was supersaturated by means of sodium oxalate addition. The urine samples contained SPS in concentrations of 10 (●), 50 (▲), and 100 (■) mg/l. A control without SPS (O) was run simultaneously.

REFERENCES

1. W. B. Gill, M. A. Silvert, and M. J. Roma, Invest. Urol. 12:203 (1974).
2. C. Y. C. Pak and K. Holt, Metabolism 25:665 (1976).
3. P. C. Hallson and G. A. Rose, Br. J. Urol. 50:442 (1978).
4. A. Ligabue, M. Fini, and W. G. Robertson, Clin. Chim. Acta 98;39 (1979).
5. F. L. Coe, H. C. Margolis, L. H. Deutsch, and A. L. Strauss, Min. Electrol. Metab. 3:268 (1980).
6. H.-G. Tiselius and A. M. Fornander, Clin. Chem. 27:565 (1981).
7. W. G. Robertson, D. S. Scurr, and C. M. Bridge, J. Cryst. Growth 53:182 (1981).
8. W. G. Robertson, F. Knowles, and M. Peacock, in:"Urolithiasis Research", H. Fleisch, W. G. Robertson, L.H. Smith, and W. Vahlensieck, eds., Plenum, New York (1976).
9. I. Thorne, and M. I. Resnick, World J. Urol. 1:138 (1983).

MAGNESIUM AND CITRIC ACID IN THE DISSOLUTION OF STRUVITE

AND HYDROXYAPATITE

A. Kroon, H. Baadenhuysen, and P. Froeling

Dept. of Internal Medicine, Division of General Internal
Medicine and Clinical Chemistry, St. Radboud University
Hospital, Nijmegen, The Netherlands

INTRODUCTION

About 20% of renal stones are composed of struvite or hydroxyapatite. The presence of these stones, which usually occur as
large staghorn calculi, may result in a reduction of kidney function
because of infection and obstruction. When surgical removal of
phosphatic stones is contraindicated or otherwise impossible, local
irrigation with citric acid-containing solutions may be used as an
alternative[1]. Magnesium may be useful in alleviating the symptoms
of irritation of the ureter and the bladder caused by citric acid
solutions[2].

Following the use of Solution G or "Suby's solution", Mulvaney
introduced Hemiacidrin (a 10% solution of Renacidin)[3-5], a solution
similar in composition to Solution R. The citric acid
concentrations in Solution G, Solution R and Hemiacidrin are 154,
286, 301 mmol/l and the magnesium concentrations 18, 292 and 325
mmol/l respectively. Solutions G and R also include 100 mg Na EDTA
and Solution R and Hemiacidrin contain 6 to 10 g gluconolactone/l.
So the concentration of magnesium in Solution R is about 15 times
higher and that of citric acid nearly 2 times higher than in
Solution G. The final pH of all the solutions ranges from 3.8 to
4.1; only Solution G is isotonic. In 1942, Suby et al[2] postulated
that the addition of magnesium to citric acid solutions enhanced the
solubility of the stones by exchange with calcium ions.

In this paper we report on in vitro studies carried out in
order to test the postulated effectivness of magnesium/citric acid
solutions in dissolving phosphate-containing stones.

899

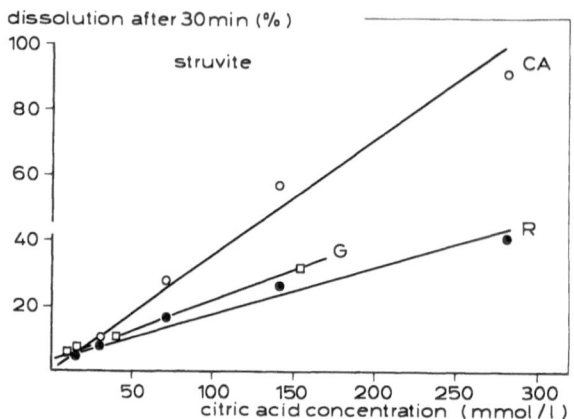

Fig. 1. The % of struvite dissolved after 30 min in relation to
citric acid concentration in pure citric acid (CA),
Solution G (G), and Solution R (R).

MATERIALS AND METHODS

    The experimental system consisted of a continuous perfusion of
tablets composed of chemically pure struvite or hydroxyapatite.
Positioned in the center of a filter-lined funnel, these tablets
were irrigated with the solution to be studied. The perfusion
fluid was analysed for calcium (in the case of hydroxyapatite) and
ammonium (in the case of struvite) in order to follow the
dissolution process. The effectiveness of Solutions R and G and of
pure citric acid solution at the same concentration and pH were
compared. The percentages of the tablets dissolved after 30 min
were calculated.

RESULTS AND DISCUSSION

    The dissolution capacities of the various solutions are shown
in Figs. 1 and 2 and the Table. These show that at citric acid
concentrations of 150 mmol/l, pure citric acid has the best
dissolution capacity both for hydroxyapatite and struvite. At this
concentration, Solution R was significantly less effective than
Solution G. Undiluted Solution R (285 mmol/l citrate) appeared to
be superior to Solution G (150 mmol/l citrate) for dissolving
struvite, whereas both solutions appeared to be equally effective
for hydroxyapatite. The effect of additives other than magnesium
in Solutions R and G seemed to be of negligible importance in the
dissolution of stones. It is known that EDTA has chelating
activity at pH values above 7 and at concentrations much higher than

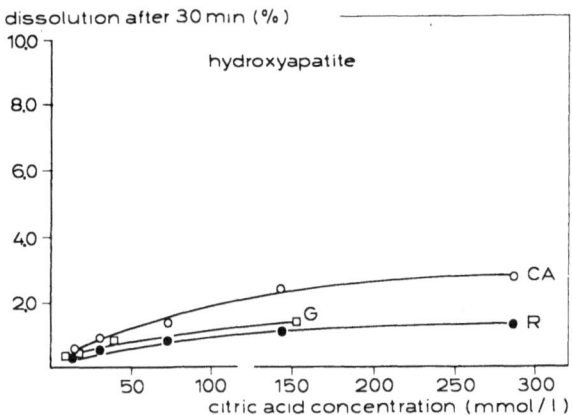

Fig. 2. The % of hydroxyapatite dissolved after 30 min in relation
to citric acid concentration in pure citric acid (Ca),
Solution G (G), and Solution R (R).

Table. Dissolution of Hydroxyapatite (HAP) and Struvite (STR) after
30 min (% $\pm$ SD; n=4).

Solutions	Citrate (mmol/l)	Mg	HAP (%)	STR (%)
(i) Citric acid	150		2.54 $\pm$ 0.06	44.80 $\pm$ 0.23
(ii) Solution R	150	154	1.12 $\pm$ 0.05	24.90 $\pm$ 1.30
(iii) Solution R	285	292	1.40 $\pm$ 0.05	42.18 $\pm$ 1.67
(iv) Solution G	150	18	1.43 $\pm$ 0.12	36.50 $\pm$ 2.19
(i) - (ii)			$P<0.01$	$P<0.01$
(i) - (iii)			$P<0.01$	$P<0.01$
(i) - (iv)			$P<0.01$	$P<0.01$
(ii) - (iv)			$P<0.01$	$P<0.01$
(iii) - (iv)			ns	$P=0.01$

used in these solutions. We have found that gluconolactone does
not influence the dissolution capacity of the solutions.

Based on Suby's suggestion of the possible exchange between
magnesium and calcium ions, one would expect that hydroxyapatite
would be more soluble in Solution R than in Solution G. Our
results, however, showed the opposite, that the addition of
magnesium decreased the in vitro dissolution capacity. This effect
was more pronounced with struvite than with hydroxyapatite. It is
clear that it is the citric acid concentration and pH which
determine the dissolution capacity.

Clinical experience, however, has shown that magnesium substantially alleviates the irritation caused by irrigation with citric acid. Therefore, the addition of magnesium is a compromise between the optimum dissolution capacity on one hand and practicability of clinical use on the other.

REFERENCES

1. H. I. Suby and F. Albright, New Engl. J. Med. 288:81 (1943).
2. H. I. Suby, R. M. Suby and F. Albright, J. Urol. 48:549 (1942).
3. W. P. Mulvaney, J. Urol. 82:546 (1959).
4. W. P. Mulvaney, J. Urol. 84:206 (1960).
5. N. J. Nemoy and T. A. Stamey, J. Urol. 116:693 (1976).

ROUND TABLE DISCUSSION ON THE COMPARISON OF MODELS FOR THE

STUDY OF INHIBITORY ACTIVITY IN URINE

H. Fleisch

Pathophysiologisches Institut, Universität Bern
Switzerland

INTRODUCTION

The processes which lead to the formation of the solid phase of urinary stones include crystal nucleation, growth and aggregation. Inhibitors are defined as substances which slow down any of these processes by a mechanism which does not depend on decreasing the concentration of crystal-forming ions, but on an action at the developing surface of the embryo or crystal itself. The panelists decided to cover only techniques involving the crystallisation of calcium phosphate and calcium oxalate. The methods presented were roughly divided into those techniques where (1) crystallisation is induced by increasing the concentration(s) of stone-forming ion(s), (2) seed crystals are added to a metastable system and (3) crystallisation is followed under conditions of constant fluid composition, although some overlap between the various systems occurs.

DR C Y C PAK (DALLAS, USA) presented a technique, first described by Dr W. Neuman, in which the minimum supersaturation required to elicit spontaneous precipitation over a given time period is determined. In order to correct for chelators, this critical supersaturation level, called the "formation product (FP)", is divided by the measured solubility product of the salt formed to yield the "formation product ratio (FPR)". Since urine invariably contains impurities, it is a measure of heterogeneous rather than homogeneous nucleation.

The experimental technique consists of increasing the concentration of calcium chloride or oxalic acid in urine to the level at which spontaneous precipitation of brushite or calcium

903

oxalate is initiated within 3 hours. The point of precipitation is determined either by the decline in the filtrate concentrations of calcium and phosphate or of calcium and oxalate, or by increased turbidity, or, in the case of brushite, by a decline in pH. Since the FPR probably represents heterogeneous nucleation, it is much less than the expected FPR for homogeneous nucleation, so that it is not necessary to reach high degrees of supersaturation.

The technique is sensitive to small and large molecular weight inhibitors, the FPR of both brushite and calcium oxalate being increased by the addition of pyrophosphate, diphosphonates, citrate, heparin and naturally occurring glycopeptides and glycosaminoglycans. It has been used for both brushite and calcium oxalate in whole urine. Inhibitory activity is low in various stone-forming groups. The FPR of calcium oxalate is increased after parathyroidectomy as well as by treatment with potassium citrate, orthophosphate and cellulose phosphate.

In summary, the advantages of the FPR-technique are: (1) It is applicable to whole urine both for brushite and calcium oxalate. (2) It demonstrates reduced inhibitory activity in stone-forming urine. (3) It is responsive to both small and large molecular inhibitors. (4) Together with the measurement of supersaturation, it provides a quantitative measure of the risk of spontaneous precipitation. This is useful in assessing the severity of stone disease and in following response to treatment. The major disadvantage of FPR is its inability to differentiate between the various crystallization processes.

DR G A ROSE (LONDON, UK) presented a technique in which the crystal forming ion concentration in the urine is increased not by adding the ions but by concentrating the urine in a rotary evaporator to a standard osmolarity. Crystal formation is determined by morphological examination of the urine under the microscope.

The technique has the following advantages: (1) The crystals formed mimic those found naturally in human urine. (2) The crystals to be studied can be selected by pH-adjustment since calcium oxalate and phosphate form at pH 5.3 and 6.8 respectively. (3) The test is performed at physiological concentrations of Tamm-Horsfall uromucoid which promotes crystal formation. (4) The test is performed in concentrated urine which is necessary for stone-formation. (5) It allows the study of the same urine sample, with and without addition or removal of test substances.

The technique has demonstrated a reduction in crystal formation with increasing concentrations of magnesium and citrate. On the other hand, pyrophosphate removal, achieved by passage of urine through a nylon coil with covalently bound pyrophosphatase, induced no difference in crystal formation either with calcium oxalate or calcium phosphate.

904

The technique is useful to assess the clinical relevance of changes in urine concentration of a given substance upon stone risk.

DR J MEYER (BETHESDA, USA) described a technique in which seed crystals are added to a metastable supersaturated solution containing the lattice ions of the crystalline phase to be formed. The method can be used to study either crystal growth or crystal aggregation. In principle, the method can be applied to any urinary stone component for which a metastable supersaturated solution can be prepared.

The reaction is initiated by adding the seed crystal and following: (1) The rate of crystal growth by measuring the lattice ion concentration remaining in solution at various time intervals; (2) the rate of crystal aggregation by inserting a Coulter counter probe into the reaction mixture and measuring crystal size distribution at various time intervals. The crystal growth of the urinary stone components can in general be described by a rate law expression. Crystal growth inhibitors act to reduce the rate constant by adsorbing to the surface of the crystal. This effect can be quantitated by plotting the kinetic data in the form of a convenient adsorption isotherm, such as that proposed by Langmuir. This plot is usually linear and the amount of inhibitor present in a given solution can be determined by noting the concentration required to produce 50% inhibition in a particular test system. No attempts to relate quantitatively crystal aggregation kinetics to surface absorption phenomena have yet been attempted.

The strengths of the methodology lie in its precision, reproducibility and relatively simple design. The major weakness of the method results from its sensitivity to the large amount of inhibitors normally present in urine. Greatly diluted systems must therefore in general be used and dilution of a physiological fluid may create artefacts of measurement.

DR H FLEISCH (BERN, SWITZERLAND) also presented a technique where seed crystals are used, but which can be utilized for non-diluted urine. It measures the amount of seed necessary to induce the precipitation of calcium phosphate from a urine with a known and constant supersaturation.

The latter is obtained experimentally by determining the solubility of brushite in urine and then bringing a second sample of the same urine to the measured equilibrium calcium and phosphate concentrations. In a third step, increasing amounts of hydroxyapatite crystals, which have a lower solubility than brushite, are added and the amount of apatite seed necessary to induce a 50% precipitation of calcium from the solution determined.

This quantity of seed is influenced by the amount of inhibitors present and will therefore reflect the inhibitory activity of the urine.

According to this technique over 75% of the inhibitory activity in urine towards calcium phosphate is due to citrate, magnesium and pyrophosphate, 25% being due to unknown inhibitors. This technique has also been developed for plasma. In this case the most powerful inhibitor is magnesium, while citrate and pyrophosphate are only of minor importance. However, if the inhibitory activity of plasma is measured by the FPR technique, as described above, pyrophosphate is by far the most important inhibitor. Thus, the relative potency of the various inhibitors could appear to depend on the test chosen.

This technique has the advantage that it can be performed on whole urine. It has the disadvantage that, so far, it has been developed only for calcium phosphate. Furthermore, by its mode of action it will tend to disfavour the inhibitors present in small amounts even if very potent in favour of inhibitors present in large quantities.

DR G H NANCOLLAS (BUFFALO, USA) presented a technique where the urinary concentration of the ions which will precipitate is kept constant (constant composition). It can be used at any urine concentration, including whole urine, and at any chosen supersaturation level within the metastable region.

Following the preparation of solutions supersaturated with respect to calcium oxalate, calcium phosphate or both, seed material is added in order to induce crystal growth. Free Ca^{2+} and/or pH are measured by means of a protected calcium electrode and/or a glass pH electrode. Changes in these parameters are automatically corrected by pumping into the solution the necessary amount of Ca and base. The decrease in oxalate and phosphate is corrected by adding these ions according to the stoichiometric ratio. The rate of titrant addition, automatically recorded, gives directly the rate of mineralisation and the nature of the solid phase formed.

In preliminary studies, it was possible to measure the inhibition of calcium oxalate monohydrate and hydroxyapatite growth by various concentrations of urine. It was important to calculate free calcium and phosphate concentrations for the assessment of the degree of supersaturation with respect to each of the calcium phosphate phases. Experiments are usually made in solutions supersaturated with respect to only one phase – the thermodynamically most stable hydroxyapatite. Problems involved in multiple precursor phase formation, such as occur in the method described by Dr. Meyer, are therefore eliminated.

The advantages of this method are as follows:
(1) Supersaturation can be kept constant and the level selected to mimic that present in vivo. (2) The sensitivity of growth rate measurement is far greater than that of any previous method, such as the conventional seeded method. (3) It can accommodate whole urine. (4) It is possible from a knowledge of the adsorption isotherms of the inhibitors to maintain a constant inhibitor concentration. (5) The solid phases formed can be characterized. (6) The method can be used to study dissolution kinetics.

DR W G ROBERTSON (LEEDS, UK) presented finally the "continuous crystallizer" system as described by Randolph and Larson. It may be used to study the effects of various constituents of urine on the crystallization kinetics of calcium oxalate. The method involves mixing calcium- and oxalate-containing solutions in an unseeded system at high levels of supersaturation, similar to those in the urines of recurrent stone-formers. Crystals are generated de novo and crystallization followed under controlled conditions of supersaturation in an environment designed to mimic urine with respect to the concentrations of all the main ions. Theoretically the system is applicable to whole urine.

The numbers and sizes of crystals are measured with a particle analyzer at frequent time intervals until a steady state is reached and then followed for approximately 2 hours. From a plot of log (particle number) against particle diameter (which should be inverse and linear in the absence of agglomeration), the crystal birth rate and linear growth rate can be calculated. Deviation from linearity usually indicates that agglomeration has occurred. The degree of agglomeration can be calculated by simulation of inter-particle collisons.

Various urinary polyanions have been shown to inhibit the urinary concentration ranges of these ions. Conversely, the nucleation rate increases to relieve the build-up of supersaturation caused by the reduction in crystal growth rate.

The system has a number of advantages over the batch and seeded growth systems: (1) It operates and is maintained at urinary levels of supersaturation. (2) As a flow system it is a better model of the kidney than a batch crystallizer. (3) Any additives are maintained at a constant concentration at levels akin to those in urine. (4) Measurements can be made of nucleation, growth and agglomeration. Studies are now under way to evaluate the usefulness of the system for studies on whole urine.

During the discussion which followed the presentations, it became apparent that it is not yet possible to recommend specifically any one of the above techniques as being superior to the others. Indeed, each has its advantages and disadvantages.

However, all the members of the panel agreed that it is of advantage to make the measurements in whole and not in diluted urine. The panel also agreed that the relative potency of the various inhibitors measured will depend upon the technique used and that it is not possible to recommend which technique is most relevant. Nor was it possible to state which of the various inhibitors described are the most important in vivo.

It was also agreed that techniques should be developed to measure not only crystal growth but also aggregation, results on which are still scanty. It was finally agreed that further research on inhibitors is necessary and should be continued, in the hope that it will be possible to define the role of inhibitors in the process of stone formation and also, perhaps, to develop a method which can be used in clinical practice to define patients at risk of stones and follow the efficacy of treatment.

MATRIX

URINARY STONE MATRIX AND URINARY MACROMOLECULES

S. D. Roberts and M. I. Resnick

Division of Urology, Case Western Reserve University
School of Medicine, Cleveland, Ohio, U.S.A.

INTRODUCTION

The role of matrix and urinary macromolecules and urinary macromolecules in the formation of urinary stones is poorly understood. Matrix has been implicated by some as a necessary substrate for crystal formation[1] and by others as a mere co-precipitant with inorganic crystals[2,3]. Several urinary macromolecules have been identified but their importance in matrix and stone formation remains obscure. The purpose of this report is to review current knowledge on these complex components of urinary calculi.

The first reference to the structural complexity of urinary stones was made in 1684 by von Heyde who noted that certain crystal elements could be removed without destroying the stone's gross structure. The substance remaining he termed "the framework" of urinary calculi[4]. The first chemical studies of the crystalline composition of urinary stones were performed by Scheele who in 1780 found uric acid in bladder stones and other constituents were identified over the next 40 years[4]. Meckel von Hemsbach stressed that stone formation was caused by precipitable material aggregating upon an organic substance which he termed "Meckel's stone-forming catarrh". Ebstein concluded that urinary calculi contained a framework of albuminous substances originating from the sloughing of epithelial cells caused by inflammation[4].

In the 1950s light microscopy investigations showed that the organic matrix had a highly organized architecture composed of fibrils and an amorphous interfibrillar material. The fibrils were parallel to one another and arranged in broad bands or circular

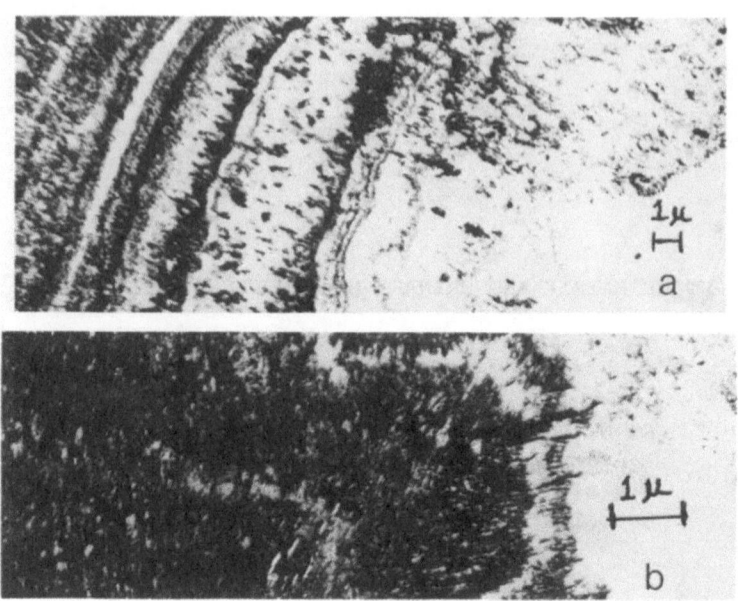

Fig. 1. (a) Electron micrograph of laminations in a demineralized
calcium phosphate and oxalate stone; (b) Electron
micrograph of end-to-side linkage of fibrils and
radial striations (with permission, W. H. Boyce).

Table 1. Analysis of Demineralized Matrix from Pools of Calculi
and Untreated Uromucoid and Matrix Substance A from
Normal Urine.

	Calcigerous Calculi (%)	Uric Acid Calculi (%)	Cystine Calculi (%)	MSA (from urine) mg/24h)	Uromucoid (mg/24h)
Matrix	3.2	10.8	2.2	23	
% Ash	13.1		14.2		4.8
% Ca in Ash	28.7		22.4		7.1
% P in Ash	13.0		1.5		21.3
Nitrogen	10.2	10.2	10.6	11.9	
Protein	63.4		76.3	74.6	64.7
Hexose	9.6	7.1	5.9	9.3	10.7
Hexosamine	4.9		1.5	6.6	5.2
Sialic Acid					3.5
Bound Water	10.9		10.2		6.3

whorls. The core of each stone was composed of one or more of these circular whorls of fibrils[5]. Later Boyce confirmed this finding and showed that there were end-to-side linkages in the fibrils with different axial orientation. Radial striations were seen oriented at right angles to fibrils, and were joined to fibrils by end-to-side linkages, extending from one concentric lamination to another (Figs. 1a,b). Within the amorphous substance of matrix were collections of microspherules (1 μm in diameter) in an electron-dense membrane[6,7].

QUANTITATIVE STUDIES

On a dry weight basis matrix accounts for approximately 2.5% of the mass of calcium oxalate or urate stones, 9% of cystine stones and up to 65% of matrix stones. The matrix content is inversely proportional to the size of the stone. Each calculus contains a surface layer of matrix and therefore, when several small stones are pooled for study a greater surface area (and hence more surface matrix) is present than if a single stone is examined[5,8-10] (Table 1). Small stones contain matrix concentrations similar to those present on the surface of large stones but of higher concentration than the interior[11]. The elemental composition of stone matrix is constant, regardless of the type of stone. It consists of approximately 10% nitrogen, 1% sulfur, 58% carbon, 7% hydrogen and 24% oxygen[5].

Carbohydrate Content

Hexose and hexosamines are the major constituents of calcigerous stone matrix. The hexose content varies considerably between stones (2.7% to 35%). The hexoses found include galactose, glucose, mannose, rhamnose and fucose. Deoxypentose has also been described[12]. Hexuronic acid, a structural component of acid mucopolysaccharides, was originally thought to be absent from stone matrix[5,9,10], but has recently been detected[12-14]. Hexosamines are present chiefly in the form of glucosamine; lesser amounts of galactosamine are also present[15]. Matrix of uric acid stones contain lesser amounts of hexose and hexosamine[16] (Table 1).

Glycosaminoglycans

Glycosaminoglycans (GAGS) are polyanionic polysaccharide chains of variable length. They consist of alternating hexuronic acid and hexosamine residues connected by alternating B1-3 and B1-4 linkages. All except hyaluronic acid are sulfated. The parent macromolecule, the proteoglycan, is a core protein to which one or more GAG chains are presumably covalently attached. Of the normal urinary GAG

913

component, approximately 60% consists of chondroitin sulfates (A and C) while heparan sulfate and keratan sulfate each account for 15%. GAGS are important components of organic matrix.

Recent evidence is most compelling for GAGS being extremely potent inhibitors of crystal growth and aggregation[17,18] and even, according to some of nucleation[19]. There is, however, strong evidence for GAGS acting as promoters of nucleation. It may be that it is the balance between nucleation-promotion and growth/aggregation-inhibition that will determine whether a person will form stones[20]. The major part of the GAG inhibitory activity lies in the chondroitin sulfates. Heparin is 25 times more effective in inhibiting growth[21] but, since it is virtually absent from urine, it is unimportant in vivo. It has been shown that the urinary GAGS of stone formers are more highly sulfated and precipitate more calcium than the less sulfated GAGS of non-stone-formers[22]. It is also thought that urate may interfere with the inhibitory properties of GAGS – possibly by binding GAGS to stabilize itself in a colloidal form[29]. Lower levels of GAGS have been reported in stone formers' urine by some while others have found no difference[21,24]. Interestingly, stone formers have a reportedly lower excretion rate of low molecular weight material containing uronic acid. Hence, degradation of GAGS may have a vital role.

The Protein Content of Matrix

Amino Acid Composition. The matrix of urinary stones is a mucoprotein of which 64% is protein[24]. Spector et al[12] analyzed the amino acid composition of one EDTA-soluble protein in matrix and confirmed an earlier report[10] that hydroxyproline and hydroxylysine were absent from calcium oxalate stone matrix. They also confirmed that matrix is rich in acidic amino acids. The amino acid composition of this protein in calcium oxalate stones was compared to an electrophoretically-similar protein found in both apatite-struvite and uric acid stones and each showed a distinct amino acid composition.

Lian et al[25] identified a protein in the EDTA-soluble, non-dialyzable fraction of calcium stones that contains residues of 𝛾-carboxyglutamic acid (Gla). This amino acid was found in calcium oxalate, hydroxyapatite and mixed stones of apatite and struvite but not in the matrices of uric acid, cystine, or pure struvite stones. In pure calcium oxalate stones about 8 times as much Gla was found in the matrix from the center of the stone than in that from the surface[26]. The Gla-containing protein has a molecular weight of approximately 17,000 daltons and about 40 Gla residues per 1,000 amino acids. Joost et al [27] measured a 2- to 3-fold increase in the daily urinary excretion of Gla in calcigerous stone formers when compared to normal controls. This increase was not significantly changed when these patients were placed on a low calcium diet, a high calcium diet, or after a 24-h fast. There was no correlation between urinary Gla and urinary calcium, c-AMP parathyroid hormone, oxalic acid, or pH. There was, however, a positive correlation between urinary Gla and uric acid; the reason for this is unclear. We have compared the urinary calcium-binding activity of active stone formers, inactive stone formers, and non-stone forming individuals[28]. Significant differences were found between the active and inactive stone formers and between the active stone-formers and controls. The precise role of Gla in this calcium-binding activity is unknown and deserves further attention.

Matrix substance A(MSA) is the most immunologically prominent matrix component[24,29] and constitutes about 85% of matrix by weight[30]. This immunologically-distinct portion of all calcigerous matrix is highly insoluble, but an immunologically-identical analogue, soluble in a variety of buffer solutions, has been found in the urine of some stone-formers. MSA has a molecular weight in the range of 30,000 to 40,000 daltons, a sedimentation constant of 2.8 (S20W) and an isoelectric point near 4.5[29]. It is approximately 75% protein, 16% carbohydrate and 5% water. Amino acid analysis showed relatively high levels of glutamic and aspartic acids. Paper chromatography showed galactose and lesser amounts of mannose to be present. Hexosamine was present chiefly as glucosamine; lesser amounts of galactosamine were detected.

MSA is present in matrix of all calculi, but its concentration in the urine of stone-formers is highly variable. In general, the amount of detectable MSA is proportional to the rapidity of stone formation. In a study of 40 urine specimens from 12 patients with rapidly recurrent renal calculi, King and Boyce measured an average of 23 mg/day of MSA. Keutel and King[31] detected MSA in the urine of 17 non-stone-formers who had a variety of diseases involving renal injury and repair. Urine infected with Aerobacter aerogenes or E.coli or both was often found to contain MSA. A substance that gives a reaction of identity with MSA has been detected in the renal parenchyma and similar reactions have been demonstrated in the renal parenchyma of patients with renal carcinoma and major arterial disease. MSA has not been immunologically identified in blood, serum, saliva or bone matrix[32]. Moore and Gowland[33] have demonstrated that MSA is not a single antigen, but an entity that may comprise 3 or 4 antigenic substances which are stone specific.

Uromucoid and Tamm-Horsfall Protein. The role of uromucoid in stone formation has received much attention. It is found in large amounts in the urine of active stone-formers and in patients who suffer from inflammatory diseases of the genito-urinary tract.

In normal urine about 25 to 50 mg are excreted per day. The matrix of many urinary calculi has been shown to contain uromucoid. This mucoprotein is thought to be immunologically identical to the urinary mucoprotein isolated by Tamm and Horsfall[34-36]. Immunofluorescent techniques have shown that it is derived from the descending limb of the loop of Henle and the macula densa segment of the distal tubule[37]. It has a molecular weight of at least 7.0 x 10[6] daltons[38,39]. Approximately 66% is protein, hexose constitutes 12% and N-acetyl hexosamine 11%. The remainder consists of fucose, sialic acid, ash, and small amounts of lipids. It is very acidic[35] with an isoelectric point of 3.5. It has been shown that uromucoids are promoters of both calcium oxalate and phosphate crystal formation[40], and may act as a template onto which aggregation of these crystals occurs. However, workers have been unable to demonstrate consistently the presence of uromucoid in kidney stone matrix.

The absence of sialic acid in stone matrix has been puzzling[5,8,10,31,41]. Although urinary uromucoid contains sialic acid, the form of this glycoprotein found in kidney stone matrix was found to have none. Malek and Boyce[30] suggested that renal sialidase or N-acetyl neuraminidase altered urinary mucosubstances by leaving sialic acid from the glucide moiety[42]. Others have found no significant differences between the neuraminidase activity of human renal tissue of stone-formers and normals[43]. Melick et al[44], however, found sialic acid in each of 12 calcium stones. Although the absolute amount of sialic acid varied considerably from stone to stone, the ratio of protein to sialic acid was relatively constant. This finding casts doubt on the validity of the above theory.

ROLE OF MATRIX

Leal and Finlayson[18] found that anionic protein adsorption on to calcium oxalate crystals was sensitive to variation in calcium ion concentration and that cationic protein adsorption was sensitive to variations in oxalate ion concentration. The protein moiety of the mucopolysaccharide was adsorbed onto the crystalline surfaces in moderate quantities and a small portion of the carbohydrate moiety was also adsorbed. Large concentrations of mucopolysaccharide were observed to inhibit crystal aggregation. The authors calculated that physical adsorption could account for part but not all of matrix deposition in calcium oxalate stones. Khan et al[45] demonstrated with scanning electron microscopy that calcium oxalate crystals from urinary stones possess an amorphous coat; they believe that this coat represents urinary macromolecules that were adsorbed onto crystal surfaces in a manner similar to that demonstrated in Leal and Finlayson's in vitro experiments. The quantitative contribution that these coats make to total matrix is uncertain but depends on the total surface area of the crystals.

These studies argue against the notion that matrix is the initiator
of stone formation and suggest that urinary macromolecular
substances have a secondary role in this process. The exact mode of
urinary stone formation is still speculative. There has been a
resurgence of interest in the role of urinary macromolecules in
urolithiasis.   It is desirable that work in this field keeps pace
with that on the crystalline aspects of urinary stones.

ACKNOWLEDGEMENT

     This work was supported in part by a Grant AM 20066 for the
National Institute of Arthritis, Metabolism, and Digestive Diseases,
National Institutes of Health and the Dudley P Allen Surgical
Scholarship Program, Department of Surgery, Case Western Reserve
University, School of Medicine.

REFERENCES

1. W. H. Boyce, Am. J. Med. 45:673 (1968).
2. C. W. Vermeulen and E. S. Lyon, Am. J. Med. 45:684 (1968).
3. B. T. Murphy and L. N. Pyrah, Br. J. Urol. 34:129 (1962).
4. A. J. Butt, "Etiologic Factors in Renal Lithiasis",
     C. T. Thomas, Springfield (1956).
5. W. H. Boyce and F. K. Garvey, J. Urol. 76:213 (1956).
6. W. H. Boyce, in:"Urolithiasis:Physical Aspects", B. Finlayson,
     L. L. Hench, and L. H. Smith, eds., National Academy of
     Sciences, Washington (1972).
7. R. S. Malek and W. H. Boyce, J. Urol. 117:336 (1977).
8. W. H. Boyce and N. M. Sulkin, J. Clin. Invest. 35:1067 (1956).
9. J. S. King and W. H. Boyce, Arch. Biochem. Biophys. 82:455
     (1959).
10. J. S. King and W. H. Boyce, Soc. Exp. Biol. Med. 95:183 (1957).
11. M. A. Warpehoski, R. J. Buscemi, D. C. Osborn, B. Finlayson, and
     E. P. Goldberg, Calcif. Tiss. Int. 33:211 (1981).
12. A. R. Spector, A. Gray and E. L. Prien, Invest. Urol. 13:387
     (1976).
13. W. G. Robertson, D. S. Scurr, and C. M. Bridge, J. Cryst. Growth
     53:182 (1981).
14. Y. Kimura, N. Kiaki, and K. Ise, Urol.Int. 31:355 (1976).
15. W. H. Boyce, in:"Proteins in Normal and Pathologic Urine",
     Y. Manue, J. P. Revillard, and H. Beutel, eds., Karger, Basel
     (1970).
16. W. H. Boyce and J. S. King, J. Urol. 81:351 (1959).
17. R. C. Boyer, J. G. Brockis, and R. K. McCulloch, Clin. Chim.
     Acta 95:23 (1979).
18. J. J. Leal and B. Finlayson, Invest. Urol. 14:278 (1977).
19. T. Kitamura, J. E. Zerwekh, and C. Y. C. Pak, Kidney Int. 21:379
     (1982).

20. G. W. Drach, S. Sarig, and A. D. Randolph, Urol. Res. 10:165 (1982).
21. R. L. Ryall, R. M. Harnett, and V. R. Marshall, Clin. Chim. Acta 112:349 (1981).
22. W. O. Foye, H. S. Hong, C. M. Kim, and E. L. Prien, Invest. Urol. 14:33 (1976).
23. R. K. McCulloch, R. C. Bowyer, and J. G. Brockis, in:"Urinary Calculus", J. G. Brockis and B. Finlayson, eds., P. S. G. Publishing Co. Littleton (1981).
24. W. H. Boyce, J. S. King, and M. L. Fielden, J. Clin. Invest. 41:5 (1962).
25. J. B. Lian, E. L. Prien, J. M. Glimcher, and P. M. Gallop, J. Clin. Invest. 59:1151 (1977).
26. J. B. Lian, J. T. Levy, and P. A. Friedman, in:"Calcium Binding Proteins:Structure and Function", F. L. Siegel, E. Carafoli, R. H. Kretsinger, D. H. Maclennan, and R. H. Wasserman, eds., Elsevier, Amsterdam (1980).
27. J. Joost, S. Silbernagl, and E. Jarosch,in:"Urolithiasis: Clinical and Basic Research', L. H. Smith,W. G. Robertson, and B. Finlayson, eds., Plenum, New York (1980).
28. M. I. Resnick, O. W. Gammon, M. B. Sorrell, and W. H. Boyce, Surgery 88:239 (1980).
29. J. S. King and W. H. Boyce, Ann. N. Y. Acad. Sci. 104:579 (1963).
30. R. S. Malek and W. H. Boyce, J. Urol.109:579 (1963).
31. H. J. Keutel and J. S. King, Invest. Urol. 2:115 (1964).
32. W. H. Boyce and J. S. King, Ann. N. Y. Acad. Sci. 104:563 (1963).
33. S. Moore and G. Gowland, J. Urol 47:489 (1975).
34. I. Tamm and F. L. Horsfall, Proc. Soc. Exp. Biol.Med. 17:108 (1950).
35. I. Tamm and F. L. Horsfall, J. Exp. Med. 95:71 (1951).
36. G. E. Perlmann, I. Tamm, and F. L. Horsfall, J. Exp. Med. 95:99 (1951).
37. J. K. McKenzie and E. G. McQueen, J. Clin. Path. 22:334 (1969).
38. M. Maxfield, Biochim. Biophys. Acta 49:548 (1961).
39. A. J. Pesce and M. R. First, "Proteinuria:An Integrated Review", Marcel Dekker, 1979.
40. P. C. Hallson and G. A. Rose, Lancet 1:1000 (1979).
41. M. Maxfield, Ann. Rev. Med. 14:99 (1963).
42. W. H. Boyce, in:"Biology of Hard Tissue", Vol. l. A. M. Budy, ed., New York Acad Science (1967).
43. T. Mutton, M. I. Resnick, and W. H. Boyce, Invest. Urol. 15:419 (1978).
44. R. A. Melick, K. J. Quelch, and M. Rhodes, Clin. Sci. 59:401 (1980).
45. S. R. Khan, B. Finlayson, and R. L. Hackett, Scan. Electron Microsc. 1:379 (1983).

ALTERNATING CRYSTALLIZATION - A PROPOSED MECHANISM FOR

LAMELLAR STRUCTURE FORMATION IN RENAL STONES

P.-T. Cheng and K. P. H. Pritzker

Dept. of Pathology, Mount Sinai Hospital
University of Toronto, Toronto, Canada M5G 1X5

INTRODUCTION

In 1936 Randall observed that while some kidney stones formed attached to ulcerative lesions on papillae without ureteral stasis, other kidney stones formed in renal pelvices with urinary stasis[1]. He also observed that the latter kind of stones were frequently laminated, being composed of different urinary salts. More recent studies indicated that partial or complete intrarenal stasis with tubular dilation could also be correlated with kidney lithogenesis, as observed in medullary sponge kidney[2], in continuous ambulatory peritoneal dialysis patients[3] and radiologically in idiopathic stone formers[4]. Moreover, both intracellular and intraluminal microliths of human nephrons have been reported to have a lamellar structure[5].

Previous studies employing polarized light and scanning electron microscopy have shown that the lamellar structure of stones consists of dense layers alternating with less dense ones. Organic matrix fibrils covered with calcium apatite crystallites constitute the dense layers and amorphous organic matrix impregnated with larger non-apatite crystals e.g. calcium oxalate, uric acid or struvite, constitute the less dense layers[6,7]. In understanding the lamellar structure formation both mineral phase and organic matrix phase must be considered.

MINERAL PHASE

Normal urine is periodically supersaturated with respect to lithogenic solutes. Although fluctuating supersaturation and decreased ambient inhibitors can account for crystal nucleation

919

and crystalluria, these phenomena appear insufficient to explain the more sporadic agglomeration that results in stone formation.

ORGANIC MATRIX PHASE

The origin of organic matrix within stones has not been established.   The possible sources include: (a) glomerular ultrafiltrate (b) surface glycoprotein on tubular cells, (c) necrotic tubular cell membranes (d) tubular cell secretion, (e) basal laminae of tubules, (f) mesenchymal matrix from interstitium and (g) bacterial cell walls. In addition to macromolecular surface nucleation of crystals, the organic matrix can promote stone formation by one or more mechanisms, which remain unclarified to date.   These include: (a) acting as a passive crystal collector, (b) catalyzing crystal agglomeration and (c) cementing crystals together.   Despite extensive efforts, the controversy of the relative importance of the mineral and organic matrix phases in the pathogenesis of renal calculi has not been resolved.   There remain two opposing theories.

Organic Matrix is a Template for Crystal Deposition

In 1928, Leduc proposed that stratified precipitations (Liesegang layers) of calcium salts in gelatin were formed by 'equipotential lines of diffusion force'[8]. Based on Leduc's theory, Lichtwitz, in 1944, proposed that all concretions were formed by incrustation of preformed organic matrices and their laminated structures were Liesegang layers[9].   Boyce expanded the Leduc-Lichtwitz theory adding that "matrix had a definitive architectural role in the morphology of all concretions"[6,10].

Organic Matrix Adsorbs Non-specifically to Crystals

In 1928, Schade proposed that concentric laminations were due to the alternate deposition of colloid and crystalloid[11]. In 1961, Finlayson and Vermeulen, having successfully produced concretions with laminations artifically, proposed that matrix was a non-essential constituent resulting from protein adsorption onto crystalline surfaces.   They concluded that stone formation was governed by crystallization phenomena rather than by matrix[12].

METHODS

We studied the ultrastructure of kidney stones from patients by correlative light and electron microscopy, X-ray and electron diffraction, and X-ray energy spectrometry.

RESULTS AND DISCUSSION

Our findings suggest that there are probably two parallel modes of kidney stone pathogenesis.

(1) Accumulation of organic matrix from cellular degradation followed by calcium apatite crystallite deposition. (2) Formation of non-apatite crystals e.g. calcium oxalate, followed by agglomeration with discrete crystals stacked together like masonry and cemented by organic matrix material.

Observation (1) supports the theory that matrix precedes mineralization but observation (2) supports the theory that crystallization is the primary event in kidney stone formation. Since both observations can originate from parallel phenomena within the same system, both major theories may be required to explain the mechanisms for genesis and growth of renal calculi.

A major difficulty with the proposed Liesegang layering mechanism for lamellar formation in renal calculi is that it fails to explain the commonly observed structure of alternating layers of calcium apatite and non-apatite crystals. We propose here an alternative mechanism involving "alternating crystallization" to explain the lamellar structure.

Under high supersaturation, calcium apatite forms only very fine crystallites spontaneously[13]. When co-precipitating with an organic matrix these fine crystallites form densely packed fibers and membranous layers which become the denser layers of the lamellar structure. Assuming slow repletion of Ca^{2+} ions, perhaps owing to local stasis, spontaneous nucleation of calcium apatite will soon cease. However, the ambient urine can be still very much supersaturated with respect to other crystals, e.g. struvite, because concentrations of other ions, e.g. Mg^{2+} and NH_4^+, have not been depleted. The non-apatite crystals are usually larger and polyhedral. Although also co-precipitated with organic matrix, they are more dispersed, forming layers less dense than the calcium apatite layers. Again, the degree of supersaturation with respect to these non-apatite crystals will be greatly reduced after their precipitation. In the meantime, the Ca^{2+} ions would have been repleted to a level high enough for a new round of nucleation of calcium apatite crystals. In turn, another round of non-apatite crystallization will follow. The concentration of any common ion, e.g. PO_4^{3-} in apatite/struvite stones, is assumed to be always sufficiently high. This alternating crystallization mechanism can theoretically explain the lamellar structure formation in most renal stones, but is unamenable to experimental verification.

ACKNOWLEDGEMENTS

   We are grateful to the Arthritis Society and the Mount Sinai
Institute for financial assistance.   We thank Mr A. Reid for
technical assistance and Miss D Federico for manuscript preparation.

REFERENCES

1. A. Randall, New Engl. J. Med. 214:234 (1936).
2. T. Ekstrom, B. Engfeldt, C. Lagergren, and N. Lindroll,
   "Medullary Sponge Kidney", Alamquist and Wiksell, Stockholm
   (1959).
3. P.-T. Cheng, K. P. H. Pritzker, and D. G. Oreopoulos,
   in:"Urinary Stone", R. Ryall, J. G. Brockis, V. Marshall, and
   B. Finlayson, eds., Churchill Livingstone, Melbourne (1984).
4. E. R. Yendt, S. Jarzylo, W. A. Finnis, and M. Cohanim,
   in:"Urolithiasis: Clinical and Basic Research", L. H. Smith,
   W. G. Robertson, and B. Finlayson, eds., Plenum, New York
   (1981).
5. R. S. Malek and W. H. Boyce, J. Urol. 117:336 (1977).
6. W. H. Boyce and F. K. Garvey, J. Urol. 76:213 (1956).
7. P.-T. Cheng, K. P. H. Pritzker, J. Tausch, A. Pittaway, and
   J. Millard, Scan. Elect. Microsc. 163:(1981).
8. S. Leduc, in:"Colloid Chemistry", J. Alexlander, ed., Chemical
   Catalogue Co. Inc., New York (1928).
9. L. Lichtwitz, in:"Colloid Chemistry", J. Alexlander, ed.,
   Reinhold Publ. Corp., New York (1944).
10. W. H. Boyce, Am. J. Med. 45:673 (1968).
11. H. Schade, in:"Colloid Chemistry", J. Alexander, ed., Chemical
    Catalogue Co. Inc., New York (1928).
12. B. Finlayson, C. W. Vermeulen, and E. J. Stewart, J. Urol.
    86:355 (1961).
13. P.-T. Cheng and K. P. H. Pritzker, Calc. Tiss. Int. 35:596
    (1983).

A MICROSCOPIC STUDY OF THE MATRIX OF SOME CALCIUM OXALATE

RENAL STONES

S. R. Khan, B. Finlayson, and R. L. Hackett

Depts. of Surgery and Pathology, University of
Florida, Gainesville, Florida, U.S.A.

INTRODUCTION

Generally over 95% of the weight of urinary stones is
crystalline material making it impossible to study the matrix,
i.e. the non-mineralized component of stones, by conventional
microscopic means without losing information concerning the crystal-
matrix interface. We have developed a procedure[1] whereby
decalcified crystals are represented as crystal ghosts, and stones
retain their architectural integrity.

METHODS

Calcium oxalate stones were fixed in half-strength Karnovsky's
fixative, and then sectioned with a diamond wafering saw.
Approximately 0.2 mm to 1 mm thick sections were collected over
water and embedded in a 1% aqueous solution of bactoagar. After
the agar hardened they were returned to the fixative at least
overnight, washed in distilled water and decalcified in 0.25 M
ethylenediaminetetracetic acid (EDTA) at pH 7.2. The decalcified
stones were processed for transmission electron microscopy (TEM),
scanning electron microscopy (SEM), and light microscopy (LM)
according to methods already described[1]. Paraffin sections were
examined after staining with hematoxylin and eosin, colloidal iron,
alcian blue (pH 0.5 and 2.5), von Kossa, alizarin red, or periodic-
acid-Schiff (PAS). An undecalcified part of every stone was also
studied by SEM.

923

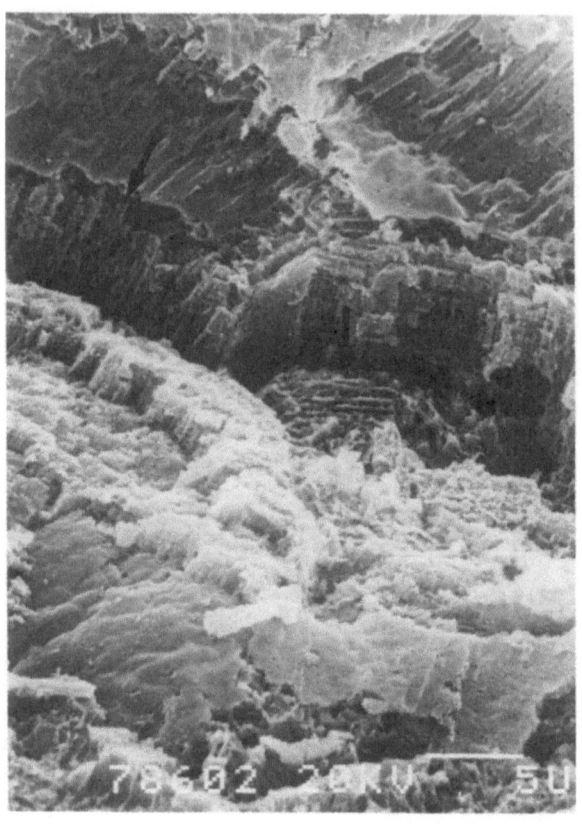

Fig. 1.   SEM of a fractured decalcified human urinary CaOx stone.
At places (arrows) the fracture has passed through plate-
like ghosts of COM crystals.   The ubiquitous nature of the
non-mineralized part of the stone and the concentric
arrangement of crystal ghosts are well pronounced.

RESULTS

     The EDTA-insoluble stone residue, representing part of the
stone matrix, maintained the original shape of the stone.   The
matrix material was ubiquitous (Fig. 1) and was composed of
amorphous and fibrillar materials, and cellular debris.   The
cellular debris consisted of blood and epthelial cells.   The
dissolved crystals were represented by crystal ghosts i.e. spaces
delimited by an electron dense layer.   This layer was probably
formed by the adsorption of urinary mucoproteins on the crystal
surfaces[2].

In paraffin sections, most of the matrix material stained positively with colloidal iron, alcian blue (pH 2.5), PAS and hematoxylin but did not stain with alizarin red or von Kossa. The staining with alcian blue at 0.5 pH was inconclusive. There were areas which appeared to stain positively while others were negative. The staining properties indicate that our decalcification procedure resulted in the loss of crystals and that the EDTA-insoluble stone residue was made of mostly non-sulfated complex carbohydrates.

DISCUSSION

In recent years there have been attempts to study the structure of decalcified stones using various microscopic techniques[3,4] which have added significantly to the information concerning the nature and morphology of stone matrix. But in those studies information on the crystal-matrix interface and precise location of matrix material in stones was lost during processing. Our study has shown that the EDTA-insoluble part of the stone matrix can be processed for conventional microscopic studies without losing its architectural integrity and thus provide important information about the nature and precise location of matrix in urinary stones.

ACKNOWLEDGMENTS

This work was supported by a National Institute of Health grant no. 20586-06. Excellent technical assistance was provided by Mr C A Cockrell.

REFERENCES

1. S. R. Khan, B. Finlayson, and R. L. Hackett, J. Urol. 130:992 (1983).
2. S. R. Khan, B. Finlayson, and R. L. Hackett, Scan. Elect. Micros. 1:379 (1983).
3. W. H. Boyce, and N. M. Sulkin, J. Clin. Invest. 35:1067 (1956).
4. W. H. Boyce, in:"Urolithiasis:Physical Aspects", B. Finlayson, L. L. Hench, and L. H. Smith, eds., National Academy of Sciences, Washington (1971).

CHEMICAL MODELS

COMMENT ON THE ROUND TABLE DISCUSSION ON THEORETICAL MODELS

RELATED TO UROLITHIASIS

B. Finlayson

Division of Urology, Dept. of Surgery, University of
Florida, Gainesville, Florida, U.S.A.

It is a sign of the times that a Round Table on theoretical
models appears on the program of this international urolithiasis
research meeting. Fields of research in clinical medicine, pure
science and engineering can interpenetrate each other more deeply
and lead to new and more precise therapeutic strategies. The body
of urolithiasis research has matured sufficiently that there is some
utility in considering stone formation models, though these models
now seem somewhat abstract. Such is the nature of models. They
are mathematical missiles manufactured and aimed at a specific
problem; only test firings reveal their exact impact. The models
under consideration are so complex that they cannot be unique. A
proper role of a model is to describe what might be and what simply
cannot be.

In urolithiasis research, the influence of physical science
and engineering is reflected by the fact that basic research
relative to stones began by viewing their formation as closely
related to a chemical engineering problem in which the kidney is
seen as a batch processor receiving metabolic inputs leading to
supersaturation with respect to salts of low solubility resulting in
nucleation and subsequent growth, vis a vis precipitation, of
crystals. These particles absorb substances present in the urine
which can inhibit the growth process. The particles aggregate to
form larger particles. Forces cause break-up of the particles.
Each aspect of this model can be treated by some aspect of physical
theory (Table 1). The primary experimental implementation of this
model is the small batch crystallizer. Historically, it has been a
tool for collecting kinetic crystal growth data and studying the
impact of growth inhibitors; aggregation was ignored. There are
other kinds of crystallizer schemes beginning to receive attention

Table 1. Aspects of the Experimental Model of Urolithiasis and
Associated Physical Theory.

Experimental Theory	Relevant Theory or Field of Study
Species equilibration and supersaturation	Debye-Hückel Solution Theory[6]
Nucleation	Velmer-Becker-Doring Theory[7]
	Spinodal decomposition[8]
	Heterogenous nucleation[9]
Crystal Growth	Catalysis spiral growth (Burton-Frank-Cabrera theory)[10]
	Birth and spread growth theory[11]
Adsorption	Adsorption theory[12]
	Electrical double layer theory[13]
	Polymer adsorption[14]
	Lattice statistical mechanics[15]
Aggregation	Derjaugin-Landau-Verwey-Overbeek theory (DLVO)[16]
Break-up	Hydrodynamics[17]
	Materials strength[18]

in urolithiasis research, such as the spontaneously nucleating crystallizers ("crash" crystallizers), continuous crystallizers and tubular flow crystallizers.

Our group at the University of Florida has been working towards a plausible numerical simulation of the kinetic consequence of a precipitation in a generalized crystallizer. This simulation can be applied to all crystallizers being used in urolithiasis research. Portions of the simulation have been written and implemented; however, the entire program has not yet been executed because of inadequate hardware and funds.

Extant models of urolithiasis-related crystallizers have thus far been concerned with processes at work within the fluid contents of the crystallizer or kidney. However, any truly comprehensive model must also account for the interaction at the wall of the container. In vitro, this amounts to accounting for wall encrustation. In vivo, one must account for the role of injury and the nature of epithelium in the formation of kidney stones as well as wall effects such as resorption of electrolytes and heterogenous nucleation on the wall. Successful theoretical modeling of experimental and clinical research in these areas will considerably extend the detailed understanding of the disease processes involved in urolithiasis.

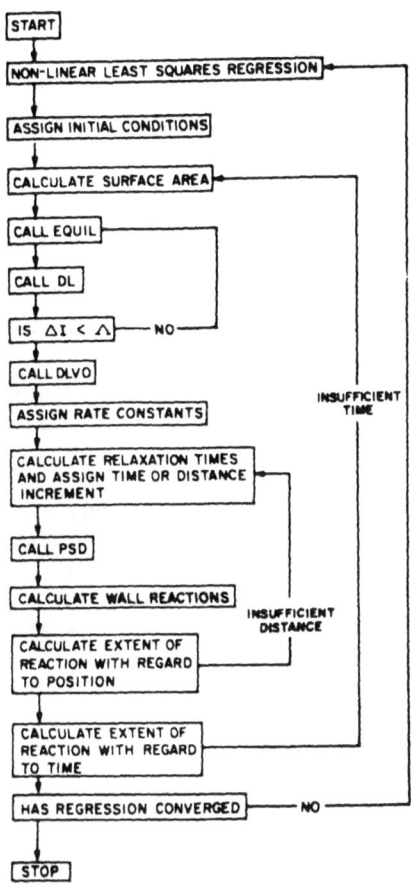

Fig. 1. Strategy for calculating dynamics in a generalized
crystallizer.

During the Round Table Discussion, a strategy for incorporating
the various theories into an overall and general simulation of
precipitation (SOAP) was presented (Fig. 1) and criticized.   The
proposal involved the solution of a large set of simultaneous
differential equations (>10,000) (Fig. 2). Solutions are taken at
time intervals along the course of the precipitation such that the
interval is 5% or less than the briefest relaxation time (τ) of any
of the simultaneous equations, i.e. for i = 1,2,3,....,>10,000,

$$\tau_i \quad {}^{f_i = f_i(t)} = f_i \left[\frac{df_i}{dt} \right]^{-1}$$

where time interval $\geqslant \tau_j$; j, an index of smallest τ_i.

nucleation:

$$dn_1/dt = \sum_{i=1}^{j} A_i \exp(-B_i/(\ln(RS))^2)$$

crystal growth:

$$dRS/dt = \sum_{i=1}^{j} K_g S_i (RS-RS_{o,i})^M$$

aggregation:

$$dn_i/dt = -\sum_{j=1}^{1} k_A(i,j)n_i n_j + \sum_{j=1}^{j<i/2} k_A(i-j,j)n_{i-j}n_j$$

break up:

$$dn_i/dt = -K_B(i)n_i + 2K_B(2i)n_{2i}$$

Fig. 2. Set of simultaneous differential equations which serve as the basis for generalized crystallizer simulation.

Conceptually, the computation strategy is trivial, but implementing and executing the numerical solution places modest demands on the programmer and the hardware. It was asserted and challenged at the Round Table that successful development of SOAP would permit a concordance of information drawn fromn the various crystallizers used in stone research.

ACKNOWLEDGEMENT

This work was supported by N.I.H. Grant AM 20586.

REFERENCES

1. J. R. Burns, C. M. Brown, and B. Finlayson, World J. Urol. 1:126 (1983).
2. Maeros User Manual, SAND 80-0822, Sandia National Laboratories, Albuquerque, New Mexico, U.S.A.
3. R. L. Ryall, C. M. Hibberd, B. C. Mazzachi, and V. R. Marshall, Urol. Res. 12:77 (1984).
4. J. Garside and F. J. Jancic, Chem. Eng. Sci. 33:1623 (1978).
5. G. W. Drach, M. D. B. Gottung, and A. Randolph, Urol. Res. 12:86 (1984).
6. S. K. Berry, S. A. Rice, and J. Rice, "Physical Chemistry", Wiley, New York (1980).
7. R. Becker and W. Doring, Ann. Physik. 24:719 (1935).
8. B. Finlayson, Kidney Int. 13:344 (1978).
9. R. F. Strickland-Constable, "Kinetics and Mechanisms of Crystallization", Academic Press, London (1968).
10. W. K. Burton, N. Cabrera, and F. C. Frank, Phil. Trans. Roy. Soc. A243:299 (1951).

11. M. Ohara and R. C. Reid, "Modeling Crystal Growth Rates from Solution", Prentice Hall, Englewood Cliffs, New Jersey (1977).

12. I. Langmuir, J. Am. Chem. Soc. 40:1361 (1981).

13. D. C. Grahame, Chem. Rev. 41:441 (1947).

14. W. Norde and J. Lyklema, J. Coll Interface Sci. 66:257 (1978).

15. C. J. Thompson, "Mathematical Statistical Mechanics", Princeton University Press, Princeton, New Jersey (1972).

16. E. J. W. Verwey and J. T. G. Overbeek, "Theory of the Stability of Lyophobic Colloids", Elsevier, Amsterdam (1948).

17. F. Charlton, "Textbook of Fluid Dynamics", Van Nostrand, Princeton, New Jersey (1967).

18. J. H. Brophy, R. M. Rose, and J. Wulff, "The Structure and Properties of Materials", Vol. II, Wiley, New York (1964).

IX. ANIMAL MODELS

MICROSTRUCTURE OF CALCIUM OXALATE FOREIGN BODY STONES PRODUCED

IN RAT BLADDER

S. R. Kahn, B. Finlayson, and R. L. Hackett

Depts. of Surgery and Pathology, College of Medicine
University of Florida, Gainesville, Florida, U.S.A.

INTRODUCTION

Implantation of a foreign body, usually a zinc disc[1], in the
rat bladder is a standard method of producing urinary calculi for
experimental studies. The diet is modified or ethylene glycol
added to the drinking water to develop a stone of the desired
composition. In order to study the microscopic architecture of
such stones, zinc is inappropriate since it cannot be sectioned.
Therefore we used discs, 4 mm to 6 mm in diameter, made of a plastic
normally used for embedding tissue for transmission electron
microscopy (TEM)[2].

METHODS

Single discs were implanted in bladders of male Sprague-Dawley
rats[3]. The rats were given drinking water containing 0.75%
ethylene glycol. After varying lengths of time the discs were
extracted, fixed in paraformaldehyde and glutaraldehyde and
processed for scanning electron microscopy (SEM)[4]. Following SEM
the encrusted discs were rehydrated, embedded in 1% agar and
immersed in 0.25M ethylenediaminetetraacetic acid (EDTA) at pH 7.2
for a week. The decalcified discs were washed in distilled water
and processed for TEM[5]. Some encrusted discs were embedded in
plastic following fixation in buffered formalin. Five to 10 μm
thick sections were cut and decalcified on a microscope slide by
treatment with either 0.1N HCl or 0.25M EDTA. The decalcified
sections were stained with toluidine blue and examined by polarized
as well as transmitted light microscopy.

RESULTS AND DISCUSSION

Encrustation of the disc surfaces started within 3 days of implantation and within a week 2/3 of the disc surfaces were covered with crystals. Within 2 weeks both surfaces of the discs as well as their margins were encrusted. Both calcium oxalate monohydrate (COM) and calcium oxalate dihydrate (COD) crystals were present. No other types of crystals were identified. The urines were free of bacteria. Kidneys showed no signs of histological damage. COM crystals consisted of plate-like crystallites (Fig. 1) arranged hemispherically of spherically around a central nucleus. COD crystals were basically bipyramidal with small crystals covering the surfaces of large COD crystals, an apparent result of growth. A number of COD crystals had etch pits that revealed internal layering. COD crystals often had plate-like crystallites of COM on their surfaces and in some cases the entire surface of a COD crystal was covered with them. On the basis of their morphology and comparison with published micrographs of human urinary stones these COD crystals are interpreted as transforming into COM crystals[6].

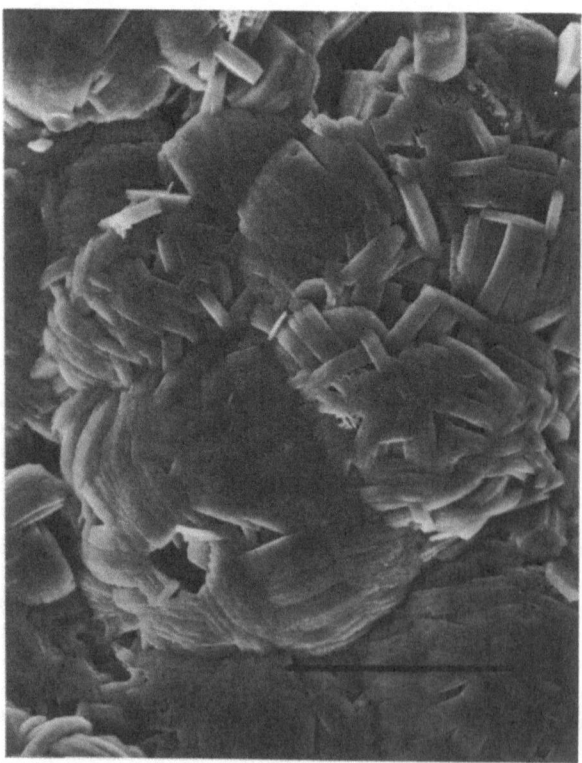

Fig. 1. SEM of the surface of spherulitic COM crystals showing edges of platelike crystallites (bar = 50 μm).

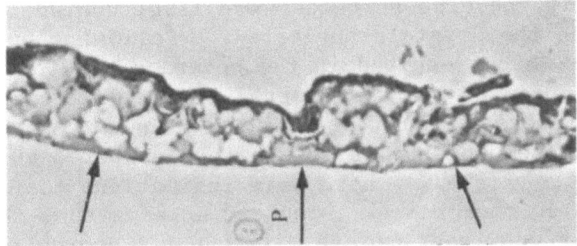

Fig. 2. LM of a cross section of the stone showing a continuous
protein layer (arrows) on the disc surface (P). Holes are
a result of the removal of crystals during decalcification.

Light microscopy (Fig. 2) and TEM showed a thin proteinaceous
layer between disc surface and crystals. TEM of demineralized
stones (Fig. 3) showed that the crystals were surrounded by an
amorphous coat and that amorphous and fibrillar materials were
present inside the crystal ghosts. Cellular debris could often be
identified in the intercrystalline areas as well as on the stone
surfaces. Cross-sections of the demineralized stones also showed
the presence of radial striations and concentric laminations.

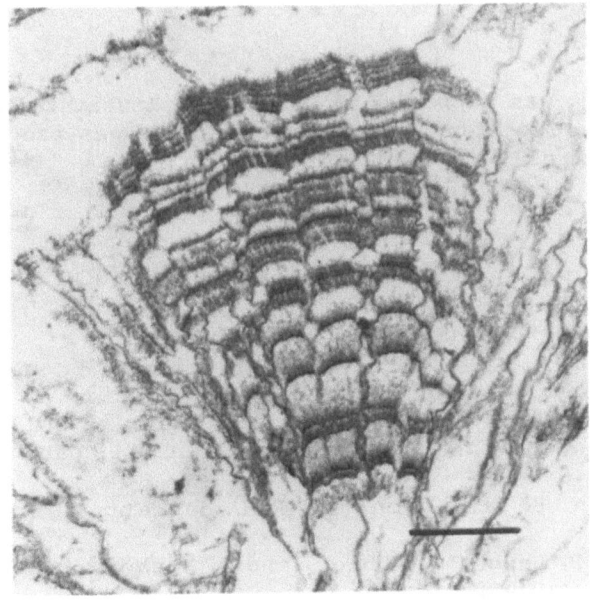

Fig. 3. TEM of a cross-section of decalcified stone showing
concentric laminations and radial striations as well as
amorphous and fibrillar materials (bar = 1 μm).

Apparently the disc surfaces were first coated by a protein layer on which the crystals nucleated. Following nucleation, crystals grew which resulted in the coverage of disc surfaces. The encrustation appeared to have started in the center of the disc surface. This initial process of nucleation and growth was followed by subsequent nucleation on the encrusted surfaces and growth of the crystals. There were indications that some crystal aggregation also took place. Thus it appears that the foreign body stones grew by confluent growth with crystal aggregation playing a minor role.

The foreign body stones described here have a number of similarities with human CaOx stones. Like human urinary stones they are made of a crystalline component and a non-crystalline component. Their surface morphology is similar to the surface morphology of human urinary stones. Internally they exhibit concentric laminations and radial striations. As with human urinary stones, they have COD crystals that appear to undergo transformation into COM. The non-crystalline component of foreign body stones is also similar to that of human urinary stones in consisting of amorphous and fibrillar materials and cellular debris. Thus it appears that a foreign body stone of the type we have studied can adequately serve as a model for the study of human urinary stone growth.

ACKNOWLEDGMENTS

This work was supported by a National Institute of Health grant no. 20586-06. Excellent technical assistance was provided by Mr C. A. Cockrell.

REFERENCES

1. C. W. Vermeulen, E. S. Lyon, W. B. Gill, and W. H. Chapman, J. Urol. 82:249 (1959).
2. A. R. Spurr, J. Ultrastruc. Res. 26:31 (1969).
3. S. R. Khan, R. L. Hackett, W. C. Thomas, and B. Finlayson, in:"Urinary Stone", R. Ryall, J. G. Brockis, V. Marshall, and B. Finlayson, eds., Churchill Livingstone, Melbourne (1984).
4. S. R. Khan, B. Finlayson, and R. L. Hackett, Lab. Invest. 41:504 (1979).
5. S. R. Khan, B. Finlayson, and R. L. Hackett, J. Urol. 130:992 (1983).
6. W. Berg, P. Lange, D. Robler, and C. Bothor, Z. Urol. Nephrol. 72:351 (1979).

URINE AND SERUM BIOCHEMISTRY RELATIVE TO THE RISK OF LITHOGENESIS

IN RATS ON AN ATHEROGENIC DIET

W. L. Strohmaier, K.-H. Bichler, I. Gaiser, E. Schulze,
H. J. Nelde, and M. Schreiber

Dept. of Urology, University of Tübingen
D-7400 Tübingen, F.R.G.

INTRODUCTION

Several animal models have been established to study the effect of dietary changes on the pathogenesis of urolithiasis. For example, an atherogenic diet (rich in cholesterol) fed to rats causes nephrocalcinosis and urolithiasis[1,2]. These changes occur within 3 to 4 weeks. The pathophysiological mechanisms, however, are not clear. Changes occur in the pancreatic islets (an increase in the total number of A-cells) which result in an increased production of glucagon and an effect on calcium metabolism and this may be the cause of the renal calcification[1,2]. The purpose of this study was to examine these interrelationships.

METHODS

Twenty male rats (CHBB:Thom, Wistar type) were kept for 8 weeks. They were divided into two groups and fed (i) an atherogenic diet (Altromin diet C 1014); and (ii) a control diet (Altromin, Lage, FRG). The animals were kept in metabolic cages in order to collect urine. The urine of each animal was pooled in weekly portions. At the end of the experiment all animals were killed. Blood samples were taken from the aorta and vena cava. The kidneys were examined for calcification and concrements. Calcium, magnesium, sodium and potassium were measured by flame photometry, inorganic phosphate and citrate by test kits (Boehringer, Mannheim, FRG), serum creatinine by the Testomar-kit (Behringwerke, Marburg, FRG), uromucoid by rocket electrophoresis[3,4] and glycosaminoglycans by the method of Blumenkrantz[5]. The Mann-Whitney U-test of statistical significance was used[6].

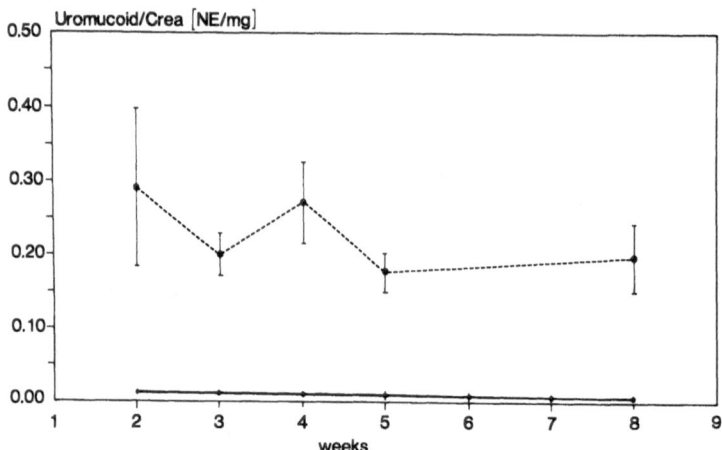

Fig. 1.   Urinary uromucoid/creatinine ratio (mean ± SD) in rats fed
an atherogenic diet (————) and in controls (-----) NE =
"Normoleinheit" (normal unit).

RESULTS

By the second week of the experiment the uromucoid excretion of
the animals fed the atherogenic diet was depressed significantly and
stayed low during the remainder of the study (Fig. 1).   The
excretions of calcium and magnesium were increased from the third
week of the experiment (Figs. 2 and 3).   The control rats excreted
higher amounts of sodium, but the difference was not significant.
The urine levels of potassium, phosphate and citrate showed no

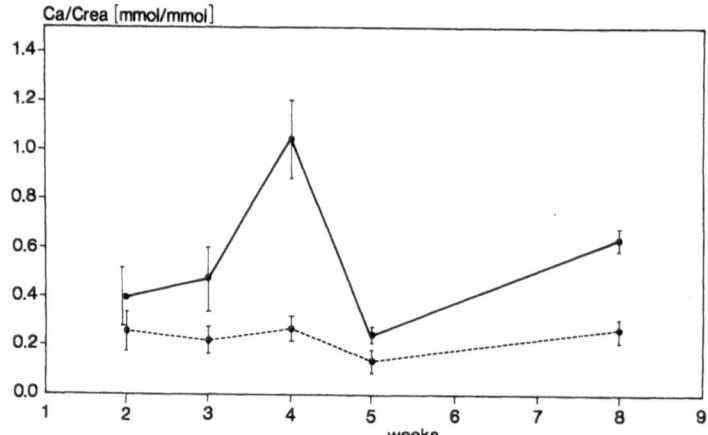

Fig. 2.   Urinary calcium/creatinine ratio in rats fed an atherogenic
diet (————) and in controls (-----).

942

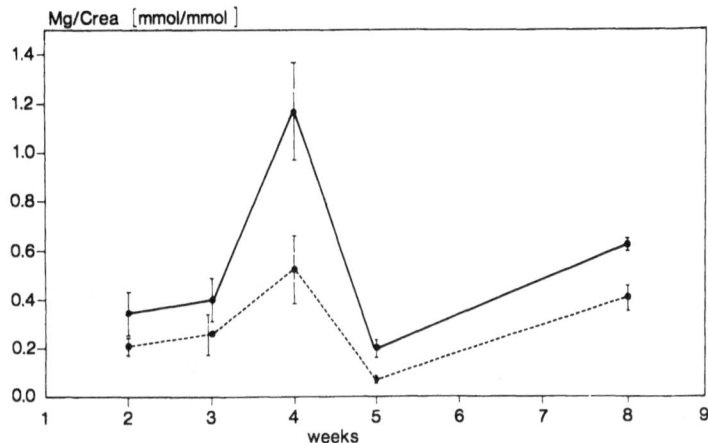

Fig. 3. Urinary magnesium/creatinine ratio in rats fed an atherogenic diet (————) and in controls (-----).

Table 1. Serum Biochemistry in Rats Fed an Atherogenic Diet and in Controls (mean ± SD).

Variable	Atherogenic diet	Control diet
Calcium (mmol/l)	2.78 ± 0.12	2.86 ± 0.14
Magnesium (mmol/l)	0.98 ± 0.12	0.85 ± 0.16
Phosphate (mmol/l)	2.37 ± 0.37	2.36 ± 0.40
Potassium (mmol/l)	4.96 ± 1.10	4.80 ± 1.02
Sodium (mmol/l)	142 ± 3.00	143 ± 2.50
Creatinine (mg/dl)*	1.77 ± 0.11	1.36 ± 0.09

*$p < 0.001$

difference between the groups. On the atherogenic diet, the serum creatinine was slightly but significantly increased (Table 1) but the serum levels of the other ions were not different in the two groups. The concrements found in the majority of the animals fed the atherogenic diet consisted of struvite and apatite.

DISCUSSION

The decrease in uromucoid production shows that the atherogenic diet alters the tubular epithelium. Earlier studies have indicated that this acid mucoprotein is synthesized in the distal tubule and its urinary excretion is decreased in chronic pyelonephritis and renal tubular acidosis[7,8]. The decrease in uromucoid production was followed by hypercalciuria although serum calcium was not different from that of the controls. Histology showed that there was calcification in the outer and inner stripes of the outer medullary zone, corresponding to localization in the distal nephron. Along with the depressed uromucoid production, the hypercalciuria seemed to be due to a primary distal tubular disorder. Although calcium reabsorption occurs largely in the proximal nephron, the fine adjustment is located in the distal region[9,10] and any disorder there may lead to a renal loss of calcium.

In contrast to the findings of Schwille et al[1,2], the urinary excretion of magnesium was increased in the present study. This increase may be due to impaired tubular reabsorption or to an increased filtered load arising from the higher serum level of magnesium. The serum creatinine demonstrates that the atherogenic diet caused an impairment of glomerular function and these animals showed a slight but significant reduction in renal function.

Possibly the atherogenic diet leads to alterations in the nutrition and metabolism of the renal epithelium caused by the hypercholesterolemia. The highly developed outer medullary zone seems to be particularly sensitive. Morphological and micropuncture investigations are necessary to clarify the pathogenesis of this form of calcification.

REFERENCES

1. P. O. Schwille and B. Viebeck, Fortschr. Urol. Nephrol. 5:166 (1975).
2. P. O. Schwille, G. Brandt, P. Brunner, D. Ulbrich, and W. Kompf, Urologe A 14:306 (1975).
3. C. B. Laurell, Analyt. Biochem. 15:45 (1966).
4. C. Kirchner and K.-H. Bichler, Urol. Res. 4:119 (1976).
5. N. Blumenkrantz and G. Asboe-Hansen, Analyt. Biochem. 54:484 (1973).
6. B. Ramm and G. Hofmann, "Biomathematik und Medizinische Statistik", Enke, Stuttgart (1976).
7. K.-H. Bichler, C. Kirchner, and V. Ideler, Br. J. Urol. 47:733 (1976).
8. S. Korn and K.-H. Bichler, Fortsch. Urol. Nephrol. 20:184 (1982).
9. W. C. Lassiter, C. W. Gottschalk, and M. Mylle, Am. J. Physiol. 204:771 (1963).
10. P. Deetjen, in:"Urologie in Klinik und Praxis", R. Hohenfellner and E. J. Zingg, eds., Thieme, Stuttgart (1978).

HISTOPATHOLOGICAL CHANGES IN THE KIDNEY OF THE RAT ON AN

ATHEROGENIC DIET

H. J. Nelde, K.-H. Bichler, W. L. Strohmaier,
E. Schulze, and I. Gaiser

Dept. of Urology, University of Tubingen
D-7400 Tubingen, F.R.G.

INTRODUCTION

We have set up a rat model to study the dependence of
nephrocalcinosis on various factors involved in stone-formation.
To induce nephrocalcinosis we fed an atherogenic diet, high in
cholesterol[1]. The position of the resulting calcification and
concrements in the different regions of the nephron was noted and
their morphology and composition determined.

METHODS

Two groups of 10 male Wistar rats were fed different diets for
a period of 8 weeks. One group was fed an atherogenic diet with a
high content of cholesterol (C 1014, Altromin, Lage, FRG) and the
other a control diet (C 1000, Altromin, Lage, FRG). To determine
the effect on various lithogenic substances in the urine, the
animals were kept in sequence in metabolic cages. At the end of
the study the rats were killed and an autopsy performed. The
kidneys and efferent urinary tract were removed, fixed in buffered
formalin (4% solution, pH 7) and embedded in paraffin after
alcoholic dehydration and clearing in methylbenzoate (avoiding
xylol[2]). Sections (7 μm thick) were subjected to various
histological tests. The histochemical method of Voigt[2] was used to
quantitate calcification. Staining with naphthalhydroxamic acid
precipitated yellow crystals which under polarised light with
crossed Nichol prisms produced a yellow luminescence. We adopted a
semi-quantitative classification of calcification based on 4 grades
(-, +, ++, +++). The concrements were analysed microscopically.
The sections were de-waxed with methylbenzoate, washed in ethanol

(100% solution) and dried. Later the sections were covered with liquids of various refractive indices (n_D) and analysed under polarised light. In order to determine the content of struvite we employed a liquid of $n_D = 1.50$, and one of $n_D = 1.662$ for calcium-phosphate (P. Cargill Laboratories Inc., Cedar Grove, New York)[3].

RESULTS

With the exception of random calcification in 2 animals, we found none in the control rats (Table 1). Rats fed the atherogenic diet, however, show marked nephrocalcinosis (Table 1, Figs. 1,2). No calcification could be seen in the cortex but numerous sites were found in the inner and outer sections of the outer medulla. Most of these were located intraluminally in the distal portion of the renal tract. The tubules were partially dilated because of these concrements. The epithelial cells seem to be reduced in height. Sporadic calcification was noted in the inner zone of the medulla and in the renal pelvis. The size of the concrements ranged from 10 to 50 µm. There was a significant difference in the extent of calcification in the two groups. Stone analysis under polarised light revealed struvite crystals, recognizable because of their characteristic white colour of lower order and indistinct birefringent under polarised light (Fig. 3). The concrements in the renal pelvis, as well as those found in the tissue sections, on average, consisted of 70% struvite and 30% calcium phosphate.

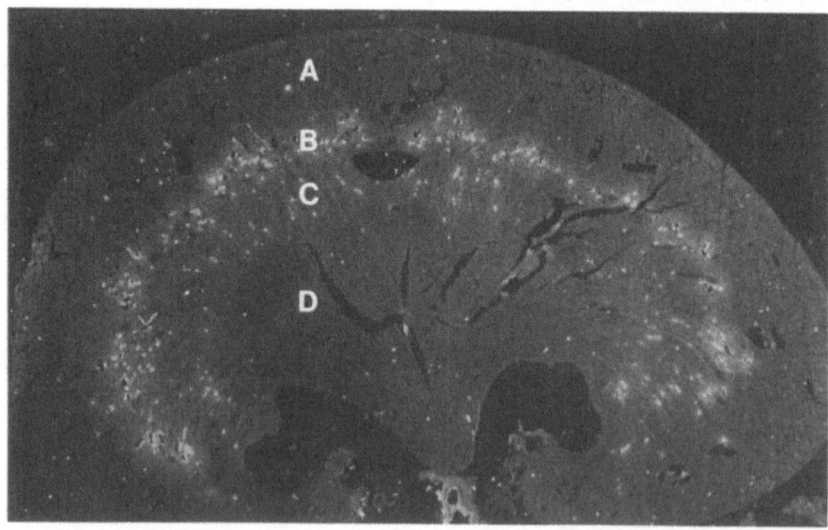

Fig. 1. Longitudinal section of a kidney of a rat fed atherogenic diet.

946

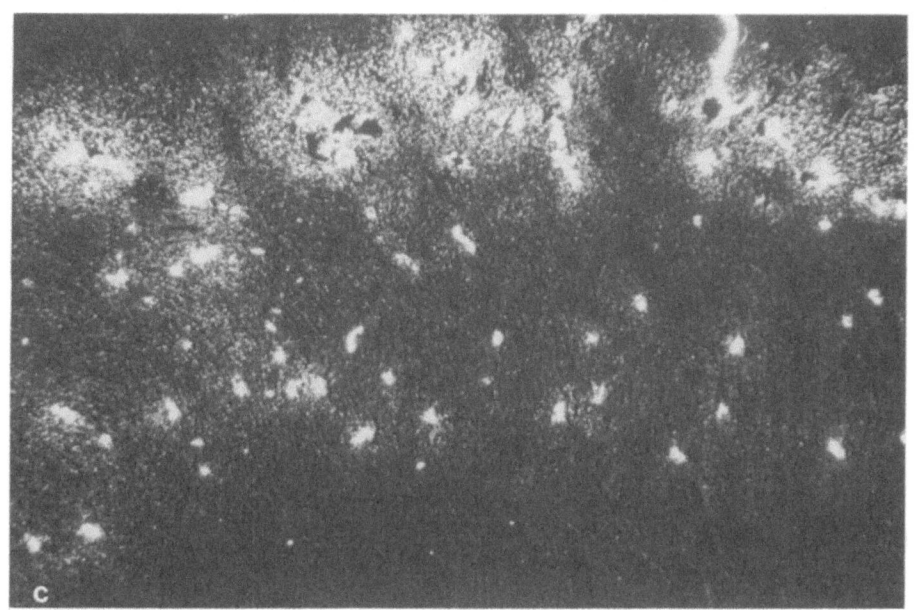

Fig. 2.   Longitudinal section of a rat fed atherogenic diet
          under polarised light.

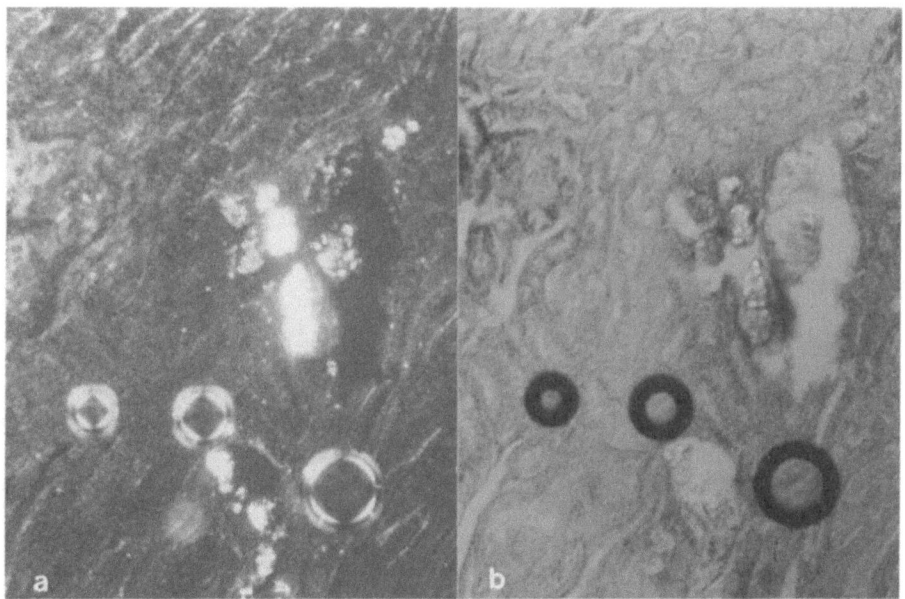

Fig. 3.   Polarising microscope analysis of concrements showing
          (a) birefringence and (b) variation in $\lambda/2$).

Table 1. Calcification in the Kidney

Animal	Control diet	Animal	Atherogenous diet
1	-	11	+++
2	-	12	+++
3	-	13	+++
4	-	14	+++
5	-	15	+++
6	+	16	++
7	+	17	++
8	-	18	++
9	-	19	++
10	-	20	+++

- no calcification; + scattered calcification;
++ moderate calcification; +++ marked calcification

DISCUSSION

In this study, we have confirmed the observations of Schwille et al[1] that within a few weeks nephrocalcinosis can be induced by an atherogenic diet and that the rats on different diets show differences in the formation of calculi. Together with the urinary data, the morphologic studies demonstrate the importance of the distal region for the formation of calculi[4,5]. On the atherogenic diet, kidney function is reduced. Earlier studies demonstrated that acid mucoproteins (e.g. uromucoid) are produced in the distal tubule and possibly protect the cells of the urothelium. Alterations in this area result in a decrease in the excretion of uromucoid in the urine. Alterations in the tubules seem to be the cause of the disturbances in this area of the kidney and may result in formation of calculi because of their effect on the tubular reabsorption of lithogenic ions.

REFERENCES

1. P. O. Schwille, Urologe A 14:306 (1975).
2. G. G. Voigt, Acta Histochem. 4:122 (1957).
3. G. Sorger and E. M. Bausch, Urologe A 10:151 (1971).
4. K.-H. Bichler, C. Kirchner, and V. Adeler, Br. J. Urol. 47:733 (1976).
5. K.-H. Bichler, C. Kirchner, H. Weiser, S. Korn, W. Strohmaier, P. Schmitz-Moormann, A. Hanck, and H. J. Nelde, Clin. Nephrol. 20:32 (1983).

^{14}C-CALCIUM OXALATE (CAOX) ADHERENCE IN THE RAT BLADDER

C. Smith

Regional Kidney Disease Program, Hennepin County Medical
Center, Minneapolis, Minnesota 55415, U.S.A.

INTRODUCTION

For clinical stone disease to occur, a nucleus must form and be
retained until a crystalline mass is attained which is sufficient to
cause clinical symptoms or be identified radiologically.   The
mechanism by which a nucleus is retained has received little
attention.   Parsons et al [1] have demonstrated that the mucin layer
of the rabbit bladder prevents the adherence of bacteria.   Gill et
al[2] showed that when crystallization of calcium oxalate was induced
in the rat bladder, few crystals adhered if the mucin layer was
intact.

The purpose of these studies was to confirm and extend the
above observations using a model of pre-formed crystals.

METHODS

Female rats were catheterized and both ureters ligated under
nembutal anesthesia.   Upon completion of the bladder treatments
outlined below, ^{14}C-CaOx crystals were instilled for 15 min.   Non-
adherent crystals were removed by multiple saline washes.   The
bladders were then excised and solubilized in NCS tissue solubilizer
and the retained radioactivity was counted in a scintillation
counter.   Data are expressed as the % of introduced radioactivity
remaining after the saline washes.

RESULTS

Histologic Studies

Two groups of rats were studied. Control (C) bladders were irrigated with saline and acid-treated (A) received 0.1 N HCl for 2 min. Study of colloidal iron-stained sections demonstrated that most of the mucin layer was removed by acid treatment.

Adherence Studies

Control (C) bladders were irrigated with saline- and acid-treated (A) with 0.1 N HCl. Table 1 demonstrates a greater than 20-fold rise in adherence following acid-treatment.

Table 1. Adherence of ^{14}Ca-CaOx Crystals in Saline-treated (C) and Acid-Treated (A) Rat Bladders (Mean $\pm$ SEM).

	C (n=0)		A (n=18)
Adherence (%)	0.6 $\pm$ 0.2	P<0.001	13.6 $\pm$ 2.2

Restoration Studies

These studies were done in acid-treated bladders to examine the ability of the test substances to restore anti-adherence factors removed by the acid treatment. Test substances included chondroitin sulphate (20 mg/ml), sialic acid (20 mg/ml), heparin (20 U/ml) and pentosan polysulphate (20 mg/ml) which were allowed to sit at room temperature for 24 h prior to use. Each was instilled for 2 min, the bladders irrigated with saline and crystal adherence studies performed. Table 2 demonstrates that chondroitin sulphate (CS) and heparin (H) fully restored anti-adherence whereas pentosan polysulphate (PPS) led to a partial reduction and sialic acid (SA) had no effect.

Table 2. The Effect of Glycosaminoglycans on Crystal Adherence in Acid-Treated Bladders (Mean $\pm$ SEM).

Test Substance	CS (n=5)	SA (n=6)	H (n=8)	PPS (n=12)
Adherence (%)	1.2 $\pm$ 0.4*	8.6 $\pm$ 3.6*	0.8 $\pm$ 0.3*	5.5 $\pm$ 1.6*[+]

* vs A, P<0.02; [+] vs C, P<0.02 .

Alteration Studies

These studies were done in mucin-intact bladders to examine alterations in crystal adherence induced by test substances, including calcium (30 mg/dl), oxalate (10 mg/dl), and phosphorus (800 mg/dl). Phosphorus was studied at pH 4, 6, and 8 as was tris buffer. Instillation of test substances was followed by saline irrigation and adherence studies as outlined above. Table 3 shows that calcium (Ca) induced an 8-fold increase in crystal adherence whereas oxalate (Ox) had no effect.

Table 3. The Effect of Ca and Ox on Crystal Adherence in Mucin Intact Rat Bladders (Mean $\pm$ SEM).

	Ca (n=10)	Ox (n=4)
Adherence (%)	4.9 $\pm$ 1.0*	0.4 $\pm$ 0.2

*vs C, P<0.02

Table 4 demonstrates increased crystal adherence in the presence of phosphorus. As the pH was increased, adherence increased but there was no statistically significant difference between the pH values. Tris buffer did not increase crystal adherence.

Table 4. The Effect of Phosphorus (P) and Tris Buffer at pH 4,6,8 on Crystal Adherence in Mucin Intact Rat Bladders (mean $\pm$ SEM).

pH	4	6	8
P	1.6 $\pm$ 0.4*	2.8 $\pm$ 0.6*	3.3 $\pm$ 0.7*
Tris	0.3 $\pm$ 0.1	0.5 $\pm$ 0.3	1.2 $\pm$ 0.4

*vs C, P<0.02

DISCUSSION

Nucleus retention within the urinary tract appears to be a necessary event if clinical stone disease is to occur. The mechanism of retention is unknown. These studies suggest that the intact uroepithelium of the rat bladder can significantly inhibit adherence of calcium oxalate crystals. This anti-adherence property appears to be associated with the mucin layer since when it is removed by acid treatment, adherence increases 20-fold.

951

Mucin is a complex substance containing a number of glycos-aminoglycans (GAGs). Three GAGs known to be present in mucin were studied for their ability to restore anti-adherence properties removed by acid treatment. A crude preparation of chondroitin sulphate restored antiadherence, as did heparin. Sialic acid had no effect. Pentosan polysulphate, a synthetic GAG, resulted in a decrease in adherence but not to control levels.

Alterations in the mucin of the uroepithelium could occur as a primary event but could also be the result of other known, predisposing factors for stone disease, i.e. hypercalciuria, hyper-oxaluria or pH. These factors were studied in the alteration experiments performed in bladders with the mucin intact. It was found that calcium increased crystal adherence as did phosphorus. The tris studies suggest that if pH has an effect, it is probably exerted through changes in the charge of phosphorus. Oxalate had no effect on adherence.

These preliminary studies support the proposal that the mucin of intact uroepithelium can prevent significant adherence of calcium oxalate crystals. A role for chondroitin sulphate and heparin as components of mucin is suggested. Adherence can be increased by calcium and phosphorus especially at high pH values, conditions not infrequently found in stone formers' urine.

REFERENCES

1. C. L. Parsons, C. Greenspan, S. W. Moore, and S. G. Mulholland, Urology 9:48 (1977).
2. W. B. Gill, K. Ruggiero, and F. H. Strauss, Invest. Urol. 17:257 (1979).

DISSOLUTION OF CRYSTALLINE CALCIUM OXALATE

K. J. Wu, X. Q. Li, Y. Dokko, B. Chen, M. A. Krupper, W. W. Chuang, S. K. Wolfson, and S. J. Yao

Surgical Research Laboratory, Montefiore Hospital and Dept. of Neurological Surgery, University of Pittsburgh Pittsburgh, PA 15213, U.S.A.

INTRODUCTION

The effects of several chemical solutions have been studied on the induction period of calcium oxalate crystallization, the in vitro rate of dissolution of calcium oxalate pellets, and calcium stone-formation in rats. These studies form a simple and reliable approach to investigations into the mechanisms of calcium urolithiasis. There is a correlation between the induction period before crystallization and the dissolution rate produced by various chemical such as α-ketoglutaric acid. In this paper we report on in vitro studies on calcium oxalate crystallization and dissolution and a new rat model for determining the relative ability of solvents to dissolve calcium oxalate stones in vivo.

METHODS AND RESULTS

For studies on the induction period of calcium oxalate crystallization, a Ca^{2+} electrode was employed to determine the onset of crystallization[1]. The standard assay medium ($37^{\circ}C$) consisted of 100 ml of 150 mM KCl, 3.0 mM HEPES buffer (pH 6.0) and 200 μM Ca^{2+}. Ca^{2+} activity was standardized by 2.5 μl additions of 1 M $CaCl_2$ to yield a final concentration of 300 μM. Aliquots of 2.5 ml of each test chemical (100 mM) were added to the medium at pH 5.0 to 6.0. Sequential additions of sodium oxalate (100 mM) with a micro pipet followed (total addition 2.5 ml). The induction periods in various solvents are tabulated in Table 1.

For the in vitro studies of artificial stones, the pellets were prepared by the method of Ziolkowski and Perrin[2]. A mixture of

953

Table 1. Induction Period (IP) of Calcium Oxalate Mineralization in Various Solvents.

Solvent	IP (min)	Solvent	IP (min)
Control[a]	12	Oxaloacetic acid	15
Citric acid	36	α-ketoglutaric acid	120
Magnesium acetate	34	Renacidin	127
Fumaric acid	12	Solution G	30
Ferric citrate	15	D-gluconic acid	14
Malic acid	11	D-gluconic acid lactone	13
Magnesium chloride	12	D-gluconic acid[b]	30
Formic acid	13	α-ketoglutaric acid	
Succinic acid	23	mixture[c]	120

[a]Calcium chloride and sodium oxalate; [b]Hemi-magnesium salt;
[c]20 mM α-ketoglutaric acid, 2.0 mM D-gluconic acid (hemi-magnesium salt), and 2.0 mM magnesium carbonate.

Table 2. Dissolution Rates (mg/min) of Artificial Calcium Oxalate Stones (Pellets) in Various Solvents using a Rotating System.

pH	Citric acid	Succinic acid	Renacidin	EDTA	α-Keto Acid	α-Keto acid mixture
6.0 to 6.5	-	0.02	0.02	0.06	0.066	-
4.0 to 4.5	0.024	-	0.03	0.03	-	0.12

20 g calcium oxalate monohydrate, 4 g of agar, and 80 ml distilled water was heated on a water bath at 90°C with constant stirring until the agar dissolved and the suspension thickened. It was then poured into a plastic Petri dish. Cylinders were cut from it with a cork borer. The cylinder of calcium oxalate was mounted on a rotating stirrer. In order to remove all loose material from the surface of a pellet, each mounted pellet was washed by rotating it in 750 ml 20 mM EDTA and 40 mM n-ethylmorpholine buffer (pH 8.0) for 5 min and then washed for 2 min in distilled water. The pellet was placed in the desired reaction solution and rotated for 30 min at a constant speed. During this time, the Ca^{2+} electrode was placed in the solution to monitor the rate of dissolution of calcium oxalate throughout the experiment. The results are shown in Table 2.

For the in vitro studies of bladder stones, a low midline abdominal incision was made on weight-matched adult Sprague-Dawley rats under intraperitoneal sodium pentobarbital anesthesia. Bilateral ureteral ligations were performed. Two polyethylene tubes (PE11) were then inserted into the urethra to the bladder and tightened. After generating urothelial injury by the injection of 0.5 ml of 0.1 N HCl for 1 min, calcium oxalate crystallization was induced by the instillation of 0.5 ml of 20 mM sodium oxalate and 0.5 ml of 20 mM calcium chloride independently through 2 separate tubes for 30 min. Then 1 ml of 20 mM sodium oxalate and 1 ml of 20 mM calcium chloride was infused continuously for 3h using an autosyringe. Finally, the bladder was drained. The infusion and drainage was repeated a second time for a total of 6 h.

After formation of mucosal crystals, the bladder was irrigated for 6 h with different solvents by continuous infusion through the same catheters. The bladder was removed from the rat and immersed in 1 N HCl for 16 h. Calcium from the crystals remaining after solvent irrigation was quantitated with the Ca^{2+} electrode. Four groups of rats (total 32) were studied in this experiment. The average amount of Ca^{2+} found in the mucosa of each group (8 bladders), after the dissolution of the crystalline calcium oxalate in 1 N HCl, is given in Table 3.

Table 3. Average Amounts of Ca^{2+} Recovered from the Mucosa.

Group	Irrigating Solution (4 ml over 6 h)	Calcium (μmol)
I	None	2.03
II	0.9% Saline	1.24
III	24 mM Renacidin	1.14
IV	24 mM α-Keto acid mixture	0.591

DISCUSSION

In vitro studies[1,3] have shown that the longer the induction period produced by the chemicals and/or solvents, the greater is the observed inhibition of calcium oxalate crystallization. Our results agree with these findings. Moreover, we have found that commercially available solvents having higher dissolution capabilities for calcium oxalate also produce longer induction periods. The induction period of crystallization can be utilized as a method, not only for studying potential inhibitors of calcium oxalate crystallization, but also for the determination of solvent dissolution capability and for screening various irrigation solvents.

Animal models to determine the ability of solvents to dissolve calcium oxalate crystals in the rat have not been previously reported. Gill[4] has shown that after chemical injury to rat bladder urothelium, calcium oxalate crystals can be induced by the injection of calcium chloride and sodium oxalate. We have increased the amounts of calcium chloride and sodium oxalate and the time period of injection in order to increase the production of calcium oxalate crystals. In the absence of urine and of bacterial contaminants, the same geometric area of the injured bladder mucosa would accumulate the same amount of calcium oxalate crystals. Since we used rats of equal weight, we assumed that they would have equal areas of injured bladder mucosa and thus the same amounts of calcium oxalate would accumulate on the mucosa.

Utilizing the principle of structural similarity, we studied the effects of various chemicals within the Krebs cycle with structures similar to that of oxalic acid. α–Ketoglutaric acid had the highest capability to dissolve calcium oxalate. With certain supporting chemicals to provide the correct ionic strength, the new solvent (20 mM α–ketoglutaric acid, 2.0 mM D-gluconic acid (hemi-magnesium salt), and 2.0 mM magnesium carbonate) appears to dissolve calcium oxalate crystals more readily than do existing irrigation solvents, such as Renacidin, which has had encouraging reports as a solvent for urinary stones[5].

In our in vivo studies, we used Renacidin for comparison purposes and found that the dissolution ability of calcium oxalate in the α–keto-acid mixture is superior to that of Renacidin. We have also found that in other experiments[6], the α–keto-acid mixture could prevent the formation of struvite stones.

ACKNOWLEDGMENT

This work was supported in part by NIH Grant AM27482. K. J. Wu is a Visiting Scholar from the People's Republic of China.

REFERENCES

1. W. P. Tew and C. D. Malis, in:"Urolithiasis, Clinical and Basic Research", L. H. Smith, W. G. Robertson, and B. Finlayson, eds., Plenum, New York (1981).
2. F. Ziolkowski and D. D. Perrin, Invest. Urol. 15:208 (1977).
3. D. J. White and G. H. Nancollas, J. Urol. 127:593 (1982).
4. W. B. Gill, K. W. Jones, and K. J. Ruggiero, J. Urol. 127:152 (1982).
5. W. P. Mulvaney, J. Urol. 84:206 (1960).
6. K. J. Wu, X. Q. Li, and S. J. Yao, in:"Urolithiasis and Related Clinical Research", P. O. Schwille, L. H. Smith, W. G. Robertson, and W. Vahlensieck, eds., Plenum, London (1985).

INDUCTION AND INHIBITION OF STRUVITE BLADDER STONES IN RATS

K. J. Wu, X. Q. Li, and S. J. Yao

Surgical Research Laboratory, Montefiore Hospital, and
Dept. of Neurological Surgery, University of Pittsburgh
Pittsburg, U.S.A.

INTRODUCTION

It have been demonstrated, both in vitro and in vivo, that
struvite stone formation is related to urinary tract infection
with urease-producing bacteria such as Proteus and Pseudomonas[1-3].
This paper presents a method for the study of the in vivo formation
and prevention of struvite in stones in rats.

METHODS

Adult Sprague-Dawley rats (300 to 350 g) were used. The
irrigation system consisted of two 85 cm lengths of soft
polyethylene tubing (size PE11) with the top end of each tube
connected to an autosyringe and the lower end inserted through the
abdominal cavity into the bladder. The tubing was tied to the
bladder with a purse-string sature. The tubes were used for
independent infusion of different test agents. To permit freedom
of movement, the tubing was threaded through a stainless steel coil
spring (50 cm) sutured to the back near the head.

In an experiment to create a calcium oxalate stone model[4], we
were able to repeat the work of others[5] in producing calcium oxalate
crystals in the mucosa of the bladder by the 1- to 6-h infusion of
sodium oxalate and calcium chloride. When the infusion time was
extended to 9 days with the hope of creating stones, small stones
did result, but analysis revealed only magnesium ammonium phosphate
stones. Simultaneous urinary tract cultures indicated the presence
of Proteus. The superimposition of bacterial contamination
(albeit unintentional) had resulted in a struvite stone model. The

model was standardized using 12 rats. Each was kept in a separate
cage and fed a normal diet. Using sterile procedures, each rat was
attached to the extracorporeal system described above. For 9 days
sodium oxalate and calcium chloride (each 200 mM) were continuously
infused into the bladder through the separate tubes at the rate of
1 ml/day. Subsequently the rat was sacrificed, a urine sample
cultured, and the bladder removed and examined for stone formation.
The stones (Fig. 1) were analyzed by Calculab (Richmond, VA,
U.S.A.). These contained 80 to 100% magnesium ammonium
phosphate and 0 to 20% calcium phosphate. According to the infusion
substance used, 24 rats were divided into 5 groups. Except for
Group III, each group contained 5 rats. Each rat was fitted with
the extracorporeal system described above. The infusion tubes were
intentionally contaminated with bacteria (e.g. Proteus, Pseudomonas,
etc.). Infusion of the various substances was continued for 9 days.

RESULTS AND DISCUSSION

With the present approach, we were able to induce the formation
of struvite stones in the rat bladder within 9 days with 65%
success. Although attempts were made to carry out the induction
experiments under sterile conditions, all rats invariably suffered
from urinary tract infection caused by the action of several kinds
of bacteria, probably due to the indwelling catheters. Cultures of

Fig. 1. Struvite bladder stone formed during 9 days of infusion
with sodium oxalate and calcium chloride.

the urine from the 8 rats with struvite stones in the bladder indicated the presence of either Proteus or Proteus and Pseudomonas. The urine pH increased to 7.5.   It is known that Proteus are strong urea-splitting bacteria which convert urea into NH_4^+ and HCO_3^-. NH_4^+ is essential for the formation of struvite stones.   None of the 8 stones formed was found to contain calcium oxalate.   It appears that whenever the rats were infected with Proteus, stones composed predominantly of struvite were obtained.

In the inhibition studies the rats were intentionally contaminated with Proteus and Pseudomonas.   In Group I, (Table 1) whenever Proteus was present in the urinary tract, struvite stones were

Table 1. Results of Inhibition of Struvite Stone Formation.

Group	Infusion (1 ml/day)	Rats	Urine Contamination (Colony count 10^5)	Rats with Stones	Urine pH	Average Stone Weight
I	Saline Chloram- phenicol (10 mg/ml)	1	Proteus and	5	7.5	29.3
II	Saline Gentamicin (10 mg/ml)	1	Proteus and Pseudomonas (resistant to gentamicin	1	7.5	20.6
		2	Gr. D Streptococcus			
		2	Staphylococcus aureus	0	6.5	--
III	Urease (60 U) Gentamicin (10 mg/ml)	2	Klebsiella	2	7.0	24.8
		2	Staphylococcus aureus			
IV	AHA (60 mg/ml) Saline	1	Proteus	1	7.0	38.0
		3	Proteus and Pseudomonas	0	6.5	--
		1	Klebsiella pneumoniae			
V	α-Keto acid mixture (2 ml/day)	3	Proteus and Pseudomonas			
		2	Gr. D Streptococcus and Klebsiella	0	5.5	--

959

produced in 100% of the rats.   When gentamicin, a bacteriocidal agent for Proteus and Pseudomonas was infused, only one rat formed a struvite stone in the presence of a Proteus resistant to gentamicin. In Group III, urease and gentamicin were infused into the bladder. Although gentamicin suppressed the growth of Proteus, struvite stones were still found in two rats, indicating that urease played an important role in struvite stone formation.

Acetohydroxamic acid (AHA) is a specific and effective inhibitor of bacterial urease. A terminal O=C-NHOH group blocks the active site on the urease molecule.   Griffith et al[6] have shown that AHA effectively inhibits alkalinization of urine by Proteus in vitro and that it can reduce bladder stone formation in rats.   In our experiment, when AHA was infused into the bladder (Group IV), struvite stone formation was reduced to 1/5 rats.

The keto-acid mixture (20 mM α-ketoglutaric acid, 2.0 mM D-gluconic acid, 2.0 mM magnesium carbonate) completely prevented the formation of struvite even under non-sterile conditions (Group V).   This is of physiological and clinical significance.   The possible reasons are: (i) the keto-acid mixture can lower urine pH to inhibit the alkalinization of urine; and (ii) presumably in the presence of a certain enzyme and its cofactors in the urine, the keto-acid mixture can aminate the NH_4^+ to form keto-glutamate, thus decreasing the possibility of producing struvite.   Infusion or irrigation of the bladder with the keto-acid mixture may be of therapeutic value for patients with struvite stone disease.

ACKNOWLEDGEMENT

This work was supported in part by NIH Grant AM27482. K.J.Wu is a Visiting Scholar from the People's Republic of China.

REFERENCES

1. C. W. Vermeulen and R. Goetz, J. Urol. 72:761 (1954).
2. D. P. Griffith and D. M. Musher, Invest. Urol. 11:228 (1973).
3. D. P. Griffith, D. M. Musher, and C. Itin, Invest. Urol. 13:346 (1976).
4. K. J. Wu, X. Q. Li, Y. Dokko, B. Chen, M. A. Krupper, W. W. Chuang, S. K. Wolfson, and S. J. Yao, in:"Urolithiasis and Related Clinical Research", P. O. Schwille, L. H. Smith, W. G. Robertson, and W. Vahlensieck, eds., Plenum, New York (1985).
5. W. B. Gill, K. W. Jones, and K. J. Ruggiero, J. Urol. 127:152 (1982).
6. D. P. Griffith, D. M. Musher, and J. W. Campbell, Invest. Urol. 11:234 (1973).

SYMPOSIUM PARTICIPANTS

Abbott, Dr R., American Board of International Medicine and
    Nephrology, 61 W. Columbia St., Orlando,Fl. 32806, USA.
Abdel-Halim, Dr El-Said, University Hospital, Urology Unit,
    P.O. Box 6615, Jeddah, Saudi Arabia.
Achilles, Dr W., Urologische Universitätsklinik, Robert-Koch-Str. 8,
    3550 Marburg, FRG.
Adler, Dr S., Dept. of Medicine, Montefiore Hospital,
    University School of Medicine, Pittsburgh, PA 15213, USA.
Ahlstrand, Dr C., University Hospital, Dept. of Urology,
    58185 Linköping, Sweden.
Anasuya, Dr A., National Institute of Nutrition, Jamai-Osmania P.O.,
    Hyderabad 500 007, India.
Arie, Dr R., Unit for Metabolism Disease, Beilinson Medical Center,
    Petah Tikva, Israel.
Arora, Dr B., M.R.C. Mineral Metabolism Unit, The General Infirmary,
    Great George Street, Leeds LS1 3EX, UK.
Asper, Dr R., Central Laboratory for Clinical Chemistry, University
    Hospital, 8091 Zurich, Sweden.
Aubia, Dr J., Hospital G.M.D. Cesperanga, Avgda Paral-Lel 141,5At.2,
    Barcelona, Spain.
Azoury, Dr R., Casali Institute of Applied Chemistry, Hebrew
    University, Jerusalem, Israel.
Baadenhuysen, Dr H., St. Radboud University Hospital, Geert
    Grooteplein Zuid 8, Nymegen, The Netherlands.
Bach, Dr D., Urologische Abteilung, Bundeswehrkrankenhaus, Oberer
    Eselsberg 40, 7900 UlM, FRG.
Backman, Dr L., Dept. of Surgery, Karolinska Institutet, Danderyd
    Hospital, 18288 Danderyd, Sweden.
Baer, Dr A., Xyrofin AG, Laettich Street 8a, 6340 Baar, Switzerland.
Baggio, Dr B., Clinica Medica 1, Policlinico Universita, Via
    Giustiniani 2, 35100 Padova, Italy.
Baghlaf, Dr A., Dept. of Chemistry, King Abdel-Aziz University,
    Jeddah, Saudi Arabia.
Baghurst, Dr P. A., Csiro, Division of Human Nutrition, Kinstore
    Avenue, Adelaide, SA 5000, Australia.
Bais, Dr R., Division of Clinical Chemistry, Institute of Medical
    Science, Box 14, Rundle Street, Adelaide, Australia.

Balagopalan, Dr N.K., Medical College Hospital, Trivandrum, S.R.F.,
    Urolithiasis R. Projekt, Kerala, India 695011.
Bastian, Dr H.P., Abt. f. Urologie, St. Josef-Hospital,
    Hospitalstr. 45, 5210 Troisdorf, FRG.
Bataille, Dr P., Service de Néphrologie, CHU Hôpital Nord,
    80000 Amiens, France.
Baumann, Dr J.M., Dept. of Urology, Regionalspital, Vogelsang 84,
    2502 Biel, Switzerland.
Bausch, Dr W.M., Institut für Geologie und Mineralogie,
    Schlossgarten 5a, 8520 Erlangen, FRG.
Bec, Dr P., Clinique Saint-Exupery, Cabinet de Consultation de
    Nephrologie, 20 Route de Revel, 31400 Toulouse, France.
Beeko, Dr R., Rehabilitationskrankenhaus, Kloskstr. 2,
    5300 Bonn-Merten, FRG.
Berg, van den, Dr C., Mayo Clinic, Division of Nephrology,
    Rochester, MN 55901, USA.
Berland, Dr Y., Service Nephrology, Hospital de la Conception, 13005
    Marseille, France.
Berlin, Dr T., Dept. of Urology, Huddinge Hospital, 14186 Huddinge,
    Sweden.
Bichler, Dr K.H., Dept. of Urology, University of Tübingen,
    Calwerstr. 7, 7400 Tübingen, FRG.
Bijvoet, Dr O.L.M., Abtlg. Endokinologie, Akad. Ziekenhuis,
    Rijnsburgerweg 10, 2333 Leiden, The Netherlands.
Biondi, Dr G., Wellcome Italia-Medical Dept., Via del Mare, 36-0040
    Pomezia, Italy.
Blacklock, Prof. N.J., University Hospital of South Manchester, Nell
    Lane, Manchester M20 8LR, UK.
Boistelle, Dr R., C.R.M.C.2, Campus Luminy, Case 913,
    13288 Marseille Cedex 9, France.
Brandl, Dr, Firma Pfrimmer & Co., Hofmannstr. 8, 8520 Erlangen, FRG.
Braun, Dr J., Dept. of Urology, TU Munich, Ismaningerstr. 22,
    8000 München, FRG.
Brielmann, Dr T., Urologische Klinik, Kantonspital Basel,
    Spitalstr. 21, 4301 Basel, Switzerland.
Brien, Dr G., Dept. of Urology, Humboldt-University, Schumannstr.
    20/21, 1040 Berlin, GDR.
Bronner, Dr F., University of Connecticut, Health Center,
    Farmington, Ct. 0603, USA.
Brown, Dr C., University of Florida, Gainesville, Florida 32610, USA.
Bruggemann, Dr V. Ch., Urologische Univ. Klinik, Hufelandstr. 55,
    4300 Essen, FRG.
Buck, Dr C., Dept. of Urology, Welsh National School of Medicine,
    Cardiff, Wales, UK.
Burckhardt, Dr P., University Hospital, 1011 Lausanne, Switzerland.
Burns, Dr J. R., Dept. of Urology, University of Alabama,
    Birmingham/Al 35209, USA.
Burr, Dr R. G., L. Guttmann Institute for Spinal Injuries, Stoke
    Mandeville Hospital, Mandeville Road, Aylesbury,
    Bucks. HP21 8AL, UK.

Butz, Dr M., St. Josef-Hospital, Dept. of Urology, 4790 Paderborn, FRG.

Caudarella, Dr R., Univ. di Bologna, Policlinico S. Orsola, Via Massarenti, 9, 40138 Bologna, Italy.

Chaussy, Dr C. Urologische Klinik der LMU, Klinikum Grosshadern, Marchioninistr. 15, 8000 München 70, FRG.

Cheng, Dr P.-T., Dept. of Pathology, Mount Sinai Hospital, 600 University Avenue, Toronto, Canada M5G IX5.

Churchill, Dr D.N., Faculty of Health Sciences, McMaster University Hamilton, Ontario, Canada.

Cifuentes Delatte, Dr L., Dept. of Urology, Fundacion Jimenez Diaz, Madrid 3, Spain.

Citron, D.J.T., Permanente Medical Group, 1425 S. Main, Walnut Creek, Ca, USA.

Cohen, Dr S.L., Dept. of Medicine, Rayne Institute, University Hospital, London WClE, 6JJ, UK

Cole, Dr F.E., Alton Ochsner, Medical Foundation, 1520 Jefferson Highway, New Orleans, La. 70121, USA.

Colussi, Dr G., Renal Unit, E.O. Ca Granda-Niguarda, Milano, Italy.

Comeri, Dr G. C., Dept. of Urology, St. Anna Hospital, 22100 Como, Italy.

Conyers, Dr R.A.J., Division of Clinical Chemistry, Institute of Medical and Veterinary Sciences, Adelaide, SA 5000, Australia.

Costello, Dr J., Renal Research Laboratory, Allegheny General Hospital, 320 East North Avenue, Pittsburgh, PA 15212, USA.

Cummings, Dr N.B., National Institutes of Health, Dept. of Health and Human Services, Bethesda, Maryland 20014, USA.

Daniele, Dr P.G., Instituto Analisi Chimica Strumentale, University, Turin, Italy.

Danielson, Dr B.G., Dept. of Internal Medicine, University Hospital, Uppsala, Sweden.

Deetjen Dr P., Institute of Physiology, Fritz-Pregl-Str.3, 6010 Innsbruck, Austria.

DiBella, Dr M.C., 9 Hospital Drive, Toms River, New Jersey 08753, USA.

Dirks, Dr J.H., University of British Columbia, Dept. of Medicine, 700 West 10 Avenue, Vancouver B.C. V5Z 1M9, Canada.

Dobbins, Dr J.W., Dept. of Internal Medicine, Yale University, New Haven, Conn. 06510, USA.

Donadio, Dr M.V., Busiri vici 16/C, 00152 Roma, Italy.

Drach, Dr G.W., Section of Urology, University of Arizona, Health Science Center, Tucson, Arizona 85724, USA.

Dulce, Dr H.J., Institut für Klinische Chemie, Universität Berlin, Hindenburgdamm 30, 1000 Berlin 45, FRG.

Edyvane, Dr K.A., Urology Unit, Flinders Medical Center, Bedford Park, SA 5042, Australia.

Entrup, Dr.M., Urolog. Abteilung, Chirurgische Universitätsklinik, Jungeblodtplatz 1, 4000 Münster, FRG.

Erickson, Dr S., Mayo Clinic, Rochester, MN 55905, USA.

Erwin, Dr D.T., Alton Ochsner Medical Foundation, 1516 Jefferson
    Highway, New Orleans, LA 70121, USA.
Ettinger, Dr B., Kaiser Permanente Medical Center, 2200 O'Farrell
    Street, San Francisco, CA 94114, USA.
Farag, Dr A., Dept. of Chemistry, Faculty of Science, King Abdulaziz
    University, Jeddah, Saudi Arabia.
Fazil-Marickar, Dr Y.M., Medical College Hospital, Trivandrum,
    Kavala 695011, India.
Fellström, Dr B., Dept. of Internal Medicine, University Hospital,
    75185 Uppsala, Sweden.
Finet, Dr M., CHU-Source Néphrologie, Hôpital Nord, 8000 Amiens,
    France.
Finlayson, Dr B., Dept. of Urology, University of Florida,
    Gainesville, Florida 32610, USA.
El Fituri, Dr M.N., Nephrology Dept., Tajoura Hospital, PO Box
    30616, Tripoli, Libya
Fleisch, Prof. H., Institut f. Pathophysiologie, Murtenstrasse 33,
    Bern, Switzerland.
Fournier, Dr A., Service de Nephrologie, CHU Hospital Nord, 8000
    Amiens, France.
Fox, Dr M., Stanford University, Stanford, California, USA.
Froeling, Dr P., Dept. of Internal Medicine, St Radboud University
    Hospital, PO Box 9101, 6500 HB Nijmegen, The Netherlands.
Füredi-Milhofer, Dr H., Rudjer Boskovic Institute, 41001 Zagreb,
    Yugoslavia.
Gaca, Dr A., Deutsche Klinik f. Diagnostik, Aukammallee 33, 6200
    Wiesbaden, FRG.
Gaiser, Dr I., Dept. of Urology, Calwerstr. 7, 7400 Tubingen, FRG.
Gallucci, Dr M., Istituto Policatteara di Urologia, via S. Godenzo
    119, 00189 Roma, Italy.
Gambaro, Dr G., Clinica Medica, Policlinico Univ., 35100 Padova,
    Italy.
Gasser, Prof. G., Krankenhaus der Stadt Wien, Wolkersbergerstr. l,
    1130 Wien, Austria.
Gault, Dr M.H., Memorial University and the General Hospital,
    St John's, Newfoundland, Alb. 3V6, Canada.
Geiser, Dr C., Medical Physiology, Ransta, 75590 Uppsala, Sweden.
Gill, Dr W.B., Dept. of Surgery, University, Box 403,950 East 59th
    Street, Chicago, Illinois 60637, USA.
Gojaseni, Dr P., Section of Urology, Ramathibodi Hospital,
    Rama VI Rd., Bangkok 10400, Thailand.
Graef, Dr V., Institut für Klinische Chemie und Pathobiochemie,
    Friedrichstr. 24, 6300 Giesen, FRG.
Green, Dr R., The University of Manchester, Oxford Road, Manchester
    M13 9PT, UK.
Greenwood, Dr S.L., Dept. of Physiology, University of Manchester,
    Manchester M13 9PT, UK.
Gregory, Dr J.G., Section of Urology, St. Louis University of
    Medicine, 1325 South Grand Avenue, St. Louis, Missouri 63104,
    USA.

Grenabo, Dr L., Dept. of Urology, Sahlgrenska sjukhuset, 413 45
    Göteborg, Sweden.
Griffith, Dr D.P., 1200 Moursound, Houston, Texas 77025, USA.
Gimaraes, Dr P., Curry Cabral Hospital, 1000 Lisabon, Portugal.
Hackett, Dr R.L., Dept. of Pathology, J.H. Miller Health Centre, Box
    J275, Gainesville, Florida 32610, USA.
Hagmaier, Dr V., Division of Urology, University Clinic, 4031 Basel,
    Switzerland.
Hallson, Dr P.C., St. Paul's Hospital, Endell Street, London WC2,
    UK.
Halse, Dr T., Bene-Chemie GmbH, Herterichstr. 1,8000 München 71,
    FRG.
Hautmann, Dr R., Dept. of Urology, RWTH Aachen, Goethestr. 27-29,
    5100 Aachen, FRG.
He, Dr J.-Y., Dept. of Urology, 2nd Affiliated Hospital, Lanzhou
    Medical College, Lanzhou, Gansu, China.
Hedelin, Dr H., Dept. of Urology, Sahlgrenska Sjukhuset, 41345
    Göteborg, Sweden.
Hegemann, Dr M., Urologische Klinik rechts der Isar, TU München,
    Ismaningerstr. 22, 8000 München 80, FRG.
Henriksson, Dr C., Dept. of Urology, Sahlgrenska Sjukhuset, 41345
    Goteborg, Sweden.
Hering, Dr F., Urolog. Klinik, Kantonsspital Basel, Spitalstr. 21,
    4031 Basel, Switzerland.
Hesse, Dr A., Urologische Univ. Klinik Bonn, Sigmund-Freudstr. 25,
    5300 Bonn, FRG.
Hofmann, Dr. R., Dept. of Urology, TU Munich, Ismaningerstr. 22,
    8000 München 80, FRG.
Holmgren, Dr K., Dept. of Urology, University Hospital, 75185
    Uppsala, Sweden.
Hopf, Dr U., Med. Wissensch. Abtlg., Deutsche Wellcome GmbH,
    Postfach 1352, 3006 Burgwedel 1, FRG.
Hosking, Dr D.H., Nephrology Res. Lab., Mayo Clinic, Rochester,
    MN 55905, USA.
Ilievski, Dr P.M., Division of Urology, Medical Center Bitola, 97000
    Bitola, Yugoslavia.
Jaeger, Dr P., Dept. of Medicine, University Hospital Lausanne, 1011
    Lausanne, Switzerland.
Jain, Dr. A.K., Dept. of Biochemistry, R.N.T. Med. College, Udaipur
    313001, India.
Jarrar, Dr K., Urologische Universitätsklinik, 6300 Giessen, FRG.
Jenkins, Dr A.D., University of Texas, Medical School, 6431 Fannin,
    Houston, Texas 77030, USA.
Jensen, Dr H., Oestra Koepmangatan 5, 37132 Karlskrona, Sweden.
Joenemar, Dr B., P.O. Box 839, 20/80 Malmö, Sweden.
Johannson, Dr G., Dept. of Internal Medicine, University Hospital,
    79185 Uppsala, Sweden.
Johny, Dr K.V., Mubarak Hospital, Kuwait.
Joost, Dr J., Urologische Universitätsklinik, Anichstr. 35, 6020
    Innsbruck, Austria.

Juhlin, Dr R., Pharmacia Infusion, PO Box 658, 751 27 Uppsala, Sweden.

Kasidas, Dr G.P., Institute of Urology, St. Peter's Hospital, 24 Endell Street, London WC2, UK.

Kau, Dr S.T., Biomedical Research Dept., Wilmington, DE 19897, USA.

Kellermann, Dr P., Dr Madaus & Co., Ostmerheimerstr. 198, 5000 Koln 91; FRG.

Khan, Dr F., Dept. of Urology, Mayo Hospital, Lahore, Pakistan.

Khan, Dr R., Dept. of Pathology, University of Florida, Box J-275, Gainesville, Fl. 32610, USA.

Kheradpir, Dr M.H., Kantonspital Bruderholz, 4101 Bruderholz, Switzerland.

Knebel, Dr L., Elisabeth-Krankenhaus, Hubertusstr. 100, 4050 Mönchengladbach, FRG.

Kok, Dr D.J., Clinical Investigation Unit, Dept. Endocrinology, Academic Hospital, Leiden, 2333 AA, The Netherlands.

Komunjer, Dr L., Ruder Boskovic Institute, 41001 Zagreb, Yugoslavia.

Koska, Dr W.W., Rochusstr. 272, 5300 Bonn 1, FRG.

Kroon, Dr A., Dept. of Internal Medicine, PO Box 9101, 6500 HB Nijmegen, The Netherlands.

Laerum, Dr E. Institute of General Practice, University of Oslo, Frederik Stangsgt. 11-12, Oslo 2, Norway.

Lang, Dr G.R., Dialysis Centers Ltd., 450 East Ohio Street, Chicago, Illinois 60611, USA.

Larsson, Dr L., Dept. of Clinical Chemistry, Linköping University, 58185 Linkoeping, Sweden.

Lemann, Dr J., Renal Section, M. County General Hospital, 9200 West Wisconsin Avenue, Milwaukee, Wi 53226, USA.

Leone, Dr M.A., II Medical Clinic-Polyclinic, Piazza G. Cesare, Bari, Italy.

Leskovar, Dr P., Urolog. Klinik rechts der Isar, TU München, Ismaningerstr. 22, 8000 München 80, FRG.

Leusmann, Dr D.B., Urologische Abteilung, Chirurg. Univ. Klinik, Jungeblodtplaz 1, 4400 Munster, FRG.

Leveille, Dr M., 1560 East Sherbrooke Street, Montreal-H3P 1X2 Quebec, Canada.

Lewi, Dr H., Dept. of Urology, Victoria Infirmary, Glasgow, UK.

Li, Dr M.K., Dept. of Urology, Washington Hospital, West Didsbury, Manchester, UK.

v. Lilienfeld-Toal, Dr H., Kreiskrankenhaus, 5220 Waldbröl, FRG.

Linari, Dr F., Osp. Mauriziano Umberto I, 10128 Torino, Italy.

Lismer, Dr L., Dept. of Urology, Sovoka Medical Center, POB 151 Beer-Sheva, Israel.

Liu, Dr F.H., Dept. of Intern. Medicine, 1425 South Main Street, Walnut Creek, Ca. 94596, USA.

Ljunghall, Dr S., Dept. of Intern. Medicine, University Hospital, 751 85 Uppsala, Sweden.

Lockefeer, Dr J.H.M., Hertog Hendriklaan 18, Oisterwijk 5062 CJ, The Netherlands.

Lovatt, Dr G.E., Wellcome Research Laboratories, Langley Court, Beckenham, Kent BR3 3BS, UK.

Lutzeyer, Dr W., Dept. of Urology, RWTH Aachen, Goethestr. 27-99, 5100 Aachen, FRG.

Lycklama à Nijeholt, Dr G.A.B., Dept. of Urology, University Hospital, Leiden, The Netherlands.

Lyrdal, Dr F., Eksjoe-Naessjoe Lasarett, 57500 Eksjö, Sweden.

Martelli, Dr A., Urological Clinic, University of Bologna, Via Massarenti 9, 40138 Bologna, Italy.

Martin, Dr X., Nephrology Research Laboratory, Mayo Clinic, Rochester, MN 55905, USA.

Massry, Dr S.G., University of S. California, Los Angeles, CA 90033, USA.

Matsushita, Dr K., Dept. of Urology, Tokai University Hospital, Bohseidai, Iseharashi, Kanagawa, Japan.

Mautalon, Dr C., Centrto de Osteopatias Medicas, Saavedra 189, 1083 Beunos Aires, Argentina.

May, Dr P., Urologische Klinik des Allgemeinen Krankenhauses, Utere Sandstr. 8600 Bamberg, FRG.

Mazzachi, Dr B.C., Dept. of Clinical Biochemistry, Flinders Medical Center, Bedford Park 5042, Australia.

Mazzachi, Dr R P., Dept. of Clinical Biochemistry, Flinders Medical Center, Bedford Park 5042, Australia.

Mazzuoli, Dr G.F., I. Semeiotica Medica, Univ. de Roma, 00161 Roma, Italy.

Mewes, Dr D., Deutsche Wellcome GmbH, Postfach 1352, 3006 Burgwedel 1, FRG.

Meyer, Dr J.L., Building 30, Room 211, National Institute of Dental Research, Bethesda, Maryland 20205, USA.

Meyer, Dr W.H., Urolog. Klinik Hamburg-Eppendorf, Martinstr. 52, 2000 Hamburg 20, FRG.

Meyer-Jurgens, Dr U.B., Inst. f. Medical Physics, Hüfferstr. 68, 4400 Münster, FRG.

Meyer-Schwickerath, Dr M., Urologische Univ. Klinik, Hufelandstr. 55, 4300 Essen 1, FRG.

Miano, Dr L., Urolog. Dept. Univ. of Rome, Policlinico Umberto I, Via S. Angela Merici, 00161 Roma, Italy.

Middleton, Dr J.E., Dept. of Chemical Pathology, General Hospital, Southampton, UK.

Monreal, Dr A., Gottfriedenstr., 5300 Bonn 3, FRG.

Monza, Dr G., Dipartimento Medico, Ciba Geigy S.p.A., Strada Statale 233 Km 20.5, 21040 Origgio (VA); Italy.

Nancollas, Prof. G.H., University of New York, Buffalo, New York 14214, USA.

Nelde, Dr H.J., Dept. of Urology, Universität, Calwer Str. 7, 7400 Tübingen, FRG.

Norman, Dr A.W., Dept. of Biochemistry, University of California, Riverside, California 92521, USA.

Norman, Dr R, MRC Mineral Metabolism Unit, The General Infirmary, Leeds LS1 3EX, UK.

Nowe, Dr P.P., Bosmanslei 17, 2018 Antwerpen, Belgium.

Nunziata, Dr V., Clinica Medica II, Universita, Via S. Pansini 5, 80131 Napoli, Italy.

Osswald, Dr H., Gödecke Aktiengesellschaft, Mooswaldallee 1-9, 7800 Freiburg, FRG.

Otnes, Dr B., Section of Urol. Akershus Central Hospital, 1316 Baerum Sykehus, Norway.

Ouimet, Dr D., Maisonneuve-Rosemont Hospital, 5415 L'Assoption, Montreal (Quebec), Canada, H1T 2M4.

Pak, Prof. C.Y.C., University of Texas, 5323 Harry Hines Boulevard, Dallas, Texas, USA.

Peacock, Dr M., MRC Mineral Metabolism Unit, The General Infirmary, Great George Street, Leeds LS1 3EX, UK.

Perlberg, Dr S, Dept. of Urology, The Hebrew University of Jerusalem, PO Box 12000, Jerusalem 91904, Israel.

Petta, Dr S., Clinica Virologica, Policlinico Umberto I, University, Roma, Italy.

Pfab, Dr R. Urolog. Klinik rechts der Isar, TU München, Ismaningerstr. 22, 8000 München 80, FRG.

Pinto, Dr B., Servico de Urologia, Hospital Valzle Hebron, Barcelona 13, Spain.

Pizzarelli, Dr F., MRC Mineral Metabolism Unit, Great George Street, Leeds LS1 3EX, UK.

Prien, Dr E.L., Massachusetts General Hospital, Boston, MA 02114, USA.

Purohit, Dr A.K., Dept. of Biochemistry, Udaipur, Rajasthan 313001, India.

Putz, Dr A., Urol. Univ. Klinik, 6020 Innsbruck, Austria.

Qunibi, Dr W.Y., King Faisal Spezialist Hospital, Riyadh, Saudi Arabia,

Rabichev, I., Bathia Mokov 14/13 Rehovoth, Israel.

Rademark, Dr C., Dept. of Urology, University Hospital, Lund, Sweden.

Rahman, Dr M.A., Dept. of Biochemistry, Jinnah Postgraduate Medical Center, Karachi, Pakistan.

Randolph, Dr A.D., Section of Urology, University of Tucson, Arizona 85724, USA.

Rao, Dr P.N., University Hospital of South Manchester, Nell Lane, Manchester M20 8LR, UK.

Rashwan, Dr H., Dept. of Medicine, Ismailia, Egypt.

Raymakers, Dr J.A., University Hospital, Deptl of Internal Medicine, Catharijnesisngel 101, 3511 GV Utrecht, The Netherlands.

Reis-Santos, Dr J.-M., Dept. of Urology, Curry Cabral Hospital, 1000 Lisbon, Portugal.

Resnick, Dr M., University Hospitals of Cleveland, 2065 Adelbert Road, Cleveland, 2065 Adelbert Road, Cleveland, Ohio 44106, USA

Reveillaud, Dr R.J., Dept. of Internal Medicine and Nephrology, Cristal Laboratory, C.H. Saint-Cloud, 92211, France.

Revusova, Dr V., Medical Bionics; Research Institute, Urological Clin., Limbova 5, 83305 Bratislava, Czechoslovakia.

Robertson, Dr W.G., MRC Mineral Metabolism Unit, The General
    Infirmary, Great George Street, Leeds LS1 3EX, UK.
Rodgers, Dr A., Dept. of Physical Chemistry, University of Cape
    Town, Cape Town 7700, South Africa.
Rodman, Dr J., Rockefeller University, 435 East 57th Street, New
    York 410021, USA.
Roehrborn, Dr C.G., Dept. of Urology, Falkeneck Hospital,
    Jägerschneise 28, 6307 Linden, Hessen, FRG.
Rogland, Dr B., Clinic of Nephrology, Lasarettet, 22185 Lund,
    Sweden.
Rombola, Dr G., Renal Unit, E.O. Ca Granda-Niguarda, Milano, Italy.
Rose, Dr G.A., Institute of Urology, St Paul's Hospital, Endell
    Street, London WC2, UK.
Rosenstein, Dr.I., Dept. of Microbiology, Royal Free Hospital, Pond
    Street, Hampstead, London NW3, UK.
Roytblat, Dr L., Ben-Gurion University of the Negev, Tabenkin Str.
    38/5, Beer Sheva, Israel.
Rüffer, Dr C., Department Anatomie IV, Org. Nr. 4140, Medizinische
    Hochschule, 3000 Hanover, FRG.
Ruemenapf, Dr G., University Hospital, Min. Metabolism and Endocr.
    Res. Lab., Maximiliansplatz, 8520 Erlangen, FRG.
Ruiz, Dr J., Ciudad Sanitaria de S.S., Barcelona 36, Spain.
Rutishauser, Dr G., Urol. Klinik, Kantonsspital, Spitalstr. 21, 4031
    Basel, Switzerland.
Ryall, Dr R.L., Dept. of Surgery, Flinders Medical Centre, Bedford
    Park, Australia 5042.
Salahudeen, Dr S.H., Dept. of Surgery, Medical College Hospital,
    Kerala, India 695011.
Sallis, Dr J.D., Dept. of Biochemistry, University of Tasmania,
    Hobart Box 252C GPO Tasmania, Australia.
Samuell, Dr C.T., St Peter's Hospital, Institute of Urology, Endell
    Street, London WC2, UK.
Sandnes, Dr T.W., Wellcome Foundation Ltd., Gml. Drammensvei 107,
    1322 Hoevik, Norway.
Sarig, Dr S., Casali Institute of Applied Chemistry, Hebrew
    University, Jerusalem, Israel.
Schaefer, Dr R.M., Urologische Universitätsklinik, Sigmund-Freud-
    Str.25, 5300 Bonn-Venusberg, FRG.
Schena, Dr F.P., 2nd Medical Clinic-Polyclinic, Piazza Cesare, Bari,
    Italy.
Schmidt, Dr K., Dept. of Surgery, University of Tübingen,
    Calwerstr. 7, 7400 Tübingen, FRG.
Schmucki, Dr O., Dept. of Urology, University Hospital, 8091 Zürich,
    Switzerland.
Schneekloth, Dr K., Deutsche Wellcome GmbII, Postfach 1352, 3001
    Burgwedel 1, FRG.
Schneider, Dr H.J., Am Ludwigsplatz 11, 6300 Giessen, FRG.
Schreiber, Dr N., Dept. of Urology, University of Tübingen, 7400
    Tübingen, FRG.

Schreiber, Dr W., Deutsche Wellcome GmbH, Postfach 1352, Burgwedel, FRG.

Schulze, Dr E., Dept. of Urology, University of Tübingen, Calwerstr. 7, 7400 Tübingen, FRG.

Schwankle, Dr G., Fa. Madaus & Co., Postfach 932001, 5000 Koln 91, FRG.

Schwille, Dr P.O., University Hospital, Min. Metab. and Endocrinol. Research Lab., Maximiliansplatz, 8520 Erlangen, FRG.

Scurr, Dr D.S., MRC Mineral Metabolism Unit, The General Infirmary, Leeds LS1 3EX, UK.

Senior, Dr F., University of Florida, Box J-126 JHMHC, Gainesville, Florida, 32610, USA.

Shepard, Dr J.E., Internal Medicine, Nephrology, and Dialysis, 1000 South Eliseo Drive, Greenbrae, California 94904-2194, USA.

Sigel, Dr A., Direktor der Urolog. Univ. Klinik, Maximiliansplatz, 8520 Erlangen, FRG.

Simmonds, Dr A., The Purine Laboratory, Guy's Hospital, London SE1 9RT, UK.

Singla, Dr S.K., Dept. of Biochemistry, Punjab Agricultural University, Ludhiana-141004, India.

Slatopolsky, Dr E., Washington University, St Louis, Missouri 63110, USA.

Smith, Dr C.L., Stone Clinic, Hennepin County Medical Center, 701 Park Avenue, Minneapolis, MN 55415, USA.

Smith, Prof. L.H., Division of Nephrology, Mayo Clinic, Rochester, MN 55901, USA.

Sörgel, Dr F., Institut f. Rechtsmedizin, Universität, 8520 Erlangen, FRG.

Sperling, Dr O., Dept. of Clinical Biochemistry, Beilinson Medical Center, Petah-Tikva, Israel.

Strohmaier, Dr W.L., Dept. of Urology, University of Tubingen, 7400 Tubingen, FRG.

Sur, Dr B., G.S.V.M. Medical College, Dept. of Biochemistry, Kanpur 208002, India.

Szabo-Foeldvary, Dr E., 1st Dept. of Surgery, University of Medicine, 4012 Debrecen, Hungar.

Tang, Dr A., Kaiser-Permanente Medical Group, 2200 O'Farrell Street, San Francisco, USA.

Tang, Dr A., Kaiser-Permanente Medical Group, 2200 O'Farrell Street, San Francisco, USA.

Thind, Dr S.K., Dept. of Biochemistry, Institute of Medical Education and Research, Chandigarh 160 012, India.

Thomas, Dr W., jr., University of Florida, Gainesville, Florida 32602, USA.

Tiselius, Dr H.-G., Dept. of Urology, University Hospital, 58185 Linkoping, Sweden.

Tomlinson, Dr B., Dept. of Medicine, University College, Rayne Institute, London WC1, UK.

Town, Dr M.H., Boehringer Mannheim, Bahnhofstr. 9-15, 8132 Tutzing, FRG.

Tricerri, Dr A., Inst. Analisi Chimica Strumentale, Turin
University, Italy.
Tschöpe, Dr W., Medizinische Universitätsklinik, Bergheimer Str. 58,
6900 Heidelberg, FRG.
Ulshöfer, Dr B.M., Urolog. Univ.-Klinik und Poliklinik,
Robert-Kochstr. 8, 3550 Marburg, Lahn, FRG.
Vahlensieck, Prof. W., Urologische Universitatsklinik, Sigmund-
Freudstr. 25, 5300 Bonn 1, FRG.
Walker, Dr W.G., Dept. of Medicine, Johns Hopkins University,
Baltimore, Maryland 21205, USA.
Walker, Dr V.R., Dept. of Medicine, University of British Columbia,
Vancouver B.C., Canada V6T 1W5.
Wallmon, Dr A., Medical Physiology, Box 572, 75123 Uppsala, Sweden.
Wandt, Dr A.E., Dept. of Physical Chemistry, University of Cape
Town, Rondebosch, Cape Town 7700, South Africa.
Weisinger, Dr J.R., Centro Nacional de Dialisis, Y Trasplante,
Apartado Postal 47365, Los Chaguaramos, Caracas 1041,
Venezuela
Werness, Dr P.G., Mayo Clinic, Rochester, MN 55904, USA.
Wikstrom, Dr B., Dept. of Internal Medicine, University Hospital,
75185 Uppsala, Sweden.
Will, Dr E.J., St James's University Hospital, Beckett Street, Leeds
LS9 7TF, UK.
Williams, Dr H.E., University of California, Dean's Office, School
of Medicine, Davis, California 95616, USA.
Willis, Dr R.G., Dept. of Physiology, University of Manchester,
Manchester M13 9PT, UK.
Wilson, Dr D.R., Dept. of Medicine, University of Toronto, Toronto,
Ontario, Canada M5G IL7.
Wilson, Dr J.W.L., Nephrology Research Unit, Mayo Clinic, Rochester,
MN 55905, USA.
Wong, Dr N.L.M., Dept. of Medicine, University of British Columbia,
Vancouver, BC V6T 1W5, Canada.
Wrong, Dr O., Dept. of Medicine, University College, London WC1E
6JJ, UK.
Wu, Dr K.J. Surgical Research Laboratory, Montefiore Hospital,
Pittsburgh, PA 15213, USA.
Wuzel, Dr H., Urologische Univ.-Klinik, Sigmund-Freud-Str.25, 5300
Bonn 1, FRG.
Yendt, Dr E., Dept. of Medicine, Queen's University, Kingston,
Ontario, Canada K1L 3N6.
Zöllner, Dr N., Medizinische Poliklinik, 8000 München 2, FRG.

INDEX

Prepared by Dr Gerhard Ruemenapf, Dept. of Surgery and Urology, University of Erlangen, F.R.G.